TURNER'S
PERSONAL AND COMMUNITY
Health

TURNER'S

PERSONAL AND COMMUNITY
Health

STEWART M. BROOKS and NATALIE A. BROOKS

SIXTEENTH EDITION

with **204** illustrations

The C. V. Mosby Company

ST. LOUIS • TORONTO • LONDON   1983

MOSBY

A TRADITION OF PUBLISHING EXCELLENCE

Editor: Nancy K. Roberson
Assistant editor: Michelle Turenne
Manuscript editor: Carolyn B. Smith
Designer: Nancy Steinmeyer
Production: Kathleen L. Teal, Judy England

Cover photograph by Jack Zehrt

SIXTEENTH EDITION

The C.V. Mosby Company
11830 Westline Industrial Drive, St. Louis, Missouri 63141

Library of Congress Cataloging in Publication Data

Turner, C. E. (Clair Elsmere), 1890-1974.
  Turner's personal and community health.

  Bibliography: p.
  Includes index.
  1. Health.   2. Public health.   I. Brooks,
Stewart M.   II. Brooks, Natalie A.   III. Title.
IV. Title: Personal and community health.
[DNLM: 1. Hygiene.   2. Public health.   WA 4 T945t]
RA776.T85   1983   613   82-7948
ISBN 0-8016-5128-X   AACR2

GC/VH/VH   9   8   7   6   5   4   3   2   1   02/A/217

To
Cameron F. McRae, M.D., M.P.H., F.A.P.H.A.,

a good friend
and
dedicated community servant

Historical note

C.E. Turner's *Personal and Community Health* first appeared in 1925 and soon established itself as a standard work in health education. Its success is easily traceable to Professor Turner's somewhat awesome career, one that spanned more than 60 active years. Professor Turner was a distinguished teacher and scholar, as well as an engaging writer. He was at one time Associate Professor of Hygiene at the medical and dental schools of Tufts University and Visiting Professor of Health Education at the School of Public Health, University of California. At the Massachusetts Institute of Technology he taught the first course in health education ever offered in a school of public health and originated the first program leading to the Master of Public Health degree in health education. When he was Director of Health Education Studies, his pioneering work and his demonstrations in schools in Malden, Massachusetts, during the 1920s laid the foundation for much of what is done in the field of school health and health education today.

During and after World War II much of Professor Turner's effort was directed toward the improvement of international health, primarily through his role as Chief of Health Education with the World Health Organization and through his work as Consultant to the United Nations Educational, Scientific, and Cultural Organization. He was the first president and chief advisor of the International Union for Health Education and honorary president of the organization from 1968 to 1974. He was also active in and honored by a host of other health-related organizations.

With the death of Professor Turner in 1974 The C.V. Mosby Company named Stewart M. Brooks and Natalie A. Brooks, a husband-wife team, as the authors of what is now *Turner's Personal and Community Health*. Professor Brooks has taught the full range of courses in the health sciences for well over a quarter of a century and, together with his wife, has authored over 40 books in science and medical history. Many of these books have achieved an international stature, and a number appear in foreign languages.

Preface

Never before have college students faced a future for which a knowledge of personal and community health is so vital. The child who was asked "what do you want to be when you grow up" was realistic, even though naive, when he answered "alive." In matters of health there are people who shout "forward" without saying either "whither" or "how." Decisions upon which the health of individuals, families, and communities rest need to be made on the basis of a factual background and with rationality and objectivity, not on emotionalism or fadism.

Today innumerable pressures impinge upon mental health. The establishment of an ideal family and exemplary parenthood requires both wisdom and greatness of character. Hygienic living must make its way in a complicated technology and a mixed if not confused culture. Community health is no longer remote from individual behavior. The pollution of air, water, and food and the disposal of domestic, industrial, radioactive, and solid wastes are significant factors in the daily life of the average citizen.

The preceding words were written by Claire E. Turner for the preface of the fourteenth edition of his textbook *Personal and Community Health*. Slightly over a decade later, they still hold true, and the issues they raise are perhaps even more critical.

This sixteenth edition of *Turner's Personal and Community Health* has been extensively rewritten and further adapted to the needs of today's college student. We have sought to present in logical form a body of knowledge from the biologic and social sciences that will stimulate a proper sense of health values and be worthy of a place in today's college curriculum. The book presents basic information concerning the care of the body and common departures from health, as well as a description of governmental and environmental health programs.

The first thirteen chapters present the various body systems in health and disease, and the remaining chapters deal with topics of special current concern, including the family, mental illness, nutrition, drug abuse, medical care, accidents and safety, school health, and the environment. Each chapter begins with a succinct Overview and Outline to guide the student through the material contained therein, and each ends with a Self-Test and Study Questions. The Self-Test may well improve the student's crossword expertise in a fun sort of way (the answers are in the back of the book), and the Study Questions should effect a better understanding of the material discussed in the text. Many of the questions seek student views on vital psychosocial issues, and some call for outside investigation.

We have placed the bibliography in an unobtrusive position at the back of the book, but we are quite serious about its contents. For each chapter we searched through all sorts of sources to find the most appropriate and up-to-date publications available. Most were used in the preparation of this book, but a number were included for their special appeal or interest over and above textual concerns. This

is particularly true of those publications dealing with historical matters.

We wish to express our appreciation to the
many teachers across the country who have
made constructive comments and suggestions
based on their use of earlier editions of this
text. Indeed, we welcome any and all remarks
that could possibly perfect future editions. We
also wish to thank a great many researchers,
authors, publishers, health organizations, and
manufacturers for their permission to use il-
lustrative materials. In particular, we would
like to note that a number of illustrations used
in this edition previously appeared in our text

*The Human Body: Structure and Function in
Health and Disease*, second edition, published in 1980 by The C.V. Mosby Co. Finally, our special appreciation for their willingness to take out time from busy schedules
to assist us in a variety of ways goes to Paul
Barlow, Peg Bradford, Marshall Brooks, Lau-
rene Fusco, Stephanie Greene, Terri Hughes,
Joanne Kent, David, Carol, and Elizabeth
Scott, Jenny Szekely, Barbara Todesco, Sally
S. Widerstrom, and Lee Wolfe.

Stewart M. Brooks
Natalie A. Brooks

A note to the student

The matching questions at the end of each chapter were carefully designed as a self-test of appropriate associations. Find the best possible (most logical) "match," but use a given letter only once. Answers to the Self-Tests are given at the back of the book.

Contents

Contents

CHAPTER 1

The meaning of health and disease

This chapter sets the stage for those that follow. Certainly we want to understand the full meaning of health and disease at the outset. *The American Heritage Dictionary of the English Language* defines health as "the state of an organism with respect to functioning, disease, and abnormality at any given time." Essentially, then, we view health in the context of disease. There are thousands of diseases, but, as we shall see, they have certain fundamental features in common. Above all, the causative factors fall into specific categories. Two of these categories—hypersensitivity and infection—will be discussed in some detail because of their vast implications. We shall also talk about immunity, or the resistance to disease, and take a general look at the very special subject of cancer.

Health and knowledge

Health values

Health progress and problems

Health potential

Student health

Health appraisal

Disease

Allergic reactions

Infection

Immunity

Cancer

As defined by the World Health Organization (WHO), health is "a state of complete physical, mental, and social well-being, not merely the absence of disease or infirmity." Certainly, health is much more than merely not being sick in bed. There are degrees of wellness, just as there are degrees of illness. Physical, mental, and social well-being are interrelated. There is, for example, a great difference between optimal nutrition and nutrition that is merely adequate to prevent obvious disease or between an athlete and a man who has only sufficient vigor to carry on a sedentary occupation.

Normal functioning of all parts of the body contributes not only to efficiency and the ability to do a full day's work without more than healthful fatigue but also to cheerfulness, attractiveness, courage, and enthusiasm for life. Conversely, mental, emotional, and social well-being contribute to physical health. In its various phases and to the degree that it is present, health makes possible a higher quality of living (Fig. 1-1). The desire for a feeling of personal worth is clearly an important driving force in our lives. Health helps us to attain this end by making possible a higher quality of service.

HEALTH AND KNOWLEDGE

Basic to the maintenance of health is an understanding of physical and mental fitness and the means by which they are secured. Sound decisions in matters of personal and community health come from logical reasoning based on a knowledge of the scientific facts involved. Better health comes, of course, not from the mere acquisition of health knowledge but from its application. In other words, health depends not only on what we know but also on what we do. Even though we know cigarette smoking causes lung cancer, many people continue to smoke. Knowledge, in itself, is not enough to make all people stop. It is a **behavioral problem** as well as an educational one. Repeated warnings—those on cigarette packages, for instance—changing social norms, the work of such groups as Smokers Anonymous, and informed decisions, such as the one to ban all cigarette advertising on television, have helped people to quit or, even more important, not to start the habit at all.

In maintaining health we are caring for a mechanism—the human body—that has no equal. One of its most remarkable qualities is the constant tendency to keep itself in physiologic balance or equilibrium. This steady state of the internal environment of the body is called **homeostasis**. Any physical or chemical drift away from normal sets in motion compensatory mechanisms that tend to correct the imbalance. In this way the body is like the automobile automatic gear shift, which makes needed adjustments by itself. When the engine approaches an uneconomic rate of operation, there is an automatic shift to a higher gear. The body likewise has innumerable automatic physiologic mechanisms. It maintains, for example, the same temperature in the desert and in the Arctic Circle. It maintains a balance of the volume and distribution of body fluids and an acid-base balance. Such compensatory mechanisms will not maintain health in spite of all possible injuries, such as from poisons, pathogenic organisms, and the abuses of unhygienic living, but it is encouraging to know that we have such mechanisms. Health is influenced by heredity, environment, and behavior, but the ability of the body to adjust automatically to changing conditions and to maintain normal functions is a powerful force in health maintenance.

HEALTH VALUES

The attention a person gives to the study and maintenance of health depends on the place of health in his system of values. Should we sacrifice health for other aims, or should

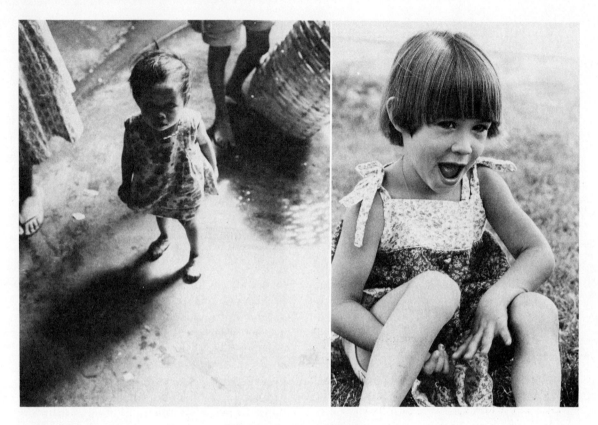

FIG. 1-1 ■ A contrast in health.

other things in life be sacrificed for health? The problem is one of relative values. The person who is struggling against sickness or disability invariably places an exceedingly high value on health. This person says, "Health is the most important thing in life." Those who have the least health value it the most. The variation in evaluation comes from the difficulty humans have appreciating what they have always possessed. Contrast sharpens vision. Things lost take on new values.

Health is certainly not the ultimate aim of life. There are more important things. Honor, integrity, justice, and freedom have been maintained at the cost of human life. Everyone has a normal ambition to perform some useful service in life. This ambition may be worthy of a sacrifice of health, but sacrificing

health does not in itself accomplish the ambition. In fact, it usually defeats it.

The health of a nation has significance beyond the relationship between the health of the individual citizen and his happiness and contentment. Disease is an economic burden that lowers both production and the standard of living. Furthermore, war has periodically thrown nations into a struggle for existence in which the physical vigor of the people has been one of the important factors determining national survival.

■■■■ HEALTH PROGRESS AND PROBLEMS

The gradual conquest of disease is dramatically reflected in military experience. The

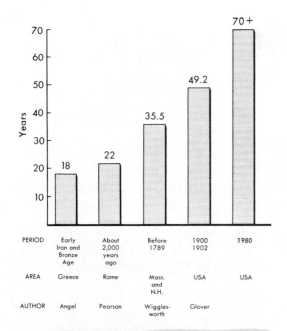

70 +

49.2

35.5

22

18

PERIOD	Early Iron and Bronze Age	About 2,000 years ago	Before 1789	1900 1902	1980
AREA	Greece	Rome	Mass. and N.H.	USA	USA
AUTHOR	Angel	Pearson	Wiggles- worth	Glover	

FIG. 1-2 ■ Life expectancy from ancient to modern times.

Redrawn from Statistical Bulletin, Metropolitan Life Insurance Co.

United States Army disease death rate per 1000 in successive wars has been as follows: Mexican War, 110 (seven times the battle deaths); the Civil War (North), 65 (twice the battle deaths); World War I, 16 (one third of the battle deaths); World War II, 0.6. World War I was the first great war in which disease deaths were fewer than battle deaths. Deaths among the wounded also dropped—from 8.3% in World War I to 4.5% in World War II to 1% in the Vietnam War. These changes reflect advances in sanitation, preventive medicine, surgery, and chemotherapy.

Public health progress in the most highly developed countries, including the United States, has been spectacular during the last century (Fig. 1-2). One communicable disease after another has been brought under control. At the same time new health problems have appeared, and the maintenance of personal and community health still presents many challenges. In these days of changing cultural patterns, continuing urbanization and industrialization, increasing speed of world transportation, and growing effects of the population explosion, society faces acute problems in mental and emotional health, poverty, healthful family living, housing, water and air pollution, disposal of urban wastes, spread of viral disease, increases in venereal disease, drug addiction, costs of medical care, and provision for expanding government health services.

These are only a few of the problems demanding study and attention. Some require community action; others depend on the individual's ability and willingness to assume responsibility for his or her own health (Table 1-1). Developments and programs in some of these fields, such as medical care, drug abuse, pollution, waste disposal, and family planning, are so active that the daily news frequently supplements basic facts in the study of personal and community health.

■ HEALTH POTENTIAL

Health potential of the individual depends on the kind of body mechanism inherited and on the care of that mechanism—somewhat as the efficiency and service of an automobile depend on the mechanism and its care. What a race horse can do depends on its inheritance, its handling, and its training. Inheritance is never the whole factor. The history of athletics tells of scores of individuals who have achieved distinction in spite of either specific handicaps or a rather frail body in early childhood.

Of course, we do not regard health and athletic achievement as synonymous. Not all healthy persons are athletes. However, speed, stamina, alertness, quick mental decisions, and neuromuscular skill reflect an efficient body mechanism. Achievement in athletics by young men and women who are willing to pay the price in effort and training shows what can be done with the body. Conversely, the wreckage of bodies or minds by abuse or lack of care

TABLE 1-1

Major causes of death in 1980 and associated risk factors

Cause	Percent of all deaths	Risk factor
Heart disease	37.8	Smoking,* hypertension,* elevated serum cholesterol* (diet), lack of exercise, diabetes, stress, family history
Malignant neoplasms	20.4	Smoking,* worksite carcinogens,* environmental carcinogens, alcohol, diet
Stroke	9.6	Hypertension,* smoking,* elevated serum cholesterol,* stress
Accidents other than motor vehicle	2.8	Alcohol,* drug abuse, smoking (fires), product design, handgun availability
Influenza and pneumonia	2.7	Smoking, vaccination status*
Motor vehicle accidents	2.6	Alcohol,* no seat belts,* speed,* roadway design, vehicle engineering
Diabetes	1.7	Obesity*
Cirrhosis of the liver	1.6	Alcohol abuse*
Arteriosclerosis	1.5	Elevated serum cholesterol*
Suicide	1.5	Stress,* alcohol and drug abuse, gun availability

From Office of Disease Prevention and Health Promotion, U.S. Department of Health and Human Services.
*Major risk factors.

shows that health is largely within our own control. We can move in either direction in health status and physical or mental output.

STUDENT HEALTH

In college the student has many aids and opportunities for health maintenance and improvement. One aid is the student health service. It provides emergency care in case of accident or sudden illness. It assesses health status through medical examination or from information supplied by the family physician. It follows through in the correction of remediable defects. Another aid to health is the physical education program. The modern college thus provides a healthful environment and assistance in varying degrees in solving food, housing, recreation, and personality problems. Physicians, nurses, dietitians, physical educators, health educators, and coaches, as well as teachers, deans, and advisers, are resources in developing physical, mental, and social well-being.

A program of building health starts with an appraisal of health. Acquainting oneself with the nature of health examinations and with the significance of the medical findings is fundamental. If these findings have implications for the college program, the necessary adjustments should be made with the advice of the physician and faculty adviser. Table 1-2 reflects the health status of typical groups of college students. The specific figures in the table are not significant, but it is interesting to see the common departures from health among

TABLE 1-2

Percentage of college students who have various physical conditions

Condition reported	Males (%)	Females (%)
Acne	17	16
Color blindness	28	—
Corrected vision	23	26
Defective vision*	52	56
Dental defects	30	28
Dysmenorrhea	—	23
Enlarged thyroid	1	1
Flatfeet	4	14
Heart abnormalities	5	6
Hernia	13	—
High blood pressure	23	4
Impaired hearing	15	12
Tonsillar defects	11	11

Data from several studies on health of college students based on the examination of a large number of students in several colleges.
*Not 20/20 in both eyes.

young people and the conditions that occur most frequently.

If a first step in the student's health program is correcting remediable conditions or adjusting to a condition that is not remediable, it is certainly not the last. Although the student's health resources are remarkable, each individual is probably more on his or her own than ever before. It is the student, with help, who is responsible for developing desirable qualities of mind, body, and personality.

A good health program is a factor in personality development. Qualities commonly listed in determining a person's strength of personality are (1) ambition, (2) industriousness, (3) persistence and patience, (4) dependability, (5) forcefulness, (6) effectiveness of speech, (7) self-confidence, (8) friendliness, (9) adaptability, (10) tact, (11) cheerfulness, (12) good judgment, (13) sensitivity to criticism, (14) ability to size up people, (15) memory, (16) neatness, and (17) health habits. The student should evaluate habits to see if they are the kind that build for

or against good health and to see how they affect his or her working ability and mental attitude day by day.

Each student has to make personal adjustments to academic life. This involves budgeting time for study, recreation, rest, eating, sleeping, and grooming. It involves following a sound schedule obtaining adequate nutrition and physical activity. It involves improving skills in listening, reading, writing, studying, and taking examinations. For example, new topics or assignments may be approached by making a brief survey of the headings and major topics in the text. The topics may suggest questions for which the student wants answers. The student should read the assigned copy and such supplementary material as will be helpful, giving attention to charts, graphs, tables, and illustrations. Difficult sections may be reread. Problems often will receive clarification in class discussions.

Alert students arrange a study place with proper lighting, chair, table, ventilation, and quiet. They secure needed source materials and plan study periods. They develop habits of serious, regular, day-by-day study with appropriate reviews instead of irregular work and all-night cramming sessions before examinations. Alert students consider with equal care the opportunities for recreational and social activity—sports, clubs, music, debate, dramatics, social functions, and religious activities. Activities suited to one's tastes and aptitudes constitute the desired balance.

HEALTH APPRAISAL

We have spoken of the appraisal of health status through an examination by a physician. A more complete picture of individual health will be obtained if we add facts about normal bodily function, indications of mental and emotional health, the appearance of the individual, and an examination of living habits.

Health appraisal, if we include not merely the absence of disease but also the broader considerations of mental health, emotional health, social health, and personality, would involve the following:

Appearance: grooming, clothing, posture, carriage, and weight

Health status: freedom from disease, correctable defects, normal bodily functions, and the health of mind and emotions

Health practices: immunization, diet, activity, sleep and rest, cleanliness, medical and dental care, recreation, control of the immediate environment, freedom from drug abuse, work schedule, interpersonal relations, and ideals of faith and service

Each of us is different. No one has perfect mental, physical, emotional, and social health. Having a permanent, uncorrectable physical defect does not mean that a person is without health if he or she has made a positive and effective adaptation to it. In large measure the individual determines whether health will be lost, maintained, or improved. The study of personal and community health should lead to wise decisions.

DISEASE

The word **disease** literally means "not at ease"; more formally, it is any deviation from the normal situation in mind or body. Like everything else, there is always an underlying reason or cause for a disease, and typically there is a **predisposing cause** as well. What is more, both the predisposing cause and the inciting cause may be multiple. This, together with the obscurities and subtleties among the processes of the living cell, easily accounts for the almost endless list of diseases of unknown cause (or **idiopathic** diseases, as physicians say). In general terms the predisposing cause either inhibits a defense mechanism or else lays the groundwork for future pathologic embellishment. The child contracts chickenpox because he or she lacks an antibody against the etiologic virus, and the adult gets a heart attack because an aging, disheveled coronary artery triggers a blood clot. Age, then, is a predisposing factor. Other obvious and well-established predisposing factors include sex, heredity, race, climate, occupation, nutrition, exposure, fatigue, stress, customs, and personal habits.

■ The disease process

The disease process amounts to cellular injury or functional alteration. The fundamental causes include (1) loss of blood supply; (2) physical agents such as heat, cold, and electricity; (3) chemical agents such as poisons and drugs; (4) hypersensitivity; and (5) infection. Hypersensitivity reactions (or allergies) and infections are alike in that both are caused by agents chemically foreign to the body. Such agents are called **antigens**, or, in the instance of allergies, **allergens**. For example, weed pollens are the causative allergens of the fall hay fever allergy, and certain viruses are the causative antigens of the common cold.

ALLERGIC REACTIONS

Allergies are hypersensitivity reactions caused by a great number and variety of allergens, including the following:

1. Certain foods (notably eggs, milk, fish, meat, and wheat)
2. Certain inhalants (notably pollens and animal dander)
3. Certain contactants that act on the skin (notably poison ivy and chemical irritants)
4. Drugs, vaccines, and antiserums
5. Insect stings

We are familiar with food allergies that produce urticarial rashes (hives) and intestinal

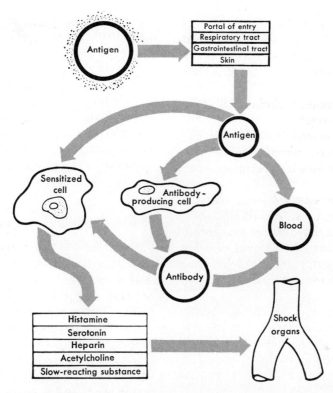

FIG. 1-3 ■ Mechanism of the allergic reaction. The reaction between antigen (allergen) and antibody at the surface of "sensitized cells" causes these cells to release histamine and other harmful agents.

With permission from Therapeutic Notes of Parke, Davis & Co. **67**:102, 1960; modified from Logan, G.B.: Am. J. Dis. Child. **97**:163, 1959.

discomfort. Hay fever and asthma are not uncommon, and we have seen both the symptoms of hay fever (inflamed membranes of eyes, nose, and throat with a watery discharge from the eyes and nose) and the sneezing and wheezing of the person with bronchial asthma. Also, we have seen the blisters produced in the allergic reaction to the toxin of poison ivy. The nature and severity of symptoms vary with different allergens and different individuals.

The mechanism of allergic reactions is not completely understood. In allergies of the **immediate type** the reaction appears within a few minutes after contact with the allergen. The release of **histamine** or histamine-like sub-

stances from certain sensitized cells seems to be involved in producing the symptoms (Fig. 1-3). This is proved in part by the fact that **antihistamines**, such as diphenhydramine (Benadryl), cause symptoms to subside in many cases. The most pronounced reactions result from insect stings. About 8 people in 1000 are allergic to insects. Symptoms range from mild to severe. But even a mild reaction is ominous, because the next time the person is stung, a moderate to severe reaction may occur. A severe reaction (**anaphylaxis**) is characterized by labored breathing, weakness, shock, and collapse. Death can result in 10 to 15 minutes.

■ Treatment

The first step in the management of an allergy is to discover the causative agent. Sometimes the individual knows very well from successive experiences what causes the allergy. This is likely to be true in the food allergies. If the allergen is not known, a restricted diet may be followed by the addition of one suspected food at a time until the culprit is found.

The cause of an inhalant or contact allergy is less likely to be obvious. If the case history does not reveal the cause, the physician can make a series of patch tests or scratch tests on the skin, applying in sequence extracts from the respective suspected allergens (Fig. 1-4). In a positive reaction a reddened area, wheal, or blister appears at the spot where the suspected allergen was applied (Fig. 1-5).

Allergies may appear in persons who have

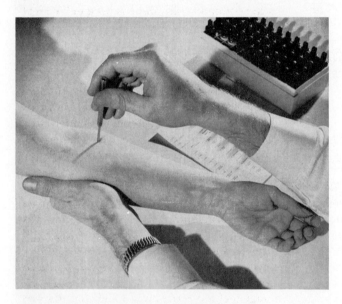

FIG. 1-4 ■ Testing for allergy by scarifying.

From Smith, A.L.: Microbiology and pathology, ed. 9, St. Louis, 1976, The C.V. Mosby Co.; courtesy Cutter Laboratories, Berkeley, California.

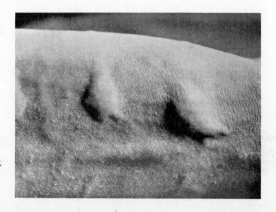

FIG. 1-5 ■ Arm showing three strong reactions for allergy.

From Vaughn and Black: Practice of allergy, ed. 3, St. Louis, 1954, The C.V. Mosby Co.

not had them before and in a few cases may disappear spontaneously. There are four possible approaches in the treatment of these conditions: avoidance, desensitization, antihistamines, and hormones.

1. Avoidance may be possible in whole or in part by change of residence, diet, or occupation, withdrawal of a drug, or removal of a household pet or an article of clothing. Avoiding trips to rural areas, using air filters, or keeping windows and doors closed may help in the case of a particular inhalant.

2. Desensitization is carried out by injecting an extract of the causative allergen in a series of gradually increasing doses. This regimen is followed in the case of pollens, dusts, spores, vaccines, and serums.

3. Antihistamines are useful for treating the symptoms of allergic reactions, including seasonal hay fever and allergic rhinitis. Also acute and chronic urticaria (hives) and certain allergic skin conditions respond well, and pruritus (itching) may be alleviated. Interestingly, the antihistamines are without effect in bronchial asthma or systemic anaphylaxis.

4. Hormones employed in the treatment and control of allergic reactions include epinephrine (Adrenalin) and corticosteroids (for example, cortisol and betamethasone [Celestone]). Epinephrine is lifesaving in anaphylaxis. Corticosteroids are employed in severe asthma (when other drugs fail) and in the management of a variety of other hypersensitivity states.

▰▰▰▰ INFECTION

Infection is the entry and development of a pathogenic (infectious) agent in the tissues of the body. The result may be inapparent (subclinical) or manifest (with signs and symptoms). The term **host** applies to humans and all other living species that give subsistence or lodgment to an infectious agent. The term **transmission** refers to the mechanism by which a susceptible species is exposed to an infectious agent. These mechanisms are either direct (for example, kissing) or indirect (for example, contaminated water). Infections are treated with **antibiotics** or injections of **antibodies** (in the form of antiserums, immune serums, and so on). For some infections, such as the common cold, there is no specific treatment available.

▰ Infectious agents

Infectious agents, or **pathogens**, include microorganisms (microbes), parasitic worms, and ectoparasites. Pathogenic microorganisms represent just about every category of microscopic life except algae. (The great bulk of all microorganisms, however, are either harmless or beneficial.) Microorganisms include **bacteria**, **viruses**, **fungi**, and **protozoa**. Bacteria are unicellular organisms, the vast majority of which do not contain chlorophyll. Viruses (and viroids) are the smallest pathogens (observable with the **electron microscope**) and reproduce only within living cells. Fungi include molds (multicellular, filamentous forms) and yeasts (relatively large, round to oval microbes). Protozoa are unicellular animals. Parasitic worms include **nematodes** (roundworms, usually pointed at both ends), **trematodes** (unsegmented flatworms), and **cestodes**, or **tapeworms** (segmented flatworms). Ectoparasites include lice, fleas, and mites.

▰ Pathogenesis

The signs and symptoms of infection develop (**pathogenesis**) from cellular destruction or intoxicating mechanisms or both. **Exotoxins**, the most deadly biologic poisons known, are responsible for a number of diseases including tetanus, diphtheria, gas gangrene, anthrax, plague, and botulism. Much less deadly, but still capable of causing violent responses, are **endotoxins**, the products released by certain rod-shaped bacteria. Exotoxins are heat-sensitive proteins readily released from the bacterial cell; endotoxins are heat-stable and not readily released. Other key differences relate to antigenicity and pyrogenicity. Exotoxins are highly antigenic, stimulating the output of neutralizing antibodies called **antitoxins**; endotoxins are weakly antigenic. Endotoxins are highly pyrogenic (fever-inducing), whereas exotoxins are not.

In addition to exotoxins and endotoxins, microbes manufacture a variety of other toxic products including hemolysin (which destroys red blood cells), leukocidin (which destroys white blood cells), coagulase (which facilitates clotting of blood), and hyaluronidase (which dissolves intercellular cement).

■ IMMUNITY

Immunity is the power of an individual to resist or overcome an infection. It may be complete, or it may be so weak as to be scarcely appreciable. Immunity relates primarily to bacterial and viral diseases, since little or no immunity develops in connection with most fungal, protozoan, and worm infections.

The invasion of the human body by a pathogen is not unlike the invasion of a country by a hostile army. If the invading army is successful, the life of the nation comes to an end. But if the invaded nation fights back and is successful, the invaders are eliminated from the territory they have overrun. Because of this experience the country sets barriers against a second invasion. These barriers, like the factors of immunity, are varied, numerous, and complex. They may consist of a new army to combat the destructive forces of the enemy, new defensive methods for the army, or a general sensitiveness and readiness of the people to respond immediately to the threat of a new attack. Likewise, the human body, in overcoming a microbial army, may create new defensive substances that remain in the blood; the tissues subject to microbial invasion may become more resistant to the particular organism; or the whole bodily reaction may be more prompt and effective at a second attack.

■ Phagocytosis and antibodies

The body has been found to react in definite ways to particular pathogens. Of special note are phagocytosis and the production of antibodies. Many kinds of pathogenic bacteria are devoured in great numbers by certain cells called **phagocytes** (Fig. 1-6). These cells are of two types: motile cells (certain white blood

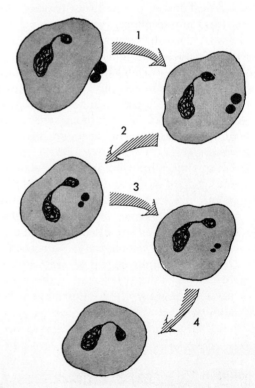

FIG. 1-6 ■ Phagocytosis. Progressive engulfment and destruction of two bacterial cells by phagocytic leukocyte.

cells) and so-called fixed-tissue cells. The motile phagocytic blood cells are attracted to bacteria at the site of infection and become an important constituent of pus.

Most infections involve what is called an **antigen-antibody reaction**. **Antibodies** are protective substances produced by the body in response to antigenic stimulation. Some antibodies (antitoxins) react with toxins to neutralize them. Tetanus antitoxin and diphtheria antitoxin, for example, neutralize, respectively, the toxins of tetanus (lockjaw) and diphtheria. Other kinds of antibodies are known to enhance phagocytosis.

■ Acquired immunity

Immunity may be either active or passive. In **active immunity** the protection against the disease results from the body's own efforts in some type of antigen-antibody reaction. A person may develop active immunity by having the disease or by being inoculated with the appropriate antigen (in the form of a **vaccine** or **toxoid**). In immunization against mumps and measles, for example, the antigen is the living attenuated (weakened) virus. In immunization against typhoid fever, cholera, and whooping cough, the antigen is a vaccine made from the killed bacterium. In immunization against diphtheria and tetanus, the neutralized exotoxin, or toxoid, is used to stimulate the production of antibodies. Both a killed virus vaccine (Salk vaccine) and an oral attenuated polio virus vaccine (Sabin vaccine) are available for immunization against poliomyelitis.

In **passive immunity** protective antibodies are either artificially transmitted to the person by injection or are transferred from mother to offspring via the placenta. For example, diphtheria antitoxin is given to susceptible persons known to have been exposed to the disease. The infant at birth usually has a passive immunity to diphtheria because of the presence of maternal antitoxin. The important thing to remember, however, is that, unlike active immunity, passive immunity is short-lived (typically, weeks versus years).

Carriers represent "immunity without eradication." Usually after a disease the body rids itself of the pathogen. Occasionally, however, this does not happen, and a condition of mutual tolerance is set up. The person continues to be a carrier of the infection without showing evidence of disease. The person and the infective organism have acquired the ability to tolerate each other. Carriers of diphtheria, typhoid fever, cholera, meningococcal meningitis, streptococcal disease, malaria, amebic dysentery, and poliomyelitis are known to exist. Many epidemics have been traced to such carriers. In some instances a lowered vitality of the carrier may result in a recurrence of active disease in the individual. In some instances the carrier has not had a recognized case of the disease but has had an inapparent infection.

Tests for immunity are very useful. For example, by the **Schick test** we can determine a person's immunity or susceptibility to diphtheria. A small amount of modified toxin is introduced into the skin. If no appreciable local reaction appears, we know that antitoxin is present in the blood and the patient is immune. The **Dick test** is a similar test for use in scarlet fever. Skin tests are also available for aid in the diagnosis of certain infections (for example, the tuberculin test).

■ Natural immunity

Somewhat over and above the body's acquired immunity is the matter of natural immunity. This type of immunity may be the heritage of a species, race, or individual. Species immunity is one peculiar to a given species (for example, humans do not have distemper, nor do dogs have measles). A racial immunity is one possessed by a race (for example, ordinary sheep are more susceptible to anthrax than Algerian sheep). Species and racial immunities are more highly developed in plants than in animals. Individual immunity is a rare condition.

▰▰▰ CANCER

Some 420,000 Americans die of cancer annually, and an estimated 1 million are diagnosed as having it. Two out of three families are affected, and often as distressing as the illness itself are the disfiguring, debilitating effects of current treatments. The financial cost of the disease is said to be over 2 billion dollars annually, but the greatest cost is in suffering and grief. In general, cancer is a disease of late maturity. Most cases occur after the age of 40, although there are many cases in children and youth.

A cancer (Gr., karkinos, crab), or **malignant tumor**, is an abnormal, seemingly unrestricted growth of cells that tend to invade and destroy surrounding tissues and to transplant themselves through the lymphatic system or bloodstream to other parts of the body (a pathologic event called **metastasis**). These cells threaten life unless removed early, and they may recur after surgical removal if any portion of the tumor remains. Cancers may affect any part of the body, but the skin, lungs, rectum, breasts, and uterus are the sites most commonly affected.

Cancers are named according to the type of tissue in which they originate. **Carcinomas** are malignant tumors originating in the epithelial tissue (skin, glands, and mucous membranes of the alimentary canal, respiratory tract, or genitourinary system). **Sarcomas** are malignant tumors originating in connective tissue, bones, tendons, fat, and muscles. Cancer of the blood-forming organs, or **leukemia**, and its increasing prevalence are mentioned in our discussion of disorders of the blood.

A tumor can also be **benign**. Such a growth is essentially harmless, although it may produce injury or even death if it presses on an important organ so as to interfere with its functioning. Examples of such interference may occur with brain tumors, tumors that hinder the circulation of the blood, or tumors that invade the tissue of the ovary, preventing ovulation. A benign tumor may become malignant, or it may soften and degenerate until it menaces health. It should be examined by a physician and removed if necessary. Once removed, it will not recur.

The overall incidence of cancer has decreased slightly in the past 25 years, but there have been sharp changes in the incidence of certain types of cancer. The occurrence of lung cancer, especially among men, has risen sharply in the last 35 or 40 years, mainly because of cigarette smoking. On the other hand, the death rate from stomach cancer has dropped over 50%. We do not know why. Furthermore, there has been an unexplained increase in leukemia but a sharp decrease in the death rate from uterine cancer. The latter relates to earlier treatment and to the wider use of the Papanicolaou vaginal smear test in detection.

Cancer reflects a disturbance in normal cell growth and reproduction that we do not yet understand. It is known, however, that some form of chronic irritation may be an inciting cause. A pigmented mole that is rubbed constantly by clothing may develop into a cancer. No suspected growth should be squeezed or manipulated. Workers in certain occupations who are exposed to irritant chemicals often develop cancer on the exposed parts of the body.

We now have a long list of cancer-producing substances (**carcinogens**) identifiable in certain tars, oils, and soots and in deposits on smoke-preserved meat and fish. Tobacco tar is a recognized carcinogen. Some substances produce cancer at the site of contact, others at distant sites. Some require metabolic conversion for activity. Studies are constantly being made of drugs, food additives, cosmetics, insecticides, and other substances to see if they contain carcinogens. Studies on human populations show that cancer is induced by various forms of radiation. Radiologists have had a higher rate of leukemia than people who are not so exposed, as has the population of Hiroshima and Nagasaki who survived exposure to the prototype atomic bomb. Persons at the early part of the century who were employed in painting watch dials with radium developed bone cancer. And perhaps above all, most forms of skin cancer (the most common cancers) are caused by the ultraviolet rays of sunlight.

Finally, there is the matter of viruses. No human cancer has been demonstrated to be caused by a virus, but viruses are implicated in uterine (cervical) cancer and in Burkitt's lymphoma. On the other hand, in various animal species at least a dozen cancers have been shown to be caused by viruses. They include leukemia, sarcomas, and skin cancers. The animals studied include mice, chickens, rabbits, guinea pigs, and monkeys. There is no single "cancer virus."

In some cases, multiple factors have been shown to be involved in the production of cancer. At the Jackson Memorial Laboratory, the transmission of breast cancer in mice was possible only if the mother came from a strain of animals having a high rate of breast cancer. Kaplan's studies at Stanford University showed that leukemia in mice could be evoked only in animals carrying a leukemia virus. Animals with the virus would not develop leukemia in the absence of radiation. Both factors were needed.

The degree of constitutional susceptibility varies greatly in persons. Likewise, the external conditions to which different persons are

---

Cancer's 7 warning signals

Change in bowel or bladder habits

A sore that does not heal *towards a month or more.*

Unusual bleeding or discharge

Thickening or lump in breast or elsewhere

Indigestion or difficulty in swallowing

Obvious change in wart or mole

Nagging cough or hoarseness

If YOU have a warning signal, see your doctor!

FIG. 1-7 ■ Cancer's seven warning signals spell CAUTION.
Reprinted by permission of the American Cancer Society, Inc.

---

subjected may vary. Many combinations of these factors occur, varying from the individual with low susceptibility who does not come into contact with irritants to the highly susceptible person who is constantly under adverse environmental influences. This may account for the great variability in the appearance of cancer and the difficulty in making generalizations about it.

The two most important steps in the control of cancer are (1) early discovery of the disease before it has had time to spread from the point of origin and scatter (metastasize) to parts of the body where it cannot be reached (Fig. 1-7) and (2) removal of the growth by surgery or destruction by radiation or chemotherapy (often used in combination). Presently, many scientists believe that an agent called **interferon** has great potential for cancer treatment. This is especially true because interferon is a natural substance (a protein) produced in virtually all human and animal cells. It is believed that interferon somehow recharges the body's own immunology system—attracting the body's natural "killer cells" to the cancerous growth, where they destroy the malignant cells. With the supply of this mysterious substance on the upswing (largely through the efforts of genetic engineering) what researchers must do now is to determine precisely how and when it can be safely used. Like all forms of chemical treatment, albeit a natural chemical, interferon does have its side effects. Most are minor, but a few give physicians cause for concern.

Still another development of a chemical-immunologic nature relates to the use of **monoclonal antibodies**. If special antigens (p. 6) can be found on cancer cells that are not present in normal cells, the lab-produced antibodies would home in on tumors without damaging normal tissue. Although such antigens have not yet been identified, monoclonal antibodies have shown some effect in

treating leukemia and lymphomas and in reducing the number of circulating tumor cells in the bloodstream. Antibodies could also be tagged with radioactive substances or chemicals to carry lethal doses directly to cancer cells while bypassing normal cells.

The American Cancer Society's Committee of Unproven Methods of Cancer Management is actively involved in strengthening and encouraging passage of state legislation to control the use of worthless cancer remedies and tests. For the most part, progress has been made in this area, with the notable exception of laetrile (a substance extracted from apricot pits). Laetrile has received exhaustive tests in animals and has never shown any effectiveness in the prevention, treatment, or cure of cancer. Nonetheless a number of states legally permit its use. In the view of the American Cancer Society and the Food and Drug Administration, "legalization of an unproven remedy can defraud the public, endanger the lives of countless persons, and open the door to a wave of worthless preparations."

SELF-TEST

1. _D_ physiologic balance
2. ____ of unknown causation
3. ____ foreign to the body
4. _K_ hay fever
5. ____ shock and collapse
6. _I_ lice and fleas
7. _m_ mode of transmission
8. ____ possesses passive immunity
9. ____ bacteria and viruses
10. _N_ stimulate active immunity
11. ____ deadly poisons
12. ____ neutralize toxins
13. ____ devour pathogens
14. _H_ blood cancer
15. ____ cancer therapy

a. anaphylaxis
b. phagocytes
c. interferon
d. homeostasis
e. exotoxins
f. newborn
g. antitoxins
h. leukemia
i. ectoparasites
j. idiopathic
k. allergy
l. antigen
m. kissing
n. toxoids
o. microbes

■■■■■ STUDY QUESTIONS

1. "Mental, emotional, and social well-being contribute to physical health." In what way(s) is this statement true? How does the process work?

2. Although communicable disease death rates have dropped precipitously since 1900, non-communicable disease death rates have actually risen. What is your explanation?

3. What do infections and allergies have in common?

4. Antihistamines, for example, diphenhydramine (Benadryl) and chlorpheniramine (Chlor-Trimeton), are helpful in hay fever, urticaria (hives), and certain other allergies. How do you explain the relief they provide, or, more formally, what is their "mechanism of action"?

5. There are four categories of microorganisms, or microbes, that cause disease. What are they?

6. All communicable (or contagious) diseases are "infections," but, strictly speaking, all infectious diseases are not "communicable." Why? Can you give examples?

7. Lasting immunity against measles arises (a) from actually having the infection or (b) through vaccination. How do you account for this?

8. For the first 4 to 6 months of life, the infant may have an immunity to measles, mumps, diphtheria, and a number of other infections. Why does this immunity not last longer or, indeed, for good? Further, why do we say "may have" rather than "has"?

9. In all recognized scientific and statistical studies pertaining to the matter, laetrile has been found to be worthless. Nonetheless, as pointed out in the text, a number of states legally permit its use. Does this make sense to you?

10. What are the very latest developments in interferon treatment of cancer?

CHAPTER 2

The human body as a whole

The human body, like all living organisms, is made up of trillions of microscopic units called cells. Stated otherwise, the cell is the fundamental unit of life. Moving our attention from the microscopic to what can be seen with the unaided eye, we discover that cells compose tissues, tissues compose organs, organs compose systems, and systems compose the body. The "living stuff" of the cell—protoplasm—is composed of water and a galaxy of organic (carbon) and inorganic (noncarbon) chemical compounds. Some of these substances constitute the structure of the cell, and others enter into complex biochemical reactions that characterize life processes. The sum total of these reactions is referred to as metabolism. Finally, there is the ultimate chemical, deoxyribonucleic acid (DNA). The information and messages contained within this awesome molecule comprise the genetic code.

The cell

Tissues and systems

Body build

Body chemistry

Metabolism

Genetic code

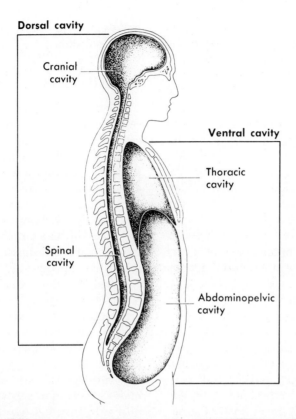

Dorsal cavity

Cranial cavity

Ventral cavity

Thoracic cavity

Spinal cavity

Abdominopelvic cavity

FIG. 2-1 ■ Body cavities. Note that the diaphragm (not labeled) separates the thoracic and abdominopelvic cavities.

The human body is a bilaterally symmetrical structure with a backbone and an array of organs housed in a **dorsal cavity** and a **ventral cavity** (Fig. 2-1). The dorsal cavity, the continuous space enclosed by the cranium and spinal canal, houses the brain and spinal cord respectively; the ventral cavity houses all the other internal organs. The **thoracic cavity**, the portion of the ventral cavity above the **diaphragm**, contains the heart, lungs, trachea, esophagus, and thymus gland (plus associated nerves, blood vessels, and so on); the **abdominopelvic cavity**, the portion of the ventral cavity below the diaphragm, contains the stomach, liver, gallbladder, pancreas, spleen, intestines, rectum, kidneys,

bladder, and sex organs. With this general plan in mind let us now consider the body's fundamental building blocks.

■ THE CELL

According to the dictionary, a cell, among other things, is "any small compartment," and this is just what Robert Hooke had in mind in 1665 when he applied the term to the empty microscopic compartments he saw in cork. More particularly, Hooke was referring to the nonliving cellulose walls—the shell of life. The idea of this empty space held sway until Dujardin in 1835 underscored the contents of the cell rather than the walls. He called the living stuff "sarcode," a term to be replaced 11 years later by Hugo von Mohl's "protoplasm." Today we think of a cell as a circumscribed mass of protoplasm with a **nucleus**.

The idea that the cell is the fundamental unit of living things—the **cell theory**—was expressed in one way or another by several biologists, including von Mohl, but most authors usually credit the revelation to the German botanist Matthias Schleiden and the German zoologist Theodor Schwann. Schleiden put forward the cell theory in terms of plant tissues in 1838, and a year later Schwann applied the theory to all living things. In Schwann's words, "all organized bodies are composed of essentially similar parts, namely cells."

■ Basic design

Cells are of various shapes and sizes, each kind designed and equipped for a particular job. Surface cells protect, muscle cells contract, nerve cells relay electrical messages, and so on. The smallest cells are as tiny as 0.1 micrometer (μm) in diameter, and the largest are the size of the largest bird's egg. Human cells have an average diameter somewhere in the vicinity of 10 μm. The ovum, the largest human cell, is about the size of the dot over an "i."

All cells are circumscribed by a cell membrane (Fig. 2-2), and plant cells are further circumscribed by an outer nonliving **cell wall**. The fundamental parts of the cell are the **nucleus**, **cell membrane**, and **cytosome** (the body of the cell apart from the nucleus). Most cells contain a single nucleus, but indeed there are notable exceptions. Some cells are without a distinct nucleus at all, whereas others are multinucleated. The classic idea of cell individuality has many exceptions, since in some tissues the cell membranes (the boundaries between the cells) dissolve away, leaving one huge cytosome with myriad nuclei throughout its substance.

■ Cell division

The human body grows as a consequence of cell division, or **mitosis**. In this complex process (Fig. 2-3) a single cell gives rise to two identical daughter cells that contain the same number of **chromosomes** as the parent cell. A chromosome is a linear body of the cell nucleus (observable only during mitosis) containing **deoxyribonucleic acid** (DNA), a chemical substance responsible for the determination and transmission of hereditary characteristics. Specifically, the DNA molecule is "blocked off" into segments called **genes**, each of which is responsible for a specific hereditary feature. Every species of plants and animals has its own characteristic chromosome number. The human chromosome number is 46.

A very special type of cell division, called **meiosis**, occurs in sexually reproducing organisms. In this division the daughter cells become **reproductive cells**, each containing one-half the species number of chromosomes. But this certainly makes biologic sense because when reproductive (sex) cells unite in the process of fertilization, the species chromosome number is restored. In humans this means that each reproductive cell—that is, each sperm and each ovum (egg)—contains 23 chromosomes. For convenience, the species chromosome number is referred to as the **diploid** number, and the reproductive cell number is referred to as the **haploid** number. Thus the human species has the diploid number 46 and the haploid number 23.

■■■ TISSUES AND SYSTEMS

A tissue is an aggregation of similar cells united for the purpose of a particular func-

Cell membrane   **Mitochondrion**

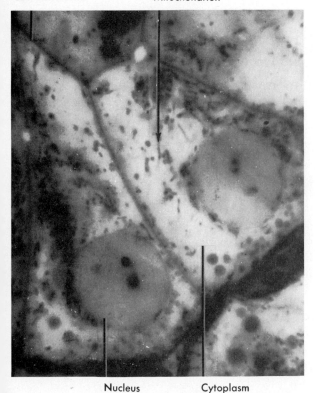

Nucleus   **Cytoplasm**

FIG. 2-2 ■ Typical animal cells (in this case liver cells from a turtle). Two complete cells can be seen. Mitochondria (sing., mitochondrion) are cytoplasmic structures associated with energy production. The dark round structures within the nucleus are called nucleoli.

From Bevelander, G., and Ramaley, J.A., Essentials of histology, ed. 8, St. Louis, 1979, The C.V. Mosby Co.

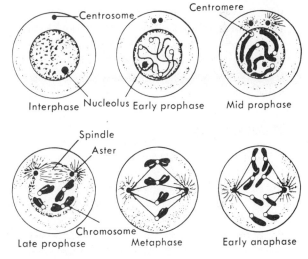

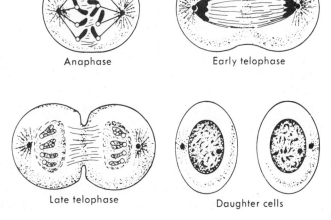

FIG. 2-3 ■ Diagram of mitosis in an animal cell with four chromosomes. Beginning with the interphase ("resting" parent cell), the division process progresses through four stages: prophase, metaphase, anaphase, and telophase. Note that between the metaphase and early anaphase the four chromosomes have split to provide each daughter cell with the same number as the parent cell. Note, too, that the chromosomes are not distinct until the mid prophase.

From Levine, L.: Biology of the gene, ed. 3, St. Louis, 1980, The C.V. Mosby Co.

tion. The body's trillions of cells are organized into four categories of tissues: epithelial, muscular, connective, and nerve. In brief, **epithelial tissues** cover and line surfaces and produce secretions; **muscular tissues** effect contraction and movement; **connective tissues** support and protect other tissues; and **nerve tissues** provide communication and response.

Cells constitute tissues, and, in like fashion, tissues constitute **organs**, those somewhat independent parts of the body that perform a special function or functions. The heart and kidneys are organs in the full sense of this definition. Further, organs constitute **systems**. A system is defined as a set of organs that function in a common purpose. The circulatory system functions to bring oxygen and nutrients to the cells; the respiratory system functions to aerate the blood; the urinary system functions to remove lethal wastes. These and other body systems—in health and in disease—will constitute the "backbone" of subsequent chapters.

■■■ BODY BUILD

Differences in body build, or physique, are apparent throughout life. Some individuals are stocky with heavy bones; others are thin with finer bones; others exhibit gradations between the two extremes. One way to charac-

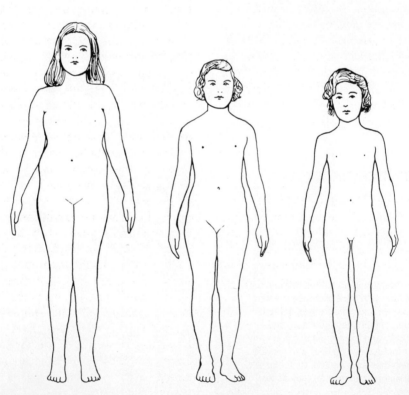

FIG. 2-4 ■ Physique differences in 10-year-old girls. From left to right, dominant endomorph (6-3-3), dominant mesomorph (4-5-2), and dominant ectomorph (2-2-6).

Courtesy Dr. Stanley M. Garn, Yellow Springs, Ohio.

terize the differences in body build was proposed by Sheldon many years ago. According to his now well-recognized scheme of classification, there are three basic **somatotypes** (body types): ectomorphic, endomorphic, and mesomorphic. The **ectomorph** is an individual who is especially tall (linear) and fragile, with a large surface area, thin muscles and subcutaneous tissues, and slightly developed digestive viscera. The **endomorph** has a relative preponderance of soft tissues throughout the body, with large digestive viscera and an accumulation of fat and with large trunk, thighs, and tapering extremities. The **mesomorph**—the well-proportioned individual—has a relative preponderance of muscle, bone, and connective tissue, usually with a heavy, hard physique and rectangular outline. Since many individuals cannot be readily categorized as belonging to one of three somatotypes, Sheldon developed a rating scheme to indicate the relative dominance of each. As an example, an extreme ectomorph would be classified as 1-1-7 (that is, endorphy 1, mesomorphy 1, and ectomorphy 7). Examples of dominant somatotypes in 10-year-old girls are presented in Fig. 2-4.

◼◼◼ BODY CHEMISTRY

Protoplasm—the "stuff of the cell"—is a jellylike substance. There is nothing unique about its constituent elements or, for that matter, many of its compounds. In other words, the chemical key to the mystery of life resides in the way all the atoms and molecules are arranged and put together.

The chief compound of protoplasm is just water (H_2O), which is usually present to an extent of about 75% by weight. The other **inorganic** constituents (carbon-free compounds) may be characterized as chemical salts. The most important are the chlorides, phosphates, and sulfates of sodium, calcium, magnesium, and potassium. These compounds are commonly referred to as **electrolytes**. The **organic** constituents of protoplasm may be categorized as **carbohydrates**, **lipids**, **proteins**, and **nucleic acids**. Carbohydrates (sugars and starches) serve as fuel for energy; lipids (fats and fatlike substances) serve as reserve fuel and, to a lesser degree, as structural elements; proteins serve as enzymes and collectively as the basic fabric or "molecular backbone" of the cell; nucleic acids (DNA and RNA) act as "chemical information" in metabolism and in the genetic code.

◼◼◼ METABOLISM

The activities of the cell and the body at large—respiration, growth, irritability, reproduction, and so on—are manifestations of **metabolism**, which may be defined as the sum of the chemical processes of protoplasm. Metabolic reactions involving the conversion of simple substances into complex substances constitute **anabolism**; those involving the breakdown of complex substances into simple substances constitute **catabolism**. In brief, anabolism is "constructive metabolism," and catabolism is "destructive metabolism."

The key anabolic event is the DNA-directed synthesis of proteins, for with new protein comes new protoplasm. Like most cellular events this process requires energy in the form of **adenosine triphosphate** (ATP), the magic molecule produced in the catabolic reactions of cellular respiration. The magic of ATP resides in its high-energy phosphate bonds, for once they are broken, their pent-up chemical energy becomes immediately available to the cell. And "immediately" is the proper word here because food energy is not immediately available. That is, the chemical bonds of food molecules are not energetic enough to be useful, and it is necessary—via cellular respiration—to concentrate and package their energy potential in fast-acting ATP.

GENETIC CODE

The chemical secret of life resides in the DNA molecule that composes the chromosomes. As noted earlier, special segments of this molecule—the genes—determine our heredity. Specifically, each gene, with the assistance of **ribonucleic acid** (RNA), directs the synthesis of a **particular protein**. Since proteins serve as protoplasmic building blocks and **enzymes** (catalytic agents that spark metabolic activities), we can well appreciate that a given cell is what it is because of its particular DNA blueprint. What is more, when a cell divides, this blueprint—or **genetic code**—is passed along to its daughter cells. This explains (1) why daughter cells are identical to the parent cell (for example, the "offspring" of liver cells are liver cells, and the "offspring" of kidney cells are kidney cells) and (2) why children resemble their parents. In the latter instance, the offspring inherits one half of its genetic code from the mother and one half from the father.

Genetic disease

Hundreds of hereditary diseases are known to be caused by **faulty genes**. The first such disease to be spelled out in pure chemical terms—right down to the last atom—was **sickle cell anemia**. The faulty gene in this case is the one that directs the synthesis of **hemoglobin**, the protein pigment of red blood cells. The result of the disease, of course, is faulty hemoglobin and sickling of the red cells (Fig. 2-5). Since these distorted cells are unable to pass through the capillaries, they plug these vessels and trigger blood clots. Further, sickled cells are more fragile than normal red blood cells and ultimately undergo dissolution (hence, the anemia). Genes, however, come in pairs (one from each parent), and in most genetic diseases the normal gene overshadows its faulty partner and is referred to as **dominant**, whereas the faulty gene is called **recessive**. This is true in sickle cell anemia; that is, the full-blown disease occurs only in those who have inherited two faulty genes. Few of these victims live beyond age 40.

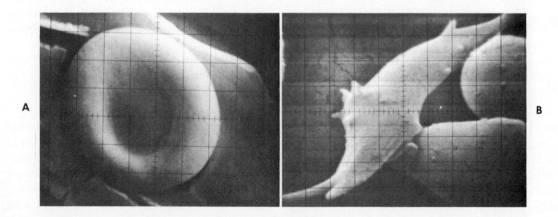

FIG. 2-5 ■ A, Normal red blood cells. **B,** Those of sickle cell anemia. (×10,000.)

Courtesy Patricia Farnsworth, Ph.D.; micrograph taken by Irene Piscopo of Philips Electronic Instruments, Mt. Vernon, N.Y., on a Philips EM 300 electron microscope with scanning attachment.

SELF-TEST

1. _____ divides abdominopelvic cavity   a. brain
2. _____ housed in thoracic cavity   b. enzymes
3. _____ housed in cranial cavity   c. gene
4. _____ unit of length   d. tissue
5. _____ biologic unit   e. cytosome
6. _____ surrounds nucleus   f. ATP
7. _____ maintains diploid number   g. lipids
8. _____ sex-cell production   h. cell
9. _____ aggregation of cells   i. carbohydrates
10. _____ group of organs   j. diaphragm
11. _____ fatlike substances   k. meiosis
12. _____ sugars and starches   l. lungs
13. _____ cellular catalysts   m. mitosis
14. _____ high-energy substance   n. micrometer
15. _____ directs protein synthesis   o. system

STUDY QUESTIONS

1. "Ventral" comes from the Latin *ventralis*, which means "pertaining to the belly." How does this fit in with the anatomic expression "ventral cavity"?
2. The abdominopelvic cavity is the division of the ventral cavity below the diaphragm. What is the diaphragm?
3. The human ovum, or egg, is about 100 μm in diameter. How many of these cells would it take to span an inch?
4. What is the distinction between "cytosome" and "cytoplasm"?
5. Sometimes meiosis is referred to as "reduction division." Why?
6. What is the relationship between a chromosome and a gene?
7. As noted in the text, there are four kinds of tissues: epithelial, muscular, connective, and nervous. Which of these types composes the skin? The spinal cord? The skeleton? The heart?
8. Body water is compartmentalized into cellular water (protoplasmic water) and extracellular water (present in the blood and in the fluid surrounding the cells). Taken together this water amounts to about 60% (by weight) of the adult human body. In the context of this value, how much water does your body contain—in pounds and kilograms, and in quarts and liters?
9. In the digestive process, carbohydrates, fats, and proteins are broken down into simpler substances (smaller molecules) that can be absorbed into the blood. Is this chemical action best characterized as metabolism, catabolism, or anabolism?
10. Galactosemia is the metabolic inability—inherited as a recessive trait—to convert galactose into glucose (galactose is a digestive product of lactose, or milk sugar). If milk feeding is not eliminated at once, the infant will either die or become mentally retarded. Based on your reading of genetic disease, what is the fundamental defect here? Are one or both parents "at fault"?

CHAPTER 3

The skeletal system

"Oh them bones, them dry bones" just about sums up first impressions. But the truth of the matter is that the skeletal system in general and the bones in particular are very much alive. Bone is a type of connective tissue, and like all tissues it is composed of cells actively engaged in physiologic pursuits. Some of these cells produce the rocklike bone substance, while others bring about the dissolution of this substance for the purpose of supplying calcium to the blood. Furthermore, certain cells in the red bone marrow manufacture blood corpuscles at a prodigious rate. It is estimated that about 1 million worn-out red blood corpuscles are destroyed every second, and quite obviously new ones must be produced to replace them. Failure of the red marrow to comply leads to anemia and, if nonreversible, ultimately to death. Finally, the skeletal system brackets all the other systems, and in so doing it serves as a logical introduction to the human body.

The names of the bones

Classification of bones

Formation and growth of bones

The skeleton

Body posture

Skeletal disorders and diseases

Sprains and fractures

The skeletal system consists of **bones** and **articulations**. Articulations are the joints between the bones; bands of fibrous tissue, called **ligaments**, serve to support and strengthen joints. The system performs or is associated with five functions: support, protection, movement, calcium metabolism, and blood cell formation. Bones serve as the supporting framework of the body in much the same way as steel girders function in supporting a building. As bony "boxes" they protect delicate structures within. In conjunction with joints (which act as fulcrums) and muscles, bones allow movement. Bones serve as the major reservoir into which **calcium** is deposited or from which it is withdrawn, the nature of the shift depending on body needs. Finally, the red marrow within the bones manufactures blood cells. In the adult, this activity, called **hemopoiesis**, is most prominent in the ribs, sternum, vertebrae, and cranial bones.

THE NAMES OF THE BONES

The anatomic name of a bone is of Latin or Greek origin. Just who did the naming is probably lost to the past, but one thing remains quite clear—they had imagination. **Coccyx**, for example, the small bone at the base of the spinal column, derives from "*kokkux*," the Greek word for cuckoo. And this bone does indeed look like a cuckoo's beak. A great many bones have acquired common names: breastbone for **sternum**; shinbone for **tibia**; heel bone for **calcaneus**; shoulder blade for **scapula**; and so on. Some anatomic names refer to a skeletal part rather than a specific bone. For example, **carpus**—the wrist—is composed of 8 carpal bones, each with its own special name.

CLASSIFICATION OF BONES

Based on shape, there are four kinds of bones: long, short, flat, and irregular. **Long** bones are found in the upper and lower extremities (the only exceptions are the bones of the wrist, the ankle, and the kneecap). A typical long bone consists of a shaft, or **diaphysis**, and the ends, or **epiphyses** (sing., epiphysis). The diaphysis is essentially a hollow tube of ivory-like compact bone with its medullary cavity filled with **yellow marrow** (Fig. 3-1). The epiphyses are composed of spongy bone and, in children, **red marrow**. **Short bones** include the wrist and ankle bones. They are more or less cuboidal in shape and consist of spongy bone covered with a shell of compact bone. **Flat bones** include the ribs, sternum, shoulder blades, and cranial bones. Relatively thin, they are composed of spongy bone sandwiched between two layers of compact bone. **Irregular bones** occur in various shapes and sizes and include all bones of the body not mentioned above. Typically, the bulky portion consists of spongy bone surrounded by a layer of compact bone. The rounded portion, or body, of a vertebra is an excellent example.

FORMATION AND GROWTH OF BONES

Bone formation, or **ossification**, is an extremely complex process, and even today there are certain unanswered chemical questions. Essentially it involves the synthesis and intercellular deposition of rocklike calcium salts by bone cells called **osteoblasts**. The molecular structure of this mineral (called hydroxyapatite) has not been positively identified, but the key elements that compose it are well known, namely, **calcium** and **phosphorus**. And, interestingly, there are other bone cells, called **osteoclasts**, that break down this mineral with the subsequent release of calcium to the blood. Bones grow in diameter by the combined action of these two kinds of cells. The osteoclasts enlarge the medullary cavity (by eating away the bone of its walls), while the osteo-

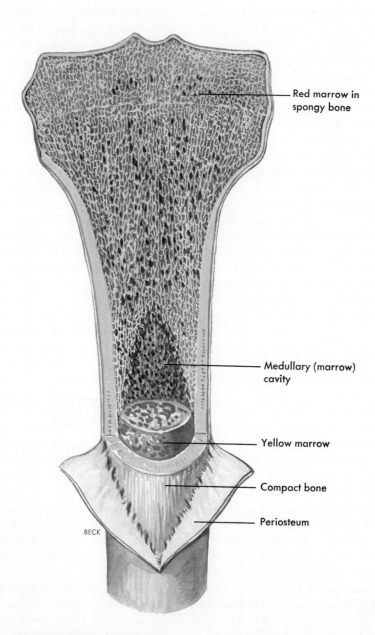

Red marrow in
spongy bone

Medullary (marrow)
cavity

Yellow marrow

Compact bone

Periosteum

BECK

FIG. 3-1 ■ Cutaway section of a long bone.

From Anthony, C.P., and Thibodeau, G.A.: Textbook of anatomy and physiology, ed. 10, St. Louis, 1979, The C.V. Mosby Co.

blasts build new bone around the outside. Throughout childhood and adolescence these opposing processes are in balance, but at about age 40 the tables turn, and from then on bone loss (**resorption**) exceeds bone gain (ossification). Gradually the bones become less resistant to the stresses of compression and bending and thereby tend to shrink or collapse, and sometimes they break. Indeed, the "giving in" of the vertebrae, even though only slightly, explains the decrease in height with advancing years.

◼ THE SKELETON

The skeleton first appears about the time the embryo becomes the fetus (2 months following conception). It is not a true skeleton, of course, but rather a cartilaginous structure whose osteoblasts are about to commence the ossification process just described. This process, to some degree, continues throughout life, but the actual growth in bones stops at about 18 years in females and at about 21 years in males. At this time bone resorption catches up with bone formation.

The adult skeleton is composed of 206 bones (Fig. 3-2). Most of these may be seen in the newborn skeleton, but during normal growth and development some bones fuse, or unite, to form just one bone where previously there had been several. By way of example, the coccyx, the tailbone, results from the fusion of four or five vertebrae. For purposes of study, the skeleton is divided into two main parts: the axial and appendicular. The **axial skeleton**, so-called because it forms the axis of the body, includes the bones of the skull, thorax, and vertebrae (Table 3-1). The **appendicular skeleton** includes the bones of the upper extremities and lower extremities. The study of bones is made more interesting if one can locate the bones in his or her own body and, insofar as possible, feel and follow their general outline.

◼ Male vs female skeleton

A growing girl at any age has reached greater maturity than a boy of the same age, and this is especially evident in the skeletal system. The pisiform bone (the bone that produces the rounded elevation on the small finger side of the wrist) affords an excellent example. X-ray assessment shows that in the female this bone is usually completely ossified at the age of 9 or 10 years, whereas complete ossification in the male does not occur until about the age of 13 years. In general appearance the male skeleton is more rugged, the bones more massive, and the bones longer. Interestingly, however, if the knee joints are examined in terms of width in proportion to height, the female has an advantage in that her wider knee joint probably provides more stability in relation to her size.

Without question the major specific distinction between the male and female adult skeleton relates to the **pelvis**, the bony basin formed by the two hipbones (os coxae), the sacrum, and the coccyx (Fig. 3-2). The female pelvis is broad and shallow, whereas the male pelvis is relatively narrow and deep. Furthermore, during pregnancy the ligaments that hold the pelvis together soften and relax (as a result of hormonal activity) and thereby permit pelvic expansion at the time of delivery.

◼ BODY POSTURE

Posture may be defined as position or bearing of the body. Good posture while standing, sitting, walking, or working is the position that enables the body to act most effectively. It does not require maintaining an unvarying position at all times. Temporary twisting, turning, stooping, and bending help to relieve strain. In good standing position (Fig. 3-3) the head is well back, the chin in, the abdomen flat, the back straight, and the knees straight and relaxed. The feet are slightly apart, with the

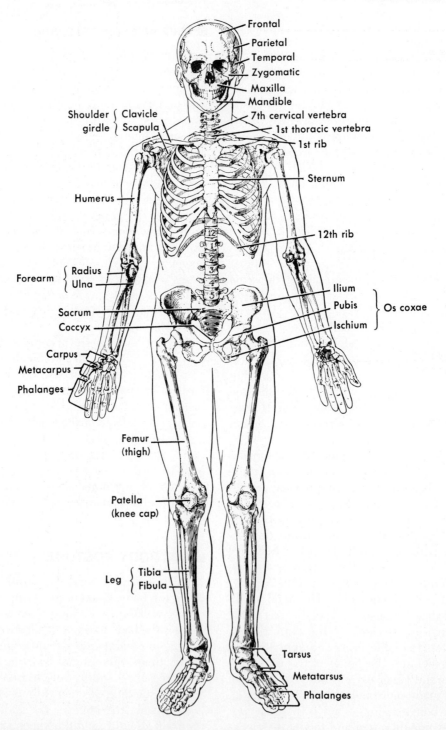

FIG. 3-2 ■ The skeleton from the front. Note that the hipbone, or os coxae, is formed by the fusion of three other bones. The two hipbones plus the sacrum form the pelvis.

From King, B.G., and Showers, M.J.: Human Anatomy and physiology, ed. 6, Philadelphia, 1969, W.B. Saunders Co.

TABLE 3-1
Bones

Bone	Single	Paired
Skull		
Cranium		
Frontal	1	
Parietal		2
Occipital	1	
Temporal		2
Sphenoid	1	
Ethmoid	1	
Face		
Nasal		2
Lacrimal		2
Maxilla		2
Inferior nasal concha		2
Zygomatic		2
Palatine		2
Vomer	1	
Mandible	1	
Vertebrae		
Cervical	7	
Thoracic	12	
Lumbar	5	
Sacrum (5 fused)	1	
Coccyx (4 fused)	1	
Thorax		
Ribs		24
Sternum	1	
Upper extremity		
Clavicle		2
Scapula		2
Humerus		2
Radius		2
Ulna		2
Carpus		16
Metacarpus		10
Phalanges of hand		28
Lower extremity		
Hip (3 fused)		2
Femur		2
Patella		2
Tibia		2
Fibula		2
Tarsus		14
Metatarsus		10
Phalanges of foot		28
Miscellaneous		
Ossicles of the ear (3 in each)		6
Hyoid	1	6
TOTAL		206

Adapted from Francis, CC: Introduction to human anatomy, ed. 6, St. Louis, 1973, The C.V. Mosby Co.

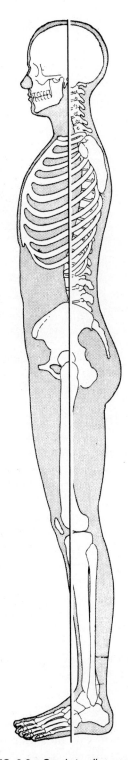

FIG. 3-3 ■ Good standing posture.

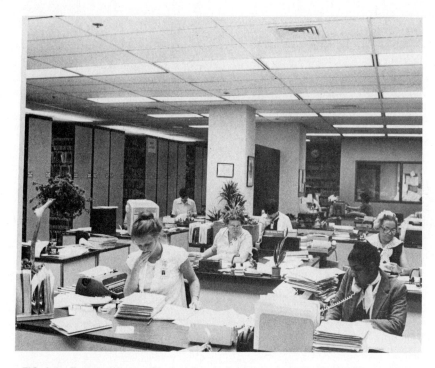

FIG. 3-4 ■ Proper sitting position is dramatically demonstrated by these office workers.

weight balanced and the toes pointed straight ahead. The chest is the point of the body that is farthest forward. It is raised as though lifted forward and upward. The buttocks are tucked under slightly. Weight is borne chiefly on the balls of the feet. A line dropped from the base of the ear would pass through the shoulder, the hip joint, the kneecap, and just in front of the ankle. The normal spine curves slightly forward at the neck and at the small of the back and backward at the shoulders and at the hips. There are no lateral curves in the normal spine.

In erect sitting posture (Fig. 3-4) the relationships of the body, neck, and head are the same as in standing posture. A straight line would pass through the ear, the shoulder, and the hip joint. The feet should not be flat on the floor because this increases pressure on the spine. It is better to cross one leg over the other, or to position them so that the knees are higher than the hips. When the person is working at a desk, as in writing, the body should be leaning forward from the hip without breaking the straight line. Proper sitting posture requires a chair so constructed that good posture is possible. The height should be such that the feet can rest squarely on the floor when the thighs are parallel to it and the knees are at right angles.

■ SKELETAL DISORDERS AND DISEASES

Disorders and diseases of the skeletal system range all the way from flatfoot to deadly bone cancer. They may be broadly categorized as (1) osteodystrophies, (2) inflammatory lesions, and (3) tumors. **Osteodystrophies** are a group of conditions in which there is an abnormality of development, form, or structure of bone. Some are congenital, and others are caused by poor posture, hormonal disturbances, or dietary deficiency. Still others are

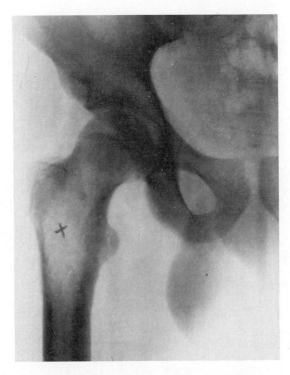

FIG. 3-5 ■ X-ray film showing cancer (*X*) of the upper femur. The lightness of the area results from bone destruction.

Courtesy Charles F. Geschickter, M.D., Georgetown University Medical Center, Washington, D.C.

of obscure or unknown origin. The better known osteodystrophies are gigantism, dwarfism, osteoporosis, rickets, spinal curvature, and flatfoot. **Inflammatory lesions** include bone infections (notably osteomyelitis) and arthritis (notably rheumatoid arthritis). **Tumors** of bone are uncommon. From the standpoint of malignancy and prognosis there are three classes: (1) benign, curable tumors, (2) tumors of borderline malignancy, and (3) malignant tumors, or cancers, many of which are incurable. Some cancers start in bone, whereas others are the result of metastasis (Fig. 3-5).

■ Curvature of the spine

One out of every 10 young people age 10 to 14 will develop some curvature of the spine.

An abnormal curvature of the spine with rearward convexity is called **kyphosis** (hunchback); an abnormal forward curvature of the spine in the lumbar region is called **lordosis** (lordoma); a side-to-side curvature is called **scoliosis**. In most cases the cause is unknown, and the condition cannot be prevented. Sometimes it runs in families. Most people with a mild curvature will only need medical observation. If the condition grows worse, a back brace is worn until bone growth stops. This does not limit most activities. Special exercise may also be included. In extreme cases, spinal surgery is performed. Failure to treat pronounced curvatures can result in medical problems later in life, including obvious physical deformity, pain and arthritic symptoms, and heart and lung disorders.

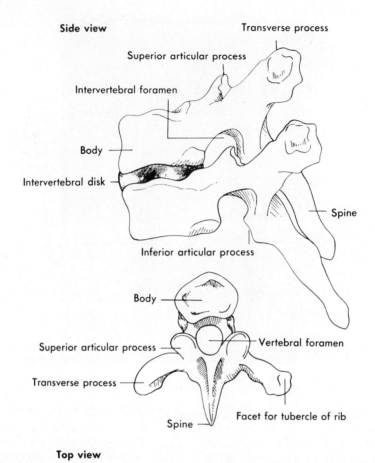

Side view

Transverse process

Superior articular process

Intervertebral foramen

Body

Intervertebral disk

Spine

Inferior articular process

Body

Superior articular process

Vertebral foramen

Transverse process

Spine

Facet for tubercle of rib

Top view

FIG. 3-6 ■ Two thoracic vertebrae and the intervertebral disk between them.

■ Low back pain

Low back pain, according to one estimate, is experienced to some degree by about one third of the population. In the typical case there is pain in the low lumbar, lumbosacral, or sacroiliac region of the back. Pain radiating down the legs commonly is present and may be more severe than the back pain. Most low back pain is related to degenerative joint disease of the lumbosacral area resulting from stress in the lumbosacral junction caused by upright posture. But other causes are almost without number, ranging from congenital defects to obesity. A very special, specific cause

of low back pain is a **herniated intervertebral disk** or, in popular language, "slipped disk." Intervertebral disks, which connect adjacent vertebrae (Fig. 3-6), contain a central core of a pulpy, elastic substance called the **nucleus pulposus**. With age the nucleus loses some of its resiliency. It then may be suddenly compressed by exertion or trauma and pushed through the disk's outer fibrous ring to enter the spinal canal. As a consequence, there is pressure against the spinal nerve roots or the spinal cord itself, resulting in severe pain.

A common cause of "slipped disk" is careless lifting. There is a right and a wrong way

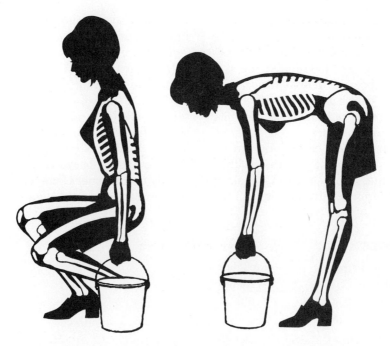

FIG. 3-7 ■ Correct (*left*) and incorrect (*right*) body mechanics in lifting an object from the floor.

to lift. The right way is to squat down, keeping the spine straight, and to lift up with the big muscles of the legs, thighs, arms, and shoulders—not with the muscles of the back (Fig. 3-7). Setting the load down is just the reverse of lifting: let the legs bend slowly, and set the load down easily.

■ Foot problems

The feet are the most abused parts of the body, a fact not difficult to appreciate when we consider that the average American walks about 115,000 miles in a lifetime—more than four times around the world! With each step, minor abnormalities in the foot structure or shoes that don't fit right, or both, can result in such ailments as corns, calluses, bunions, and hammer toes. The never ending introduction of foot-distorting shoe styles for women is the chief culprit. High heels can be deadly, literally. Many painful afflictions of the feet can

be avoided entirely or their more serious consequences averted by simple preventive measures. The experts recommend shoes with low heels, well-cushioned soles, and supportive arches. It is crucial that shoes be at least half an inch longer than the longest toe. Furthermore, shoes and socks should be changed daily, and once or twice a day the feet should be cleansed, dried carefully, and dusted with foot powder. A 10-minute soak in warm water may be the best remedy for tired feet. Foot problems that do not yield to simple ministrations should be attended to a by a podiatrist. "Bathroom surgery" can be dangerous, especially in persons prone to infection.

■■■ SPRAINS AND FRACTURES

A band of fibrous tissue that connects bones or cartilage, serving to support and strengthen joints, is called a **ligament**. An injury that results in a partial or complete tear through one or more ligaments at a particular joint site is called a **sprain**. Besides immediate pain, there is eventual swelling around the sprain because of the leakage of blood under the skin and also possibly because of bone dislocation. Severe sprains, especially sprained ankles, should be x-rayed to determine if there are dislocations or broken bones.

Minor injuries to bone cause localized inflammation of the periosteum (periostitis). More severe injuries may cause a break or **fracture**. In children relative elasticity of the bone may allow bending without a complete break (green-stick fracture). In elderly persons bones are relatively brittle and fracture with slight trauma. Fractures are said to be **compound** when they produce an open wound in the skin and **simple** when they do not produce such a wound. Understandably, compound fractures are often complicated by infection. Healing of bone is slower than healing of other tissues because of the limited blood supply to the bone. Complete return to structural integrity takes about a year.

■■■■■ **SELF-TEST**

1. __E__ red bone marrow
2. _____ articulation
3. _____ formation of bone
4. __G__ dissolution of bone
5. _____ bone covering
6. _____ yellow bone marrow
7. _____ vertebral column
8. _____ flat bones
9. __I__ appendicular skeleton
10. _____ hipbones plus sacrum
11. _____ shinbone
12. _____ bone infection
13. _____ malignant tumor
14. _____ torn ligament
15. _____ broken bone

a. ossification
b. fracture
c. tibia
d. cancer
e. epiphysis
f. periosteum
g. resorption
h. osteomyelitis
i. extremities
j. sprain
k. pelvis
l. joint
m. diaphysis
n. ribs
o. spine

■■■■■ **STUDY QUESTIONS**

1. Certain forms of radiation inhibit or destroy bone marrow. What is the effect of this action?
2. What is the relationship between a joint and a ligament?
3. Give the common name for each of the following bones: sternum, tibia, calcaneus, scapula, and clavicle.
4. What is the relationship among the terms skull, cranium, and face?
5. In regard to the hand, what bones compose the wrist, the palm, the fingers?
6. We all know the phalanges of the foot by another name. What is it?
7. Appendicular, according to the dictionary, pertains to "appendage." What does this tell us about the "appendicular skeleton"?
8. When the calcium level in the blood starts to drop, the body responds by releasing calcium (stored as bone mineral). What bone cells bring about this release?
9. The expression "slipped disk" is somewhat of a misnomer. Why?

10. The word periosteum comes from the Greek *peri*, meaning "around," and *osteon*, meaning "bone." Referring to Fig. 3-1, do you think this is an apt name?

11. Some osteodystrophies are caused by dietary deficiency. Based on what you know about the process of ossification, what two dietary mineral elements are involved?

12. What is the difference between a sprain and a fracture?

13. Why are compound fractures more dangerous than simple fractures?

14. The bones of children are relatively more elastic than the bones of adults. Why?

15. Some bone cancers are the result of metastasis. What does this mean?

CHAPTER 4

The muscular system

There are three kinds of muscle tissue: smooth, cardiac, and skeletal. Smooth muscle occurs in the walls of such viscera as the stomach, the intestines, and the urinary bladder; cardiac muscle composes the heart; and skeletal muscle composes the muscle masses attached to the bones. Our skeletal muscles are the subject of this chapter. Taken together they contain over one third of all body protein and make up 40% to 50% of body weight. Skeletal muscles cover the skeleton, give shape to the body, maintain posture, and in concert with the bones (which act as levers) effect locomotion. Furthermore, they are a powerhouse of chemical and mechanical activity, serving as the body's main source of heat.

Structure and action of muscles

Individual muscles

Disorders and diseases of the muscular system

The skeletal muscles make up the bulk of the human body (Figs. 4-1 and 4-2). They are the muscle masses that attach to bones for the purpose of movement and posture. Skeletal muscle contractions produce movements either of the body as a whole (**locomotion**) or of its parts. The continued partial contraction of many muscles makes possible standing, sitting, and other maintained positions of the body. Contraction, of course, requires considerable energy, which means that muscle cells are actively engaged in the synthesis of **adenosine triphosphate** (ATP). This high-energy compound, we shall recall, fuels cellular activities—notably, contraction in the case of muscle. But interestingly, only a fraction of the energy released in the breakdown of ATP actually goes into contraction—all the rest appears as heat! Indeed, most of our body heat arises from skeletal muscle contraction.

Skeletal muscle tissue, regardless of its body location, looks the same under the microscope. As we see in Fig. 4-3, it is composed of cells in the form of fibers, each of which bears characteristic stripes, or striations. (This is why skeletal muscle is often referred to as **striated muscle**.) When a nerve impulse arrives at a muscle fiber, it sets off a chain of chemical events that terminates in the release of ATP energy and the consequent shortening of the fiber. The shortening of muscle fibers en masse produces muscle contraction.

■ STRUCTURE AND ACTION OF MUSCLES

Muscles vary greatly in size and shape, ranging from the tiny stapedius of the middle ear to the bulky gluteus maximus of the buttock. The typical muscle has a main part (called the **body**) and two extremities (called the **origin** and **insertion**), both of which are attached to bone or cartilage. When such an attachment terminates as a strong white cord, we call it a **tendon**. By convention, the origin is

the extremity attached to the stationary bone (during contraction), and the insertion is the extremity at the "movable end." In not a few instances, however, the origin and insertion are interchangeable, depending on the particular movement. The muscle whose contraction actually produces the desired movement is called the **agonist**, whereas the muscle that concomitantly relaxes (to permit the movement) is referred to as the **antagonist**. Only rarely is a single muscle responsible for a given movement, and for the sake of smoothness the agonist is aided by neighboring muscles called **synergists**. For instance, in extending the leg four large muscles are called into play.

Skeletal muscles are customarily characterized according to their principal action. **Flexors** decrease the angle of a joint; **extensors** increase the angle of a joint; **abductors** move a part away from a median line; **adductors** move a part toward a median line; **supinators** turn the palm upward; **pronators** turn the palm downward; **levators** raise, or lift, a part upward; **depressors** lower a part; **rotators** cause a part to pivot on its axis; **tensors** stiffen, or tense, a part; **sphincters** reduce the size of an opening; **dorsiflexors** pull the foot backward; and **plantar flexors** pull the foot downward.

■ INDIVIDUAL MUSCLES

There are over 600 muscles in the human body, each with its own special Latin name. Surprisingly, these names are quite easy (and can be fun) to learn if we keep in mind that a given name tells us something. This "something" includes one or more of the following features about the muscle: direction of fibers, overall shape, number of subdivisions, location and points of attachment, and principal action. For example, **triceps brachii** is a three-part muscle acting on the arm; **biceps brachii** is a two-part muscle acting on the arm; **pectoralis major** is a large muscle of the chest;

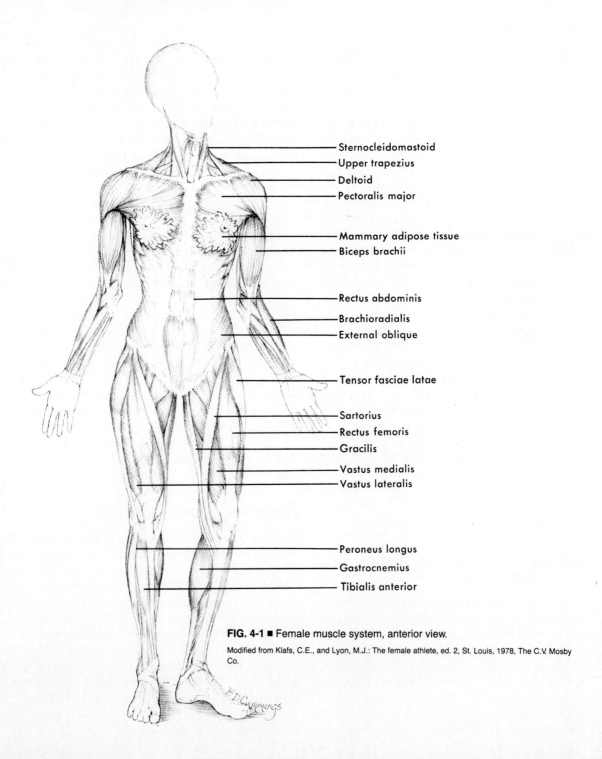

Sternocleidomastoid
Upper trapezius
Deltoid
Pectoralis major

Mammary adipose tissue
Biceps brachii

Rectus abdominis
Brachioradialis
External oblique

Tensor fasciae latae

Sartorius
Rectus femoris
Gracilis
Vastus medialis
Vastus lateralis

Peroneus longus
Gastrocnemius
Tibialis anterior

FIG. 4-1 ■ Female muscle system, anterior view.

Modified from Klafs, C.E., and Lyon, M.J.: The female athlete, ed. 2, St. Louis, 1978, The C.V. Mosby Co.

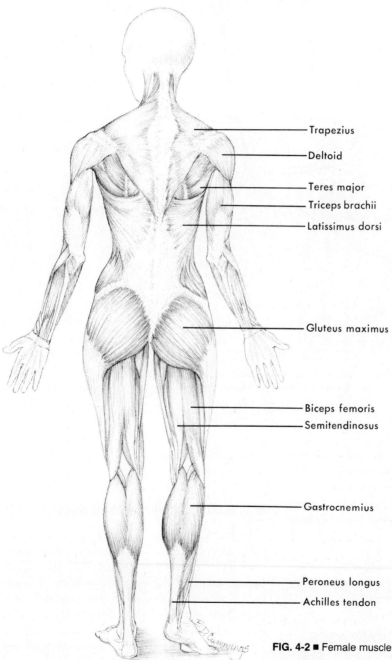

Trapezius

Deltoid

Teres major

Triceps brachii

Latissimus dorsi

Gluteus maximus

Biceps femoris

Semitendinosus

Gastrocnemius

Peroneus longus

Achilles tendon

FIG. 4-2 ■ Female muscle system, posterior view.

From Klafs, C.E., and Lyon, M.J.: The female athlete, ed. 2, St. Louis, 1978, The C.V. Mosby Co.

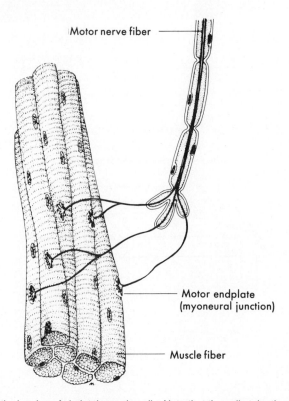

Motor nerve fiber

Motor endplate
(myoneural junction)

Muscle fiber

FIG. 4-3 ■ Schematic drawing of skeletal muscle cells. Note that the cells take the form of multinucleate fibers with cross striations. Seven fibers are shown, together with their associated nerve supply.

pectoralis minor is a smaller muscle of the chest; and **transversus abdominis** is an abdominal muscle with transverse fibers.

From a practical standpoint the muscles are conveniently categorized on the basis of their "body performance," ranging from muscles of facial expression to muscles acting on the foot. The major extensors and flexors of the head, spine, forearm, and thigh are presented in an animated fashion in Figs. 4-4 to 4-7.

■ DISORDERS AND DISEASES OF THE MUSCULAR SYSTEM

Disorders and diseases of the muscular system include muscular atrophies and dystrophies, myasthenia gravis, tennis elbow, ten-

dinitis, bursitis, gas gangrene, and trichinosis, to name the more common.

■ Muscular atrophies and dystrophies

In the language of clinical medicine, **muscular atrophy** refers to muscular weakness and wasting (of tissue) because of some pathologic involvement of the nervous system. A number of muscular atrophies are recognized. One important example is **Werdnig-Hoffmann disease**. This disease appears in infants and is frequently familial. It is characterized by weakness from degeneration of motor nerve cells in the spinal cord and brainstem.

In contrast to atrophy, **myopathy** is muscu-
Text continued on p. 45.

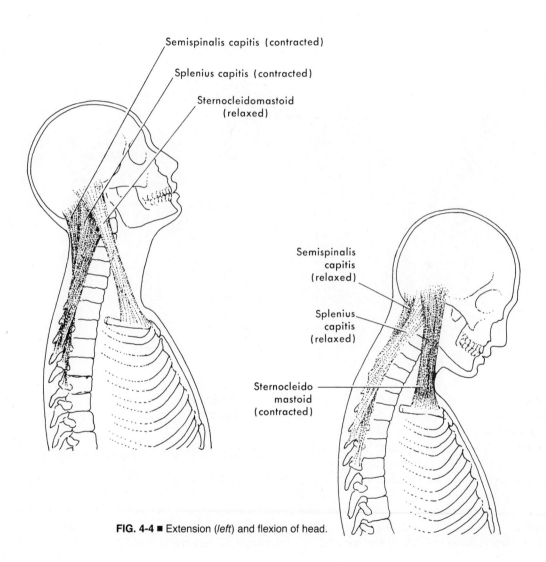

Semispinalis capitis (contracted)

Splenius capitis (contracted)

Sternocleidomastoid
(relaxed)

Semispinalis
capitis
(relaxed)

Splenius
capitis
(relaxed)

Sternocleido
mastoid
(contracted)

FIG. 4-4 ■ Extension (*left*) and flexion of head.

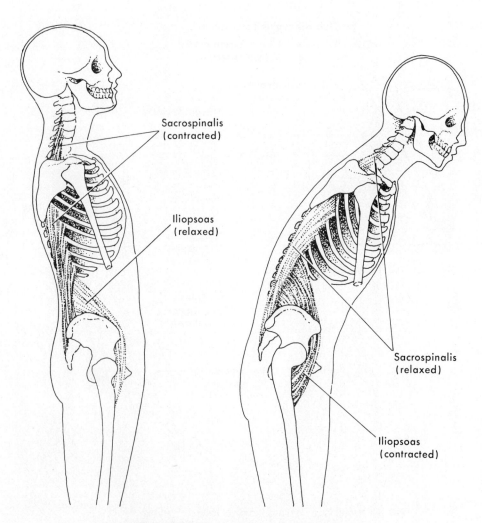

Sacrospinalis
(contracted)

Iliopsoas
(relaxed)

Sacrospinalis
(relaxed)

Iliopsoas
(contracted)

FIG. 4-5 ■ Extension (*left*) and flexion of spine.

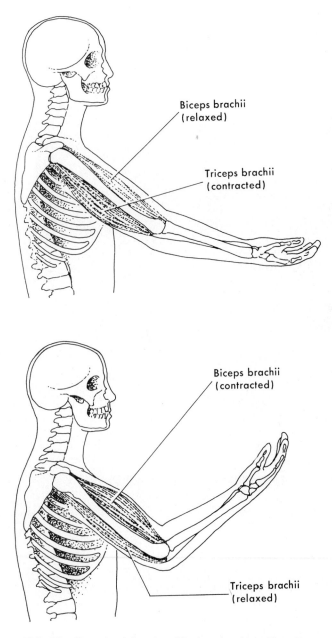

Biceps brachii
(relaxed)

Triceps brachii
(contracted)

Biceps brachii
(contracted)

Triceps brachii
(relaxed)

FIG. 4-6 ■ Extension (*above*) and flexion of supinated forearm.

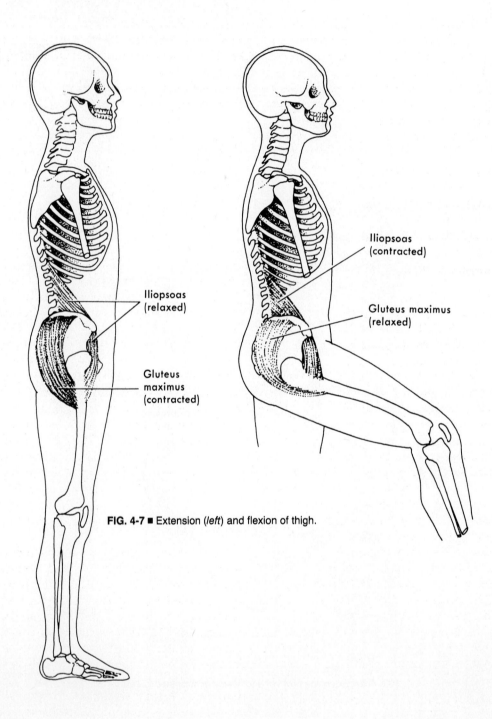

Iliopsoas
(relaxed)

Gluteus
maximus
(contracted)

Iliopsoas
(contracted)

Gluteus maximus
(relaxed)

FIG. 4-7 ■ Extension (*left*) and flexion of thigh.

lar weakness and wasting without evidence of neural involvement; it may arise in muscle or relate to some distant biochemical derangement. The best known myopathies are the **muscular dystrophies**, a class of hereditary diseases characterized by progressive weakness because of degeneration of the muscle fibers. Two major varieties are recognized: the **Duchenne** form, which affects mostly males, and the **Landouzy-Déjerine** form, which affects both sexes about equally.

There is no specific treatment or cure for any of the atrophies or dystrophies. Physiotherapy and good nursing care are essential.

■ Myasthenia gravis

Myasthenia gravis is a disease characterized by fatigue and exhaustion of the muscles and is almost always improved by drugs that mimic the action of nerve stimulation. Characteristically, there is progressive paralysis without atrophy or sensory disturbance. Although any muscle may be affected, those of the head and the neck are most commonly involved. This accounts for the expressionless face and drooping eyelids of the person who has this disorder. The nerve impulse fails to cross at the **motor endplate** (Fig. 4-3). Present evidence indicates this defect is caused by some sort of "autoimmune disease" involving the thymus gland. About one third of persons with myasthenia gravis have either an abnormal persistence of the gland, which normally disappears during childhood, or a thymoma (thymus tumor). Also, about one half of the persons with thymoma display the signs and symptoms of myasthenia gravis. In such cases removal of the gland (thymectomy) may afford some relief. For the most part, though, the treatment centers on drug therapy.

■ Tennis elbow

Tennis elbow, with the colorful medical name **radiohumeral epicondylitis**, is a strain of the lateral forearm muscles attached to the lateral epicondyle of the humerus (that is, the part of the humerus near the elbow). It is caused by repetitive strenuous supination of the wrist against resistance, as in manual screwdriving, or by violent extension of the wrist with the hand pronated, as in tennis. In mild cases, avoiding the pain-producing movement results in gradual improvement. Moderate to severe cases, in which the pain can be disabling, call for strapping, hydrocortisone injection, and sometimes surgery.

■ Tendinitis

Tendinitis is inflammation of a tendon; tenosynovitis, inflammation of the **tendon sheath** (called the tenosynovium), generally occurs simultaneously. The cause of this inflammation is not known. Localized tenderness of variable severity is present; it may be severe and associated with disabling pain on movement. Calcium deposits may occur both in the tendon and its sheath. Relief is provided by resting the affected part, applying heat or cold (whichever benefits the person), and administering antiinflammatory and analgesic drugs. In severe cases hydrocortisone injections and sometimes surgery (to remove calcium deposits) may be necessary.

■ Bursitis

Bursae (sing., bursa) are sacs or saclike cavities filled with a thick fluid and situated at places in the tissues at which friction would otherwise develop, notably where tendons pass over bony prominences. Acute or chronic inflammation of a bursa is called **bursitis**. The most commonly affected bursa is the subdeltoid of the shoulder. Miner's elbow and housemaid's knee are other common forms of bursitis. The cause of most bursitis is unknown although trauma, acute infection, arthritis, or gout may be a factor. Acute bursitis is marked by pain, tenderness, and limitation of movement. Injection of hydrocortisone into the bursa is the treatment of choice.

◼ Gas gangrene

Gas gangrene is a serious infection caused by certain soil bacteria (called **clostridia**) that thrive when introduced into the tissues, especially muscle tissues. This explains the common occurrence of the infection in dirty, lacerated wounds. As indicated by the name, death of cells occurs en masse (gangrene), and there is formation of considerable amounts of noxious gas in the affected area. Both effects result from the destructive toxins and enzymes produced by the bacteria. Thorough cleansing of wounds is essential, and gas gangrene antitoxin and penicillin are given as soon as possible.

◼ Trichinosis

Trichinosis is an infection caused by one of the smallest of parasitic worms, a roundworm called *Trichinella spiralis* (Fig. 4-8). When contaminated pork is eaten, the larvae of this worm are released in the intestine, and at maturity they copulate. The female worm later gives birth to about a thousand new larvae that migrate to the skeletal muscles via the blood vessels and lymphatic vessels. The early signs of the infection include fever, nausea, abdominal pain, and diarrhea. Later, when the larvae take up residence in the muscles, the person experiences stiffness, pain, and swelling; insomnia is also a prominent feature. Treatment centers largely around good nursing care, and in most cases recovery is good. The drug thiabendazole is highly effective against the parasite in host animals, but in humans the response has been variable. Still, most physicians believe the drug is worth a try in the acute stage of the disease. The answer to trichinosis, of course, lies in prevention. All pork products should be thoroughly cooked, and all garbage fed to hogs should be sterilized.

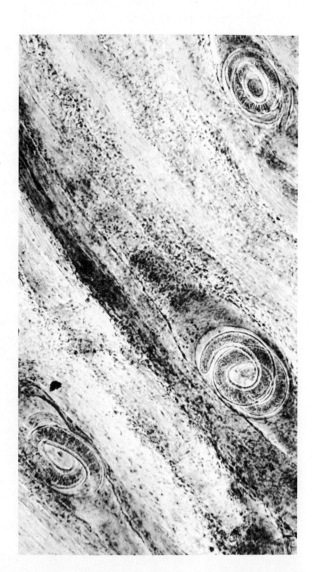

FIG. 4-8 ◼ Photomicrograph showing larvae of *Trichinella spiralis* in muscle tissue. Three larvae (spiral structures) stand out clearly.

From Hickman, C.P., Sr., Hickman, C.P., Jr., and Hickman, F.: Integrated principles of zoology, ed. 6, St. Louis, 1979, The C.V. Mosby Co.

■■■■ SELF-TEST

1. __D__ cardiac muscle
2. __K__ smooth muscle
3. __N__ body movement
4. __L__ body position
5. __I__ fuels muscle contraction
6. __J__ muscle cell
7. __m__ "movable end"
8. __H__ "stationary end"
9. __E__ "work together"
10. __O__ decrease joint angle
11. __G__ increase joint angle
12. __B__ turn palm up
13. __F__ turn palm down
14. __A__ close openings
15. __C__ white chord

a. sphincters
b. supinators
c. tendon
d. heart
e. synergists
f. pronators
g. extensors
h. origin
i. ATP
j. fiber
k. viscera
l. posture
m. insertion
n. locomotion
o. flexors

muscles contract

■■■■ STUDY QUESTIONS

1. Smooth muscle is sometimes referred to as visceral muscle and involuntary muscle. Why?
2. Skeletal muscle is sometimes referred to as striated muscle and voluntary muscle. Why?
3. The chemical energy of food molecules fuels cellular activities, such as contraction, but only indirectly. Why do we say "indirectly"? What is the direct, or immediate, source of energy?
4. Muscle contraction relates to "muscle shortening." Explain.
5. What is the difference between a ligament and a tendon?
6. When we flex the arm, the biceps brachii is the agonist and the triceps brachii is the antagonist. What about when we extend the arm?
7. Synergism means "working together." What is the connection between this term and synergistic muscles (synergists)?
8. What are the antonyms for the following terms: flexor, abductor, supinator, levator, dorsiflexor?
9. Three muscles of the front thigh have the following names: vastus lateralis, vastus medialis, and vastus intermedius. What does this tell us about their location?
10. Based on what we see in Fig. 4-2, what muscles do we sit on?
11. What abdominal muscle must be especially strengthened to establish a "firm, flat stomach" (Fig. 4-1)? What type of exercise would strengthen this muscle?
12. Muscle exercise does not increase the number of muscle fibers. What does it do then?
13. In extreme cold we shiver, and for good reason. Explain the reason.
14. What is the fundamental distinction between muscular atrophy and muscular dystrophy?
15. Fever, pain, and soreness of the muscles are characteristic clinical features of trichinosis. What is the explanation for these signs and symptoms?

CHAPTER 5

The circulatory system

The circulatory system, in its broadest sense, embraces the cardiovascular system and the lymphatic system. Together, these two systems serve the overall purpose of "transportation." The cardiovascular system is composed of the heart, blood vessels, and blood. The right side of the heart pumps blood to the lungs (to pick up oxygen), and the left side pumps oxygenated blood to all parts of the body. In addition to oxygen, the blood transports nutrients, wastes, and an endless variety of other substances including hormones and antibodies. Furthermore, the blood destroys microorganisms and plays a key role in temperature control. The lymphatic system circulates lymph, a watery fluid that would otherwise accumulate in the tissues and cause swelling. This system also filters out and destroys tissue debris, including pathogenic microbes, and produces protective antibodies. Diseases and disorders of the circulatory system are of major consequence. Heart disease is the leading cause of death in the United States, and about one out of every five Americans has high blood pressure. Major lymphatic diseases include mononucleosis ("mono") and a variety of cancers, such as Hodgkin's disease.

The heart

Blood vessels

Blood pressure

Blood flow

The blood

Lymphatic system

Disorders and diseases of the circulatory system

The circulatory system encompasses the cardiovascular and lymphatic systems. The cardiovascular system is composed of the heart and blood vessels and the blood, and the lymphatic system is composed of the lymph, the lymphatic vessels, and the so-called lymphoid tissues. First we shall take a good look at the cardiovascular system, starting with the heart; then we will consider the lymphatic system.

◼◼ THE HEART

The heart is a sac-enclosed muscular pump located directly behind the sternum. It is somewhat pear shaped, with the apex directed to the left (about 3 inches from the sternum), and it is about the size of the person's fist. The enclosing sac, called the **pericardium**, is a tough, fibrous structure with its base attached to the diaphragm below. Essentially, the heart is a mass of cardiac muscle (**myocardium**) organized into four chambers: the two **atria** (sing., atrium) above and the two **ventricles** below (Fig. 5-1). The atria, much smaller than the ventricles and with relatively thin walls, are marked by an ear-shaped, or auricular, appendage (hence the use of the word **auricle** for atrium). Between the two atria there is a small oval depression (the **fossa ovalis**) marking the site of an opening (the **foramen ovale**) in the fetal heart. The right atrium receives blood from the **venae cavae** (the great veins returning blood to the heart) and empties into the right ventricle through an opening guarded by the **tricuspid valve**. The left atrium receives the four **pulmonary veins** carrying blood from the lungs and empties into the left ventricle via the **bicuspid** (or mitral) **valve**. The left ventricle, the larger of the two ventricles, forms the apex of the heart.

The secret of the beating heart resides in the **sinoatrial** (SA) **node** sequestered in the wall of the right atrium. This tiny bit of nervous tissue, commonly dubbed the "pacemaker," emits electrical impulses at a rate of about 72 per minute, each impulse causing the atria and ventricles to contract. The atria contract first (**atrial systole**), and then the ventricles contract (**ventricular systole**), the impulse reaching the lower chambers via a special conduction system.

The highlights of the cardiac cycle (the "beat") are dramatically portrayed by the **electrocardiogram** (ECG). The **P wave** and the **QRS complex** of the ECG (Fig. 5-2) correspond to the electrical impulse passing through the atria and ventricles, respectively; the **T wave** represents electrical recovery of the cardiac fibers. Accompanying the ECG are the heart sounds disclosed by the stethoscope. The first sound ("lubb") is caused by the sudden closing of the heart valves when the ventricles contract, and the second sound ("dup") is caused by the blood's bumping back against the **aortic valve** and the **pulmonary artery valve** (Fig. 5-1) when the ventricles relax.

The heart's phenomenal automatism notwithstanding, a number of highly influential extracardiac factors influence that organ's activities. Perhaps foremost is blood volume. According to Starling's law, the volume of blood pumped by the heart is normally determined by the volume of blood returned to the heart. This is because cardiac muscle contracts with greater force the more it is stretched—up to a point, of course. Other extracardiac factors are hormones and the autonomic nervous system. The adrenal hormone epinephrine, for example, increases both the rate and strength of contraction.

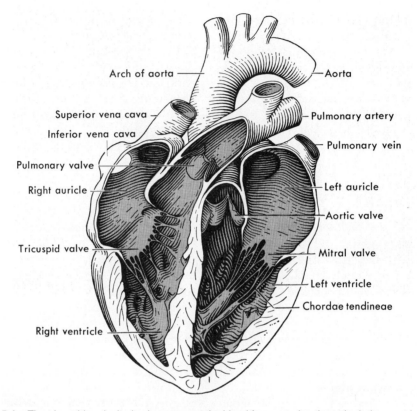

FIG. 5-1 ■ The tricuspid and mitral valves prevent the blood from entering the atria during ventricular systole, and the pulmonary valve and aortic valves prevent the blood from leaking back into the ventricles during ventricular diastole. Note that only parts of the valves are shown because of the nature of the cut. For example, only one cusp (or "flap") of the mitral (bicuspid) valve is shown.

From Haggard: Man and his body, courtesy Harper & Row, Publishers, Inc.

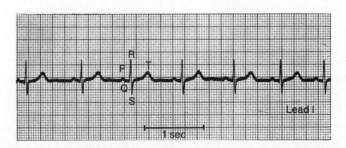

FIG. 5-2 ■ Normal electrocardiogram (ECG) and electrical events of a single cardiac cycle. P wave represents atrial systole; QRS complex represents ventricular systole; T wave represents electrical recovery of heart muscle during ventricular diastole.

From Schottelius, B.A., and Schottelius, D.D.: Textbook of physiology, ed. 18, St. Louis, 1978, The C.V. Mosby Co.

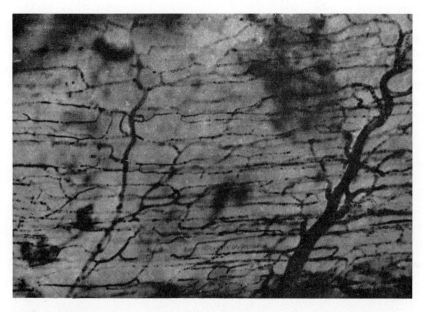

FIG. 5-3 ■ The capillaries (magnified 200 times) as they appear in skeletal muscle.

Courtesy Dr. Benjamin W. Zweifach, University of California, San Diego.

BLOOD VESSELS

The blood vessels include the arteries, arterioles, veins, venules, and capillaries. **Arteries** are the vessels that carry blood from the heart; **veins** are vessels that carry blood to or toward the heart. Both types of vessels are composed of three coats in differing proportions: tunica intima, tunica media, and tunica externa. The tunica intima, the smooth inner lining, runs uninterrupted throughout the vascular system and thus forms the lining of all the vessels; variable amounts of elastic tissue and smooth muscle occur in the other two coats. The larger blood vessels possess tiny vessels (called **vasa vasorum**) within their walls for nourishment. The walls of veins are quite a bit thinner than those of arteries. Unlike arteries, veins are collapsed when empty, and those of the lower extremities are equipped with valves to prevent backflow. As suggested by their names, the **arterioles** and **venules** are the smallest arteries and veins, the former leading blood into the capillaries and the latter leading it from the capillaries. And, most important, the arterioles have relatively large amounts of smooth muscle, a fact accounting for their pronounced ability to alter their caliber when the occasion demands. The **capillaries** (Fig. 5-3) are an interlacing network connecting the arterioles and venules. In a very real sense, these microscopic vessels are the "heart" of the cardiovascular system, for through their one-celled walls nutrients and wastes are exchanged between the blood and tissue fluid (the fluid that nourishes the cells). The capillaries are the ultimate element, as it were, in the maintenance of fluid balance, because the volume of fluid (water, for the most part) leaving the capillaries is rather evenly balanced by the fluid entering them. This accounts in large part for the constant volumes of blood and tissue fluid.

BLOOD PRESSURE

The blood pressure reaches its highest point during cardiac **systole** and its lowest point during **diastole** (Fig. 5-4). The normal pressure for young adults measures about 120 millimeters of mercury (120 mm Hg), systolic, and 80 millimeters of mercury (80 mm Hg), diastolic; that is, "120 over 80." What is called the **pulse pressure** equals the difference between the two, that for young adults averaging about 40 mm Hg. As the blood travels away from the heart, there is a dampening of the blood pressure, and in the venae cavae the pressure drops almost to zero.

Of the many factors influencing blood pressure, strenuous exercise tops the list. In a matter of minutes the systolic pressure can easily go to a height of 200 mm Hg. Furthermore, except in the well-trained athlete, this rise in pressure is accompanied by a marked increase in heart rate (easily up to 150 to 200 beats per minute). Actually, an inordinate increase in heart rate tells us we are "out of shape," especially when it is high following a bout of mild to moderate exercise.

BLOOD FLOW

The purpose of the cardiovascular system is to circulate the blood throughout the tissues

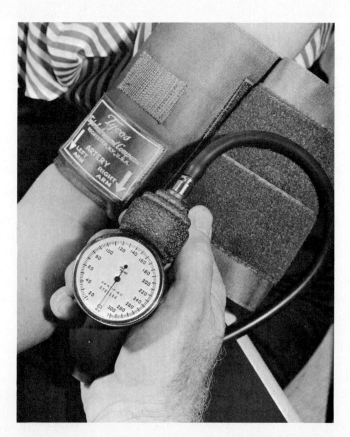

FIG. 5-4 ■ Blood pressure is measured in millimeters of mercury.

Courtesy Taylor Instrument Co.

(Fig. 5-5). At rest each ventricle pumps about 5 liters per minute, but during exercise the value can be seven to eight times as much. Of the blood leaving the heart, approximately 25% flows through the kidneys, 25% through the muscles, 15% through the abdominal region, 10% through the liver, 8% through the brain, 4% through the heart muscle, and 13% through the remaining areas.

The highlights of the actual circulation are as follows: Blood enters the heart's right atrium via the inferior and superior venae cavae and from there flows into the right ventricle. Ventricular systole now follows, and the blood is

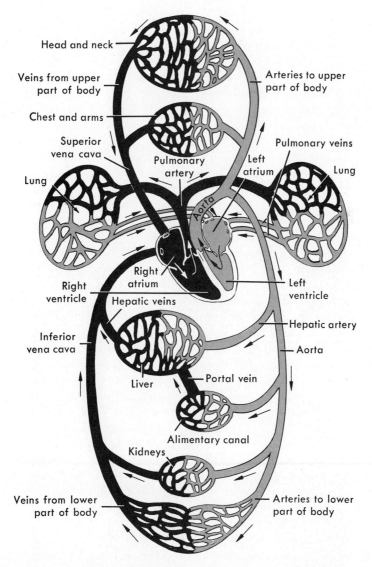

FIG. 5-5 ■ Diagram showing general circulation of the blood. Oxygenated blood is shown in gray; nonoxygenated blood is shown in black.

From Schottelius, B.A., and Schottelius, D.D.: Textbook of physiology, ed. 18, St. Louis, 1978, The C.V. Mosby Co.

forced into the lungs via the pulmonary artery; from the lungs it returns to the heart—to the left atrium—via the pulmonary veins. This circuit, the flow of blood between the lungs and the heart, comprises the **pulmonary circulation**, the purpose being to get rid of carbon dioxide (CO_2) and pick up oxygen (O_2). From the left atrium the blood flows into the powerful left ventricle, whose contraction forces it out through the aorta to the body at large (the so-called **systemic circulation**). The aorta divides into countless branches, the latter, in turn, dissolving into myriad arterioles and capillaries. The capillaries merge into venules; the venules merge into veins; the veins finally gather together to form the venae cavae.

THE BLOOD

The blood is the bright red fluid that nourishes the tissues, carts away wastes, fights infection, and has much to do with the regulation of temperature and fluid balance. The amount of blood in the body averages about 70 milliliters (ml) per kilogram of body weight. Blood is actually a type of connective tissue composed of cells, or **corpuscles**, suspended in a clear, almost colorless fluid called **plasma**. In males, the cells normally compose about 45% (by volume) of the blood, and in females the figure is normally in the vicinity of 40%. (For convenience, blood cell volume is referred to as **hematocrit**.)

Plasma and cells

The plasma is about 90% water, in which are dissolved inorganic salts, proteins, lipids, glucose, waste products, vitamins, hormones, enzymes, antibodies, and gases, to name the main components. With the exception of proteins, whose molecules are largely confined to the circulation, these various substances easily diffuse into the tissue fluid surrounding the cells; by the same token cells' waste products diffuse into the blood.

Blood cells include the **red cells**, **white cells**, and **thrombocytes** (Fig. 5-6). The red cells (**erythrocytes**), normally ranging between 4.5 and 5.5 million per cubic millimeter (mm^3) of blood, are characterized by the absence of a nucleus and the presence of an iron-bearing, red pigment called **hemoglobin**. In the fetus the red cells are manufactured in the liver, spleen, and red bone marrow, but by the time of birth the job is confined exclusively to the marrow, especially the marrow of the flat and irregular bones. Needed for the manufacture and proper development of red cells are, among other factors, iron, folic acid, and vitamin B_{12}. Oxygen, too, plays a role in a negative sort of way; that is, an increase of oxygen slows the output of red cells, and a decrease accelerates their production. The function of the red cells is to transport oxygen. Specifically, oxygen reacts with hemoglobin to form the unstable compound called **oxyhemoglobin**; in the tissues oxyhemoglobin breaks down into hemoglobin and oxygen.

The white cells (**leukocytes**) normally number in the neighborhood of 8000/mm^3 of blood; they are dubbed "white" for no better reason than their lack of any kind of pigment. Classification of white cells is based on the presence or absence of granules in the cytoplasm. Granulocytes include neutrophils, eosinophils, and basophils; agranulocytes include lymphocytes and monocytes. Except for the lymphocytes, produced by the lymphatic system, white cells are formed in the red bone marrow right along with red cells. The main function of white cells is to fight infection. Thrombocytes, or **platelets**, number about 250,000/mm^3. They play a key role in the coagulation of blood.

Clotting

The clotting, or **coagulation**, of the blood seems to involve an endless chain of molecular gymnastics, and the experts appear to be in agreement only on the overall fundamental

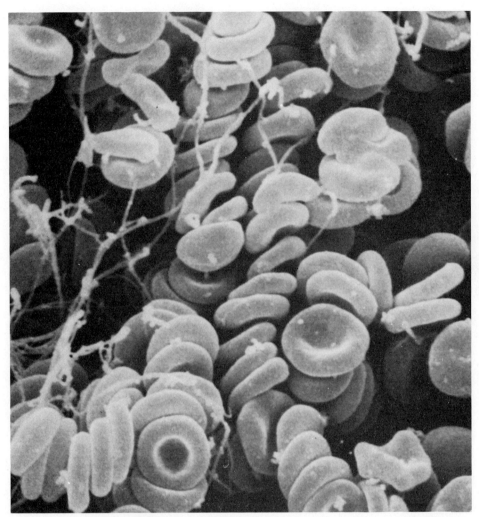

FIG. 5-6 ■ Red blood cells magnified 4200 times by means of scanning electron microscope.

From Kessel and Shih: Scanning electron microscopy in biology, Springer-Verlag.

steps. One thing is for certain: injury (to the vessels) sets off the process. Further, the last step involves the conversion of the soluble plasma protein **fibrinogen** into the insoluble **fibrin**. A sticky, thready substance, fibrin entraps blood corpuscles and thereby establishes the **clot**. As a safeguard against intravascular clotting, the blood contains a number of anticoagulants. One such agent, **heparin**, is present in most tissues throughout the body.

Very tiny clots may form, however, and when this occurs there is a back-up mechanism of blood and tissue enzymes that digest and dissolve clots.

■ Blood types

The blood of all human beings falls into one of four major **types** (A, B, AB, and O) depending on whether the red cells do or do not con-

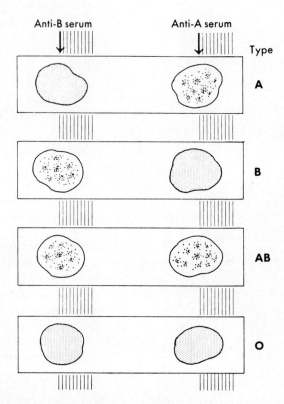

Anti-B serum   Anti-A serum

Type

A

B

AB

O

FIG. 5-7 ■ In blood typing two drops of blood are placed on a glass slide. To one drop is added a drop of anti-A serum (which contains alpha agglutinins) and to the other a drop of anti-B serum (which contains beta agglutinins). Note that there are four possible results, each corresponding to a particular blood type. For example, in the top slide clumping, or agglutination, occurs only with anti-A serum, which means that the red cells contain agglutinogen A—hence the blood is type A.

tain one or both of two protein factors called **agglutinogens** (Fig. 5-7). Specifically, type A blood contains agglutinogen A; type B contains agglutinogen B; type AB contains both agglutinogens; and type O contains neither. Additionally, in their plasma, types A, B, and O contain agglutinating antibodies called **agglutinins**. Type A blood contains **beta** agglutinins; type B contains **alpha** agglutinins; type O contains both alpha and beta agglutinins; and type AB contains neither. The reason for this distribution of agglutinogens and agglutinins is that alpha agglutinins clump, or **agglutinate**, red cells containing agglutinogen A, and beta agglutinins agglutinate red cells con-

taining agglutinogen B. Thus different blood types do not "mix" because cross agglutination occurs, the resulting "clumps" plugging the small vessels and causing trouble in other ways. Obviously, in blood transfusions donor blood and recipient blood must be of the same type (Fig. 5-8).

In addition to blood types A, B, and O, there are a number of other classifications, but by far the most important concerns the **Rh factor**. Blood whose red cells contain this factor (about 85% of the population) is said to be **Rh positive**, and blood without it is said to be **Rh negative**. When Rh-positive blood is given to persons whose blood is Rh negative, it stimu-

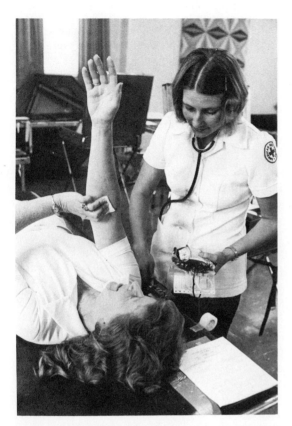

FIG. 5-8 ■ Taking blood for the blood bank. Technician is holding plastic bag containing blood.

lates their immunity cells to produce anti-Rh agglutinins. No reaction occurs on the first encounter, but a subsequent infusion results in agglutination and a severe response or even death. The classic Rh incompatibility is a destructive blood disorder of the newborn, called **erythroblastosis fetalis**, that occurs in about one out of every 50 babies born to Rh-negative mothers and Rh-positive fathers. If the fetus inherits the Rh factor from the father (thereby becoming Rh positive), its red cells will provoke the output of anti-Rh agglutinins when they enter the mother's circulation. This is most likely to happen at or near the time of delivery. The first child is usually unaffected,

but because the mother's immunity cells are now sensitized, subsequent pregnancies shoot the agglutinin concentration higher and higher, causing a severe case of erythroblastosis fetalis in the child. A way around the dilemma is to give the mother a shot of **anti-Rh antibody** (RhoGAM) at the time of delivery (at each pregnancy). This "neutralizes" the Rh factor (in the event fetal red cells have escaped into the maternal circulation) and prevents it from sensitizing the mother.

■■■■ LYMPHATIC SYSTEM

The lymphatic system (Fig. 5-9) includes the **lymph**, **lymphatic vessels**, and **lymph nodes**—the system proper—and an assortment of structures and glands marked by the presence of **lymphocytic cells**: the spleen, tonsils, thymus gland, and lymphatic nodules (Peyer's patches) of the intestine. The lymphatic vessels originate among the cells as microscopic lymph capillaries that come together to form progressively larger vessels, much as twigs on a tree coalesce into branches. And finally these larger vessels join together to form two main channels, the **thoracic duct** and the **right lymphatic ducts**. The thoracic duct originates in the lumbar region as a tiny sac (the cisterna chyli), works its way up the trunk, and finally terminates at the juncture of the left internal jugular and subclavian veins. The right lymphatic ducts (sometimes there is just one) join the venous system at the juncture of the right internal jugular and subclavian veins. Except for the right arm, right upper chest, and right side of the head, which are drained by the right lymphatic ducts, all lymph flows into the thoracic duct.

Located along the lymphatic vessels, especially in the groin, neck, and axillary ("arm pit") regions of the body, are the lymph nodes, tiny glands through which the lymph must pass on its way to the bloodstream. Lymph itself is nothing more than tissue fluid that has left the

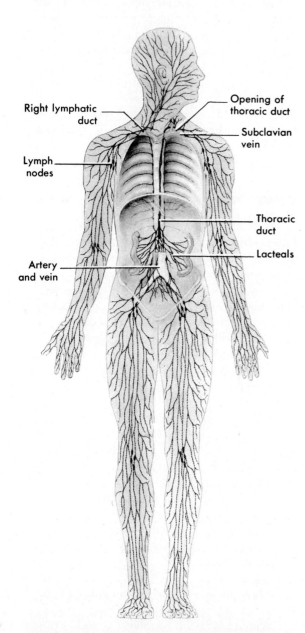

Right lymphatic duct

Opening of thoracic duct

Subclavian vein

Lymph nodes

Thoracic duct

Lacteals

Artery and vein

FIG. 5-9 ■ The lymphatic system. Note the points where the thoracic duct and the right lymphatic duct enter the bloodstream. Note also the areas of the body where lymph nodes are concentrated.

tissue spaces and entered the lymphatic vessels. Once within these vessels it is massaged onward by the pressing of the muscles against the vessel walls. Clearly, lymph flows at a snail's pace, with only about a fraction of an ounce passing through the system per minute.

From the foregoing discussion we can see that the lymphatic system functions to remove excess tissue fluid. But this is far from all that it does. Dead cells, bacteria, and other intercellular debris are filtered out and destroyed (phagocytized) in the lymph nodes; the protein continuously escaping from the blood capillaries is returned to the circulation; the lymph nodes and spleen manufacture **lymphocytes** (a type of white cell); and certain special lymph node cells (plasma cells) bolster body immunity by producing **antibodies** against microbial invaders.

■ Tonsils

The tonsils are aggregates of lymph tissue situated in the oral cavity and throat. Of chief concern are the **palatine tonsils** and **pharyngeal tonsil**. The tonsils produce monocytes, lymphocytes, and other scavenger cells that serve to protect the mouth, nose, and throat against bacterial attack. When people speak of the tonsils, they usually mean the palatine, or **faucial**, tonsils, easily seen at the entrance to the throat. The pharyngeal tonsil is on the upper surface of the throat and "out of sight." Enlargement of the pharyngeal tonsil is called **adenoids**.

■ Spleen

The spleen is an ovoid organ located directly below the diaphragm on the left side of the body. Microscopically, it resembles a lymph node and is characterized by numerous venous sinuses. Because of these tiny sinuses, the spleen can swell up with blood to a volume of approximately 1 liter and, conversely, shrink to a volume as low as 100 ml. In this way the spleen serves as a reservoir, removing blood from the circulation during times of quietude or plenty and releasing it in times of stress and deprivation. The spleen also functions to cleanse the blood. Throughout the pulp and lining of the sinuses there are special phagocytic cells that devour bacteria and the debris remaining from the breakdown of old red cells. Finally, the spleen aids in the production of lymphocytes and, in the fetus, the production of red cells.

■ Thymus

The thymus is a flat, pinkish gray, two-lobed gland lying high in the chest behind the sternum. Large in relation to the rest of the body in fetal life and in early childhood, by the age of puberty it has stopped growing and started to atrophy, or degenerate. The thymus makes possible the production of the immunity cells of the lymph nodes that are involved in delayed hypersensitivity and rejection of skin grafts. Infants born without the gland develop no delayed hypersensitivity in response to various antigens and sometimes completely fail to reject a graft of skin from an unrelated donor.

■ DISORDERS AND DISEASES OF THE CIRCULATORY SYSTEM

Disorders and diseases of the circulatory system involve the heart, the blood vessels, the blood, and the lymphatic tissues. Diseases of the heart and blood vessels are collectively referred to as **cardiovascular** diseases. Generalized cardiovascular diseases include atherosclerosis, hypertension, shock, and embolism. Specific cardiovascular diseases include coronary artery disease, congestive heart failure, cardiac arrhythmias, congenital heart disease, endocarditis, and peripheral vascular

disorders. Diseases and disorders of the blood (and bone marrow) include anemia, polycythemia, agranulocytosis, leukemia, and hemophilia. Well-known diseases of the lymphatic tissues (lymphatic system) include lymphadenitis ("swollen glands"), tonsillitis, infectious mononucleosis, and Hodgkin's disease.

■ Atherosclerosis

Atherosclerosis is a very common form of **arteriosclerosis** ("hardening of the arteries") in which deposits of fatty plaques (**atheromas**) are formed within the lining of the large and medium-sized arteries (Fig. 5-10). The great medical importance of atherosclerosis is due to its predilection for coronary, cerebral, and peripheral arteries. Its complications are the major causes of death in the United States; deaths classified as resulting from **coronary artery disease** represent 33% of deaths from all causes, and **cerebral vascular disease** is the third most common cause of death in the United States after heart disease and cancer.

Specifically what sets off the formation of atheromas is not known. But it is known that the likelihood of atherosclerosis is increased in the presence of certain biochemical, physiologic, and environmental factors known as **risk factors**. The presence of one or more of these risk factors increases the possibility that a person will suffer from atherosclerosis and its complications. It is also suggested that removal or modification of the risk factors in a population will diminish the incidence of the complications of atherosclerosis, such as coronary artery disease. The major risk factors are (1) **hypertension**, (2) **elevated blood lipids** (especially cholesterol), (3) **cigarette smoking**, (4) **diabetes mellitus**, and (5) **obesity**. Other presumed risk factors include physical inactivity, certain types of personality and patterns of behavior, hardness of the drinking water, and a family history of premature atherosclerosis. Additionally, there is the matter

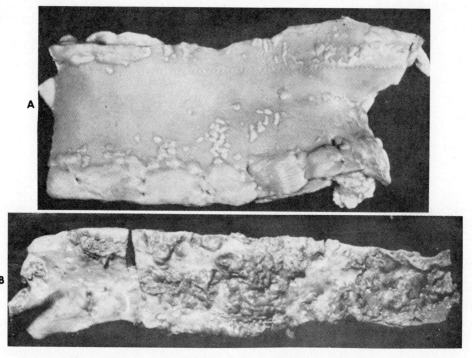

FIG. 5-10 ■ Atherosclerosis. Two sections of aorta opened lengthwise to show early, **A,** and advanced, **B,** "takeover" of otherwise smooth lining by atheromatous plaques.

From Anderson, W.A.D., editor: Pathology, ed. 4, St. Louis, 1961, The C.V. Mosby Co.

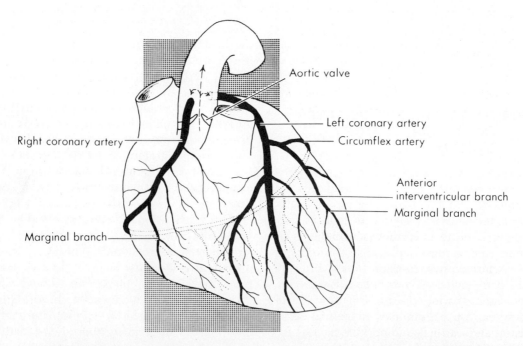

FIG. 5-11 ■ Coronary circulation. Note the two main coronary arteries arising from the aorta just above the aortic valve. An occlusion of one of these or of a major branch could spell instant death.

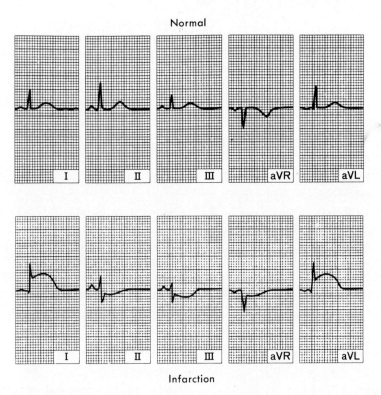

Normal

Infarction

FIG. 5-12 ■ Electrocardiogram (*lower view*) taken a few hours after myocardial infarction. The Roman numerals and aVR and aVL (referred to as "leads") indicate different positions of the ECG connectors. Normal ECG is shown for comparison. Note that most drastic changes occur in leads I and aVL.

Courtesy Merck, Sharp, and Dohme, West Point, Pa.

of age and male sex, both of which may be considered "natural risk factors." The death rate from coronary artery disease for 60-year-old white men is 10 times that for 30-year-old white men. Furthermore, in the age bracket 35 to 44 the death rate from coronary heart disease among white men is six times that of white women.

In many societies the incidence of atherosclerosis is much lower than in ours, and attempts to prevent the disease by focusing on the risk factors makes common sense. For the most part, risk factors can either be eliminated or controlled. The treatment of atherosclerosis is directed at its complications, such as coronary artery disease and heart failure.

■ Coronary artery disease

Narrowing, or **occlusion**, of the coronary arteries (Fig. 5-11) causes an imbalance between blood supply and myocardial demands; the underlying cause is usually atherosclerosis. The result is **myocardial ischemia** (deficiency of blood in the heart muscle) and, commonly, damage (infarction). A short period of relatively mild ischemia is called **angina pectoris**; a severe and prolonged ischemia with heart muscle damage is called **myocardial infarction** (MI), the classical "heart attack" (Fig. 5-12). Whether or not the victim survives the attack depends on the size of the vessel involved and the speed of the occlusion. In the event of recovery, the heart is weakened for several months and often for life. The treatment of myocardial infarction is designed to (1) relieve the patient's distress, (2) reduce cardiac work, (3) prevent complications, and (4) treat complications. Since 50% of all deaths occur within 2½ hours of onset of the attack, the first few hours are obviously crucial.

■ Cardiac arrhythmias

The average adult heart generally beats 72 to 78 times per minute. However, from birth to old age, the rate progressively decreases. Normal rhythm in the infant is 110 to 150. Cardiac **arrhythmias** are changes in heart rhythm (Fig. 5-13) relating to disturbances of the pacemaker, or conduction, system. **Ventricular fibrillation** ("quivering ventricles") is the most ominous of the arrhythmias. Here the blood pressure falls to zero, and the outcome is commonly sudden death. The causes include myocardial infarction, overdosage of digitalis and certain other drugs, cyclopropane anesthesia, and certain surgical procedures, notably those involving the heart. Ventricular fibrillation may be the cause of death in electrocution. The treatment is largely preventive and consists of using every precaution in giving drugs known to incite arrhythmias. If fibrillation begins, **electrical defibrillation** by external electric countershock may be lifesaving. If this is not available, intravenous chemical defibrillators, such as lidocaine or procainamide, are given. Artificial respiration and external cardiac massage are also essential to maintain cardiac output.

■ Heart blocks

Heart blocks are conditions in which the spread of the electrical impulse through the heart muscle is slowed or interrupted in a portion of the normal conduction pathway. The cause is usually an underlying heart problem, including coronary artery disease, rheumatic heart disease, congenital heart disease, or myocardial infarction. Some types of heart blocks cause no symptoms, while others result in dizziness, fainting, or even convulsions. The more serious conditions call for an artificial pacemaker.

■ Rheumatic heart disease

The relationship between rheumatic heart disease and **streptococcal infections** has now been established. The basic problem concerns the **valves**, generally the mitral and aortic. If they become puffy and their openings thereby narrowed, there is damming of blood in the lungs with the result that the elevated pressure in the capillaries forces fluid into the

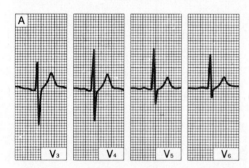

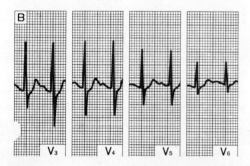

FIG. 5-13 ■ Cigarette smoking and ECG. **A,** Normal resting pattern. **B,** After smoking. Rate has increased from 80 to 130.

Courtesy Merck, Sharp, and Dohme, West Point, Pa.

alveoli or air sacs. Thus the person drowns in his or her own water. On the other hand, if the valves fail to close properly because of erosion, there is a leaking backward of blood (producing a characteristic murmur). The heart, in attempting to correct itself by beating harder and faster, becomes strained and weakened. The prompt use of penicillin in all streptococcal ("strep") infections is now recognized as the best defense against rheumatic heart disease.

■ Congenital heart disease

In contrast to the high incidence of acquired heart disease, serious congenital heart diseases are, fortunately, relatively uncommon. These conditions, caused by failure of normal development during the fetal period,

are marked by poor circulation and poor oxygenation. The more common and important congenital disorders of the heart are **pulmonary stenosis**, **septal defects**, and **tetralogy of Fallot**. The first condition, a narrowing of the opening between the pulmonary artery and the right ventricle, decreases the flow of blood through the lungs, on the one hand, and the return of blood to the heart, on the other. The septal defects (openings in the walls of the heart chambers) sabotage the circulation by permitting the blood to flow directly between the atria and between the ventricles. The tetralogy of Fallot entails four defects: pulmonary stenosis, patent interventricular septum, enlargement of the right ventricle, and displacement of the aorta to the right. Other congenital defects relate to faulty valves and absence of valves. Such defects typically cause **heart**

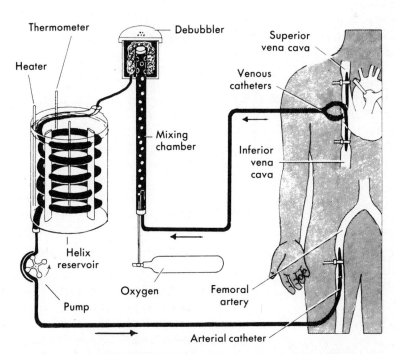

FIG. 5-14 ■ Heart-lung machine. Blood flows from two catheters inserted in venae cavae to bottom of mixing chamber. Bubbles of oxygen rising through chamber are removed in debubbler. Blood then flows into helix reservoir and is pumped into femoral artery of patient.

murmurs and sometimes prove extremely serious.

In no other area of cardiovascular research have there been more fruitful or more dramatic results than in the surgical management of congenital heart disease. The surgeon can now repair and replace defective valves and patch openings between the chambers. Indeed, even the tetralogy of Fallot has yielded to the needle and scalpel. Such procedures demand an artificial heart and an artificial lung to keep the body alive during the operation. The essentials of the heart-lung machine are shown in Fig. 5-14.

Congestive heart failure

The term "congestive heart failure" is applied to the inability of the heart to pump at top efficiency. Although the condition can result from more blood returning to the heart than the heart can pump out (for example, overloading the circulation with intravenous fluids), the usual cause stems from heart damage; either the valves are faulty, as in rheumatic heart disease, or the muscle has been weakened by coronary artery disease or other injury.

The signs and symptoms of congestive heart failure are related to poor circulation. A rapid, weak pulse, bluing of the skin, shortness of breath, fatigue, and edema (tissue fluid accumulation) are the classic features. The treatment of congestive heart failure centers on the use of digitalis preparations to strengthen the heart muscle, the use of diuretics to flush out the water and salt held in the tissues, and the implementation of a salt-free diet.

Endocarditis

Endocarditis is an inflammation of the heart lining and heart valves and is usually caused by streptococci or staphylococci. This situation is dangerous and often fatal. The use of penicillin or related antibiotics is essential to treatment.

Hypertension

High blood pressure, or **hypertension**, refers to a systolic pressure above 140 mm Hg and a diastolic pressure above 90 mm Hg. The disease occurs in about one out of every five persons, causing misery and, not infrequently, death. Hypertension kills by rupturing a vessel in a vital organ or by causing the heart or kidneys to fail. In about 9 out of 10 cases the cause is unknown. Known causes of hypertension include certain brain abnormalities, kidney disease, and an excessive output of epinephrine. The treatment of hypertension centers on the use of diuretics to reduce body sodium and blood volume and vasodilators to relax constricted blood vessels. A salt-free diet is also highly important.

Varicose veins

Varicose veins are veins that are weak and dilated. Although factors that elevate the venous pressure, such as continuous standing and congestive heart failure, are usually associated with the disease, there may be an inherited weakness of the walls or valves. External elastic support ameliorates the symptoms, which usually include leg fatigue and pain. Severe manifestations—edema, eczema, and skin ulcers—may call for surgical intervention.

Embolism

Embolism is the sudden blocking of an artery by a blood clot that originated in another vessel. If the lung is affected, death is often instantaneous. Embolism is always a threat in peripheral vascular diseases that predispose to the formation of blood clots. Treatment centers on the use of anticoagulants to halt the growth of the clot.

■ Shock

Shock is perhaps the most baffling medical emergency. The ominous signs (hypotension, pallor, clammy skin, weak and rapid pulse, decreased respiration, anxiety, and often unconsciousness) are frightening even to the seasoned physician. Morbidly interesting, shock is triggered not by one situation but by many. A severe blow, a burn, a hemorrhage, a heart attack, an unpleasant experience, or even a bee sting may result in shock and death. Shock relates to the circulation, and most cases can be explained, at least in part, on the basis of circulatory dynamics. In a severe hemorrhage or burn, for example, the reduced blood volume leads to reduced cardiac output. A severe heart attack causes a drastic cut in cardiac output because the pump is damaged.

In mild shock the body does a remarkable job of protecting itself by constricting the vessels and the venous reservoirs. Thus, even though blood may be lost, the constricted vessels facilitate venous return and cardiac output. If more than a liter of blood is lost, however, this mechanism cannot cope with the task, and cardiac output starts to fall. The treatment demands speed and the proper choice of restorative measures. To correct a volume deficiency, blood plasma or a plasma substitute (for example, dextran) is used. Digitalis preparations are given if the heart has been weakened. Drugs that constrict blood vessels (vasopressors) may be necessary in the emergency treatment of shock from any cause when the systolic pressure is below 80 mm Hg, but these drugs are not used until blood volume has been restored.

■ Anemias

Anemia may be defined as a deficiency in red blood cells or hemoglobin or both. Anemia is serious because of the impaired ability of the blood to carry oxygen. As a result the cells degenerate, especially those of the nervous system. This explains such early symptoms as disinterest, fatigue, and loss of energy.

There are various kinds of anemia. For example, **blood loss anemia** is a result of hemorrhage or the chronic loss of blood. Although the bone marrow may be able to maintain a nearly normal red blood count, the iron stores of the body become progressively decreased. Accordingly, this type of anemia is marked not only by a decrease in the number of red blood cells but also by a severe drop in hemoglobin.

Iron deficiency anemia results from the insufficient intake of iron. Although the red cell count is usually nearly normal, the concentration of hemoglobin in each cell is reduced greatly, hence the expression **hypochromic** ("lack of color") anemia. This condition is quite common and is treated successfully with iron compounds such as ferrous sulfate.

Hemolytic anemias involve excessive destruction of red blood cells. The more common forms include sickle cell anemia, erythroblastosis fetalis (Rh incompatibility), and poisoning from drugs and chemicals. Sickle cell anemia is a hereditary disease characterized by distorted red blood cells. Since the membranes of these cells are fragile, they are easily damaged and destroyed. In erythroblastosis fetalis the pregnant female builds up destructive antibodies against the red blood cells of the fetus. Consequently, the baby is born with a severe anemia.

Pernicious anemia, which proves fatal if not treated, results from a deficiency of a so-called **intrinsic factor** normally present in the lining of the stomach. Since this factor is needed for the absorption of vitamin B_{12} (the **extrinsic factor**), a deficiency will severely curtail the manufacture of red blood cells in the marrow. (Vitamin B_{12}, we recall, is an essential raw material in the manufacture of red cells.) The treatment of pernicious anemia is highly specific and calls for periodic shots of vitamin B_{12}.

Aplastic anemia is a fatal condition stemming from destruction of the bone marrow. The usual causes are drugs, poisons, and overexposure to x rays, gamma rays, or certain other forms of radiation.

Polycythemia

An increased red blood cell count, or **polycythemia**, is a normal response during strenuous exercise and at high altitudes. In the condition called **polycythemia vera**, however, the elevated count results from tumorous bone marrow. A tremendous number of red blood cells are poured into the circulation, and, as a result, the blood gets thicker and thicker. Actually the blood "flows like molasses," and there is a tendency for clot formation or **thrombosis**. The treatment includes phlebotomy ("blood letting") and the use of anticoagulants and radioactive phosphorus.

Thrombosis

A common cause of death is thrombosis, or the formation of an intravascular clot. Such a clot, or **thrombus**, may remain where it is, or it may be swept away by the blood. In the latter event the clot is called an **embolus**, and the condition is termed **embolism**. Death results from the obstruction of blood to a vital area or organ. A classic example is pulmonary embolism. Thrombosis of the peripheral vessels is most often traceable to sluggish blood flow, particularly in the legs. Since some of the platelets have a tendency to adhere to the walls of the veins anyway, they are even more likely to do so in areas of poor circulation. In so doing, the platelets rupture, and clotting ensues. Other predisposing factors include atherosclerosis, phlebitis, and varicose veins. The treatment and prevention of thrombosis and embolism centers on the use of heparin and other anticoagulants.

Lymphadenitis

The inflammation of one or more lymph nodes is called **lymphadenitis**. Just about any microbe can be responsible, but the usual pathogens are staphylococci and streptococci. The infection may be local and mild or widespread and severely toxic. The nodes may enlarge greatly and become extremely painful and tender. The surrounding tissues often become inflamed and give way to abscesses. Treatment centers on the removal of the underlying cause of the infection and the use of antibiotics.

Lymphangitis

Inflammation of the lymphatic vessels, or lymphangitis, may be caused by any pathogen, but again the usual culprits are staphylococci and streptococci. As the infection creeps along the vessels from the portal of entry, its path becomes red, swollen, and painful, and there is almost invariably lymphadenitis. Ulcers may develop along the path of the infection, and the pathogen may even enter the blood to cause septicemia ("blood poisoning"). Fever, chills, headache, malaise, and generalized aching are prominent systemic features, even without blood poisoning.

Tonsillitis

Tonsillitis is an inflammation of the tonsils, especially the palatine (faucial) tonsils. The acute form, usually caused by certain streptococci, can be a severe infection in which the tonsils become red, swollen, painful, and filled with noxious debris and pus. The person's throat is severely sore, and swallowing is agonizing. Systemically, the repercussions include muscular pains, malaise, fever, and chills. Bed rest, aspirin, and antibiotics are generally prescribed. Although tonsillectomy was at one time the fashion of the day, this is no longer the case. Since the tonsils are apparently a natural defense mechanism (perhaps much more so than has been realized), many authorities believe that they should be removed only in instances in which they are a chronic focus of infection.

■ Infectious mononucleosis

Infectious mononucleosis ("mono") is an acute disease caused by the Epstein-Barr virus (EBV). Sporadic attacks occur chiefly between the ages of 15 and 30, and epidemics occur for the most part in children. College students appear likely candidates, and "deep kissing" is often cited as the reason. Infectious mononucleosis is extremely varied in its severity. The incubation period may run from a few days to several weeks. Typically, the initial features include fever, malaise, sore throat, and headache. In almost all cases the lymph nodes are enlarged, especially those of the neck and armpit regions. In about one half of these cases the spleen is tense and swollen, and the liver is enlarged. Signs and symptoms persist for 2 to 8 weeks and sometimes last for several months. Rarely, death may occur as a result of an overwhelming infection, a ruptured spleen, a damaged heart, or suffocation from swollen vocal cords obstructing the windpipe. The treatment is essentially a matter of relieving the symptoms; rest is essential.

■ Hodgkin's disease

Hodgkin's disease is a cancer of the lymphatic system. About 56% of the cases of the disease occur between the ages of 20 and 40; less than 10% occur before the age of 10 and less than 10% after age 60. More than 7000 Americans develop Hodgkin's disease each year; about 2600 die from it annually. The actual cause is not known, but there seems to be a connection between the development of Hodgkin's disease and the presence of an abnormal immune state.

The most common first sign of Hodgkin's disease is a swollen lymph gland, usually in the neck, less often in the armpit or the groin (Fig. 5-15). If left unchecked, the cancer

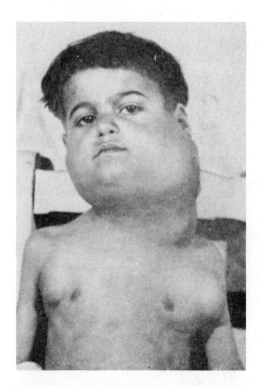

FIG. 5-15 ■ Hodgkin's disease.

From Goodale, R.H.: Nursing pathology, ed. 2, Philadelphia, 1956, W.B. Saunders Co.

spreads throughout the entire lymphatic network; eventually the lungs, adbominal organs, and bones will be involved. With early diagnosis the prognosis is good to excellent. The disease can be cured in up to 90% of cases through the use of expertly administered **supervoltage radiation**. Many patients are now alive and well 10 years after treatment. Even in advanced cases, chemotherapy (sometimes with radiation) can cure more than half the patients, with two thirds living at least 5 years and 58% alive 10 years later.

■ Leukemia

Leukemia is the lawless proliferation of white blood cells. These cells are immature and abnormal, and they often literally flood the bone marrow and lymphatic tissues. Paradoxically, the white blood cell count of the circulating blood is not always elevated and on occasion may actually be decreased! The disease accounts for about half of all cases of cancer in persons between the ages of 3 and 14. The precise cause is unknown, but two facts stand out: (1) certain viruses cause animal leukemia, and (2) radiation is definitely one cause of human leukemia. Leukemias are classified on the basis of the speed of the disease (**acute** or **chronic**) and the type of cell chiefly involved. For the acute form, chemotherapy is often spectacularly effective, and cures are being reported. Among the drugs (**antineoplastics**) of major value are 6-mercaptopurine (6MP), methotrexate (amethopterin), and corticosteroids.

SELF-TEST

1. __B__ venae cavae
2. __H__ pulmonary artery
3. __N__ pulmonary veins
4. __m__ aorta
5. __A__ encloses heart
6. __I__ displays cardiac cycle
7. __K__ heart rate
8. __O__ watery fluid
9. __E__ exchange of CO_2 and O_2
10. __L__ 120 mm Hg
11. __G__ 80 mm Hg
12. __J__ red blood cells
13. __D__ white blood cells
14. __F__ clotting of blood
15. __C__ blood types

a. pericardium
b. right atrium
c. agglutinogens
d. leukocytes
e. capillaries
f. thrombocytes (platelets)
g. diastolic pressure
h. right ventricle
i. ECG
j. erythrocytes
k. pacemaker
l. systolic pressure
m. left ventricle
n. left atrium
o. lymph

STUDY QUESTIONS

1. Normally the human body averages about 70 ml of blood per kilogram of body weight. How much blood does your body contain?
2. One usually says that arteries carry oxygen-rich blood and that veins carry oxygen-poor blood. Cite two major exceptions.
3. Suppose that the QRS complex of the electrocardiogram did not appear normal. What part of the heart is most likely to be in trouble?
4. Throughout the tissues of the body, there is an ongoing exchange of nutrients and wastes between the tissue fluid and the blood. Specifically, where does this exchange, or diffusion, occur, and in which direction?
5. With each beat the left ventricle pumps out about 70 ml of blood to the general circulation. (This is called the stroke volume.) If the heart is beating at a rate of 72 times per minute, how much blood (in liters and quarts) is pumped out every minute?
6. Other things being equal, persons in good physical shape tend to have low pulse rates and high stroke volumes (refer to above question). Assuming a heart rate of 60 and a stroke volume of 100 ml, how much blood is pumped per minute? How does this compare with the value obtained in Question 5?
7. What is your systolic pressure? Diastolic pressure? Pulse pressure?
8. In arteriosclerosis (hardening of the arteries) the systolic pressure increases more than the

diastolic. What effect then does this condition have on the pulse pressure?

9. According to Starling's law the volume of blood pumped by the heart is normally determined by the volume of blood returned to the heart. This is certainly the way any good pump should work. In the case of the heart how do you explain this action?

10. It is well known that exercise strengthens the heart. What is the physiologic explanation for this fact?

11. The fluid that surrounds the cells of the tissues is called intercellular fluid, or tissue fluid. Chemically, this fluid is just about identical to lymph. Why is this so?

12. Follow the path of a molecule of oxygen from the air in the lung to the interior of a cell.

13. Persons with anemia lack energy. Why?

14. If a person has anemia, would you expect the hematocrit to rise or fall?

15. What is the major function of erythrocytes? Leukocytes? Platelets?

16. In a blood transfusion the blood type of the donor must match the blood type of the person receiving the blood. Otherwise, a serious or perhaps fatal reaction ensues. By way of example, what would happen to the red cells if type A blood were given to a person with type B blood?

17. The disease of the newborn called erythroblastosis fetalis occurs only when the mother is Rh negative and the father Rh positive. Why is this so?

18. What do all anemias, regardless of their cause, have in common?

19. The pain experienced in angina pectoris is caused by myocardial ischemia. What does this mean?

20. Other things being equal, what pathologic fact determines whether or not a heart attack victim survives?

21. Pulmonary embolism often arises from diseased blood vessels in the legs. How do you account for this, or what is the connection?

22. Anticoagulants, such as heparin and warfarin (Coumadin), are used in the treatment of thrombosis and embolism. Inasmuch as these agents do not dissolve clots, how do you account for their lifesaving action?

23. A common feature of congenital heart disease is cyanosis, or bluing of the skin. This is due to poor oxygenation. Explain why there is poor oxygenation.

24. What would happen if for some reason the lymph vessels in the extremities were to be obstructed?

25. Hodgkin's disease is usually first manifested in the neck, armpit, or groin. Why these areas?

CHAPTER 6

The respiratory system

The overall purpose of the respiratory system is to bring about the exchange of oxygen (O_2) and carbon dioxide (CO_2) between the atmosphere and the cells of the body. The processes involved include ventilation (inspiration and expiration), the diffusion of oxygen from lung air into the blood and of carbon dioxide from the blood into lung air, and the transport of oxygen to and carbon dioxide from the body cells. Thus the respiratory system and the circulatory system work hand in hand to provide the body with life-giving oxygen. The structural features of the respiratory system include the nose, pharynx, larynx, trachea, bronchi, lungs, and the so-called respiratory muscles, namely, the intercostal muscles (between the ribs) and the diaphragm. One should also keep cellular respiration in mind, a topic discussed earlier in conjunction with metabolism. Cellular respiration, we shall recall, is the process cells use to produce energy-rich adenosine triphosphate (ATP). Oxygen, of course, is central to this process.

Respiration encompasses the exchange of gases in the lungs between the blood and the air, the exchange of gases between the blood and the tissues, and the transport of gases (by the blood) between the lungs and the tissues. The exchange that occurs in the lungs is called **external respiration**, and that which occurs in the tissues is termed **internal respiration**. Structurally, the respiratory system includes the respiratory tract and the muscles of respiration. We will first take a look at the tract proper and then go on to functional matters. Following this we will consider the major disorders and diseases affecting the system.

RESPIRATORY TRACT

The respiratory tract includes the **nose**, **pharynx** (throat), **larynx** (voice box), **trachea** (windpipe), **bronchi** (sing., bronchus), and **lungs**, in this order. Lining the tract is a special ciliated epithelium. The nasal cavities are fashioned into tortuous passageways, and the trachea and primary bronchi (Fig. 6-1) are composed of cartilaginous rings strung together by connective tissue and smooth muscle. We also find smooth muscle throughout the small bronchi and bronchioles. The terminal bronchioles enter alveolar ducts, and these in turn enter alveolar sacs, each of which resembles a bunch of hollow grapes. Each "grape" of the sac, continuing with the analogy, is called an **alveolus**, and because the alveolar wall is only one cell thick, gases easily diffuse across it between the air within and the blood in the surrounding capillaries. The terminal bronchioles, the alveolar sac, and the associated vessels together make up what is called a **pulmonary unit**; millions of these units compose the substance of the lungs (Fig. 6-2).

The lungs are spongy, cone-shaped organs filling the lateral, or pleural, cavities of the chest. Separated from each other by the heart and other chest structures, their bases rest on the diaphragm, and their pointed ends extend slightly above the clavicles, or collar bones. Through fissuring, the left lung is partially divided into two lobes, and the right lung is divided into three lobes. A thin membrane, the visceral pleura, envelops each lung, and a similar membrane, the parietal pleura, lines the chest. The two pleura are always in immediate contact and move against each other when we breathe, the movement being facilitated by a small amount of watery fluid.

BREATHING

The chest, or thorax, is a marvelous piece of engineering. When the **external intercostal muscles** (between the ribs) and the **diaphragm** contract, the bony cage increases in all dimensions, almost beyond expectation. As a result, the pressure within drops, and the lungs are "sucked out," causing an inrush of air. This is called **inspiration**. To effect **expiration** the body merely relaxes these muscles; that is, the diaphragm returns from a stretched-out horizontal position to its normal rounded dome shape, and the intercostal muscles drop the ribs. Forced breathing calls other muscles into play: the rhomboid muscles and levator scapulae muscles in the case of forced inspiration, and the innermost intercostals and abdominal muscles in the case of forced expiration. The volume of air moving to and fro during quiet, normal breathing averages about 0.5 liter. This is called **tidal air**. The greatest volume of air that one is able to expel after the greatest possible inhalation averages about 4.5 liters. This is called **vital capacity**.

Interestingly, the thoracic pressure is always negative (below atmospheric), meaning that during inspiration it becomes more negative and during expiration less negative. This is important to keep in mind because an opening in the chest wall (as from an injury) causes air to rush in and thereby collapse the lung (a situation called **pneumothorax**).

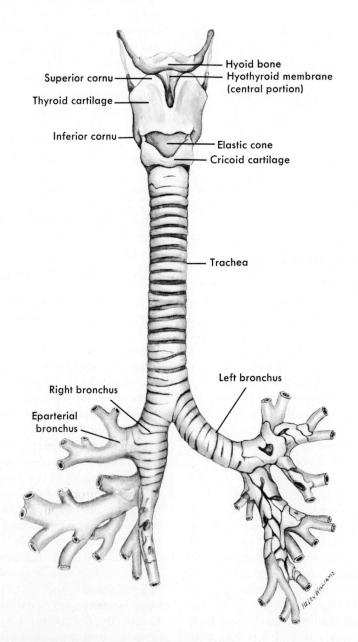

Superior cornu

Thyroid cartilage

Inferior cornu

Hyoid bone

Hyothyroid membrane
(central portion)

Elastic cone

Cricoid cartilage

Trachea

Left bronchus

Right bronchus

Eparterial
bronchus

FIG. 6-1 ■ Respiratory tract viewed from the front.

From Francis, C.C, and Martin, A.H.: Introduction to human anatomy, ed. 7, St. Louis, 1975, The C.V. Mosby Co.

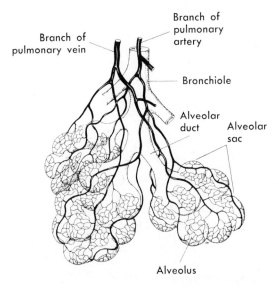

Branch of pulmonary vein

Branch of pulmonary artery

Bronchiole

Alveolar duct

Alveolar sac

Alveolus

FIG. 6-2 ■ Pulmonary units of the lung. Note especially the blood supply.

EXCHANGE AND TRANSPORT OF OXYGEN AND CARBON DIOXIDE

At the end of inspiration the air pressure within the lungs averages 760 mm Hg (atmospheric pressure), of which 100 mm Hg is due to oxygen (O_2) and 40 mm Hg is due to carbon dioxide (CO_2). Venous blood entering the lungs has oxygen and carbon dioxide pressures of 40 and 46 mm Hg, respectively. Because of these differences in pressure, oxygen diffuses from alveolar air into the blood, and carbon dioxide diffuses from the blood into the alveolar air. The events in the tissues take the opposite direction; that is, blood oxygen diffuses into the tissue fluid, and carbon dioxide diffuses into the blood.

The mechanism by which oxygen and carbon dioxide are transported (by the blood) between the lungs and the tissues is complex chemistry, to say the least. In brief, oxygen combines with hemoglobin (in the red cell) to form an unstable compound called **oxyhemo-globin**, and carbon dioxide reacts with blood plasma to form **sodium bicarbonate**. In the tissues oxyhemoglobin breaks down into hemoglobin and oxygen, the latter entering the tissue fluid and ultimately the cells; in the lungs sodium bicarbonate breaks down into carbon dioxide, which is then exhaled.

Because of the gaseous exchange taking place in the lungs, alveolar air (1) loses oxygen and (2) gains carbon dioxide. This explains why the air we exhale contains less oxygen and more carbon dioxide than atmospheric air. On the average, atmospheric air contains about 21% oxygen and 0.04% carbon dioxide. In contrast, exhaled air contains about 15% oxygen and 5% carbon dioxide.

RESPIRATORY REGULATION

The respiratory rate is regulated primarily through the respiratory centers situated in the brain. The normal rate is 12 to 18 respirations per minute. The regulation of normal, quiet breathing involves what is called the **Hering-Breuer reflex**. In this reflex, at the end of inspiration "stretch receptors" among the alveoli are stimulated and accordingly transmit inhibitory impulses to the respiratory center, relaxing the respiratory muscles and thereby effecting expiration. But as the lungs deflate, the stretch receptors become "less tense," and fewer inhibitory stimuli arrive at the center; as a result the respiratory muscles are caused to contract, thereby effecting inspiration. And so on.

The most potent stimulant of respiration is an increase in blood carbon dioxide. As the pressure of carbon dioxide rises above 40 mm Hg, the respiratory center is directly stimulated. Blood oxygen also plays a role. A decrease in the pressure of the gas stimulates the respiratory center directly. Other stimulants to respiration include irritant chemicals, strong light, sudden pain, heat and cold, and emotion.

THE LARYNX AND PHONATION

The larynx, or "voice box," located at the top of the trachea, is composed of nine pieces of cartilage and abundant skeletal muscle woven together by connective tissue into a tough, wedge-shaped box. Its anterior portion (formed by the thyroid cartilage) is known to us all as the **Adam's apple**. To prevent food and drink from going down the "wrong way," a tonguelike structure, called the **epiglottis**, closes off the larynx from the throat during swallowing. The lining of the larynx is thrown up into two prominent horizontal folds called the **false vocal cords**; below these are the **true vocal cords**, which are actually fibrous bands. The utterance of vocal sounds (**phonation**) is brought about by ejecting bursts of air from the lungs, thus causing the vocal cords to vibrate and causing the air throughout the respiratory passageways, cavities, and bone sinuses to resonate. The pitch of the voice is controlled by the tension placed on the cords by the laryngeal muscles, tense and relaxed cords yielding high-pitched and low-pitched sounds, respectively. The quality of the voice depends on the number and nature of the overtones, which in turn relate to the structure of the nose, mouth, pharynx, and sinuses.

DISORDERS AND DISEASES OF THE RESPIRATORY SYSTEM

Because the respiratory tract is in immediate contact with the outside air, it is little wonder that there are so many serious respiratory problems, the most serious of which relate to pathogenic microbes, pollutants, and cigarette smoking. Following are brief descriptions of the common and important disorders and diseases.

■ Pneumonia

Pneumonia is an acute infection of the alveolar spaces of the lung. As a result these spaces become filled with mucus, and not enough oxygen enters the blood to meet the requirements of the body. Death is not an infrequent occurrence in this ominous infection. Pneumococcal pneumonia is the most common bacterial pneumonia. The pathogen, *Streptococcus pneumoniae*, gains entrance to the body through the nose or mouth. Although it may be transmitted indirectly by food or contaminated objects (fomites), most cases result from droplet infection. The treatment of pneumonia centers on the use of antibiotics and the administration of oxygen. Vaccination is recommended for older persons and others at high risk.

■ Legionnaires' disease

Legionnaires' disease, which first appeared in 1976 (at an American Legion convention in Philadelphia), is a severe form of pneumonia caused by *Legionella pneumophila*, a previously unknown bacterium (Fig. 6-3). Interestingly, there are no distinctive clinical features to distinguish pneumonia caused by this organism and that caused by other well-established infectious agents. Perhaps the most valuable clue is the progression of pneumonia despite treatment with penicillin or a cephalosporin, drugs ordinarily effective in most bacterial pneumonias. Gentamicin, erythromycin, and rifampin are antibiotics that produce the best results in the treatment of Legionnaires' disease.

■ The common cold

The signs and symptoms of the common cold (acute coryza) are well known, as is the cause—a special class of microbes called rhinoviruses. Hundreds of these viruses have been identified. The infection may be limited to the upper respiratory tract or may extend to the larynx, trachea, and middle ear. Often, however, the latter involvements are the result of bacterial complications. The treatment of the

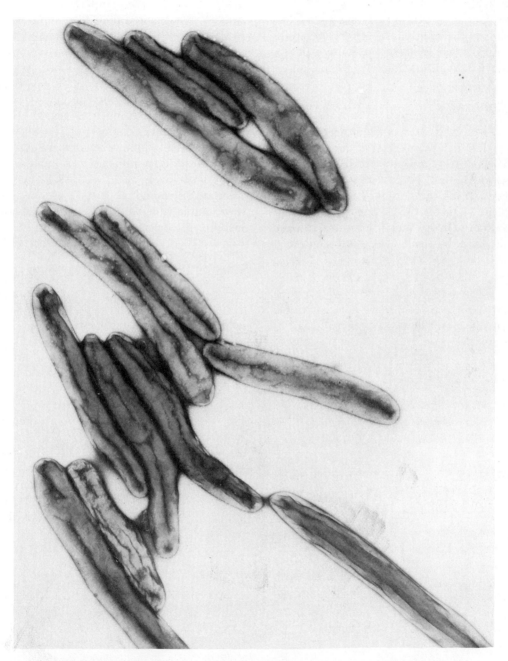

FIG. 6-3 ■ *Legionella pneumophila*, the cause of Legionnaires' disease, magnified 30,000 times.

Courtesy Centers for Disease Control, Atlanta, Ga.

common cold remains purely symptomatic, and its prevention is still an unsolved problem. Because of the multiplicity of pathogens, the prospects for an effective vaccine are not especially bright at this time.

■ Influenza

On a worldwide basis influenza, or the "flu," is our most deadly enemy. In the great pandemic (worldwide epidemic) of 1918 the death toll was close to 20 million! Lesser pandemics occurred in 1957 ("Asian flu"), in 1968 ("Hong Kong flu"), and in 1973 ("London flu"). Pandemics occur every 1 to 4 years and develop rapidly, since the incubation period is only from

1 to 3 days. The flu pandemic of 1980–1981 caused an estimated 60,000 to 70,000 deaths in the United States.

Influenza is caused by a class of viral microbes (called myxoviruses), which are categorized into types A, B, and C (Fig. 6-4). Type A viruses continue to be the major problem because of their strong tendency to mutate, or undergo genetic change. The signs and symptoms of influenza include inflammation of the respiratory mucous membranes, aches and pains, fever, and prostration. In severe cases fever (as high as 104° F) may last 4 or 5 days, and fatigue, weakness, and sweating may last 4 or 5 weeks. Treatment is purely symptomatic (bed rest and fluids) except for use

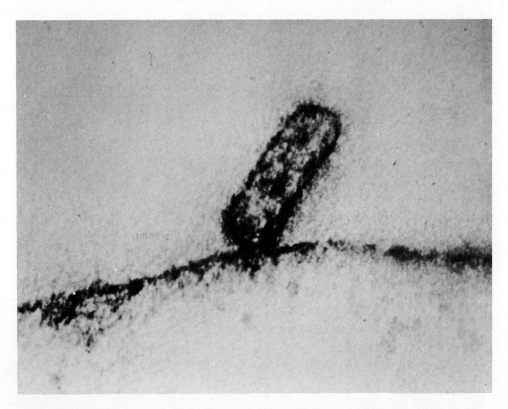

FIG. 6-4 ■ Influenza virus, showing a single virus particle (magnified 90,000 times) attached to cell membrane.

Courtesy Eli Lilly & Co., Indianapolis, Ind.

of antibiotics in the event of bacterial complications such as pneumonia. Almost always the flu kills via bacterial complications. Vaccination is effective against prevalent strains but clearly affords little or no protection against major mutations.

■ Tuberculosis

Although chemotherapy has drastically reduced the death rate, tuberculosis still remains a major threat to human welfare, particularly in underprivileged areas. The infection is caused by *Mycobacterium tuberculosis*, a rod-shaped bacterium (commonly referred to as the tubercle bacillus). Tuberculosis is usually spread by contact with "open cases" through coughing, sneezing, and kissing. The organism may also enter the body through milk or other contaminated foods. Pasteurization and the removal of infected cattle, however, have almost eliminated, in the United States at least, milkborne tuberculosis. Pulmonary (lung) tuberculosis is the most common form of the disease (Fig. 6-5). From the initial lesion, or primary focus, tubercle bacilli migrate throughout the body and, if unchecked, may overrun the body's defenses.

Treatment of tuberculosis centers on the use of antimicrobial drugs, including isoniazid (INH), streptomycin (SM), *para*-aminosalicylic acid (PAS), and ethambutol. Prevention centers on early diagnosis through chest x-ray examination and the **tuberculin skin test**. The tuberculin skin test is based on the fact that a person previously or presently infected with the tubercle bacillus becomes sensitized to tuberculin, an extract derived from the organism. Since a positive reaction can mean an inactive as well as an active lesion, it cannot be interpreted as unequivocal evidence of clinical (active) tuberculosis except in infants and young children. Vaccination with BCG vaccine has been recommended for tuberculin nonreactors who have been heavily exposed to tuberculosis. For "new reactors,"

isoniazid will prevent the development of tuberculosis.

■ Emphysema

Pulmonary emphysema is a disease of the lungs characterized by abnormal enlargement of the air spaces and by destructive changes in the alveolar walls. The alveoli are distended and disrupted, with a decrease in the amount of elastic tissue and in the number and size of vascular channels. Wheezing, chronic coughing, and labored breathing are prominent features. In the United States the incidence of emphysema has increased alarmingly. According to one survey, 27% of men over 40 years old demonstrate some evidence of the disease. The incidence is four to five times greater among men than among women. Heavy cigarette smoking is the usual cause. Symptomatic benefit and measurable improvement in pulmonary function usually follow intensive therapy for airway obstruction. This is accomplished best by the use of bronchodilators and intermittent positive pressure breathing. Above all, the person who has emphysema should not smoke and should avoid all respiratory irritants.

■ Bronchial asthma

Bronchial asthma is a distressing disease marked by recurrent attacks of labored breathing, wheezing, and coughing caused by spasmodic contraction of the bronchi and bonchioles. An acute attack leads to a deficiency of oxygen in the body and often to sudden death. The cause usually can be attributed to such external factors as pollens, animal danders, lint, and the like ("allergic asthma") or to respiratory infections (infective allergy). Secondary factors that greatly influence the frequency and severity of attack include temperature, humidity, noxious fumes, fatigue, endocrine changes, and emotional stress. Specific treatment is directed to the basic

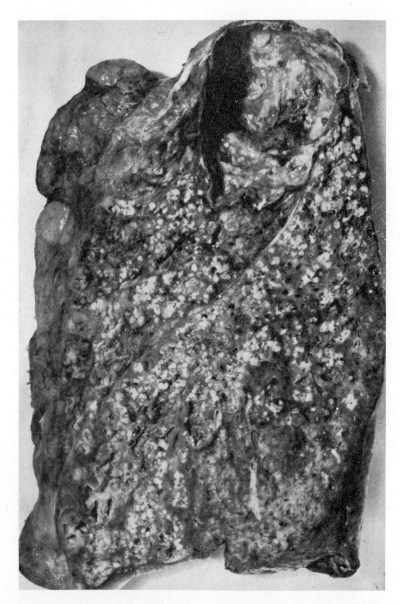

FIG. 6-5 ■ Pulmonary tuberculosis showing a lung section peppered with grayish white spots, each one representing a "colony" of the tubercle bacillus.

From Anderson, W.A.D., and Scotti, T.W.: Synopsis of pathology, ed. 10, St. Louis, 1980, The C.V. Mosby Co.

cause, and symptomatic treatment includes the use of bronchodilators (epinephrine, isoproterenol, aminophylline, or related agents), corticosteroids, cough depressants, and sedatives.

Atelectasis

Atelectasis is the collapse, or failure of expansion, of a part or all of the lung. The condition may be acquired or congenital. Acquired atelectasis may result from intrapulmonary obstruction by secretions accumulated postoperatively or by tumors of the bronchi. Also, outside pressure (as from pleural effusions or pneumothorax) may cause atelectasis. The signs and symptoms depend on the rapidity of onset; in acute episodes labored breathing and cyanosis are cardinal signs. Treatment includes giving oxygen and correcting the underlying cause.

Pleurisy

Pleurisy is inflammation of the pleura commonly arising from some unrecognized subpleural infection; the condition often accompanies pneumonia. In the acute form the membranes become reddened and often covered with a thin, watery secretion; the inflamed surfaces tend to unite by adhesions. The symptoms are a "stitch," or severe pain, in the side, chills, fever, and dry cough. Chronic pleurisy is long continued and characterized by dry surfaces, pus formation, adhesions, and even calcification. Treatment is both specific (when the cause is known) and symptomatic (mainly relief of pain).

Pneumoconioses

Pneumoconioses are chronic fibrous reactions in the lung provoked by inhalation of dust particles. The lungs characteristically become hard and pigmented, but the precise clinical picture depends on the nature of the dust. The more important dusts are coal, silica, asbestos, and beryllium. For the most part, treatment is symptomatic.

Lung cancer

Lung cancer is the leading cause of male cancer deaths, and the rate is now 15 times what it was at the turn of the century. In 1982, for men, the estimated new cases and deaths were a staggering 88,000 and 77,000, respectively. Lung cancer in women is on the rise, ranking second along with colorectal cancer as the greatest cancer killer among women. Of 34,000 estimated new cases for 1982, there were 28,000 deaths! (Breast cancer, the number one cancer killer in women, accounted for 36,800 deaths.) The statistical evidence against cigarettes is overwhelming, and at the laboratory level researchers have induced lung cancer in dogs using methods simulating hu-

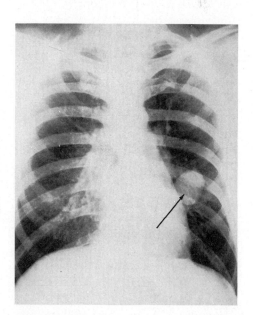

FIG. 6-6 ■ Well-delineated cancer (*arrow*) of the left lung.
From Maier, H.C., and Fischer, W.W.: J. Thorac. Surg. **16**:392-398, 1947.

man smoking. Additionally, the probability of lung cancer is increased in persons who work with asbestos, uranium ore, nickel dust, chromates, and certain other industrial materials. Prolonged exposure to air pollution is also believed to be a factor.

Common early features of this morbid involvement are coughing (often with blood), wheezing, hoarseness, and persistent fever; advanced features relate to the outright destruction of lung tissue and to metastasis (to lymph nodes, liver, bones, kidney, brain, or heart). The diagnosis involves x-ray examinations (Fig. 6-6), exploratory surgery, and biopsy. The only curative treatment, in curable cases, is the removal of a lobe or an entire lung. Radiation is helpful preoperatively and in the treatment of the inoperable patient. Only about 5% of all cases are curable because of the advanced standing of the tumor on diagnosis; metastases underscore a negative prognosis. Cancers confined to the lung are more hopeful; almost half the patients who have such cancers and are operated on live up to 5 years longer, or more. The chances of developing lung cancer can be reduced by smoking less; quitting altogether is by far the best safeguard.

■ Cystic fibrosis

Cystic fibrosis is a hereditary disease of the **exocrine glands** that affects the pancreas, respiratory system, and sweat glands. It usually begins in infancy and is characterized by chronic respiratory infection, pancreatic insufficiency, and susceptibility to heat. It is inherited as a recessive trait and has a 1 in 4 chance of developing in a child (of either sex) if both parents are carriers. The disease has an incidence of about 1 in 2000 and appears predominantly in Caucasians. No cure is known, but health can be maintained and life usually extended by preventing pulmonary complications and by treating them promptly if they occur. Of patients diagnosed in early infancy and treated in special care centers, about three fourths reach adulthood.

■■■■■■ SELF-TEST

1. _j_ Adam's apple
2. _o_ throat
3. _i_ vocal cord vibration
4. _n_ trachea
5. _h_ respiratory epithelium
6. _b_ exchange of gases
7. _m_ envelop lungs
8. _a_ lungs collapse
9. _k_ lungs expand
10. _c_ lungs deflate
11. _l_ pressure measurement
12. _g_ red cell
13. _e_ respiratory center
14. _d_ exhaled air
15. _f_ inhaled air

a. pneumothorax
b. alveoli
c. expiration
d. 5% CO_2 (Carbon Dioxide)
e. brain
f. 21% O_2 (Oxygen)
g. oxyhemoglobin
h. cilia
i. phonation
j. larynx
k. inspiration
l. mm Hg (mercury)
m. pleura
n. windpipe
o. pharynx

■■■■■ **STUDY QUESTIONS**

✳ In its journey from atmospheric air to a cell of the big toe a molecule of oxygen passes through the following structures: tissue fluid, blood, nose, trachea, larynx, bronchus, pharynx, alveolus, and bronchiole. These are not in order. What is the proper order?

2. The lining, or epithelium, of the respiratory tract is warm (because of the rich blood supply beneath) and moist, and it possesses cilia (microscopic hairlike structures). What do you think are the purposes of these features?

3. A small object, such as a safety pin, swallowed the wrong way is more likely to lodge in the right bronchus than in the left bronchus. Referring to Fig. 6-1, explain.

4. The human lung floats in water. Why?

5. In the lung oxygen enters the blood and carbon dioxide leaves the blood. Why is it not the other way around?

6. In the tissues carbon dioxide enters the blood and oxygen leaves the blood. Why is it not the other way around?

7. A bullet wound in the chest results in the entrance of atmospheric air into the pleural space (chest cavity) and the subsequent collapse of the lung (pneumothorax). Why, precisely, does air enter through the wound?

8. Carbon monoxide is poisonous because it reacts with hemoglobin to form a compound called carboxyhemoglobin. The cause of death is anoxia (lack of oxygen in body tissues). Why, precisely, is there a lack of oxygen?

9. Breathing into a paper bag (with the nose closed) causes an increase in the respiratory rate. Why?

10. In mouth-to-mouth resuscitation the victim is kept alive by expired air. How is this possible? Where's the oxygen?

11. Pneumonia causes death by asphyxia. Explain.

12. Vaccination is effective against prevalent strains of the flu virus but affords little protection against new strains. Why is this so?

13. How do you explain the fact that a person in perfectly good health and with a negative chest x-ray report has a positive reaction to the tuberculin skin test?

14. An acute attack of asthma can result in sudden death. What is the precise cause of death?

15. Lung cancers occur in persons who have never smoked. How do you account for this?

CHAPTER 7

The urinary system

All metabolic activities ultimately result in the production of wastes that must be removed from the body. Carbon dioxide, a volatile waste, is eliminated in exhaled air; solid food residues are eliminated by way of the large intestine; excess water is eliminated through all channels of excretion. All other wastes—urea, sodium chloride, acids, and a variety of other soluble substances—are eliminated by the urinary system. Specifically, the kidneys, the central organs of the system, remove these wastes from the blood and then concentrate them into urine. But the production of urine is not merely a matter of waste removal. That is to say, the kidneys monitor and regulate body fluids and maintain acid-base balance. In a very real sense the composition of the blood is determined not by what we eat but rather by what the kidneys retain.

Structural features

Formation and composition of urine

Water balance

Acid-base balance

Disorders and diseases of the urinary system

The fundamental purpose of the urinary system is the maintenance of the constancy of the body's internal environment by removing and excreting wastes and by conserving useful substances. Additionally, the kidneys influence red cell production and blood pressure and play a key role in water and acid-base balance.

STRUCTURAL FEATURES

The urinary system is composed of the **kidneys**, **ureters**, **bladder**, and **urethra** (Fig. 7-1). The kidneys are bean-shaped organs, weighing about 200 g, embedded in the back abdominal wall on either side of the vertebral column; through the hilus (or opening in the concave side of each organ) pass the renal artery and vein, lymphatic vessels, nerves, and ureter. Cut longitudinally the kidney discloses two regions (an outer cortex and an inner medulla) and a cavity, or **renal pelvis**, from which the ureter is an outlet (Fig. 7-2). Leading off the pelvis are a number of cup-shaped recesses (**calices**), each calix enclosing the apex, or papilla, of a triangular structure called the **pyramid**; each pyramid is composed of collecting tubules that open at the papilla.

The ureters are fibromuscular tubes, about 28 cm in length and 1.2 cm in diameter, that convey urine from the renal pelvis to the bladder. Situated immediately before the vagina in the female and immediately before the rectum in the male, the urinary bladder is a tough, muscular sac. Leading urine from the bladder to the exterior is the urethra, a membranous tube about 3.5 cm in length in the female and about 20 cm in length in the male.

Urination is effected through contraction of the bladder musculature and relaxation of the sphincters guarding the opening into the urethra (Fig. 7-1). The urge to urinate starts when about 250 ml of urine has accumulated in the bladder. When about 600 ml has accumulated, a sensation of pain may be aroused, and

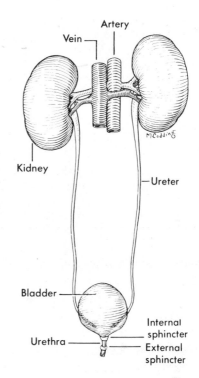

FIG. 7-1 ■ The urinary system.

urination becomes urgent. Delaying urination until this point can have damaging effects, especially if it becomes a practice to do so.

FORMATION AND COMPOSITION OF URINE

Making up the substance of the kidney are some one million **nephrons**, the chief features of which are the renal corpuscle (or malpighian body) and the renal tubule (Fig. 7-3). The corpuscle is composed of a tuft of capillaries (the **glomerulus**) enclosed within a double-walled membrane known as **Bowman's capsule**. This is the invaginated blind end of the proximal convoluted renal tubule; the distal convoluted renal tubule enters a collecting duct of a pyramid. Because the vas afferens (leading blood into the glomerulus) is of greater

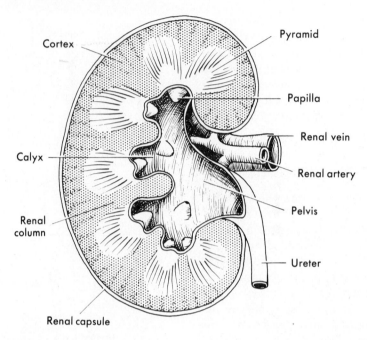

Cortex

Pyramid

Papilla

Renal vein

Renal artery

Calyx

Renal column

Pelvis

Ureter

Renal capsule

FIG. 7-2 ■ The kidney and associated structures. Note that the renal pelvis is actually an expansion of the upper end of the ureter.

caliber than the vas efferens (leading blood out of the glomerulus), enough pressure builds up to force water and water-soluble substances out of the blood into Bowman's capsule. (Blood cells and blood proteins are not forced through.) As this aqueous solution (the so-called **glomerular filtrate**) makes its way through the renal tubule, almost all of the water and essential solutes are reabsorbed back into the blood by the cells lining the tubule. Consequently, by the time the filtrate reaches the collecting duct, it has become a relatively concentrated solution of wastes—that is, **urine**. Extrarenal ("outside") factors having a bearing on kidney function include, among others, blood pressure and the hormones **aldosterone** and ADH (**antidiuretic hormone**). An increase in blood pressure causes an increase in the output of glomerular filtrate; ADH (secreted by the pituitary gland) stimulates the reabsorption of water by the renal tubule; and

aldosterone (secreted by the adrenal gland) causes the tubules to increase their uptake of sodium and their rejection of potassium.

Freshly voided urine is a clear, pale yellow and has a faint but characteristic odor. On standing it becomes cloudy and develops a strong odor as a result of the bacterial conversion of urea into ammonia. The pH varies from about 4.5 to 7.5 (depending on the diet), and the specific gravity averages about 1.020. (By comparison plain water has a pH of 7 and a specific gravity of 1.) In a 24-hour period the total volume of urine from one individual averages 1200 ml, with a range anywhere from 600 to 2500 ml. Aside from urea, the main waste product, urine contains sodium chloride, creatine, creatinine, uric acid, and an assortment of other organic and inorganic substances. **Urochrome**, a pigment derived from bile, is responsible for the color of urine.

A number of conditions can be detected by

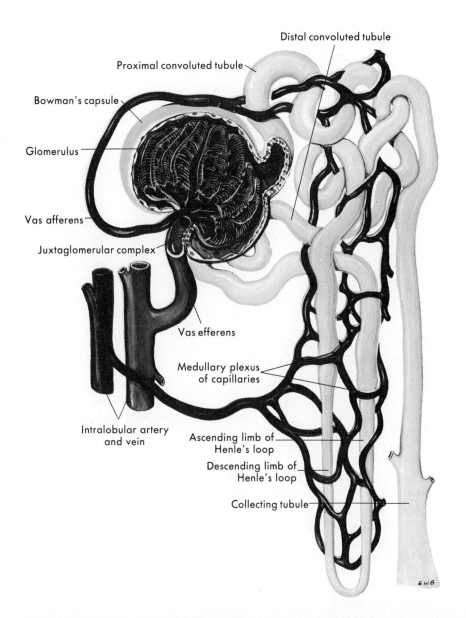

Distal convoluted tubule

Proximal convoluted tubule

Bowman's capsule

Glomerulus

Vas afferens

Juxtaglomerular complex

Vas efferens

Medullary plexus of capillaries

Intralobular artery and vein

Ascending limb of Henle's loop

Descending limb of Henle's loop

Collecting tubule

FIG. 7-3 ■ The nephron. High pressure within the glomerulus forces out a fluid, called the glomerular filtrate, that works its way through the convoluted tubules. As a result of tubular reabsorption this filtrate becomes a concentrated solution of waste products (urine) by the time it reaches the collecting tubule.

From Schottelius, B.A., and Schottelius, D.D.: Textbook of physiology, ed. 18, St. Louis, 1978, The C.V. Mosby Co.

chemical examination of the urine (**urinalysis**). The habitual presence of glucose in the urine (**glucosuria**) suggests diabetes mellitus. The habitual presence of protein, namely albumin (**albuminuria**), may indicate kidney disease. (Traces of protein in the urine may signal early "silent" heart and blood vessel disease.) Urine is also tested easily for hemoglobin, bile, specific gravity, and acidity (pH). When a specimen of urine is centrifuged, a sediment is produced that can be examined under the microscope. It may reveal blood corpuscles, bacteria, pus, renal tubular debris (casts), or other evidence of disease.

WATER BALANCE

Plants and animals vary tremendously in their water requirements. Intake increases with size and, interestingly enough, in a mathematical way. Also of interest is the time required for a given member of a species to imbibe a quantity of water equal to its own weight. A mouse takes 5 days; a cow, 2 weeks; a camel, 3 months; a tortoise, 1 year; a human being 1 month; and a cactus, 29 years! Regardless of the amount of water taken in, however, the body normally balances the gain with an equivalent loss. Conversely, the body balances a loss with an equivalent gain. Either way, the central idea is balance. Humans possess phenomenal balance; in a 24-hour period a person's weight may vary less than 250 g.

■ Intake

A person's daily intake of water is said to average about 2.5 liters. This water comes not only from fluids but also from **preformed water** (water trapped in food) and **oxidative water** (water resulting from cellular respiration). The respective volumes from these sources are shown in Fig. 7-4. Obviously, food intake has a great bearing on the need for imbibed

fluid. The kangaroo rat, a desert creature, never takes a drink as long as it lives, deriving its water solely from solid food! We could do the same if we lived on cucumbers and lettuce.

■ Output

As noted, the daily output of water balances the daily intake (Fig. 7-4). The kidneys carry the heaviest load, excreting up to about 1.7 liters. The other channels, though not so apparent, are no less vital. From the skin and lungs, about 0.5 liter and 0.4 liter of water are lost, respectively. About 0.2 liter leaves the body in the feces. Water escapes from the lungs as vapor. Water lost from the skin is usually vapor (**insensible perspiration**), but it builds up into sweat when the body becomes overheated. Perspiration is about 99% water, with traces of salt (sodium chloride) and urea. In certain diseases other constituents may appear, such as bile pigments, albumin, and sugar.

ACID-BASE BALANCE

The blood and tissue fluid have an average pH of 7.4, which means that they are just very slightly basic (or alkaline). (Solutions with a pH below 7 are acidic, and those with a pH above 7 are alkaline.) A blood pH below 7 (**acidosis**) or a blood pH above 8 (**alkalosis**) may spell death unless corrected. Accordingly, the maintenance of the magic number of 7.4, or "acid-base balance" (Fig. 7-5), is crucial, especially when we consider that a single drop of acid or base (alkali) can significantly alter the pH of a whole gallon of water. Put another way, why aren't dill pickles lethal? The answer is complex chemistry, involving the lungs, the blood, and the kidneys. The kidneys bear the greatest burden in acid-base balance because they are the ultimate regulators. Spe-

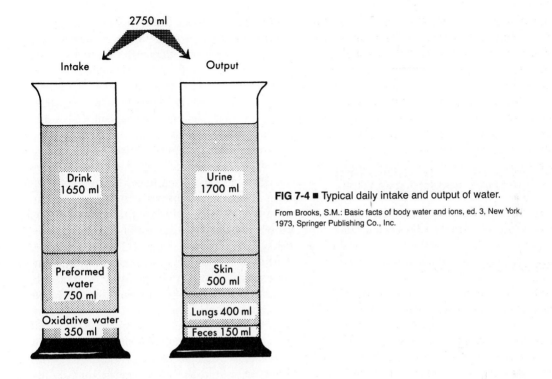

FIG 7-4 ■ Typical daily intake and output of water.

From Brooks, S.M.: Basic facts of body water and ions, ed. 3, New York, 1973, Springer Publishing Co., Inc.

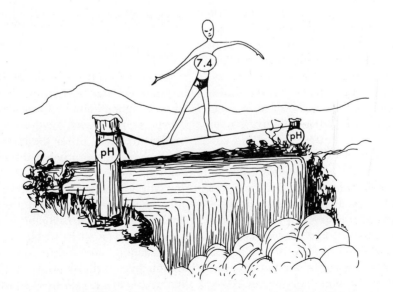

FIG. 7-5 ■ Tightrope walking can prove fatal, as can an alteration of body pH.

cifically, when the blood's chemical buffers become overtaxed, and the pH starts to change, the kidneys respond by excreting acid or base; they excrete acid in the event of acidosis and base in the event of alkalosis. Since most metabolic wastes are acidic, the usual trend of body pH is downward, which explains the acidosis of renal (kidney) failure.

◼◼◼◼ DISORDERS AND DISEASES OF THE URINARY SYSTEM

Disorders and diseases of the urinary system are the result of either infection or degenerative changes. Both eventualities can result in renal failure and sometimes death.

◼ Urinary tract infections

Genitourinary (GU) tract infection is the most common type of bacterial infection that affects the human body; likewise urinary tract infection is the most common disease process that affects the GU tract. Urinary tract infections are about ten times more frequent in girls and women than in boys and men. During infancy bacteria enter the GU tract most often from the blood or lymph; in older children and in adults the main route of infection is an ascending one (from the vagina-urethra-bladder). The majority of urinary tract infections are caused by so-called **gram-negative bacteria**, especially the organism *Escherichia coli* (responsible for about 85% of the cases).

Urinary tract infections are named according to the site of the infection. From the lower tract on upward these include urethritis (urethra), cystitis (bladder), ureteritis (ureter), and pyelonephritis (kidney). Pyelonephritis is the most serious infection, and cystitis is by far the most common, especially among women. Most cases of cystitis in women are caused by an **ascending infection** from the vagina through

the urethra, often following sexual intercourse. Women who develop recurrent urinary tract infections differ from normal women in that they harbor (in the vagina) large numbers of abnormal organisms for long periods of time. Apparently there is a lack of some form of vaginal defense mechanism that would prevent the colonization of these organisms. At present the best way to prevent recurrent cystitis in those women who have four or more infections a year is long-term, continuous, low-dose antibacterial therapy. In most cases the drug combination trimethoprim-sulfamethoxazole (Bactrim, Septra) produces excellent results.

Cystitis in men generally results from an infection of the urethra or prostate or occurs as a result of urethral instrumentation (for diagnostic purposes). The most common cause of recurrent cystitis in men is chronic bacterial infection of the prostate (prostatitis). Most antimicrobial drugs do not produce a lasting cure for prostate-linked cystitis because they do not diffuse into the prostate from the blood. That is, once therapy is stopped the prostatic pathogen eventually reinfects the bladder.

◼ Renal failure

Renal failure is the inability of the kidneys to perform their normal excretory and regulatory function. The hallmark of the condition is **uremia**, which may be defined as the retention of urea and other metabolic wastes and the toxic effects produced thereby. These effects include nausea, vomiting, headache, dizziness, dimness of vision, coma, and convulsions. There are a multitude of underlying causes of renal failure, including hemorrhage, poisoning, enlarged prostate, kidney stones, and inflammation of the glomeruli (glomerulonephritis). If these are correctable, the outlook is good to excellent. The removal of kidney stones, for example, is clearly the answer

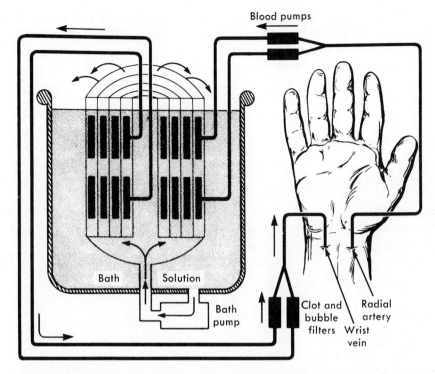

Blood pumps

Bath Solution

Bath pump

Clot and bubble filters

Radial artery

Wrist vein

FIG. 7-6 ■ Simplified diagram of twin-coil apparatus for hemodialysis (artificial kidney).

Courtesy Travenol Laboratories, Inc., Artificial Organs Division, Deerfield, Ill.

to renal failure of this origin. When the cause is not correctable, or when the limits of effectiveness of conventional therapy have been reached, long-term **dialysis** or **transplantation** must be considered.

Dialysis is a fundamental process of physics, whereby smaller molecules are separated from larger molecules in a solution by means of selective diffusion through a semipermeable membrane. Medically speaking, "dialysis" refers to the removal of waste products from the blood by means of an artificial semipermeable membrane (the so-called **artificial kidney**) or by means of the peritoneum that lines the abdominal cavity (**peritoneal dialysis**). In both cases wastes, which are relatively small molecules, diffuse into a cleansing solution or bath while blood cells and blood proteins—because of their large size—remain in circulation (Fig. 7-6). In other words, the blood is cleared of wastes but not at the expense of its vital elements. More than 50,000 Americans have their blood cleansed daily by artificial kidney machines, and a few thousand or so are on peritoneal dialysis.

Even at its best dialysis is a stopgap measure that can prolong life but not overcome an underlying fatal disease. Only kidney transplantation can "cure" chronic renal failure by replacing the diseased kidney with a healthy one. More than 10,000 Americans live with the aid of someone else's kidney, and 15,000 to 20,000 more are waiting for a suitable organ to become available for transplantation.

Because of a shortage of donated kidneys, only between 4000 and 5000 patients receive transplants each year. Among patients who receive a kidney from a living relative, about 90% are alive and well 2 years later and are likely to go on being so. Among patients whose kidneys come from cadaver donors, 50% to 60% survive.

■■■■■ **SELF-TEST**

1. __D__ conveys urine to bladder
2. __J__ male urethra
3. __L__ female urethra
4. __m__ relaxation of sphincters
5. __O__ tuft of capillaries
6. __I__ renal tubule
7. __K__ solution of wastes
8. __C__ diabetes mellitus
9. __n__ insensible perspiration
10. __h__ preformed water
11. __E__ oxidative water
12. __g__ drop in blood pH *7.4*
13. __A__ rise in blood pH *< 7.0*
14. __B__ kidney disease
15. __F__ intake vs. output

a. alkalosis *release* *protein - blood*
b. albuminuria
c. glucosuria
d. ureter
e. cellular respiration
f. balance
g. acidosis
h. food
i. reabsorption
j. 20 cm
k. urine
l. 3.5 cm
m. urination
n. skin
o. glomerulus

14 many OH
few H

↑ balance
H+ OH-

few OH
O many H+

■■■■■ **STUDY QUESTIONS**

1. A molecule of water passes through the following structures on its journey from the blood to voided urine: ureter, urethra, glomerulus, collecting duct, renal tubule, renal pelvis, bladder, and renal calix. These are not in order. What is the proper order?
2. The male urethra is about six times the length of the female urethra. Why?
3. What is the difference between glomerular filtrate and urine?
4. In shock there is a sudden, drastic drop in blood pressure. Based on your knowledge of renal (kidney) physiology, what effect do you think this has on urinary output? Why?
5. In the disease called diabetes insipidus there is a lack of antidiuretic hormone (ADH). Based on your knowledge of renal physiology, what effect do you think this has on urinary output?

6. Excess salt, or sodium, in the body tends to increase blood pressure, and a lack of salt, or sodium, tends to lower blood pressure. Armed with this fact plus your knowledge of renal physiology, what happens to the blood pressure in Addison's disease (where there is a lack of the hormone aldosterone)?
7. Large amounts of albumin in the urine (albuminuria) point to a defect in the renal nephrons. Specifically, what part of the nephron?
8. The specific gravity of urine is always above one, although ever so slightly. Why?
9. On the usual American diet the pH of the urine is normally on the "acid side," just below seven. Why?
10. When for some reason the pH of the blood starts to drop, how do the kidneys respond? What would be proof of this response?

11. Cystitis is much more common in females than in males. Why?
12. Urinary tract infections in older children and adults are usually of an "ascending nature." What does this mean?
13. The bacterial species *Escherichia coli* is normally present throughout the colon and rectum. What is the relationship between this fact and urinary tract infections?
14. In the artificial kidney machine the bath solution (Fig. 7-6) contains a carefully controlled concentration of various chemical substances. Inasmuch as blood wastes easily diffuse into plain water, why the solution?
15. The reason the body tends to reject tissue and organ transplants is because they are "chemically foreign." How does this fit in with the results noted in kidney transplantation?

CHAPTER 8

The digestive system

The need for food is adequately underscored by the fact that the digestive organs make up the bulk of the abdominal viscera. The digestive apparatus includes the gastrointestinal (GI) tract proper and a number of accessory organs. Physiologically, the system has a simple enough purpose, that is, the physical and chemical extraction of nutrients from the diet and their absorption into the blood through the intestinal mucosa. Digestion, or the breaking down of food, is brought about by digestive juices that contain potent enzymes. These enzymes split food into molecules small enough to edge their way into the intestinal villi. Such absorbable nutrients include water, minerals, vitamins, amino acids (from protein), glucose (from carbohydrates), and glycerol and fatty acids (from fats). Once in the blood these substances are transported throughout the body and ultimately enter the complex machinery of the cell where they are burned for energy or forged into the materials of life.

Basic structure

Digestion and absorption

Feces and defecation

Regulation

Disorders and diseases

The digestive system includes the gastrointestinal tract and associated organs and glands; its purpose is to convert food molecules—carbohydrates, fats, and proteins—into smaller molecules capable of being absorbed into the blood. This chapter discusses the system's structure, the digestive process proper, and certain major disorders and diseases affecting the system.

◼ BASIC STRUCTURE

The gastrointestinal tract proper is formed by the **mouth**, **pharynx**, **esophagus**, **stomach**, and **intestine**, in that order (Fig. 8-1). Bounded on the sides by the cheeks, above by the hard and soft palates, and below by a sheet of muscle, the mouth opens into the pharynx, or throat. The tongue, a highly agile, muscular organ located at the floor of the mouth, is covered by a mucous membrane thrown up into a number of nipple-shaped elevations called papillae; distributed among these structures are microscopic barrel-shaped receptors called **taste buds**. The jaws give rise to 20 **deciduous (milk) teeth** and 32 **permanent teeth**.

The pharynx (throat), a musculomembranous structure interconnecting the nose, mouth, larynx, and esophagus, serves as a common passageway for air and food, leading air into the larynx and food into the esophagus. The esophagus is a muscular tube, 28 cm in length, running behind the trachea and entering the stomach just beneath the diaphragm, which it pierces.

The healthy empty stomach has a small cavity and thick tough muscular walls formed into deep wrinkles (**rugae**) on the inside. This telescoped surface permits great distention and accounts for the fact that the adult stomach can accommodate a volume of up to 3 or 4 liters. Its mucous lining secretes an abundance of gastric juice in response to both neural and hormonal stimulation. The terminal portion of the stomach, the pylorus, opens into

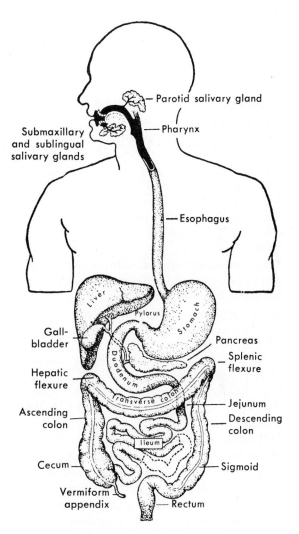

FIG. 8-1 ◼ The digestive system.

the duodenum, the first of the three somewhat arbitrary divisions of the **small intestine**; the other two divisions are the jejunum and ileum. The overall length of the small intestine averages about 6 m.

Attaching the small intestine to the back abdominal wall is the **mesentery**, a fan-shaped fold of peritoneum of two layers between which run blood and lymphatic vessels and nerves. And characteristically the inner lining (mucosa) of the small intestine sends up an enormous number of fingerlike projections called **villi**, each villus possessing a capillary network and a large lymphatic vessel called a **lacteal**.

The **large intestine** is about 1.6 m in length, extending from its juncture with the small intestine to the anus, and comprises the cecum, colon, and rectum; there are no villi, and the walls are puckered into incomplete sacculations, or pouchlike structures, called haustra. Branching from the lower cecum is the apparently worthless **vermiform appendix**—a blind, wormlike tube varying in length from 7 to 15 cm.

The "accessory organs" of the digestive system include the **salivary glands**, the **liver**, the **gallbladder**, the **pancreas**, and a number of endocrine glands. Arranged in pairs about the face, the salivary glands (the parotid, sublingual, and submaxillary) secrete saliva into the mouth in response to the presence of food or merely seeing, smelling, or thinking about food. Saliva aids in chewing and swallowing and, to a minor degree, in the actual digestive process.

The liver is a dark-red organ situated in the upper part of the abdomen on the right side. It is dome-shaped from fitting in under the diaphragm and has a double blood supply from the hepatic artery and the portal vein. Chemically speaking, the liver is involved in just about everything going on in the body. It acts on carbohydrates, fats, and proteins; it stores vitamins and minerals; it detoxifies poisons and potentially harmful substances; it bolsters body immunity; and last, but certainly not least, it manufactures **bile**, a yellowish green secretion essential to the digestion and absorption of fats. Once formed, bile trickles down the hepatic duct to the common bile duct and then backs up the cystic duct into the gallbladder, a pear-shaped pouch partially embedded in the undersurface of the liver. Here in the gallbladder bile is stored and concentrated.

The pancreas is a pinkish, fish-shaped organ running horizontally between the stomach and back abdominal wall; its head and neck are nestled in the C-shaped curve of the duodenum, and its tail just touches the spleen. Aside from a potent digestive juice, the pancreas also secretes **insulin**, a hormone essential to the proper utilization of carbohydrate and fat. Pancreatic juice makes its way into the duodenum via a special duct that meets the common bile duct (Fig. 8-1).

■■■■ DIGESTION AND ABSORPTION

Absorbable nutrients include the simple sugars **glucose**, **fructose**, and **galactose** from carbohydrates; **glycerol** and **fatty acids** from fats; and **amino acids** from proteins. These, in brief, are derived as follows: Salivary amylase (ptyalin), saliva's sole enzyme, splits (breaks down) about 40% of ingested starches into the double sugar maltose, the remaining 60% entering the small intestine as intermediates (dextrins) and unaltered molecules. In the small intestine pancreatic amylase converts this assortment into maltose. Intestinal maltase then delivers the coup de grace by splitting all maltose into glucose. Ingested sucrose (regular table sugar) is split by intestinal sucrase into glucose and fructose; lactose (milk sugar) is split by intestinal lactase into galactose and glucose. Fats and oils are first emulsified by bile and then split by pancreatic lipase into glycerol and fatty acids. In the stomach proteins are first broken down by the enzyme pepsin into a mixture of digestive intermediates. Then in the intestine the job is completed through the action of trypsin and chymotrypsin, components of the pancreatic juice, in concert with certain enzymes of the intestinal juice.

Thanks to the digestive enzymes (Table 8-1), **chyme**, the mushy mixture moving through the gastrointestinal tract, contains a rich assortment of nutrients destined for absorption (into the blood) by the myriad microscopic projections (**villi**) lining the small intestine.

TABLE 8-1

Major digestive enzymes

Organ	Digestive juices and important enzymes	Where produced	Acts on	Resulting products	Substance absorbed
Mouth	Saliva Salivary amylase (ptyalin)	Salivary glands	Starch	Maltose	None
Stomach	Gastric juice	Stomach lining			Practically none (except alcohol)
	Rennin* Pepsin†		Milk and proteins	Milk curds Proteoses and peptones	
Small intestine	Bile (contains no enzymes)	Liver	Fats and oils	Emulsified fats and oils	Amino acids, simple sugars, fatty acids, glycerol, vitamins, and minerals

	Pancreatic juice
	  Trypsin and chymotrypsin‡
	  Pancreatic lipase (steapsin)
	  Pancreatic amylase (amylopsin)
		Pancreas	Proteins
			Emulsified fats
			Starch
				Polypeptides
				Fatty acids and glycerol
				Maltose	

	Intestinal juice	Intestinal lining			
	Peptidases Sucrase		Polypeptides Sucrose	Amino acids Glucose and fructose	
	Maltase Lactase		Maltose Lactose	Glucose Glucose and galactrose	
Colon	None				Water

*Rennin not present in adult gastric juice.
†Secreted as inactive pepsinogen (and activated by hydrochloric acid).
‡Secreted as trypsinogen and chymotrypsinogen (and activated by enterokinase).

■■■■ FECES AND DEFECATION

The main functions of the large intestine are absorption of water and elimination of the wastes of digestion. As the chyme is propelled along, it becomes progressively less watery and eventually becomes a semisolid material called **feces,** an excrement composed of nondigestible food residues (roughage or fiber), bacteria, and intestinal secretions. Its characteristic chocolate color is attributable to the pigments formed by the action of the digestive enzymes on bile. Defecation, or discharge of feces, is initiated by the passage of fecal material into the rectum. Sensory impulses are relayed to the spinal cord, and intestinal movement is thereby stimulated; simultaneously, the internal anal sphincter is relaxed to aid passage through the anal opening. The external sphincter is relaxed voluntarily to complete the act. The abdominal muscles also play a role in defecation, for when contracted, they compress the intestinal contents downward against the rectum and stimulate the sensory endings in the rectum.

In this manner defecation is both initiated and promoted.

◼ REGULATION

The emptying of the stomach, the opening and closing of valves, the contraction of the gallbladder, the wormlike movement of the intestinal tract (**peristalsis**), and the manufacture and secretion of digestive juice are very carefully regulated and integrated through the cooperation of neural and hormonal mechanisms. The major events are as follows: psychic and physical factors reflexly stimulate the secretion of saliva and gastric juice; protein provokes the release of the hormone gastrin (by the stomach mucosa), which in turn stimulates the secretion of gastric juice; the presence of chyme in the duodenum reflexly causes the contraction and closing of the pyloric sphincter; distention and acidity reflexly initiate peristalsis; the hormone secretin (released by the duodenum in response to the presence of chyme) stimulates the production of bile and pancreatic juice; and the hormone cholecystokinin (produced by the duodenum in response to fatty chyme) causes contraction and emptying of the gallbladder.

◼ DISORDERS AND DISEASES

Disorders and diseases of the digestive system are almost without number. Considering the length of the digestive tract (some 20-odd feet!) and the great bulk of the overall system, this hardly comes as a surprise. For the most part, digestive disorders are functional in origin, whereas digestive disease is either organic (degenerative) or the result of infection. Following are highlights of the more common and serious disorders and diseases.

◼ Constipation

Constipation (a "crowding together") is a delayed movement of intestinal contents. It may result in infrequent evacuation or in a stool that is dry or reduced in amount or difficult in passage. Normal frequency of movement ranges from 3 times a day to once in 3 days. Many persons incorrectly believe that daily defecation is crucial to normalcy. Furthermore, many believe that a daily movement of a certain color or consistency is essential. As a result of these beliefs, the colon is abused by laxatives, suppositories, and enemas, which can lead to a real problem, called **spastic colon**. In this condition the colon is subject to persisting spastic contractions that inhibit normal peristalsis. The final outcome is constipation (spastic constipation) and abdominal pain. However, some cases of spastic constipation (Fig. 8-2) arise from stress and emotional conflict. The usual underlying factors are marital discord, anxiety related to children, loss of a loved one, and obsessional worries over trivial everyday problems (for instance, bowel movement).

Aside from spastic colon, other causes of constipation include **inactive colon** and some form of **obstruction**. Inactive colon (atonic constipation) occurs in the aged person, invalid, or the person confined to bed by illness. Feces accumulate because the colon does not respond to the usual stimuli promoting evacuation. Obstruction is principally of a mechanical nature. A major example is cancer.

The treatment of constipation includes measures to relieve the immediate complaint (using bulk laxatives and stool softeners) and appropriate attention to the underlying cause. Diet is highly important, and an increased intake of roughage or fiber, such as bran, is often all that is needed.

◼ Diarrhea

Diarrhea is an increase in volume, fluidity, or frequency of bowel movement relative to the usual pattern for a particular person. Since water makes up 60% to 90% of stool weight, diarrhea is mainly the result of excess fecal

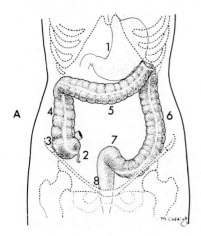

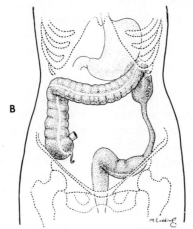

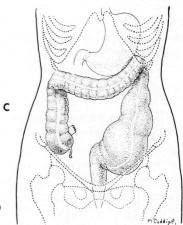

FIG. 8-2 ■ A, The normal large bowel or colon in the proper position in relation to other structures: *1*, stomach; *2*, appendix; *3*, cecum; *4*, ascending colon; *5*, transverse colon; *6*, descending colon; *7*, sigmoid flexure; *8*, rectum. **B,** The colon in spastic constipation. **C,** The colon in atonic constipation.

water. Acute diarrhea is generally encountered in three forms: (1) in an epidemic of viral origin, (2) in food poisoning, and (3) in isolated cases in which no infectious agent is apparent (dietary indiscretion, misuse of laxatives, food allergy, emotional upset, and so on). Common to all three forms is "speedy peristalsis" resulting from excessive stimulation of the intestinal musculature. That is, there is not sufficient time for normal absorption of intestinal fluid to occur. The consequences of diarrhea are electrolyte loss (namely, sodium and potassium), dehydration, shock, collapse, and sometimes death. Collapse may develop rapidly in persons who are very young, who are elderly or otherwise debilitated, or who have severe diarrhea (for example, those with cholera).

The treatment of diarrhea includes the use of medications to decrease peristalsis and reduce the fluidity of watery stools and, of course, specific measures directed at the underlying disorder, such as the use of antibiotics in the case of infection. Severe diarrhea may require urgent fluid and electrolyte replacement to correct dehydration, electrolyte imbalance, and acidosis. Simply correcting the water loss (dehydration) without replacing the lost electrolytes can prove fatal, because intestinal fluid lost to the stool contains vital electrolytes, namely sodium, potassium, magnesium, and bicarbonate. The loss of bicarbonate (which is an alkaline substance) is responsible for the acidosis.

■ Food poisoning

The most common cause of food poisoning is the **toxin** produced by certain strains of the pathogen *Staphylococcus aureus*. The usual events, which begin 2 to 4 hours after ingestion of food, include nausea, severe vomiting, abdominal cramps, diarrhea, and prostration. But despite the violence of the acute attack, the symptoms usually subside after about 6 hours. Symptomatic treatment with replacement of fluids is generally all that is required. Inasmuch as staphylococcal food poisoning is actually caused by a toxin, many authorities refer to it as a type of **food intoxication**. The most common type of food poisoning caused by the organism per se (so-called **food infection**) is **salmonellosis**, a gastrointestinal infection involving dozens of species of *Salmonella*, the same group to which belong the pathogens of typhoid and paratyphoid fever. Many of these species are natural pathogens of domestic animals, and thus meats, fish, milk, eggs, and milk and egg products are the usual culprits. Also, foods may become contaminated during processing by human carriers and by infected rats and mice that inhabit food plants, warehouses, and kitchens. The treatment of salmonellosis centers on the replacement of water and electrolytes and the use of antibiotics.

The most deadly food poisoning, **botulism**, is caused by *Clostridium botulinum*, a bacterium that produces one of the most potent biological poisons known. It has been estimated that as little as 60 micrograms of the poison may be lethal. Botulism is almost always contracted by eating contaminated food, especially uncooked or improperly processed sausage, ham, fish, and vegetables. Many cases have been caused by canned food prepared in the home. Diagnosis is made by injection of the suspected food into mice or by isolation of the pathogen from the food, feces, or vomitus. Botulism antitoxin is of limited value once signs and symptoms develop, but it is generally regarded as highly effective if given before the onset of symptoms. All exposed persons should be given the antitoxin immediately.

■ Infection

Infections of the digestive system encompass the full spectrum of pathogenic microbes plus many species of parasitic worms. Major

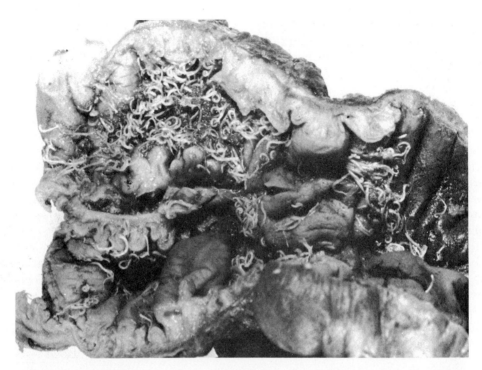

FIG. 8-3 ■ Massive whipworm infection in young child that resulted in severe hemorrhagic diarrhea and death. Segment of colon opened to show worms on inner mucosal surface.

From Anderson, W.A.D., and Kissane, J.W.: Pathology, ed. 7, St. Louis, 1977, The C.V. Mosby Co.

bacterial infections include *Salmonella* food poisoning, typhoid fever, bacillary dysentery, cholera, and peritonitis; major **viral infections** include mumps, yellow fever, and hepatitis. The most common and important infection caused by a protozoan is **amebiasis** (amebic dysentery), and the most common and important fungal infection is **candidiasis** (thrush). Except in the instance of viral infections treatment centers on the use of antimicrobial drugs. Prevention involves good sanitation and, for some infections, vaccination. Effective vaccines are available for typhoid fever, cholera, mumps, yellow fever, and hepatitis B (serum hepatitis).

The presence of parasitic worms in the intestinal tract is the most common form of **hel-**minthiasis (worm infection) (Fig. 8-3). Intestinal worms harass the host by causing obstruction, faulty digestion, inflammation, and anemia. Intestinal worms encountered in the United States include hookworm, roundworm, pinworm, whipworm, beef tapeworm, pork tapeworm, and fish tapeworm. These worms range in length from the very small pinworm (1.2 cm) up to the giant fish tapeworm (9 m). A number of drugs (anthelmintics) are available to treat worms. **Pinworm infection** (enterobiasis) is by far the most common worm infection, especially among children. Adult pinworms reside in the lower colon and rectum. At night, about 9 o'clock, the female worm wiggles through the anal opening and deposits eggs in the surrounding area.

This produces itching, scratching, and contaminated fingernails, thereby ensuring reinfection via the oral route. The anthelmintic mebendazole (Vermox) is highly effective against pinworm.

■ Malabsorption syndrome

Impaired absorption of nutrients from the small intestine results in a varied and complex array of signs and symptoms ranging from minor and subtle complaints, such as lassitude and fatigability, to major ones, such as bleeding and convulsions. Most cases are characterized by loss of fecal fat. Possible underlying causes of malabsorption syndrome are manifold. Established causes include, among many others, radiation injury, hormonal disorders, infection, liver disease, and enzyme deficiencies. Treatment is symptomatic and, whenever possible, specific.

■ Peptic ulcer

Peptic ulcers are erosions of the mucosal lining exposed to pepsin and hydrochloric acid; most occur in the stomach and in the first portion of the duodenum. The cause is obscure, but hypersecretion of gastric juice and emotional tension are clearly involved. The signs and symptoms include pain, heartburn, nausea, vomiting, loss of appetite, weight loss, diarrhea, and anemia. Perforation, massive hemorrhage, and obstruction (of the outlet of the stomach) are grave complications. Medical treatment centers on mental and physical rest and the suppression of hyperacidity and gastric activity. If these measures fail, surgery must be considered.

■ Diverticulosis

Diverticulosis refers to the presence of outpouchings (**diverticula**) that are prone to develop in weakened areas of the intestinal wall.

The lower colon is especially susceptible to the condition. When fully developed, diverticula are spherical pouches connected with the intestine by narrow necks; commonly, these necks become obstructed and infected, giving rise to inflammation (**diverticulitis**). Diverticulosis is often of little consequence, and no treatment is required. Diverticulitis, on the other hand, calls for antibiotics. In the event of complications, surgery is indicated. Common complications are abscess formation, intestinal obstruction, and hemorrhage. A large congenital outpouching of the intestine is called **Meckel's diverticulum**. This may become infected (Meckel's diverticulitis) and rupture (simulating acute appendicitis) or continue in a chronic form and cause obstruction. The treatment is surgical.

■ Ulcerative colitis

Ulcerative colitis involves the large intestine, with the rectum and lower colon affected earliest and most severely; in one third or less of cases the lower small intestine may also be involved. First, there is inflammation and swelling of the mucosa, followed by ulceration. Hemorrhage and perforation (with **peritonitis**) account for about 40% of the deaths. The incidence of colorectal cancer among persons with colitis is about 10 times that of the rest of the population. The cause of ulcerative colitis is unknown, and there is no specific treatment. Resting the bowel as much as possible and providing supportive therapy is the best that can be done. If these measures fail, or if the condition grows progressively worse, the removal of the rectum and the colon is recommended.

■ Hemorrhoids

Of the several annoying and painful anorectal disorders, hemorrhoids (piles) are the most common and perhaps the most excruciating.

Hemorrhoids are actually **varicose** (distended) veins situated beneath the mucosa of the anus and lower rectum. Complications include inflammation, local thrombosis, and bleeding. Precipitating causes include pregnancy, straining at the stool, obesity, coughing, sneezing, cirrhosis of the liver, and abdominal tumors. Also, as in all cases of varicose veins, there is apparently a hereditary element of susceptibility. Small hemorrhoids usually do not require treatment beyond efforts to correct the underlying cause. Large, protruding hemorrhoids and those that result in disabling pain call for surgical excision.

■ Cirrhosis

Cirrhosis, the eighth leading cause of death in the United States, is a fibrosis, or scarring, of the liver that is progressive and not simply the stationary, healed, end stage of an injury. It is a chronic disease, and all parts of the liver are involved. There are several varieties of cirrhosis, which differ in cause, nature, form, and effects. Accordingly, classifications and terminologies abound, and there is a fair amount of confusion. Generally agreed on, however, are three forms of the disease based on what is seen under the microscope: postnecrotic, biliary, and portal. Postnecrotic cirrhosis results from liver infection (hepatitis); biliary cirrhosis is associated with gallbladder disease; and portal cirrhosis, the best known form of the disease, is generally associated with **alcoholism** and **malnutrition**. The effects and complications of the disease include faulty liver function, obstruction of the portal circulation, gastrointestinal hemorrhage, and, possibly, cancer. Treatment is essentially symptomatic.

■ Hernia

A very different type of disorder involving the digestive tract is hernia or "rupture." This is a protrusion of part of an organ through an abdominal weak spot. An **inguinal hernia** occurs when a loop of the intestine makes its way through the inguinal canal in the groin. This is the canal that carries the spermatic cord in the male. A **femoral hernia** passes through the femoral canal, which carries the blood vessels to the leg. These canals may be congenitally wider than normal, and strain, such as lifting or hard coughing, may create enough pressure within the abdominal wall to push a part of the intestine into the canal. Occasionally hernia (**umbilical**) occurs through the umbilicus or navel. The danger of hernia is that the protruded part of the intestine may become strangulated or pinched in such a way as to shut off its blood supply—a condition that requires immediate operative attention.

■ Gallstones

Gallstones are concretions, or "stones," formed in the gallbladder or in a bile duct. Ten percent of the population in the United States and 20% of those over 40 years of age have gallstones. Most of the stones are composed of **cholesterol**, and there is strong reason for believing that enhanced body synthesis of this fatty chemical is a predisposing factor in the development of the condition. But most authorities believe that other factors are necessary, including dietary, hormonal, and hereditary predispositions. Signs and symptoms range from none at all to severe attacks. Abdominal discomfort, bloating, intestinal gas, and food intolerance are typical complaints. Complications include inflammation of the gallbladder and cancer of the gallbladder. Troublesome cases call for the surgical removal of the gallbladder or the oral use of bile salts to dissolve the stones. The use of bile salts (which must be given over a period of several months) is especially helpful in the treatment of the elderly or other persons who are poor surgical risks.

■ Jaundice

Jaundice is a condition marked by elevated levels of **bilirubin** (a bile pigment) in the blood and its deposition in the skin, mucous membranes, and whites of the eyes. The latter is especially noticeable, even in mild cases. In severe cases the person literally "turns yellow." The causes of jaundice are many and varied, each being related in some way to bilirubin. Well-known causes include liver disease, bile duct obstruction, and hemolytic anemia. It is important to keep in mind that jaundice is not a disease but a sign—a sign that something is wrong. What that something turns out to be will obviously dictate the treatment. Hopefully it is correctable.

■ Appendicitis

Appendicitis, or inflammation of the vermiform appendix (Fig. 8-1) varies from mild involvements to those with serious and fatal results. The condition is most common in adolescents and young adults, with a peak incidence between ages 15 and 24; it is the most common reason for abdominal surgery in in-

fants and children. The full cause is not known, but there is general agreement that obstruction of the opening between the appendix and the cecum is the underlying cause (Fig. 8-4). In most cases the obstruction is believed to be a **fecalith**, or dried fecal concretion. According to the "obstruction theory," appendiceal mucus is prevented from emptying into the cecum, resulting in the buildup of pressure of sufficient intensity to squeeze the walls of the appendix and the blood vessels within. This cuts off the blood supply and thereby lowers resistance to attack by fecal bacteria. Inflammation, gangrene, perforation (rupture), and peritonitis follow, typically in that order. Peritonitis (inflammation of the peritoneum) is the classic cause of death. An acute attack of appendicitis calls for an immediate appendectomy.

■ Cancer

Cancers of the gastrointestinal tract and associated organs and glands are a common threat to life. **Colorectal** cancers, the "number-one gastrointestinal killer," number about 122,000

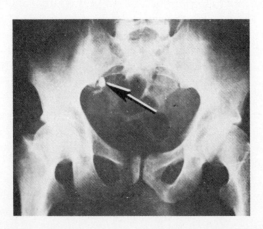

FIG. 8-4 ■ X-ray film showing .22 caliber bullet (*arrow*) lodged in appendix. Patient, who accidentally swallowed bullet, had typical signs and symptoms of appendicitis, a fact supporting the "obstruction theory" of the disease.

Courtesy Drs. M.W.H. Friedman and W.C. MacKenzie.

new cases yearly, and colorectal cancer deaths number some 55,000 per year. About half of these cancers involve the rectum, and about a fourth involve the lower colon. Stomach cancer averages about 24,000 new cases a year. This number is about half of what it was at the turn of the century. Other malignancies of special note involving the digestive system are cancers of the mouth and throat, the pancreas, the liver, and the gallbladder. In the United States liver cancers are predominantly secondary, or **metastatic** (Fig. 8-5). The causes of all these cancers are essentially unknown, but there is evidence that smoking is responsible for oral cancer and the chemical benzpyrene for stomach cancer. Benzpyrene, a proved carcinogen in animals, has been isolated from smoked meat and fish, which are dietary staples in Iceland and Japan, the countries leading the world in stomach cancer. Treatment of all the cancers mentioned centers for the most part on irradiation and surgery. The prognosis in colorectal cancer is unexpectedly good. Cure rates of 80% to 90% are possible with early diagnosis and prompt surgery.

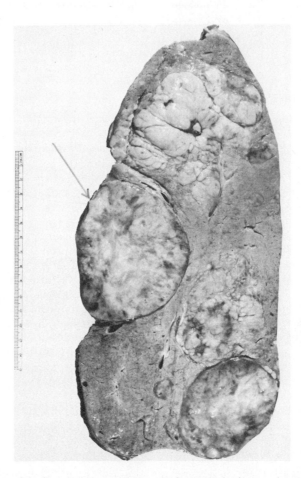

FIG. 8-5 ■ Cancer of the liver, in this case, the result of metastasis. Arrow points to one of the four growths.

Courtesy Dr. W.A.D. Anderson, Miami, Fla.

■■■■ **SELF-TEST**

1. _J&_ food and air   a. peristalsis
2. _O_ deep wrinkles   b. gallbladder
3. _m_ opens into duodenum   c. saliva
4. _A_ wormlike movement   d. lipase
5. _K_ attached to cecum   e. villi
6. _B_ stores bile   f. liver
7. _H_ manufactures insulin   g. glucose
8. _C_ parotid gland   h. pancreas
9. _F_ manufactures bile   i. chyme
10. _L_ "splits maltose"   j. pharynx
11. _N_ "splits proteins"   k. appendix
12. _D_ "splits fats"   l. maltase
13. _G_ simple sugar   m. pylorus
14. _I_ mushy mixture   n. pepsin
15. _E_ absorption   o. rugae

■■■■ **STUDY QUESTIONS**

1. A molecule of cellulose (plant fiber) on its journey from the mouth to the rectum passes through the following structures: esophagus, duodenum, descending colon, ascending colon, ileum, transverse colon, jejunum, and stomach. This is not the proper order. What is the proper order?
2. When the stomach is full, the rugae disappear. Explain.
3. Compare the small and large intestines in regard to both structure and function.
4. What is the relationship of bile to the gallbladder and liver?
5. A number of drugs are contraindicated (cannot be used) in the presence of liver disease. Based on your knowledge of liver function, why is this so?
6. The pancreas is often referred to as a "dual gland." Why?
7. Starch and double sugars (sucrose, maltose, and lactose) are converted (in the digestive process) into glucose, fructose, and galactose. Why is this necessary?
8. What are the end products of fat and protein digestion?
9. Galactosemia is a genetic defect in which the body cannot utilize galactose. Unless milk is excluded from the diet during the first 3 years

of life, the condition leads to mental retardation. Why milk?
10. The gallbladder, liver, and pancreas are not part of the GI tract proper. How do they "know" when to participate in the digestive process?
11. An atonic colon and a spastic colon both result in constipation. How do you account for this?
12. Staphylococcal food poisoning results in severe abdominal pain and profuse diarrhea. How do you explain the pain? The diarrhea?
13. Botulism antitoxin is much more effective prophylactically than it is therapeutically. How can this be explained?
14. Why is pinworm so common among children?
15. Cimetidine (Tagamet) is a drug that inhibits the production of hydrochloric acid. How does this fit in with its use in peptic ulcer?
16. Based on your reading of the text, do you think you can have diverticulitis without diverticulosis?
17. According to statistics, what type of tumor is relatively common in persons with ulcerative colitis?
18. Pregnancy and straining at the stool are common causes of hemorrhoids. Based on your reading of the text, how do you account for this?

19. What are some possible explanations for blood in the stool?
20. Alcoholism is not listed as a major cause of death, but in a sense it is. How so?
21. Lifting heavy furniture can precipitate a hernia. What is the explanation?
22. The sudden onset of abdominal pain could signal appendicitis. Taking a laxative at this time could result in your death. Precisely, why?
23. Over the years there has been a substantial drop in stomach cancer. Do you have a theory as to why?
24. Most liver cancers are "secondary or metastatic." What does this mean?
25. There is evidence that a low bulk diet is a factor in the development of colorectal cancer. Do you have a theory as to why?

PANCRES - PRODUCES digestive juices - hormones

ASE - ENZYME

CHAPTER 9

The nervous system

The human body contains a dozen billion nerve cells (neurons) interwoven into what we call the brain and spinal cord. These organs together with their extensions (the nerves) make up the nervous system. This is the system that controls the other body systems. Furthermore, it enables us to respond to events occurring in the environment and, perhaps above all, forms the basis for the various mental processes of thought, learning, and memory. It is little wonder, then, that physicians consider the absence of brain waves as the paramount sign of death. For purposes of study, the nervous system is thought of in terms of two subsystems, the central and the peripheral systems. The central nervous system—the brain and spinal cord—functions to correlate and integrate. The peripheral nervous system consists of nerve fibers that connect the central nervous system to sensory cells (receptors) and to muscles and glands (effectors), which perform the actual adjustive actions of the body.

Neurons and nerves

Stimulus, response, and the nerve impulse

Spinal cord and spinal nerves

Brain and cranial nerves

Autonomic nervous system

Neurotransmitters

Sleep

Pain

Disorders and noninfectious diseases

Infections

The nervous system is an extensive and complicated organization of structures by which internal reactions of the individual are correlated and integrated and by which the individual's adjustments to the environment are controlled. Although the system is well integrated structurally and functionally, it is, for convenience of study, considered to fall into two major divisions, the **central nervous system** and **peripheral nervous system**. The central nervous system (Fig. 9-1) includes the brain and spinal cord, and the peripheral nervous system includes the nerves, ganglia, and receptors, which are distributed throughout the body.

■■■■ NEURONS AND NERVES

The basic unit of the nervous system is the **neuron** (Fig. 9-2), which consists of a cell body and branched extensions, or processes. **Dendrites** are those processes conducting nerve (electrical) impulses to the cell body, and **axons** are those processes conducting nerve impulses away from it. **Sensory neurons** conduct nerve impulses to or toward the central nervous system; **motor neurons** conduct nerve impulses to the muscles, glands, and organs; and **connector neurons** conduct impulses from sensory to motor neurons. Whereas the sensory neuron typically has long dendrites and a short axon, the motor neuron has short dendrites and a long axon; connective neurons generally have short processes. The junction between the terminal endings of the axon of one neuron and the dendrites of another is referred to as a **synapse**.

Nerves are made up of **nerve fibers**, a nerve fiber referring to a dendrite or axon extending from the brain or spinal cord out into the body proper, sometimes for many inches. **Myelin**, a white fatty substance, envelops most of these fibers. Some nerves are "pure motor" (composed solely of the axons of motor neurons); some are "pure sensory" (composed

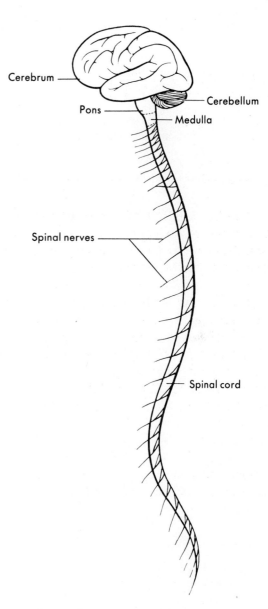

FIG. 9-1 ■ Central nervous system in overview.

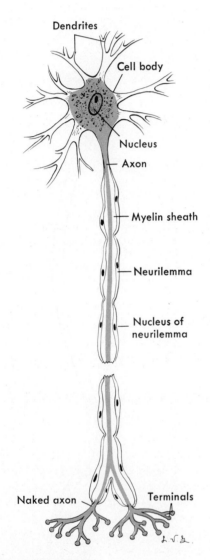

Dendrites

Cell body

Nucleus

Axon

Myelin sheath

Neurilemma

Nucleus of
neurilemma

Naked axon   Terminals

FIG. 9-2 ■ Motor neuron.

From Schottelius, B.A., and Schottelius, D.D.: Textbook of physiology, ed.
18, St. Louis, 1978, The C.V. Mosby Co.

solely of sensory dendrites); and some nerves are "mixed" (composed of both types of fibers).

STIMULUS, RESPONSE, AND THE NERVE IMPULSE

The response to a stimulus may be voluntary or involuntary. The former response is under conscious control and generally involves the more highly developed areas of the brain, and the latter—the so-called **reflex**—is automatic and executed unconsciously. A reflex in its simplest form calls into play a sensory neuron, a motor neuron, a receptor, and an effector. On stimulation the **receptor** initiates a nerve impulse that travels via the sensory neuron and motor neuron (in this order) to the **effector** (muscle or gland), causing the effector to respond. Reflexes associated with experience and training are said to be **conditioned**; that is, they do not occur naturally but are developed by regular association of some physiologic function with an unrelated outside event, such as the ringing of a bell or flashing of a light.

SPINAL CORD AND SPINAL NERVES

The spinal cord (Fig. 9-3) is a two-way avenue between the brain and peripheral nerves. It is an ovoid structure, about 45 cm long, occupying the spinal canal from the opening in the floor of the cranium to the first lumbar vertebra. Enveloping the cord are three membranes (the **meninges**), which are continuous with those covering the brain. Between the innermost of the three (the pia mater) and the middle membrane (the arachnoid) is a space (the subarachnoid space) filled with watery **cerebrospinal fluid**. In cross section the cord has an H-shaped area of gray matter surrounded by white matter, the latter being organized into nerve **tracts** named according to

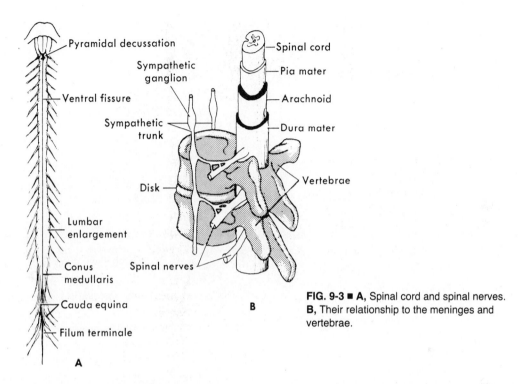

Pyramidal decussation

Sympathetic ganglion

Ventral fissure

Sympathetic trunk

Disk

Lumbar enlargement

Conus medullaris

Spinal nerves

Cauda equina

Filum terminale

A

Spinal cord

Pia mater

Arachnoid

Dura mater

Vertebrae

B

FIG. 9-3 ■ A, Spinal cord and spinal nerves. **B,** Their relationship to the meninges and vertebrae.

their origin and destination. **Ascending,** or sensory, tracts convey nerve impulses to the brain; **descending,** or motor, tracts convey nerve impulses from the brain.

Along its length the spinal cord gives birth to 31 pairs of nerves, which emerge through the openings between the vertebrae and are named according to the vertebrae from which they emerge. There are 8 pairs of cervical nerves, 12 pairs of thoracic nerves, 5 pairs of lumbar nerves, 5 pairs of sacral nerves, and 1 pair of coccygeal nerves. Each spinal nerve has an anterior branch and a posterior branch. The posterior branches run uninterrupted to the skin of the back and shoulders and to muscles of the neck and back that have an up-and-down movement; most of the anterior branches fuse into complex networks called **plexuses.** The cervical plexus, for example, is formed by the anterior branches of the cervical nerves; secondary branches (emerging from the plexus) supply the diaphragm (via the

phrenic nerve), the neck muscles, and the skin on the back part of the skull. Other major plexuses are the brachial, lumbar, and sacral.

■ BRAIN AND CRANIAL NERVES

The brain (Fig. 9-4) is a 3-pound mass of nervous tissue representing some 12 billion neurons organized and interconnected in a manner defying description. A computer with just a fraction of the brain's ability might possibly be the size of the Empire State Building. According to the most severe classification, the brain, or **encephalon,** is divided into the telencephalon, diencephalon, mesencephalon, metencephalon, and myelencephalon. The **telencephalon,** or **cerebrum,** the largest part, has a gray outer surface (cortex) formed into "hills" (gyri) and "valleys" (sulci) and is divided lengthwise into hemispheres by the **longitudinal fissure.** The interior contains both white and gray matter, the

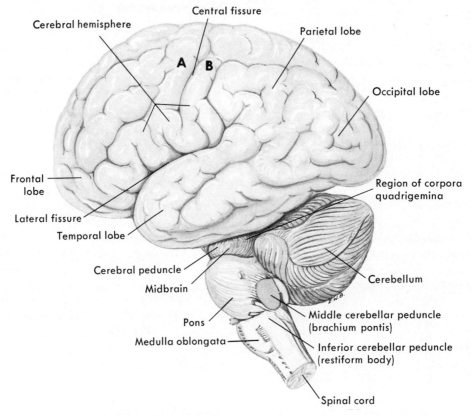

FIG. 9-4 ■ Human brain. **A,** General motor area. **B,** General sensory area.

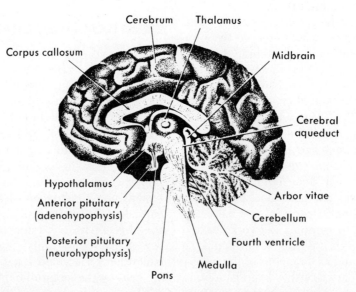

FIG. 9-5 ■ Brain as seen in cut through longitudinal fissure (corpus callosum connects the cerebral hemispheres).

former constituted by myelinated fibers and the latter by neuron cell bodies. Recognized functional areas of the cerebrum include the motor area (sends nerve impulses to skeletal muscles and makes voluntary movement possible), somesthetic area (receives the sensations of touch, pain, heat, cold, and body movement), and the areas (or centers) of taste, hearing, smell, speech, and vision. **Cognition**—learning, memory, reasoning, language, and the like—is generally regarded as a function of the cerebral cortex.

The **diencephalon** (tween-brain) is divided into the **thalamus** and **hypothalamus** (Fig. 9-5), the former structure acting as a relay center for sensory impulses on their way to the cerebral cortex and the latter structure acting as a control center for autonomic activity, temperature regulation, hormone production, appetite, and possibly sleep. The **mesencephalon** (midbrain) is a link between the lower and higher areas of the brain and coordinates muscular movements related to visual and auditory stimuli. The **metencephalon** is divided into the **pons variolii** and **cerebellum**. An egg-shaped mass situated just above the medulla, the pons variolii, or simply "pons," connects the cerebrum and cerebellum and gives rise to certain cranial nerves. The cerebellum, or "little brain," is a large mass of nervous tissue lying beneath the back part of the cerebrum. Among other things the cerebellum maintains balance, or equilibrium, and reinforces and refines impulses transmitted by the cerebral motor areas. The **myelencephalon**, or **medulla oblongata**, is just below the pons and appears as an enlargement of the spinal cord. It gives rise to four pairs of cranial nerves and acts as the control center for the circulatory and respiratory systems.

Within the brain there are four interconnected spaces, or **ventricles** (Fig. 9-6), that

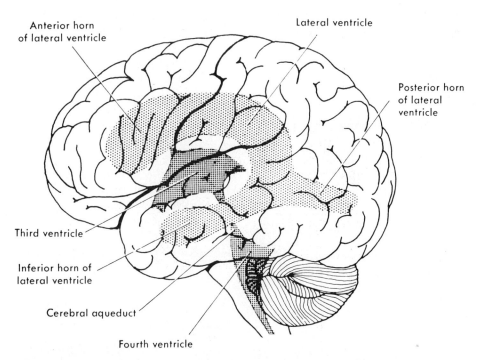

Anterior horn
of lateral ventricle

Lateral ventricle

Posterior horn
of lateral
ventricle

Third ventricle

Inferior horn of
lateral ventricle

Cerebral aqueduct

Fourth ventricle

FIG. 9-6 ■ Brain ventricles. Note that all four ventricles (right lateral not shown) are interconnected. Cerebral aqueduct connects third and fourth ventricles.

communicate with the subarachnoid space surrounding the brain and spinal cord. The largest are the two **lateral ventricles** of the cerebral hemispheres. The **third ventricle** is a single irregular space lying below the lateral ventricles and between the thalami; the **fourth ventricle** is a diamond-shaped space immediately before the cerebellum. Filling the ventricles and subarachnoid space is the **cerebrospinal fluid** produced by capillary networks situated in the roof of each ventricle. The cerebrospinal fluid protects the brain and spinal cord from mechanical injury by acting as a watery shock absorber. It also serves as a "middleman" in the exchange of nutrients and wastes between the bloodstream and nerve cells.

Emerging from the undersurface of the brain are 12 cranial nerves. In order and function these are the **olfactory** (smell), **optic** (vision), **oculomotor** and **trochlear** (eye movements and size of pupil), **trigeminal** (mastication and sensations of head and face), **abducens** (abduction of eye), **facial** (facial expression, salivary secretion, and taste), **acoustic** (hearing and equilibrium), **glossopharyngeal** (swallowing, secretion of salvia, and taste), **vagus** (parasympathetic regulation of abdominal and thoracic viscera), **spinal accessory** (motor fibers to shoulder and head), and **hypoglossal** (tongue movements). In the event the student for one reason or other wishes to commit the cranial nerves to memory, the following mnemonic device is recommended:

On **O**ld **O**lympic **T**owering **T**ops, **A** **F**inn **A**nd **G**erman **V**iewed **S**ome **H**ops.

◼◼◼ AUTONOMIC NERVOUS SYSTEM

The autonomic nervous system (Fig. 9-7) is a division of the peripheral nervous system and includes those nerves associated with the control of the heart, lungs, abdominal viscera, and glands of secretion; characteristically it operates automatically and, by and large, involuntarily. There are two divisions of the system involved, the **parasympathetic** and **sympathetic**, and in the usual instance a given structure or organ is supplied by both in an antagonistic fashion. That is to say, if parasympathetic stimulation produces one response, sympathetic stimulation produces the opposite. As a rule of thumb, the parasympathetic division prevails in times of quietude, and the sympathetic system prevails in times of stress, preparing the body for "fight or flight." By way of example, parasympathetic stimulation slows the heart and sympathetic stimulation speeds the heart.

◼◼◼ NEUROTRANSMITTERS

Neurotransmitters are chemical agents released at nerve fiber (axon) terminal endings. In the central nervous system they serve to relay nerve impulses across synaptic gaps; in the peripheral nervous system they serve to relay nerve impulses across the microscopic gaps between nerve fiber endings and effectors (muscles and glands). Major neurotransmitters include acetylcholine, epinephrine, dopamine, and serotonin. Interestingly, some neural chemicals act as negative neurotransmitters. For example, a class of agents called **endorphins** inhibits the transmission of dull, chronic pain—the same type of pain relieved by morphine. A number of disorders of the nervous system are in some fashion related to neurotransmitters. For example, a lack of **dopamine** is responsible for Parkinson's disease, and a lack of **norepinephrine** may possibly be the cause of psychotic depression.

◼◼◼ SLEEP

Sleep is a period of rest for the body and mind, during which volition and conscious-

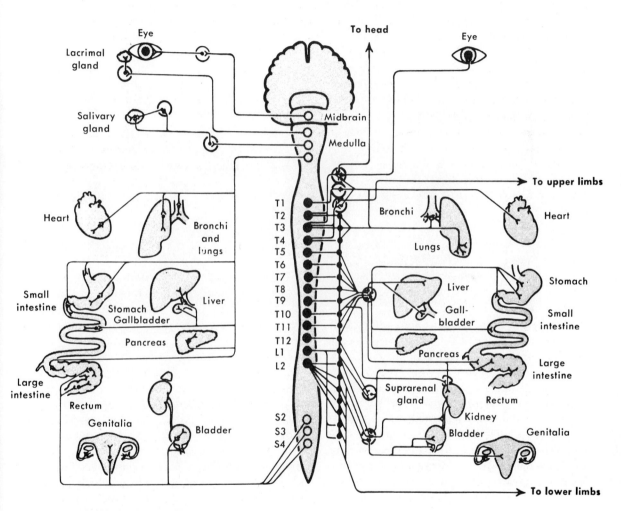

PARASYMPATHETIC NERVES   SYMPATHETIC NERVES

FIG. 9-7 ■ Autonomic nervous system in overview. Note that organs are supplied by both sympathetic and parasympathetic nerves.

From Goth, A.: Medical pharmacology: principles and concepts, ed. 10, St. Louis, 1981, The C.V. Mosby Co.; redrawn from a Sandoz Pharmaceuticals publication.

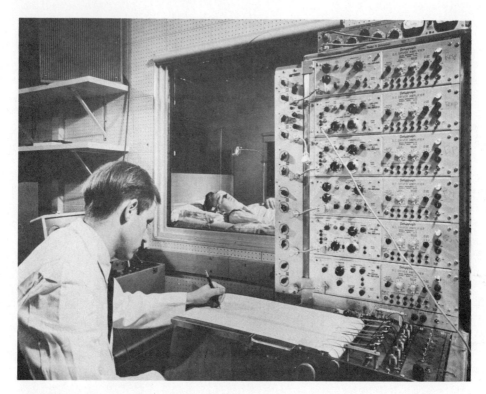

FIG. 9-8 ■ Sleep studies. Using the electroencephalograph it is possible to get recordings of brain wave changes during different stages of sleep.

Courtesy National Institutes of Health.

ness are in partial or complete abeyance and body function partially suspended. As to its true nature or to what is really going on within the brain during sleep, there are clearly more questions than answers. Most authorities seem to agree, however, that sleep relates to a so-called **wake center** in the hypothalamus. Presumably the center functions as part of an arousal or alerting mechanism when it is "turned on." Accordingly, drowsiness and sleep ensue when the wake center is "turned off." Clinical evidence that somnolence characterizes certain hypothalamic disorders supports this theory.

Sleep has several stages related both to brain waves (as recorded by the electroencephalograph, or EEG) and to eye movement (Fig. 9-

8). Two of the best known stages are those called **slow-wave sleep** (SWS) and **rapid eye movement** (REM) sleep. SWS takes its name from the slow-frequency, high-voltage **delta waves** that identify it. Sometimes called "delta sleep," SWS is a deep sleep from which a person is not easily aroused; it is almost entirely dreamless. REM sleep, on the other hand, is associated with dreaming. It occurs five to six times during a normal night's sleep and accounts for 20% to 25% of the total sleep. Many **hypnotic drugs** ("sleeping pills") tend to depress REM sleep, and a number of studies show that abrupt withdrawal of such drugs results in a pronounced temporary increase in both REM sleep and nightmares.

Most of us tend to feel and work better if our sleep schedule can be kept fairly constant; sleep is indeed an important physiologic and psychologic need. As far as the amount of sleep needed each night, 8 hours has been widely recommended (especially for the young), but average amounts of habitual sleep can vary from 5 to 10 hours. Some persons are quite rested with 2 to 3 hours. Age is a factor that can affect sleep. As we grow older, we require less sleep, especially past age 55 (and women appear to require less than men). Many authorities recommend some of the following in order to get a good night's sleep on a regular basis: (1) exercising routinely during the day (not at night), (2) establishing a regular bedtime if possible and going to bed only when tired, (3) using the bedroom only for sleep and sexual relations (not for watching television, reading, eating snacks, or working), (4) avoiding alcoholic beverages and beverages containing caffeine (tea, coffee, cola) just before bedtime, and (5) avoiding mental stimulation just before bedtime.

Some problems associated with sleep include **insomnia** (inability to sleep), **narcolepsy** (sudden attacks of sleep), bed wetting, and sleepwalking. There are an estimated 75 million Americans afflicted with insomnia who spend millions of dollars each year on over-the-counter sleeping aids and prescription sleeping pills. The majority of these persons are adults. Insomnia may be acute or chronic, and its cause is poorly understood, but researchers have been scrutinizing the problem with great intensity in recent years. As far as a cure is concerned, the only thing agreed on is that there is no one solution that works for everybody and that sleeping pills, at best, provide only a temporary solution.

◼◼◼ PAIN

Pain is a more or less localized sensation of discomfort, distress, or agony, resulting from the stimulation of specialized sensory nerve endings. These endings are probably stimulated by pain-triggering substances—**bradykinin** is one—released when cells are injured. Once stimulated, these nerves transmit the pain message through the spinal cord to the brain, which processes the information and tells us that we are hurt. Most often pain is a protective signal, calling attention to some underlying disease or else inducing the sufferer to remove or withdraw from the source. Pain is either acute or chronic. **Acute pain** is usually the result of injury, infection, internal disorder, or surgery that will heal within a reasonable time. **Chronic pain** is persistent, lasting months or even years. It has outlived its usefulness as a warning and has become all-consuming and life disrupting. Sometimes chronic pain results from an incurable disease. Or it may be emotional in origin. But whatever the cause, the longer the pain lasts, the more important the psychologic factors become.

The perception of pain is influenced by a number of factors, which is not surprising when we consider that the "pain message" is interpreted by the brain. Indeed, the **pain threshold**—the point at which a person reports pain—can be raised almost 50% by hypnosis or by loud noise or other distractions. Further, a sugar pill, if the sufferer believes it to be a "pain killer," is often dramatically effective. Religious attitudes are also of interest. Those who accept pain as a just punishment for sin or even view it as an opportunity to share the suffering of Jesus may hurt less than those who regard pain as undeserved. Finally, there is the matter of age and sex. The pain threshold tends to rise with advancing years, and women tend to have a lower pain threshold than men.

Pain, although not necessarily curable, as in severe chronic cases, may be relieved by any number of avenues, depending on the situation involved. Obviously, the first approach is to remove the underlying cause, if possible. Since the beginning of history humans have sought relief from pain by using resources provided by nature. The first recorded treatment of pain dates back to 2250 BC, when a mixture of henbane seeds and gum mastic was used to relieve toothache. The ancient Egyptians, Greeks, and others had their drug compendium. The use of plants and herbs has evolved through the centuries into modern chemotherapy, the treatment of pain and disease by chemical means. Today, drugs running the gamut from aspirin to narcotics are prescribed for pain, although physicians keep possible side effects in mind. **Anesthesia** is well established. It may be local or general; local anesthetics are used in the dentist's chair, general anesthetics in the operating room.

Other options in pain control include severance of nerve pathways, acupuncture, transcutaneous nerve stimulation, hypnosis, biofeedback, yoga, meditation, and behavior modification, to name a few. Before treating severe pain or pain of long duration with self-prescribed methods, a person should seek professional help. There are many reputable pain clinics throughout the United States that provide treatment and relief. The consumer should avoid the assistance of any unqualified person or the clinic that has not been recommended by a physician. Quackery abounds!

■■■■ DISORDERS AND NONINFECTIOUS DISEASES

A functional or organic disorder of nervous tissue, especially one involving the brain and spinal cord, is often serious. Many times little can be done other than treating the symptoms and hoping for the best. Such is usually the case in pathologic situations in which nerve cells are destroyed. Since these cells are not replaced, the damage is irreversible. Manifestations of neurologic disorders include pain, headache, dizziness, tics, hiccups, recurrent attacks of sleep (narcolepsy), tremors, convulsions, unconsciousness, and disorders of memory and language function. Major highlights of some specific disorders and diseases follow.

■ Unconsciousness

Unconsciousness is a state of insensibility that is normal only during sleep. It may range in depth from stupor or semiconsciousness to **coma,** a profound unconsciousness from which the victim cannot be aroused even by powerful stimulants. Because unconsciousness is a manifestation of an underlying injury or disease, its duration and intensity naturally depend on the basic cause. Among the variety of causes are simple fainting, acute alcoholism, head injury, cerebrovascular accidents, depressant poisoning, epilepsy, diabetic acidosis, infections, heart failure, severe anemia, shock, uremia, hepatic failure, hysteria, heat stroke, exposure to extreme cold, eclampsia, and Addison's disease.

Unconsciousness is an emergency situation. Pending diagnosis of the underlying disorder, the physician directs his or her skills toward maintenance of respiration and circulation. This includes such measures as controlling hemorrhage, giving oxygen, and applying artificial respiration. In the event of depressant poisoning (barbiturates, opiates, and the like), specific measures are available.

■ Epilepsy

Epilepsy, or "seizure," is a recurrent paroxysmal disorder of cerebral function marked by sudden, brief attacks of altered consciousness, motor activity, sensory phenomena, or

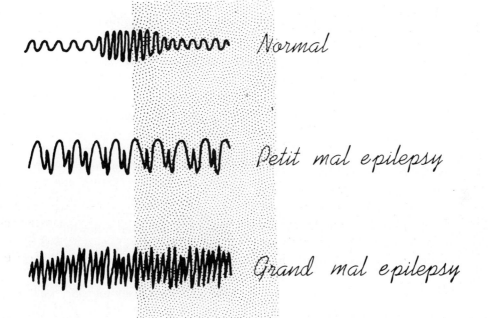

Normal

Petit mal epilepsy

Grand mal epilepsy

FIG. 9-9 ■ Brain wave tracings (electroencephalogram) in two forms of epilepsy. Normal tracing also shown for comparison.

inappropriate behavior. One of every 100 Americans has it. Although in most cases no significant underlying cause is revealed, in other instances a tumor or a cerebral lesion of some magnitude may be present. This may have resulted from injury or from another morbid process.

There are several types of epilepsy. Most familiar are **grand mal** epilepsy and **petit mal** epilepsy (Fig. 9-9). In approximately 70% of the patients only one type of seizure occurs; the remaining 30% have two or more types. It is most important to understand that most epileptic individuals are normal between attacks. Indeed, three fourths of the noninstitutionalized epileptic persons are mentally competent, and when there is mental deterioration, it generally is related to accompanying brain damage. Many famous people have had epilepsy, including Socrates, Julius Caesar, Dostoevski, Lord Byron, Berlioz, Handel, Van Gogh, Alfred Nobel, and Alexander the Great.

The treatment of epilepsy is multidimensional. It includes correction of the causative or precipitating factor (for example, surgery to remove a tumor or relieve pressure on the brain), physical and mental hygiene, and drug therapy. Drugs that are effective in controlling and preventing one type of seizure often fail to control or prevent the others. Phenytoin (Dilantin), for instance, yields good results in grand mal epilepsy but fails to control the petit mal form. This indicates, of course, that these forms of epilepsy have different causes.

■ Cerebral palsy

Cerebral palsy is a nonprogressive motor disorder resulting from injury at birth or from intrauterine brain damage. The most common manifestation is spastic weakness of the extremities, characterized by scissor gait and exaggerated tendon reflexes. In the most severe cases the extremities are stiff, and there is great difficulty in swallowing. Though most patients afflicted with cerebral palsy exhibit some degree of mental retardation, this poor showing may well result from difficulty in self-expression. Drugs to relieve spasticity and control convulsions, if and when they occur, special courses, and vocational guidance are essential if the patient is to live out his or her years in a meaningful way, especially those persons with milder forms of the disorder for whom the potential for a normal way of life exists. As indicated, many cerebral palsy victims are much brighter than they appear.

■ Multiple sclerosis

Multiple sclerosis is marked by myelin-free patches throughout the brain and spinal cord; clinically, it is characterized by progressive weakness, incoordination, jerking movements, abnormal mental exhilaration, and disturbances of speech and vision. The cause remains unknown. Possible causes include autoimmune mechanisms, "slow viruses" (agents producing symptoms after a prolonged incubation period), certain poisons, and trauma. The duration of the disease averages about 12 years following onset, but the course is highly variable. In some cases attacks are frequent; in others, there may be remissions of as long as 20 years or more. At present, there is no specific therapy. The patient is made as comfortable as possible, and the physician may recommend such measures as physiotherapy and psychotherapy. Moving to a warmer climate may help. Multiple sclerosis is relatively uncommon in the tropics.

■ Parkinsonism

Parkinsonism (also referred to as "Parkinson's disease," "paralysis agitans," and "shaking palsy") is a chronic disorder marked by tremor, muscular rigidity, and slowness of movement. Most cases are of unknown cause ("idiopathic"), but the disorder may be produced by various agents, including carbon monoxide, manganese poisoning, and certain tranquilizers. Postencephalitic parkinsonism commonly occurred following attacks of epidemic encephalitis between 1919 and 1924.

The discovery that parkinsonism is accompanied by a decrease in the level of **dopamine**, a neurotransmitter concentrated in some areas of the brain, led to the therapeutic use of levodopa (Larodopa), the metabolic precursor of dopamine. Although this drug is not always effective and may provoke serious side effects, it does represent a definite breakthrough in treatment. Surgical destruction of certain areas of the thalamus by cryotherapy has effected cures in selected cases.

■ Stroke

A stroke, or cerebrovascular accident (CVA), results from hemorrhage, thrombosis, embolism, or other vascular problems within the brain. It is the most common neurologic disability in Western countries. Common CVA symptoms include headache, vomiting, convulsions, and coma. The specific symptoms will naturally depend on the site of the lesion. In cerebral hemorrhage, for example, the lesion is usually well within the brain substance, and the characteristic features are **hemiplegia** and **hemianesthesia** (paralysis and loss of sensation, respectively, of one side of the body).

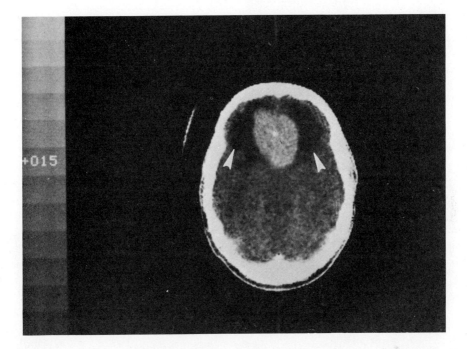

FIG. 9-10 ■ CAT scan of patient with brain tumor. Brain is outlined in white (skull bones); forehead is at top. Tumor appears as grayish white mass (behind forehead) surrounded by zone of edema (*arrowheads*).

From Daffner, R.H.: Introduction to diagnostic radiology, St. Louis, 1979, The C.V. Mosby Co.

The specific treatment depends on the cause. If the diagnosis is thrombosis or embolism, anticoagulants are given in the hope of preventing further enlargement of the clot. General measures include skillful nursing care, physiotherapy, and operative removal of the blood clot if there is increased intracranial pressure. If only a small vessel is involved, almost complete recovery can be expected sometime within a year. Massive brain damage, however, generally results in death a week or so following the attack.

■ Tumors

Cancers of the brain and central nervous system kill about 12,000 Americans annually.

Of chief concern are the intracranial growths, perhaps a third of which are metastatic. Primary intracranial tumors arise from brain tissue itself or from lesser structures (namely, blood vessels, cranial nerves, meninges, and the pituitary gland). Nearly half of all primary tumors are **gliomas**, or growths involving the neuroglia (brain connective tissue). In the adult the most common glioma—and the most common brain cancer—is the rapidly expansive, invasive, and deadly **glioblastoma multiforme** of the cerebral hemispheres. Intracranial tumors in children occur almost exclusively in the cerebellum. The most common are the benign **astrocytoma** and the highly malignant **medulloblastoma**.

Actual manifestations of brain tumors are

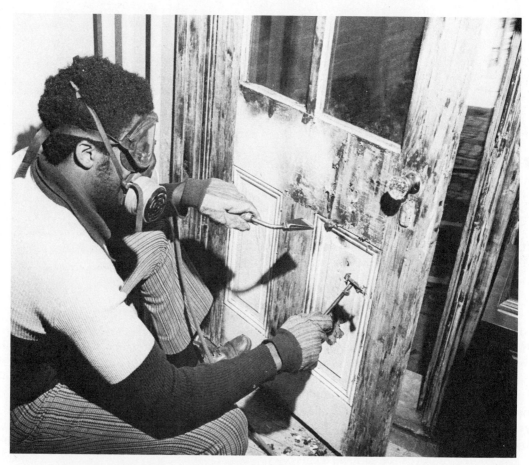

FIG. 9-11 ■ Lead poisoning control worker removes hazardous paint from a home interior.

Courtesy Philadelphia Department of Health, Philadelphia, Pa.

best thought of in terms of pressure and location. The pressure arises because the cranium does not give and because the tumor generally interferes with the drainage of cerebrospinal fluid. Symptoms caused by pressure include, among others, headache, vomiting, and failing vision. Other signs and symptoms relate to the function of the brain region involved. Frontal lobe tumors cause a change in personality, occipital lobe tumors cause visual hallucinations; and so on. Diagnosis involves a number of procedures, especially CAT scans (Fig. 9-10). Treatment centers on surgery; in the curable case, surgical removal remains the one and only avenue.

■ Mental retardation

Mental retardation is subaverage intellectual ability. About 3% of the total population are said to be mentally retarded, but only about half of these individuals are actually identified. The birth rate of children with IQs under 50 is in the vicinity of 4 in 1000 live births. Although the cause of mental retardation is not known in three fourths of the cases, there are indeed a great many established causes. These causes may occur in the prenatal, perinatal, and postnatal periods.

Prenatal causes of mental retardation may be chromosomal abnormalities, genetic defects, or infectious diseases. The best known chromosomal disorder is **Down's syndrome**, in which the person has 47 chromosomes instead of the normal 46; others include Edward's syndrome, Patau's syndrome, Klinefelter's syndrome, Turner's syndrome, and the so-called fragile X chromosome. Genetic defects (where typically only a single gene is involved) number in the dozens, the better known including phenylketonuria (PKU), galactosemia, maple syrup urine disease, Tay-Sachs disease, Niemann-Pick disease, Gaucher's disease, and Hurler's syndrome. Infec-

tions identified as prenatal causes of mental retardation include rubella (German measles), toxoplasmosis, and syphilis.

Perinatal causes of mental retardation occur between the fifth month of pregnancy and 1 month after birth. These include bleeding, breech or instrument delivery, asphyxia, malnutrition, and prematurity. Premature infants who weigh less than 1.5 kg have a 10% to 50% chance of being retarded, depending on the quality of care provided. **Postnatal causes** of mental retardation include infection, lead poisoning (Fig. 9-11), and severe head injuries.

The management of mental retardation entails family support and counseling and requires the services of a wide range of medical and paramedical specialists. Speech pathologists and audiologists, for example, are helpful with major language delays or with suspected hearing loss. The prevention of mental retardation centers on genetic counseling, in utero diagnosis (amniocentesis), infection control, and continuing improvements in obstetric and neonatal care.

■ Dyslexia

Dyslexia is a common neurologic disorder that, for reasons not yet clearly understood, makes it difficult for children, no matter how high their IQs, to learn in the standard educational environment. They have problems reading, for example, not because they do not understand words but because they cannot focus on a single word or sentence. They reverse letters and fail to grasp critical concepts of time, space, and sequence. Presumably there is a brain defect having to do with the organization of graphic symbols. A family history of language problems is common, and boys are affected more often than girls.

Early diagnosis (using psychologic tests) is

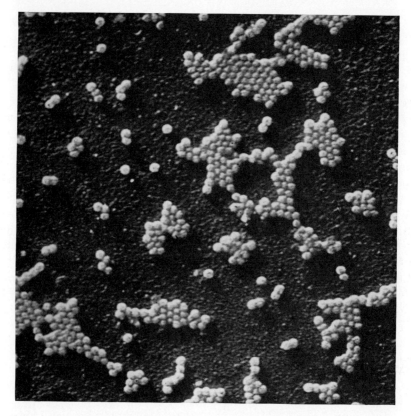

FIG. 9-12 ■ Poliovirus as it appears under electron microscope (magnified 80,000 times).

Courtesy Parke, Davis & Co., Detroit, Mich.

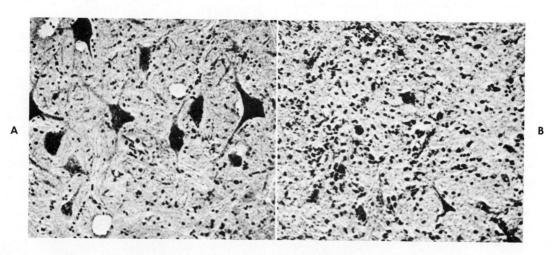

Fig. 9-13 ■ Poliovirus attacking nerve tissue. **A,** Normal spidery nerve cells of monkey spinal cord before attack. **B,** After attack.

From Burrows, W.: Textbook of microbiology, ed. 17, Philadelphia, 1959, W.B. Saunders Co.

highly important, since the prognosis is much better if the defect can be identified and treated before a pattern of frustration and failure is established. Because there is no way to correct perceptual deficits, the treatment of dyslexia is a matter of remedial education. Remedial steps are aimed at teaching around the problem, using the child's abilities and intact capabilities to compensate for the areas of weakness.

■ Mental illness

Mental illness is clearly a disorder of brain function, but by convention it is considered a special area of study, an area known as **psychiatry**. Accordingly, we shall reserve this topic for Chapter 17.

■ INFECTIONS

Any infection of the nervous system is potentially serious and, not uncommonly, may prove fatal. Major infections include tetanus, encephalitis, meningitis, poliomyelitis, and rabies. **Tetanus**, or lockjaw, is caused by the bacterium *Clostridium tetani*, an inhabitant of soil and feces—hence the danger of dirty wounds. Muscle spasms and convulsions highlight the infection. Unless tetanus antitoxin is given immediately, the outlook is grim; even with only a 24-hour delay a person's chances are no better than 50-50. Actually, no one need die of tetanus: vaccination (with tetanus toxoid) is 100% effective.

Poliomyelitis (infantile paralysis or polio) is an acute viral infection of the central nervous system (Figs. 9-12 and 9-13). Somewhat contrary to popular belief, relatively few of those affected develop significant signs and symptoms. These include, in a full-blown infection, fever, headache, stiffness, and paralysis. Less than one quarter of those who develop paralysis sustain permanent disability. Death can occur as a result of respiratory failure.

Vaccination has proved extremely effective in the prevention of polio, and the oral (Sabin) vaccine is recommended for all infants and children.

Rabies, or hydrophobia, a viral involvement of the brain, is the most deadly infection known to mankind. The virus—present in the saliva of rabid animals—enters the body via bites, scratches, and sometimes licks. Highlights of infection include fanatic excitement, painful muscle spasms, and paralysis. Death has been considered inevitable—once the signs of infection appear—but around-the-clock treatment has reportedly saved the lives of three or four victims. Prevention and control of rabies demands a wide approach: (1) dog restraint, (2) immunization of dogs and cats, (3) systematic reduction of skunks, foxes, raccoons, and bats in high-risk areas (farms, campgrounds, and so on), (4) immediate soap and water cleansing of all lacerations or wounds inflicted by dogs, cats, and wild animals, and (5) immediate vaccination in high-risk situations, such as in cases of wild animal bite.

Encephalitis, or inflammation of the brain, encompasses hundreds of viral infections throughout the world. **Encephalomyelitis** is the same disorder affecting spinal cord structures as well as the brain. For the most part these infections are mosquito borne and appear only during warm weather. There is no specific treatment, but there is clearly a specific preventive remedy—mosquito control.

Meningitis, or inflammation of the meninges, is caused by many species of bacteria and a variety of viruses. Antibiotics have greatly reduced the fatality rate of acute bacterial meningitis, but they must be given without delay. Even with prompt diagnosis and treatment meningitis in infants or in the elderly is still frequently fatal. The best that can be done in the way of prevention is to be on guard, namely, to identify, isolate, and treat new cases with dispatch.

■■■■ SELF-TEST

1. __L__ encephalon
2. __O__ autonomic system
3. __B__ nerve fiber junction
4. __H__ unconscious response
5. __A__ muscles and glands
6. __N__ sensory neuron
7. __G__ enveloping membranes
8. __K__ cerebrospinal fluid
9. __m__ spinal cord
10. __C__ longitudinal fissure
11. __J__ temperature regulation
12. __E__ medulla oblongata
13. __I__ maintains equilibrium
14. __F__ olfactory nerve
15. __D__ acoustic nerve

a. effectors
b. synapse
c. hemispheres
d. hearing
e. respiration
f. smell
g. meninges
h. reflex
i. cerebellum
j. hypothalamus
k. ventricles
l. brain
m. tracts
n. receptors
o. viscera - guts -(deep)

■■■■ STUDY QUESTIONS

1. What is the structural difference between a sensory neuron and a motor neuron? What is the functional difference?
2. What is the difference between a nerve and a nerve fiber?
3. What is the difference between a receptor and an effector?
4. If a particular reflex involved three neurons—a sensory neuron, a connective neuron, and a motor neuron—how many synapses would be involved?
5. Sometimes, a spinal injury involves only ascending tracts and sometimes only descending tracts. What difference does it make?
6. How do nerve impulses reach the body's muscles and glands?
7. The nerve impulses responsible for the voluntary movement of the toes involve the peroneal nerve, cerebral cortex, toe muscles, and spinal cord. What is the proper sequence or the path the nerve impulses take from "start to finish"?
8. Certain brain injuries can result in the loss of temperature control; that is, the body temperature does not stay at 98.6° F. What part of the brain is most likely involved here?

9. If a brain injury results in a pronounced loss of balance or equilibrium, what part of the brain is involved?
10. A sharp blow to the medulla oblongata can result in sudden death. Why, specifically?
11. Of the 12 cranial nerves, which ones are purely sensory?
12. Remembering that the sympathetic nervous system prepares the body for "fight or flight," what is the effect of sympathetic stimulation on the pupil?
13. The autonomic nervous system is a division of the peripheral nervous system. Elaborate on this statement.
14. What is the relationship between neurotransmitters and synapses?
15. Aspirin has been shown (in the laboratory) to inhibit the action of a tissue chemical called bradykinin. Based on your reading of the text, what is the significance of this fact?
16. A so-called phantom limb pain is pain felt as though arising in an absent (amputated) limb. What does this tell us about the perception of pain?
17. A given drug may be effective in one type of epilepsy but worthless in another type. What

does this tell us about the cause of this brain disorder?

18. A cerebral hemorrhage typically produces paralysis on only one side of the body, which is quite understandable if we consider the anatomy of the cerebrum. Explain.

19. An unexplained loss of the sense of taste may signal a brain tumor. Explain.

20. Mental retardation relates to prenatal causes, perinatal causes, and postnatal causes. Which of the three is the special concern of "genetic counseling"?

21. There is no known relationship between intelligence and dyslexia. What does this tell us about the functioning of the brain?

22. A dog bite (or other animal bite) through clothing, such as a pant leg, is potentially less serious than say on the bare hand. Why, specifically?

23. Antibiotics are ineffective in the treatment of encephalitis, rabies, and polio. This underscores something about the general usefulness of these agents. What is it?

24. If the victim of a severe wound has had a tetanus booster within the past 3 years, another booster (of tetanus toxoid) is considered adequate protection. Otherwise the situation calls for tetanus antitoxin. Why?

25. Meningitis may involve the spinal cord, the brain, or both the spinal cord and the brain. Explain.

Sympathic chain - Autonomic Nervous system.

CHAPTER 10

The sense organs

The sense organs provide our contact with the world around us. Written and spoken communication and our appreciation of food, fragrances, color, music, scenery, and the nature of the surfaces we touch are made possible by receptors, whose messages to the brain produce awareness and sensations—pleasurable and otherwise. The health and effective functioning of the sense organs, especially the organs of sight and hearing, are of basic importance to the enjoyment of life. The receptors in the skin and the chemical receptors of taste and smell are relatively simple in structure and function. The eye and the ear, on the other hand, are highly complex and subject to various kinds of disease and derangement. A basic understanding of their function and conservation is important.

Cutaneous sensations

Taste and smell

The eye

The ear

The body has millions of sense organs, or **receptors**. Some are merely the free endings of sensory neurons, and others are specialized structures attached to such endings. Either way, stimulation initiates a nerve impulse that the brain reads and registers as a sensation. Receptors may be thought of as superficial, deep, visceral, and special. **Superficial receptors**, located in the skin and upper connective tissues, give rise to sensations of touch, pressure, warmth, cold, and pain. **Deep receptors**, located in muscles, tendons, and joints, give rise to sensations of position, deep pressure, and pain. **Visceral receptors**, located in the viscera, give rise to sensations such as hunger, nausea, and visceral pain. **Special receptors** located in the eye, ear, nose, and mouth give rise to vision, hearing, smell, and taste, respectively.

CUTANEOUS SENSATIONS

The skin contains receptors or nerve endings that, when stimulated, give rise, respectively, to five cutaneous sensations: cold, warmth, touch, pressure, and pain. Those of each type can be located as "spots," pinpoint or larger in size, and can be mapped on the skin. Pain receptors are the most numerous, whereas those for heat are least numerous. Because of such variations in the number of receptors, not all parts of the body are equally sensitive. An area that has few receptors is relatively insensitive; sensitive areas have large numbers of receptors. Any form of stimulus evokes pain if it is sufficiently strong. The warnings of pain are a powerful aid in preserving a person's life.

TASTE AND SMELL

Gustatory receptors, or **taste buds**, of four types initiate the sensations of the basic tastes (sour, salty, sweet, and bitter) from taste-producing substances in solution. The taste buds are unevenly distributed on the tongue, with the sensation of bitter taste more readily perceived at the base, sweet at the tip, and sour at the sides. The taste of many "finer flavors" includes not only combinations of these fundamental taste sensations but also sensations of smell. Raw onion eaten with the nose shut tastes somewhat like raw potato.

Receptors for the sense of smell (olfaction) are located in the mucosa of the upper nasal cavity. These receptors are surrounded by supporting cells and glands. The latter secrete a fluid that absorbs and dissolves molecules of volatile odorous substances; only volatile substances in solution can stimulate olfactory receptors. If the change in concentration of an odorous substance in the air is sufficiently rapid, it serves as a stimulus; otherwise, it does not. This explains why we quickly become unaware of an odor that does not change in intensity.

THE EYE

The eye is situated in the socket ("orbit") of the skull and cushioned there by a thick bed of fat (Fig. 10-1). The six ocular muscles originating at the back of the orbit attach to the outside and enable the eye to move in all directions. The three coats of the eye are (1) the outer **sclera**, which covers the entire eyeball except in front where it becomes transparent and is called the **cornea**; (2) the blood-rich middle coat, or **choroid**; and (3) the inner light-sensitive **retina** (Fig. 10-2). Behind the cornea is the **iris**, the colored, doughnut-shaped piece of muscle that regulates the amount of light entering the eye through the **pupil** (the "hole in the doughnut"). Just behind the pupil is the **lens**, a crystal clear elastic disk critical to focusing. The anterior cavity of the eye, which divides into the anterior and posterior chambers, is filled with a watery fluid called the **aqueous humor**; the much larger posterior cavity of the eyeball proper is filled with

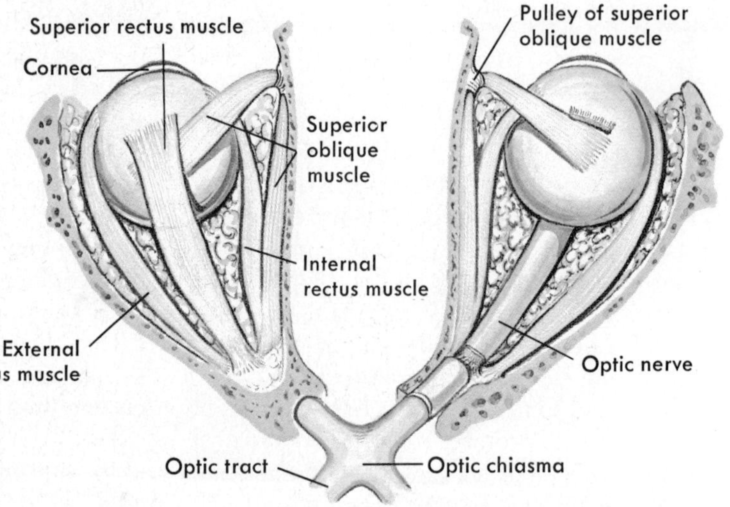

FIG. 10-1 ■ The eye in its socket, showing eye muscles and optic nerve. Superior rectus muscle of right eye has been cut away to show optic nerve as it arises from eyeball.

From Schottelius, B.A., and Schottelius, D.D.: Textbook of physiology, ed. 18, St. Louis, 1978, The C.V. Mosby Co.

a clear jellylike material called the **vitreous humor**.

The retina is made up of countless light-sensitive receptors called **rods** and **cones**. The nerve fibers emerging from the retina gather at the **optic disk** (blind spot) (Fig. 10-3) and leave the eyeball as the **optic nerve**. Curving inward, the two optic nerves meet at the **optic chiasma** (Fig. 10-1), where there is a 50% crossover of nerve fibers; more precisely, the nerve fibers originating from the inner half of the retina cross over to the optic nerve of the opposite side, while the nerve fibers from the lateral portion pass directly into the optic nerve on the same side. It is because of this crossover that each of the two **visual areas** of the brain "sees with both eyes."

Vision depends on focusing, light control, and photochemical reactions. As light rays travel through the cornea, the aqueous humor, the lens, and the vitreous humor, in this order, they are bent, or **refracted**, so that the normal eye brings into clear focus on the retina an object 20 or more feet away. To bring into focus an object closer than this, the ciliary muscle removes tension on the lens, causing the lens to become more convex and more refractive (Fig. 10-4). This adjustment for near objects is referred to as **accommodation**. The intensity of light is controlled by the iris, which contracts to constrict the size of the pupil in bright light and relaxes to dilate the pupil in darkness.

Light striking the retina initiates nerve impulses as a consequence of photochemistry. Vision in dim light is made possible through the photosensitivity of **rhodopsin** ("visual purple"), the rod pigment synthesized from vitamin A. Vision in full light involves three types of **cones**, each of which is charged with a photosensitive pigment responsive to a primary color. Thus we experience red, green, or blue when red, green, or blue cones are stimulated by the corresponding light wavelengths. Other color sensations arise from an interplay of the three cones. Yellow stems from stimulation of an equal number of green and red cones plus a very few blue cones. We see white when all three are equally stimulated.

■ Eyelids and lacrimal apparatus

The eyes are protected in front by the **eyelids**, the two movable folds of skin containing muscle and a border of thick connective tissue

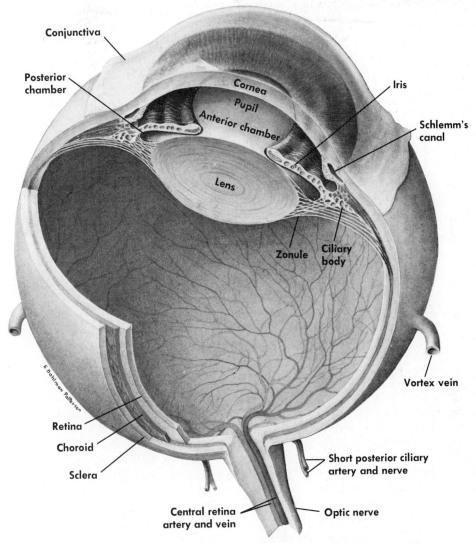

Conjunctiva

Posterior chamber

Cornea

Pupil

Anterior chamber

Iris

Schlemm's canal

Lens

Zonule

Ciliary body

E. Dahlman Patterson

Retina

Choroid

Sclera

Vortex vein

Short posterior ciliary artery and nerve

Central retina artery and vein

Optic nerve

FIG. 10-2 ■ The human eye.

From Newell, F.W.: Ophthalmology: principles and concepts, ed. 5, St. Louis, 1982, The C.V. Mosby Co.

FIG. 10-3 ■ Demonstration of the blind spot. With left eye closed, hold figure about 12 inches in front of right eye and, while focusing on white circle, slowly move book toward eye until white cross disappears. When this occurs, the image of the cross falls on the optic disk, or blind spot (which contains no rods or cones).

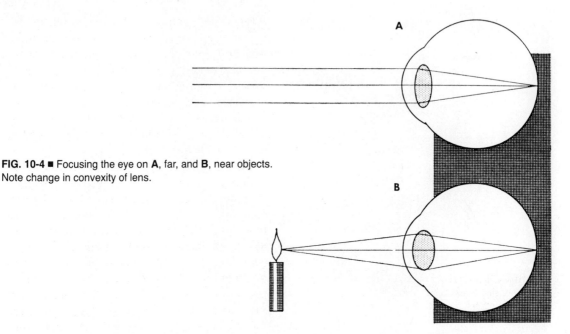

FIG. 10-4 ■ Focusing the eye on **A**, far, and **B**, near objects. Note change in convexity of lens.

from which project the **eyelashes**. There are a number of sweat and oil glands in the lids that empty by minute openings along the free border. Though we tend to think of the eyelashes in terms of cosmetics, they do indeed serve as a valuable protective device against the entrance of foreign bodies. The inside surface of the eyelids is lined with a transparent mucous membrane, the **conjunctiva**, which also continues over the surface of the eyeball. The **lacrimal apparatus** is composed of the lacrimal (tear) glands (situated in a depression in the frontal bone at the upper, outer margin of the eye socket) and a number of small ducts. The lacrimal ducts lead tears onto the surface of the conjunctiva, and the nasolacrimal duct (one per eye) drains the tears into the nose. Tears function to moisten the exterior part of the eye, to lubricate the eyelids, and to wash down any debris on the conjunctival surface.

■ Visual acuity and optical defects

If a person can read letters at 20 feet that are readable at that distance to all people with

normal vision, that person's **visual acuity**, or "eyesight," is said to be 20/20. If, on the other hand, a person is barely able to read letters at 20 feet that are readable at 40 feet to all people with normal vision, that person's visual acuity is said to be 20/40. Worse yet, if a person is barely able to read letters at 20 feet that are readable at 100 feet to all with normal vision, that person's visual acuity is 20/100, and so on. The more common optical defects that relate to visual acuity are discussed as follows.

Astigmatism. Astigmatism, probably the most common defect of the eye, is a condition characterized by "blemished vision"; that is, instead of light rays striking the retina in sharp focus, they spread out over a more or less diffuse area (Fig. 10-5). Interestingly, the word astigmatism (of Greek origin) means "without point." Astigmatism is caused by the unequal curvature of either the cornea or the lens, sometimes both. Because the cornea and lens are never optically perfect, most of us experience some degree of astigmatism. If this were not true, stars would appear as small bright dots instead of star-shaped bodies (that is,

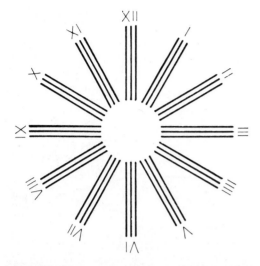

FIG. 10-5 ■ To normal eye, all black lines will appear of same intensity. To astigmatic eye, some will appear darker than others.

bright centers with radiating short lines). The natural imperfection of the refractive apparatus of the eye also explains why a light in the darkness appears to come to the eye in radiating beams. To correct astigmatism, the ophthalmologist prescribes glasses that compensate for the faulty curvatures of the refracting surfaces.

Myopia. Myopia, or **nearsightedness**, is an eye condition in which the focus falls in front of the retina (Fig. 10-6). To put the image on the retina where it belongs, the myopic person must look at an object at closer range than does the normal, or **emmetropic**, person. The cause of myopia may be either that the refractive power of the eye is too great or that the eyeball is too long. To remedy the defect, the ophthalmologist prescribes glasses with concave lenses that diverge the light rays hitting the cornea just enough "to force" the focus back on the retina.

Hyperopia. In contrast to the myopic eye, the hyperopic eye sees objects most clearly at far range; that is, hyperopia is **farsightedness**. Thus instead of the focus falling in front of the retina, as in myopia, it falls behind it (Fig. 10-6). The usual cause of hyperopia is a flattened lens or cornea (with a consequent loss of refractive power) or an eyeball that is too short. To correct the condition, the refractive power of the eye must be increased by a convex lens, which causes parallel light rays to converge before entering the eye and, therefore, to come to a focus sooner.

Color blindness. Color blindness is the inability to distinguish differences in color; it is generally partial and is seldom, if ever, complete. Usually hereditary and rarely seen in women, the condition is said to affect about 8% of all men. In **dichromatism**, the most common variety, the person does not see red or green but only yellow and blue or combinations thereof. Apparently, the retina lacks the photosensitive chemicals sensitive to these fundamental colors. Since color blindness may lead to serious accidents in driving motor vehicles and in all occupations in which colored signals are used, it is of utmost importance that the condition be detected at an early age.

Glaucoma. Glaucoma, a leading cause of blindness in the United States, results from faulty drainage of aqueous humor. Because the inflow and outflow of the fluid are normally balanced, the result of faulty drainage is a rise in the **intraocular pressure**, sometimes four times the average range (15 to 25 mm Hg). Indeed, the affected eye may feel as hard as a marble. In the acute condition there is intense pain, fogged vision, and lights ringed with halos, whereas in the chronic type, in which the pressure rises over long periods of time, the symptoms are transitory and mild. In either circumstance, however, the prolonged elevation of pressure ultimately leads to retinal damage. With early treatment (with drugs and/or surgery) loss of sight from glaucoma can be prevented. But any damage that has occurred before the disease is detected cannot be corrected. Periodic eye tests make common sense.

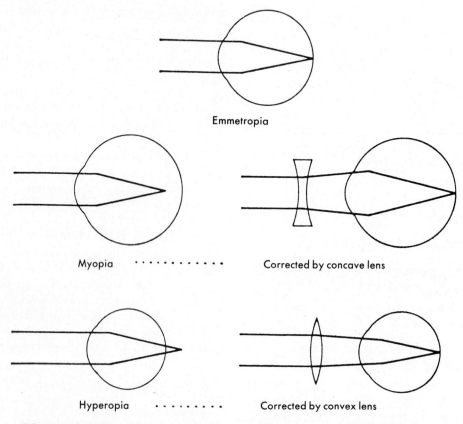

FIG. 10-6 ■ Refraction of light in emmetropia (normal vision), myopia (nearsightedness), and hyperopia (farsightedness) and correction of these defects.

Modified from Schottelius, B.A., and Schottelius, D.D.: Textbook of physiology, ed. 18, St. Louis, 1978, The C.V. Mosby Co.

Cataract. A cataract is an **opacity** of the lens of the eye. The so-called developmental cataracts seen in young persons result from infection of the mother in the first trimester of pregnancy, or they may be hereditary. Degenerative cataracts, on the other hand, occur in elderly persons ("senile cataracts") and in persons exposed to excessive radiation and heat. Degenerative cataracts make up the bulk of all cases. When there is considerable impairment of vision, operative removal of the lens is essential.

Infections. The tissues and various structures of the eye are fertile ground for a variety of pathogens. The more common infections

include **sty** (involvement of one or more glands of the eyelids); **blepharitis** (involvement of the margin of the eyelids); **conjunctivitis** (involvement of the conjunctiva); **keratitis** (involvement of the cornea); and **iritis** (involvement of the iris). Gonorrheal conjunctivitis in the newborn infant is easily prevented by the instillation of 2 drops of 1% silver nitrate solution into each eye at the time of delivery.

Strabismus. Strabismus means ocular deviation; that is, one eye is "not in line" with the other. There are two forms: paralytic and nonparalytic. Paralytic strabismus results from paralysis of one or more ocular muscles; nonparalytic strabismus usually results from unequal muscle tone. Nonparalytic strabismus may be convergent (cross-eye), divergent (walleye), or vertical (eye turns up or down). Ocular deviation, if constant, should be investigated shortly after birth; if intermittent, by age 6 months. If muscle imbalance alone is responsible, strabismus should be treated early with corrective lenses, eye drops, eye exercise, patching of the normal eye, or surgery. Permanent visual loss can occur if the disorder is not treated before age 4 years.

■ Eye care

Eyestrain and other problems of vision occur most commonly in near vision, as when using the eyes for reading or other close work. In distant vision very little, if any, strain occurs. Students should take special care in the use of their eyes and have periodic checks of visual acuity.

Most of us fail to realize the tremendous amount of precise, rapid, and coordinated muscular activity involved in reading. The external muscles must move the eyes so that they follow along each line. This is done in a series of jumps, since the region of clear vision is short. The eye must then jump back to the beginning of the next line. If difficulties are encountered, other movements are added. At the same time, constant effort is necessary to keep the two eyes exactly centered on the same point with every movement. The very delicate ciliary muscles controlling the convexity of the lens must be kept in constant tension in order to keep the visual images clearly focused on the retina. This is also true of the muscles controlling the regulation of light through the iris. The efficiency with which these muscles do their work is remarkable, and the fact that eyestrain follows when they are required to labor under unfavorable conditions is not surprising. Flickering lights and sharp contrasts in illumination of the work area should be avoided. Both cause excessive activity of the eye muscles.

Eye fatigue is fatigue of the muscles of the eye. They rest during sleep. When one is doing close work, it is restful to look away to a distant object from time to time. Many persons look at television so long as to produce fatigue. Television viewing for a limited time in a partially lighted room and with a screen of good size presenting a clear image will not damage the eyes.

A person should avoid glare—any light shining into the eye that causes discomfort and interferes with clear vision. A light from an unshaded source, paper that is too glossy, or a bright reflection from a highly polished surface tends to produce eyestrain. Direct sunlight reflected from a printed page is particularly injurious. The iris reacts to this light and, by contracting, reduces the visibility of the object being studied. Light should be strong and steady. It should fall on one's work from above and slightly behind or beside a person, not from directly in front.

Caution should be used in protecting the retina from direct rays of the sun. If a person looks directly at the sun, the lens of the eye serves as a burning glass, and the rays of the sun may actually destroy portions of the seeing area of the retina, just as the same rays brought to a focus on a bit of paper would scorch it. Protective sunglasses should be worn while on the beach and when driving.

When a foreign body, such as a bit of dirt, gets in the eye, it should be removed with care. Tears may wash it out of the eye. You can sometimes help this process if, after washing your hands, you lift the upper lid by the eyelashes and pull it over the lower lid two or three times. If the speck is on the lower part of the eye, you can press your finger against the cheek just below the lower lid and remove the dirt with the corner of a clean handkerchief. If the particle of dirt is over the pupil or iris, or if it is not easily removed, keep the eye at rest and seek medical aid.

Corrective lenses. Three professions are involved in the fitting of corrective lenses. The terms ophthalmologist, oculist, optometrist, and optician are often confused by the public. An **ophthalmologist**, or **oculist**, holds the degree of M.D., and the practice includes treatment of eye diseases. Many ophthalmologists are diplomates of the American Board of Ophthalmology, which requires postgraduate training beyond internship. The **optometrist** is licensed by the state as a specialist in vision and, if graduated since 1955, is required to have training in a school or college of optometry approved by the American Optometric Association to be eligible for a state examination. The optometrist tests vision and fits corrective lenses. The **optician** fills prescriptions for corrective lenses but is not licensed to examine eyes or test vision, just as a pharmacist fills prescriptions for drugs but is not licensed to diagnose or treat illness.

Corrective lenses should be worn as prescribed and should be kept spotlessly clean and free from scratches. Bifocal lenses allow the wearer to look through the center of the upper lens for distant vision and through the lower lens for near vision. Lenses should be changed when periodic eye examinations indicate that a change is needed.

Contact lenses are worn by over 12 million persons in the United States (approximately 8½ million of whom are women), and their use among the 110 million persons who wear corrective lenses of all kinds is steadily growing. Made of specially prepared plastic, there are four basic types: (1) hard contact lenses (the first available—in the late 1940s), (2) soft contact lenses, (3) intraocular lenses (IOLs), and (4) extended-wear soft contact lenses. The hard and soft contact lenses are usually worn for cosmetic purposes by those who need corrected vision. The IOLs and extended-wear soft contact lenses are designed specifically for cataract patients. All four types have advantages and disadvantages, and each has health, care, and safety factors to be considered.

Safety measures for protecting vision. On the average, every 11 minutes one person in the United States becomes blind. Eye injuries are a major threat to vision, even though accidental damage to vision is nearly always preventable. Of all eye injuries, 41% occur at home. Precautions should be taken at home, in school, and in industry. Protective glasses should be worn at all times when indicated, for example, when working in the chemistry laboratory, when using sun lamps, when working in the home workshop, when using power law mowers, and when using garden insecticides. Providing adequate lighting for the job at hand, reading instructions carefully on labels of strong cleaning agents and chemicals, and keeping such products out of reach of young children are all safety measures that should not be ignored. Also, the person who uses glasses for corrective purposes should habitually wear the glasses to protect his vision, especially if one eye has lost its sight or if one eye is a "lazy eye."

◼◼◼ THE EAR

The ear, the organ of sound and balance, is divided into the outer, middle, and inner parts (Fig. 10-7). The **outer ear** consists of the auricle (or pinna) and the auditory canal. The **middle ear**, a small chamber lying within the temporal bone and separated from the outer ear by the **eardrum** (tympanic membrane), houses the **ossicles** (three tiny bones bearing the names malleus, incus, and stapes) and communicates with the upper throat via the **eustachian tube**. The **inner ear** consists of the outer osseous labyrinth enclosing the inner membranous labyrinth, whose parts are the cochlea, semicircular canals, utricle, and saccule. A watery fluid, the perilymph, fills the space between the osseous and membranous labyrinths, and another watery fluid, the endolymph, fills the membranous labyrinth. The **organ of Corti**, the actual receptor of sound, is situated within the cochlea.

Sound waves striking the eardrum cause that structure to vibrate; this, in turn, causes the

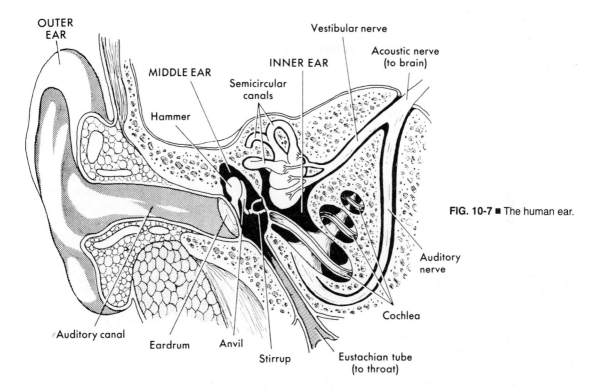

FIG. 10-7 ■ The human ear.

malleus (hammer), incus (anvil), and stapes (stirrup) to vibrate, in that order. Since it is attached to the membranous oval window at the beginning of the inner ear, the vibrating stapes disturbs the perilymph and endolymph sufficiently to stimulate the organ of Corti. The impulses thus generated make their way to the brain's auditory center via the **auditory branch** of the acoustic nerve and are interpreted as sound. To ensure free movement of the eardrum, the air pressure on its inner and outer sides is equalized—via the eustachian tube.

Balance, or equilibrium, is maintained through the combined operation of the semicircular canals, the utricle, and the saccule. In brief, the three canals possess hairlike receptors that initiate a nerve impulse in response to the movement of the endolymph. Because the canals lie in three different planes, any particular movement causes more stimulation in one canal than in the others, and the resulting nerve impulse (carried by the **ves-**

tibular branch of the acoustic nerve) is sensed and "acted on" in the cerebellum. The receptors of the utricle and saccule, triggered mainly by the position of the head, likewise transmit impulses to the cerebellum.

■ Deafness

About 10% of the population of the United States suffers some degree of hearing loss. Deafness is lack or loss, complete or partial, of the sense of hearing. It is said to be either conductive or sensorineural. **Conductive deafness** is caused by some defect in the sound-conducting system, that is, the auditory canal, eardrum, ear bones, and eustachian tube. In children, most cases of conductive deafness result from the presence of excessive lymphoid tissue in and about the eustachian tube's openings in the nasopharynx. This interferes with proper ventilation of the middle ear, thereby upsetting the normally equalized pressures on either side of the eardrum. As a result, eardrum vibrations are inhibited, and hearing is impaired. The treatment is surgical removal of the lymphoid obstruction. In adults the usual causes of conductive deafness are **impacted earwax** and **otosclerosis**. The latter is a chronic disease caused by ossification of the ligament that attaches the stapes to the oval window. Earwax is easily removed in the doctor's office, and otosclerosis is usually correctable through surgery.

Sensorineural deafness results from disorders of the cochlea, auditory nerve, cerebral pathways, or auditory center. The causes include infection, tumors, psychogenic disturbances, injuries, and certain drugs (for example, quinine and streptomycin). Treatment is directed at the underlying cause, and every attempt is made to eradicate the cause. If the condition is irreversible, careful rehabilitation—hearing aid, lipreading—is essential.

The nature and extent of hearing loss can be determined by the audiometer, an instrument that can produce sounds of known loudness (decibel levels) at specific pitches. When the person cannot hear a specific pitch at the normal decibel level, we can find out how much louder that sound must be to enable the subject to hear it. Thus we can learn how serious the hearing loss is and whether it is greater at the higher tones or the lower tones.

The outlook for the hard-of-hearing person is more optimistic than it was a generation or so ago, largely because of surgery, drugs, and the modern hearing aid. Once surgical or medical treatment is ruled out or completed, the ear specialist (otologist) may advise the patient to have tests done by an audiologist or to seek hearing aid evaluation directly from a hearing aid dispenser (a person who sells, leases, or rents hearing aids). In most states these persons are licensed under standards of competence and a strict code of ethics. An FDA regulation (1977) imposed conditions for the sale of hearing aids to help misrepresentation and to assure adherence to proper medical standards. There are four types of hearing aid (a miniature amplifying system):

1. The all-in-the ear unit fits directly into the ear and extends partway into the ear canal. It is lightweight, has no external wires, and is most suitable for compensating mild hearing losses.
2. The behind-the-ear aid is small and fits snugly behind the ear. Its microphone, amplifier, and receiver are in one unit connected to the ear by a short plastic tube. It is suitable for losses ranging from mild to severe.
3. The eyeglass aid is similar to the behind-the-ear unit but is built into an eyeglass frame.
4. The body aid (Fig. 10-8) has a larger microphone, amplifier, and power supply in a pocket case connected by a cord to the receiver, which is attached directly to the ear mold. This type of hearing aid is most suitable for those persons with severe hearing loss.

Organizations such as the American Speech and Hearing Association, National Hearing Aid Society, and National Easter Seal Society for Crippled Children and Adults provide help to persons with problems of deafness. In many areas of the country speech and hearing centers associated with universities and hospitals can provide assistance. Services may include hearing aid evaluation, lipreading instruction, speech correction, voice improvement, audiometer testing, recreation with other hard-of-hearing persons, and encouragement for newly afflicted individuals.

■ Tinnitus

Tinnitus is an annoying symptom characterized by hissing, ringing, buzzing, thumping, whistling, or roaring in the ears. The underlying cause can be an infection, drug intoxication, obstruction of the auditory canal, obstruction of the eustachian tube, or a dental disorder. When this symptom occurs, there-

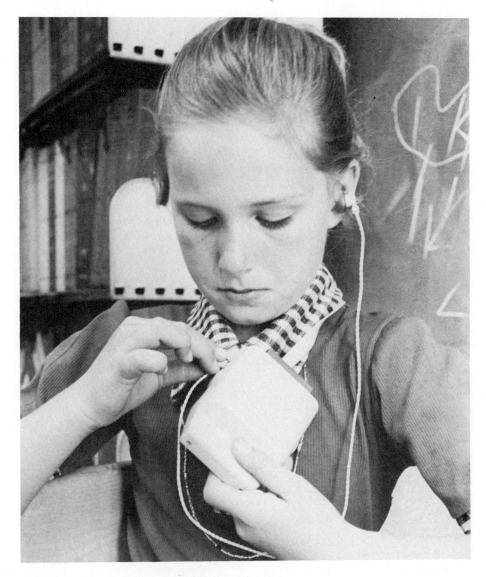

FIG. 10-8 ■ The body hearing aid for deafness.

From Gearheart, B.R., and Weishahn, M.: The handicapped child in the regular classroom, St. Louis, 1976, The C.V. Mosby Co.

fore, the physician has to consider every possibility in searching for the cause.

■ Ménière's disease

Of the various labyrinthine (inner ear) disturbances, Ménière's disease is perhaps the most common. Possibly of an allergic nature, it is marked by bouts of deafness, tinnitus, vertigo (dizziness), nausea, and vomiting. Antihistamines and tranquilizers help in some cases but not in others. When these drugs fail, a variety of surgical procedures are available.

■ Infection

From the standpoint of a general threat to health, infection (particularly the acute form) is probably the most serious ear condition. Infection of the outer ear (**otitis externa**) involves the auricle or auditory canal. Since the area is relatively easy to reach, the use of appropriate antiinfective drugs usually brings about a swift cure. **Otitis media**, or middle ear infection, however, is always potentially dangerous. Acute otitis media is a bacterial or viral infection common in young children. Microorganisms migrate from the nasopharynx to the middle ear via the eustachian tube. Often the infection occurs in the wake of scarlet fever, measles, mumps, pneumonia, and influenza. The principal danger is mastoiditis (an infection of the temporal bone). Mastoiditis may lead to infection of the brain and sudden death. Treatment with antibiotics must be immediate and vigorous.

■ Noise

Noise has gained status in the past decade as a source of environmental pollution. In 1972 the United States Congress enacted the Noise Control Act, which required the Environmental Protection Agency to identify and regulate major sources of noise. The decibel levels of power lawnmowers, jackhammers, air conditioners, trucks, bulldozers, motorcycles, vacuum cleaners, and other sources of noise were (and still are) being studied. There are now federal limitations on the noise produced by loud violators such as garbage trucks, railroad trains, motorcycles, semitrailers, and portable air compressors. Standards have been set for control and abatement of aviation noise. However, since there is still much to be done to alleviate the noise that is a contributing factor to hearing loss, various industrial and trade organizations and technical and scientific societies are concerned with acoustics. Researchers want to determine just how much exposure to outdoor noise and indoor noise can be tolerated by the human ear. The student should keep in mind that one study found that the background noise level from rock music is often high enough to cause hearing loss, for the intensity of sound reaches around 100 decibels, with peaks of 115 to 120 decibels! By comparison, a whisper is about 20 decibels.

■ SELF-TEST

1. _____ taste buds
2. _____ nasal receptors
3. _____ cutaneous receptors
4. _____ rods and cones
5. _____ regulates light
6. _____ posterior chamber
7. _____ posterior cavity
8. _____ "blind spot"
9. _____ "bending of light"
10. _____ "visual purple"
11. _____ lacrimal glands
12. _____ tympanic membrane
13. _____ organ of Corti
14. _____ semicircular canals
15. _____ ear bones

a. iris
b. tears
c. balance
d. eardrum
e. ossicles
f. gustation
g. retina
h. vitreous humor
i. vitamin A
j. sound receptor
k. olfaction
l. optic disk
m. touch
n. refraction
o. aqueous humor

■■■■■■ **STUDY QUESTIONS**

1. A pimple near the lips can be quite painful, whereas elsewhere on the body it may go unnoticed. How do you account for this?
2. Often times a room smells musty when one first enters it, and then in a minute or so the smell "disappears." Why?
3. It is well known that a bad cold robs us of our "sense of taste." Why is this true?
4. By looking in the mirror we can easily see the iris, pupil, and sclera ("white of the eye"). Why can't we see the cornea?
5. Why is the pupil of the eye dark?
6. Why is the optic disk "blind"?
7. With advancing years all of us tend to get hyperopic. What effect does this have in a person with myopia as a youngster?
8. Is it possible to have both myopia and astigmatism?
9. Dichromatism can easily cause an auto accident. Explain.
10. In dim light or twilight the eye does not detect color. Why?
11. Nyctalopia (night blindness) is one of the first signs of a vitamin A deficiency. Explain.
12. Why do the eyes tend to water when we have a stuffy nose?
13. In glaucoma the eyeball may get as hard as a marble. Why?
14. Enlargement of the pupil normally tends to decrease the drainage of aqueous humor. How do you connect this finding with the fact that sitting through a long movie may precipitate an acute attack of glaucoma in predisposed persons?
15. During excitement do the pupils constrict or dilate? Which autonomic system—the sympathetic or parasympathetic—is responsible for this?
16. Why is the lens of the eye removed in a cataract operation?
17. Conjunctivitis involves the eyelids as well as the eye. Why is this so?
18. The "path" of a sound from its source to the brain involves the acoustic nerve, oval window, auditory center, hammer, eardrum, anvil, organ of Corti, and stirrup. This is not the proper sequence. What is the proper sequence?
19. Of the two types of deafness—conductive deafness and sensorineural deafness—which is usually the more serious?
20. What is the simpler and more easily corrected form of deafness?
21. The acoustic nerve is actually two nerves. Explain.
22. Of the two types of ear infection—otitis externa and otitis media—which is more common and easier to treat?
23. Ménière's disease is characterized by bouts of deafness, tinnitus, dizziness, nausea, and vomiting. What accounts for these signs and symptoms?
24. The buzz or hum noted in the ear as a result of a fast ride in an elevator can be corrected easily by swallowing a few times. Can you account for the cause? For the cure?
25. What steps would you recommend for the control of noise pollution in your community?

CHAPTER 11

The skin

Everything considered, the skin, or integument, as some say, is clearly an awesome organ. To begin with it is the body's largest organ. Indeed, in terms of surface area—about 16 square feet in the adult—it is as large as the body itself. Aside from its obvious role of protection, the skin performs a number of ancillary functions, including excretion, fluid balance, temperature control, and sensory perception. Additionally, the skin chemical 7-dehydrocholesterol is converted into vitamin D by the ultraviolet rays of sunlight. Vitamin D deficiencies are common in the tropics because of the swaddling of infants and confinement of women and children to the home.

Epidermis and dermis

Subcutaneous tissue

Hair and nails

Glands

Skin receptors

Disorders and diseases

Maintaining healthy skin

Cosmetics

The skin is the body's largest organ. Its functions are numerous, diverse, complex, and crucial to survival. The skin shields us from infection and injury, informs us of changes in our external environment, plays a vital role in fluid and electrolyte balance, and aids in maintaining body temperature.

EPIDERMIS AND DERMIS

The skin is composed of two distinct layers—the superficial layer, called the **epidermis**, and the deep layer, called the **dermis** (Fig. 11-1). The epidermis receives no blood vessels and must rely on the nutrient fluids derived from the vascularized dermis below. The color of skin depends basically on its content of **melanin**, the dark pigment formed by special epidermal cells called melanocytes. The skin of the black person and the darker areas on the white person (for example, about the nipple) contain large amounts of this pigment. In most whites the color of the skin is influenced by the blood. The white pallor of someone who has fainted is striking evidence of this.

In the areas where the epidermis is thickest (palms of the hands and soles of the feet), it is made up of five strata. The outermost stratum, the stratum corneum, consists of several dozen layers of dead scalelike cells composed of a water-repellent protein called **keratin**; the most superficial layers are continually flaking off, a process called exfoliation. The stratum basale is composed of a single layer of cells that undergo rapid mitosis. New cells are produced in this deepest stratum at a rate equal to the loss of cells from the stratum corneum. The new cells push upward into each successive layer and eventually flake off.

The dermis, or corium, is composed of connective tissue, blood vessels, lymph vessels, nerves, and accessory glandular structures. Characteristically, it thrusts itself upward into peglike structures called papillae that lock together the two layers of skin. The papillae produce the fingerprints at the fingertips. Fingerprints differ, even in identical twins.

SUBCUTANEOUS TISSUE

Subcutaneous tissue, or **superficial fascia**, is an extensive fibrous membrane that underlies the skin and forms a continuous sheet throughout the body. It is composed of connective tissue interlaced with fat, vessels, nerves, receptors, and glands. This tissue nourishes, supports, and cushions the skin, and its fat serves as a food reserve. Fat is deposited and distributed according to a person's sex, and this, together with muscle and bone development, explains differences in body shape between the sexes. When we overeat, fat piles up beneath the skin; when we diet, excess fat is burned, the skin resumes its normal texture and contour, and we "get our shape back."

Beneath the subcutaneous tissue lies what is called the **deep fascia**, a thin layer of dense connective tissue without fat that covers the muscles and passes toward the body's interior to form intermuscular partitions. In certain areas the deep fascia thickens to produce ligaments and tendons.

HAIR AND NAILS

The so-called accessory organs of the skin include hair, nails, glands, and receptors. Except for the palms of the hands and the soles of the feet, hair adorns the entire body. Over the eyes and in the nose and the ears, it screens out insects, dust, and other airborne debris, and elsewhere it serves as a solar screen and a valuable sensory structure.

A shaft of hair grows upward as a consequence of extensive cellular multiplication at the **papilla**, a structure located at the base of the root (Fig. 11-1). The root (the portion of the hair embedded in the skin) and its coat of connective tissue constitute the hair follicle.

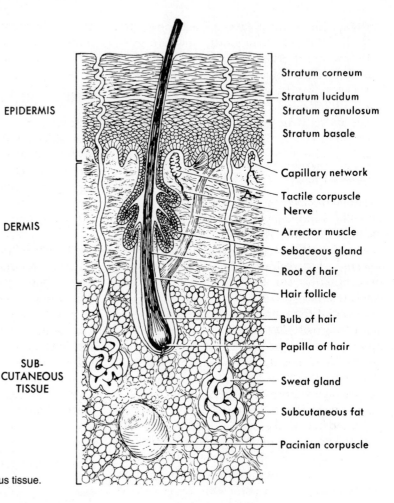

EPIDERMIS

DERMIS

SUB-
CUTANEOUS
TISSUE

Stratum corneum

Stratum lucidum
Stratum granulosum

Stratum basale

Capillary network

Tactile corpuscle
Nerve

Arrector muscle

Sebaceous gland

Root of hair

Hair follicle

Bulb of hair

Papilla of hair

Sweat gland

Subcutaneous fat

Pacinian corpuscle

FIG. 11-1 ■ The skin and subcutaneous tissue.

As long as the cells near the papilla remain alive, a hair will continue to grow and regenerate. As we know, "hair stands on end" and goose pimples appear in response to fright or to cold. These somewhat primitive responses are caused by contractions of the tiny muscles (arrectores pilorum) attached to the hair follicles. Also around the follicle are **sebaceous glands** that oil the hair (Fig. 11-1). The color of hair is due to the presence of varying amounts of melanin within the shaft. White hairs have no pigment; when they are mixed with pigmented hairs, the "mixture" that results is called **gray hair**.

The nails are horny distal appendages of the fingers and the toes. They are composed of keratin and develop from the epidermal cells of the stratum lucidum lying under the **lunula**, the white crescent-shaped structure situated at the base of the nail.

■ GLANDS

For each hair there are at least two sebaceous, or oil, glands that secrete about the shaft an oily substance called **sebum**. Sebum keeps the hair supple and the skin soft and pliant.

Sudoriferous, or sweat, glands (Fig. 11-1)

are distributed over the entire body, especially on the palms, the soles, and the forehead and in the axillary regions. In these areas there are thousands per square inch of skin. Sweat glands soften the stratum corneum and regulate body heat. To a minor degree they help rid the blood of wastes. Sweat is about 99% water, but it also contains dissolved salt, traces of urea, and miscellaneous other substances. When the body becomes overheated, the sudoriferous glands step up the production of sweat, which evaporates to cool the skin. In the tropics 10 to 15 liters of water may be lost daily through perspiration. The sweat glands are governed by autonomic nerves, which presumably are under the direction of a "sweat center" in the brain. When the temperature of the blood rises in response to external temperature or muscular activity, the center is triggered and sends impulses to the glands, causing the production of sweat. In addition to sweat, water seeps through the epidermal layers and leaves the surface as water vapor (**insensible perspiration**). On a typical day about 0.5 liter is lost this way.

Ceruminous glands are modified sweat glands located in the auditory canal of the external ear. Instead of sweat, they secrete **cerumen**, a waxlike substance that aids the hairs in trapping dust, insects, and the like. This action serves to protect the eardrum.

SKIN RECEPTORS

The skin's extreme sensitivity is effected through sensory nerve endings and specialized structures called **receptors**. These microscopic receivers are distributed over the entire body, but they are more concentrated in some areas than in others. The back, for instance, has fewer receptors per unit area than the fingertips. **Pain receptors** are naked nerve endings found throughout the skin and within the body. They are the most numerous of all the receptors. Temperature and touch also stimulate these endings. **Meissner's corpus-**

cles are encapsulated receptors located in the fingers, the toes, the lips, the mammary glands, and the external genitals. They are tuned to the sense of delicate touch. **Pacinian corpuscles** are ovoid receptors found in the deeper parts of the skin covering the hands and the feet. They also occur throughout the subcutaneous tissue and in the muscles, the mesentery, and the mesocolon. Each contains a granular central bulb enclosing a single terminal nerve ending sensitive to pressure.

DISORDERS AND DISEASES

When we consider that the skin covers such an intricate and sensitive mechanism as the human body, it is little wonder that most of us cannot go through life without an occasional flare-up of this expansive organ. Such flareups may be caused by a microbial, physical, or chemical attack from without or by some microbial or metabolic attack from within. In the latter connection, it is important to appreciate that a skin disease of internal cause often relates not only to forces in the skin itself but also to extracutaneous mechanisms.

Infections involving the skin

Infections involving the skin are almost without number, and they range in severity from pimples to life-threatening conditions. In some cases the infection is confined to the skin, whereas in others the skin is only one feature of a generalized infection. The causal pathogens span the full microbial spectrum: bacteria, viruses, fungi, and ectoparasites. **Bacterial** infections include pimples, sties, boils, carbuncles, impetigo, infected wounds, scarlet fever, plague, rabbit fever, anthrax, Rocky Mountain spotted fever, and leprosy (Fig. 11-2). **Viral** infections include measles, German measles, cold sores, shingles, chickenpox, and warts. **Fungal** infections include the various ringworms, so-called because the typical lesions are ringshaped. The most common form

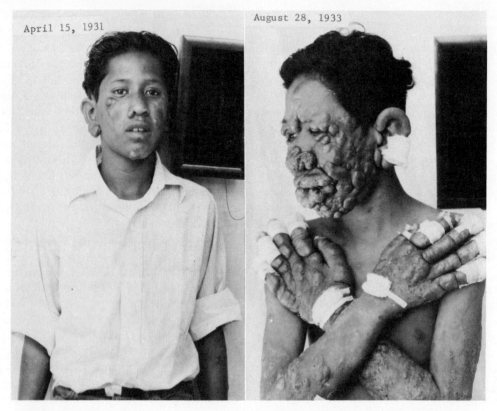

April 15, 1931

August 28, 1933

FIG. 11-2 ■ Leprosy. Progressive disease in a teenaged Filipino. Note dates. This occurred before sulfone (not sulfa) drugs were available.

Courtesy Dr. C. Binford, Washington, D.C.

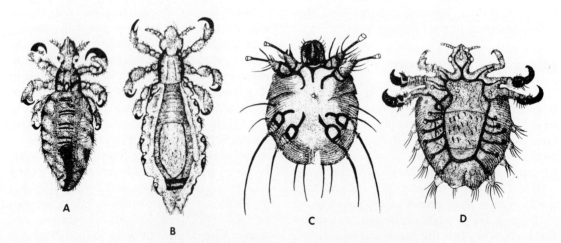

A

B

C

D

FIG. 11-3 ■ Ectoparasites. **A,** Head louse. **B,** Body louse. **C,** Itch mite. **D,** Pubic or crab louse.

Modified from Sutton, R.L., Jr.: Diseases of the skin, ed. 11, St. Louis, 1956, The C.V. Mosby Co.

of ringworm involves the scalp and feet (**athlete's foot**). **Ectoparasite** infections, usually referred to as **infestations**, include pediculosis and scabies. **Pediculosis** is an infestation with lice, namely, the head louse, the body louse, and the crab louse; **scabies** involves the itch mite (Fig. 11-3).

The treatment of skin infections generally centers on the use of antimicrobial drugs. For example, penicillin is a sure cure for scarlet fever, and gamma benzene hexachloride (Kwell) is a sure cure for pediculosis. Prevention is often possible, however, and, in a sense, certainly supercedes treatment. For example, vaccination is 100% effective in the prevention of measles and German measles, and almost always the prompt soap and water washing of a wound or laceration prevents subsequent infection. Again, extra care in drying the feet after bathing and a daily change of light socks (dusted with a medicated foot powder) will usually prevent athlete's foot. If one has possibly come in contact with a case of head lice (pediculosis capitis), a prompt shampooing (with a medicated product) will easily stem the tide.

■ Acne

Acne is a common, self-limited disease involving the **sebaceous glands**, usually first noted in the teenage years. In girls it may begin as early as age 8 to 10, or it may begin as late as age 20 to 30 in women. An interaction between hormones, sebum, and bacteria somehow determines the course and severity of the disease. Those with severe acne frequently have oily skin. Factors that worsen acne include menstruation, emotional upset, exposure to heavy oils and greases, seasonal changes, certain drugs, fondling or pinching lesions, and habitual resting of the chin in the hand while reading. Acne lesions predominate on the face but are also common on the chest and upper back; they include "blackheads," "whiteheads," small reddish skin elevations, cysts, and abscesses. If left alone acne tends to disappear slowly in the early twenties in men and somewhat later in women, but in all cases appropriate treatment will either decrease its severity or effect a cure. According to some authorities, an environmental change—to a warm, sunny climate with absence of high heat and humidity—may be more beneficial than medical treatment. The same, however, cannot be said for dietary changes. If certain foods are found to aggravate the condition, they should, of course, be avoided, but strict diets are probably worthless at best.

■ Dry skin

Mild to severe itching resulting from dry skin is one of the most common and uncomfortable dermatologic problems, although its cause is unknown. Dry skin can appear after exposure to soaps, to irritating cleaning products (disinfectants, cleansers, etc.), and to dry air in overheated rooms. (It is often called "winter itch.") It is important to use lotions to prevent severe itching because the scratching that may follow can lead to infection or long-term skin irritation. Many different kinds of moisturizers are available, ranging from heavy creams to light, nongreasy lotions. Although products vary greatly in price, the most expensive is not necessarily the best. The most important factor in choosing a moisturizer is the way it feels on your skin. Highly perfumed products should be avoided.

■ Corns and calluses

Corns and calluses are not necessarily minor complaints, especially "when you have them." They can be disabling. Both relate to the thickening of the **stratum corneum** (Fig. 11-1) at sites subject to prolonged friction, pressure, or shearing stress. Generally corns are better demarcated than calluses, and they are more painful; the favorite site is the top of the fifth toe. Additionally, small (seed) corns may be found anywhere on the sole of the foot. Calluses are more diffuse thickenings—painful on pressure—present most commonly on the upper sole behind the first and fifth toes. They are also seen as occupational marks, for example, the callused hands of a laborer or the callused fingers of a violinist. Removal of corns and calluses (by a podiatrist) treats only the result and not the cause of the problem. Poorly fitted footwear, foot malformations, faulty weight distribution, and the like must be corrected, or otherwise the painful growths will rapidly recur. Shoe supports, x-ray studies for anatomic defects, and referral to a podiatrist or orthopedic surgeon are essential measures in difficult cases.

■ Psoriasis

Psoriasis is a chronic and recurrent skin disease of unknown cause. It is characterized by dry, well-circumscribed, silvery, scaling lesions. The usual sites are the back and buttocks and the exterior surfaces of the elbows and knees. Some persons develop a joint involvement similar to rheumatoid arthritis. Heredity is a factor in about one third of the cases, and the disease is uncommon in blacks. Acute attacks usually clear up, but complete and permanent remission is rare. No therapeutic measure assures a cure.

■ Lupus erythematosus

Discoid lupus erythematosus (DLE) is a skin condition characterized by disklike patches with raised, red edges and depressed centers. These patches are covered with scales that eventually fall off, leaving a white scar. **Systemic** lupus erythematosus (SLE) is more serious. It is a chronic and often fatal disease with systemic repercussions involving collagen, the main supportive material of connective tissue. Typically, a morbid redness of the face spreads across the nose in a butter-

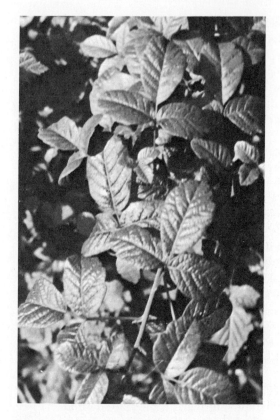

FIG. 11-4 ■ Poison oak, showing typical arrangement of leaves.

fly pattern. About 90% of cases occur in women and most of these before the menopause. Corticosteroid drugs are helpful but not curative.

■ Contact dermatitis

Contact dermatitis, as its name suggests, is an inflammation of the skin produced by substances in contact with the skin. Such substances appear without number. Well-known offenders include acids, alkalis, solvents, soaps, detergents, cosmetics, poison ivy, and poison oak (Fig. 11-4). Appropriate dermatologic preparations are highly effective, but common sense tells us that any kind of treatment is ineffective unless the offending substance is identified and removed. Further, contact dermatitis is often "photosensitive," which means that exposure to light is to be avoided as well.

■ Sunburn

Sunburn results from overexposure to the sun or sunlamps. (Sunlamps can produce skin damage, and dermatologists warn that they must be used with great caution.) Sunburn can occur even on cloudy days because **ultraviolet rays**, the causative component of sunlight, can filter through the clouds. Furthermore, since ultraviolet rays reach the skin through reflection (from snow, sand, or sidewalks), hats and umbrellas do not provide complete protection. Those with less melanin pigment—blue-eyed persons, redheads, blondes, freckled persons—withstand sunlight exposure poorly, burn easily, and suffer the chronic effects of sunlight exposure earlier in life. Studies have shown that mild sunburn will develop in fair-skinned persons after 15 to 20 minutes of noonday sun at latitude 40° N (Philadelphia, Toledo, Denver, northern California); 2 hours of such exposure can produce a severe burn. Certain drugs enhance the effect of sunlight on the skin, including thiazide diuretics, tetracycline antibiotics, phenothiazine tranquilizers, sulfa drugs, and oral medication for diabetes. Though most cause only a small amount of photosensitivity, thiazide diuretics (often prescribed for high blood pressure) and tetracycline can cause a severe sunburn.

Treatment of sunburn calls for plenty of fluids, aspirin, cool baths, and talcum powder dustings. Spray-on painkillers containing benzocaine provide temporary relief but can cause allergic reactions. Blistering, especially if widespread, should be seen by a physician. But the very best treatment is prevention—namely, gradual exposure to the sun, avoiding the early afternoon hours. The best cover-up available is a chemical one—any of the popular brand name **sunscreens** that contain either PABA (para-aminobenzoic acid) or a benzophenone derivative. These preparations absorb ultraviolet rays and allow gradual tanning. Another type of chemical protection, the **sunblock**, allows no tanning at all. It deflects the ultraviolet rays totally and is most useful in shielding lips, nose, and other extra-sensitive or already burned areas. A well-known sunblock is zinc oxide, an opaque white ointment often used by lifeguards and others whose jobs require constant exposure to the sun. Still another effective protection is clothing—cool, loose-fitting beach robes, caftans, long-sleeved shirts, and wide-brimmed hats.

■ Burns

Burns vary in degree, and their severity is measured by how deeply they penetrate and by the size of the area they cover. They range from a simple sunburn to one that can be life threatening. A **first-degree** burn is one with reddening and pain with no blister formation. A **second-degree** burn is one in which blisters do form, but underlying tissue damage does not occur. A **third-degree** burn inflicts deep tissue damage, and there is a lack of pain (because nerve endings are destroyed). A first-degree burn can almost always be treated at home. A second-degree burn, if it does not cover a large or critical area—hands, face, joints, or genitals—can usually be treated at home. Second-degree burns covering a large area and all third-degree burns are medical emergencies. Burns covering 50% or less of the body generally are not considered fatal, but those involving larger areas may result in death even under the best of circumstances. The immediate cause of most burn deaths is infection.

■ Cancer

Cancer of the skin outnumbers all other cancers. The estimated number of new cases per year is about 400,000, compared to some 120,000 new cases for cancer of the lung. Sunshine and its ultraviolet rays are considered

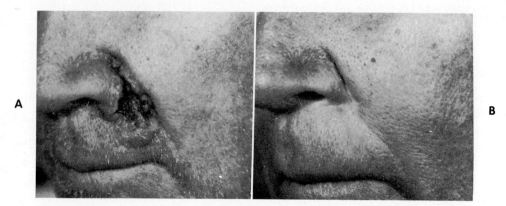

FIG. 11-5 ■ Cancer of nasolabial fold. **A,** Before treatment. **B,** Following x-ray therapy.

From del Regato, J.A., and Spjut, H.J.: Ackerman and del Regato's cancer: diagnosis, treatment, and prognosis, ed. 5, St. Louis, 1977, The C.V. Mosby Co.

the major cause. There is much support for this view. In the United States, for instance, skin cancer is three times more common in the southern part of the country than in the northern part. The "big three" among skin cancers are basal cell carcinoma, squamous cell carcinoma, and malignant melanoma. **Basal cell carcinoma,** which involves the basal cells of the deeper strata of the epidermis, accounts for well over three fourths of all malignancies of the skin but kills few of its victims because it does not metastasize. The upper half of the face (Fig. 11-5) and head is the classic site. The early lesion, usually a pale, pearly, raised nodule, slowly enlarges and eventually ulcerates. **Squamous cell carcinoma** is a true cancer in every sense of the word, above all, because it metastasizes to near and distant parts of the body. The lower lip is a favorite site, and pipe smoking may be a predisposing factor. **Malignant melanoma** is essentially a cancer of the melanocytes (the cells that produce melanin). It is about twice as common among whites as among blacks, and redheads and blondes are especially susceptible. Typically, the tumor begins as a black to brown nodule surrounded by a reddish halo of inflammation; soon small satellite lesions appear about

a half inch or so away. The nodule then enlarges, ulcerates, and progressively takes over adjacent tissues by direct extension and metastasis. These cancers are unpredictable. Some kill in a matter of months, whereas others smolder for years.

There are five ways to treat skin cancer: radiation, surgery, electrodesiccation (tissue destruction by heat), cryosurgery (tissue destruction by freezing), or application of drugs in the form of ointments or lotions (especially the drugs 5-fluorouracil and dimethyl sulfoxide [DMSO]). Additionally, immunotherapy (stimulating the patient's immune reaction) has been used successfully for patients with a number of extensive, superficial cancers as well as for those with precancerous lesions. For basal cell carcinoma and squamous cell carcinoma, cure is virtually assured with early detection and treatment. For malignant melanoma the outlook is not nearly as good. The 5-year survival rate for persons with this disease is 63% compared with 95% for persons with other kinds of skin cancer. In regard to prevention the American Cancer Society stresses the following: (1) avoid repeated overexposure to the sun (especially between 10 AM and 3 PM), (2) use sunscreens and sunblocks, and (3) wear protective clothing. Above all, remember that the immediate key to saving lives is the early detection and prompt and adequate treatment of a skin abnormality.

MAINTAINING HEALTHY SKIN

Consumers spend millions of dollars each year on wrinkle creams, skin bleaches to fade "age spots," oils, and other cosmetics in order to keep their skin looking young. At the same time they spend not only money but countless hours trying to tan the skin, in the belief that a tan will make them look healthy and more attractive. Unfortunately, most people do not realize that long periods of sun exposure are the major reason that skin looks wrinkled before old age. Signs of aging rarely appear in protected skin until sometime after the age of 50, and even then aging progresses very slowly. Tips for maintaining healthy, young-looking skin are as follows:

1. Wear sunscreens when skin is exposed to the sun and avoid the use of devices that can result in overexposure. Once skin shows signs of aging, the damage cannot be reversed, but further damage can be prevented.
2. To prevent dryness wear protective gloves when washing dishes and when using strong cleaning agents or other chemicals. Use mild soaps. Use petroleum jelly or other moisturizers as often as necessary, especially after bathing.
3. Wear soft clothing. Avoid strong detergents in the washing machine. Some fabric softeners can also cause skin irritation and itching.
4. Treat with caution the abrupt onset of generalized itching, for it can be a sign of certain diseases. If itching persists after taking preventive measures, check with your doctor.
5. Remember that many age-related skin changes, as well as most skin cancers, are

surgically correctable. Anyone over the age of 65 who has had skin cancer should see a dermatologist annually.

COSMETICS

Cosmetics are regulated by the Food and Drug Administration (FDA), U.S. Department of Health and Human Services, under the authority of the Food, Drug, and Cosmetic Act of 1938. This law was passed to prohibit the movement in interstate commerce of adulterated or misbranded foods, drugs, cosmetics, and medical devices. Another law affecting cosmetics is the Fair Packaging and Labeling Act. Its purpose is to ensure that packages and labels provide consumers accurate information about the identity of the product, the net contents, and the name and address of the manufacturer or distributor.

The Food, Drug, and Cosmetic Act defines cosmetics as articles that may be "rubbed, poured, sprinkled, or sprayed on, introduced into, or otherwise applied to the human body for cleansing, beautifying, promoting attractiveness, or altering the appearance without affecting the body's structure or functions." The law specifically excludes soap from the definition of a cosmetic, and ordinary soap is not regulated by the FDA. Some products most people consider cosmetics—and which often are promoted as cosmetics—actually are classified as drugs because they do affect the structure or functions of the body. These include antiperspirants, antidandruff shampoos, bleaching creams to lighten the skin, and products that prevent sunburn.

For the person buying a certain product, probably the most significant difference between an item classified as a cosmetic and one classified as a drug is that drugs must be proven safe and effective before they are put on the market. Premarketing proof of safety is not required of cosmetics, but the Food and Drug Administration can have a cosmetic removed from the market if it proves unsafe in actual use. Although not required by law to do so, most cosmetic manufacturers do test their products for safety. Even products that have been tested, however, can cause adverse reactions in persons who are allergic to the ingredients used in them.

In recent years the FDA has taken a number of important actions to protect the consumer. Most of these deal with labeling that must include adequate instructions for the safe use of the product and warnings about potential hazards. For example, products that use aerosol propellants have been labeled as possibly explosive with the danger of accidental discharges into the eyes. A special warning is required on feminine deodorant sprays to help prevent such adverse reactions as itching, burning, and blistering. The message cautions users, among other things, to "spray 8 inches from the skin." A proposal to label a warning on bubble bath products has been introduced, since prolonged or excessive use of bubble bath, particularly by children, is believed to contribute to cracking of the skin and subsequent inflammation or infection.

The FDA now requires that the ingredients used in cosmetics be listed on the product label. An ingredient listing can help a person avoid adverse reactions and can assist in the comparison of products. If you know you're allergic to a certain ingredient, you can check the label and avoid using products that contain it. If a certain cosmetic or type of product causes you problems, you and your doctor can check the ingredients and perhaps determine what is causing the trouble.

For many years companies have been producing items that they claim are "hypoallergenic" or "safe for sensitive skin" or "allergy tested." These statements have suggested that the products making the claims are less likely to cause allergic reactions than competing brands. But there has been no assurance that this actually is the case. At present there is no regulation by the FDA specifically defining or governing the use of "hypoallergenic" or similar terms. A person concerned about allergic reactions from cosmetics should understand one basic fact: There is no such thing as a "nonallergenic" cosmetic, that is, a cosmetic that can be guaranteed never to produce an allergic reaction. Furthermore, the basic ingredients in so-called hypoallergenic cosmetics usually are the same as those used in other cosmetics sold for the same purposes. Years ago some cosmetics contained harsh ingredients that had a high potential for causing adverse reactions. But these ingredients are no longer used. According to the FDA, no scientific studies exist to show that "hypoallergenic" cosmetics or products making similar claims actually cause fewer adverse reactions than competing conventional products.

Most cosmetic labels give directions for use, and sometimes this can be the most important part of the label. A product may be safe when used correctly but hazardous when not used according to directions. For example, a dipilatory cream may be safe when left on the skin for a few minutes but unsafe when left on too long. Some key points to remember about using cosmetics are:

1. Keep containers closed when they are not in use; this helps prevent contamination or decomposition of the product.
2. Do not use another person's cosmetics; they may be contaminated.
3. Do not use cosmetics on irritated or injured skin.
4. Keep cosmetics away from children.
5. When an adverse reaction occurs, discontinue using the product; if the problem persists, see a physician and give the doctor the cosmetic container and any labeling and directions that came with it.
6. Report any adverse reaction to the manufacturer.

▬▬ SELF-TEST

1. _____ corium
2. _____ vitamin D
3. _____ stratum corneum
4. _____ skin pigment
5. _____ deep fascia
6. _____ hair root base
7. _____ sebaceous glands
8. _____ sudoriferous glands
9. _____ insensible perspiration
10. _____ ceruminous glands
11. _____ "white crescent"
12. _____ Meissner's corpuscles
13. _____ pacinian corpuscles
14. _____ naked nerve endings
15. _____ subcutaneous tissue

a. sunlight
b. vapor
c. fat
d. lunula
e. pain
f. sweat
g. pressure
h. ligaments
i. touch
j. dermis
k. oil
l. keratin
m. wax
n. papilla
o. melanin

▬▬ STUDY QUESTIONS

1. Disorders and diseases of the skin are caused by factors either from within or from without. Explain what this means and give some examples.
2. Of the infections involving the skin that are cited in the text, how many are preventable by vaccination?
3. Ringworm infection has nothing to do with worms. Explain fully.
4. The prompt and thorough cleansing of a skin wound with soap and water is much more important than simply applying an antiseptic. Think of a number of reasons why this is true.
5. Pediculosis is caused by an insect (the louse), and scabies is caused by an arachnid (the itch mite). What is the fundamental difference between an insect and an arachnid?
6. There are three forms of lice infestation: pediculosis capitis, pediculosis corporis, and pediculosis pubis. These involve the crab louse, the head louse, and the body louse. Match up the infestation with the causative parasite.
7. Moisture, heat, and poor foot hygiene predispose to athlete's foot. Why?
8. "An interaction between hormones, sebum, and bacteria somehow determines the course and severity of acne." What clinical features of this disorder support this statement?
9. Keratolytic agents (for example, salicylic acid) soften or dissolve keratin. In what type of foot problem(s) would these agents be useful?
10. The cause of SLE (systemic lupus erythematosus) is not known, but its predominance in young women does point to at least one possible predisposing chemical factor. What could this be?
11. A case of poison ivy and a reaction to a "new kind" of hair spray are examples of what dermatologic disorder?
12. If a sunburn results in both reddening and blistering of the skin, what degree of burn is involved?
13. Based on their mode of action, what is the difference between a "sunscreen" and a "sunblock"?
14. What factors other than the degree of a burn are important in assessing severity?
15. Skin cancer outnumbers all other forms of cancer. Why?

CHAPTER 12

The endocrine system

The activities of the various tissues and organs of the body are subject to control by a system of chemical messengers as well as by the nervous system. These messengers, which are produced by endocrine glands, are called hormones. The effects they produce are many. Their varied and specific functions influence metabolism, growth, reproduction, sexuality, appearance, mental activity, expenditure of energy, development, maturation, aging, and general well-being. Overproduction or underproduction of certain hormones produces specific dysfunction and disease. The removal of certain endocrine glands is fatal unless corrective treatment is given. Hormones are so intimately related to health as to be of real interest to students who are attempting to understand themselves and others. Even the slightest variation in the activity of an endocrine gland may affect appearance, efficiency, or personality.

Thyroid gland

Parathyroid glands

Adrenal glands

Pituitary gland

Pancreas

Pineal gland

Gonads

Thymus

Prostaglandins

Enkephalins and endorphins

The endocrine, or **ductless**, glands of the body include the thyroid, the parathyroids, the thymus, the adrenals, the pituitary, the pineal, the pancreas, and the sex glands. They are shown in solid black in Fig. 12-1. The **hormones** they produce are picked up and carried away by the bloodstream. Unlike **exocrine** glands, such as the salivary glands and tear glands, they do not secrete through a duct. The products of the endocrine glands were named hormones (Gk. horman, to urge on, to stir up) because those first discovered had the effect of stimulating physiologic action. The name is not entirely suitable because some hormones "depress" rather than "excite," and others have still other functions. Although produced in extremely small quantities—"trace" amounts—they have remarkable effects in the regulation of bodily functions (Table 12-1). Functionally, the endocrine glands are related. Indeed, some hormones have the effect of stimulating the secretion of others or of supplementing their activities.

■ THYROID GLAND

The thyroid gland consists of two lobes connected by an "isthmus," and it weighs about 30 grams. Located in front of the larynx, it produces thyroxine and triiodothyronine, hormones rich in iodine. In fact, the thyroid is the principal reservoir for iodine in the human body. The amount of iodine in the gland varies from 50 times to several hundred times the amount found in the blood. The principal factor in maintaining enough iodine in the

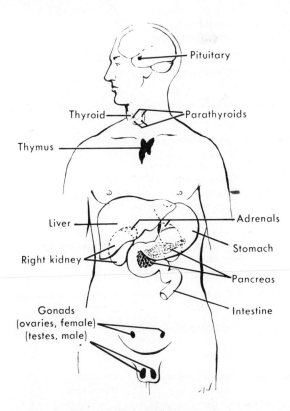

FIG. 12-1 ■ The endocrine system.

TABLE 12-1

The principal endocrine glands

Gland	Hormones	Main function	Hypofunction	Hyperfunction

Adrenals	1. Corticoids
	  a. Glucocorticoids
	    (cortisol)
	  b. Mineralocorticoids
	    (aldosterone)
		Mainly stability of body
		  state
		Help regulate metabolism
		Regulate water-mineral
		  balance
			Addison's disease	Cushing's syndrome
				Adrenogenital syndrome

	2. Epinephrine	Reserve mechanism for emergencies	No effect observed	Hypertension
	3. Norepinephrine 4. Androgens	Constricts blood vessels		Masculinization

Ovaries	1. Estrogens	Regulate reproductive
		  system
			Ovarian deficiency: in-
			  fantilism, decreased
			  fertility
				Precocious maturity

	2. Progesterone	Regulates menstruation,
		  lactation, and repro-
		  ductive system		

Pancreas	1. Insulin	Controls carbohydrate metabolism	Diabetes mellitus	Hypoglycemia
	2. Glucagon	Raises blood sugar		

Parathyroid	Parathyroid hormone	Regulates calcium and
		  phosphorus metabo-
		  lism
			Tetany	von Recklinghausen's
				  disease

Pineal	Melatonin	Sex cycle?	?	?

Pituitary	1. Anterior lobe
	  a. Growth hormone
	  b. Thyrotropin
	  c. Gonadotropins
	  d. Prolactin
	
	  e. Adrenocorticotropin
	    (ACTH)
	2. Posterior lobe
	  a. Vasopressin
	  b. Oxytocin
		Promotes growth
		Stimulates thyroid
		Regulate sex glands
		Regulates mammary
		  glands
		Helps regulate metabo-
		  lism
		
		Regulates body water
		Stimulates uterine con-
		  traction
			Dwarfism
			
			Diabetes insipidus
				Gigantism
				Acromegaly

Testes	Testosterone and others	Regulate male reproduc-
		  tive system
			Imperfect sex develop-
			  ment
				Precocious maturity

Thymus	Thymic hormone (?)	Aids in formation of white
		  blood cells and in im-
		  munity
			?	?

Thyroid	Thyroxine and triiodothy-
	  ronine
		Influences metabolism
		  and growth
			Cretinism
			Myxedema
				Thyrotoxicosis

thyroid gland is the amount of iodine that a person absorbs from daily food, and this in turn depends largely on the iodine content of the soil in the region. We get iodine mainly from fruits, grains, vegetables, and seafood. There seem to be some differences in the abilities of people to absorb and metabolize iodine when the food contains only limited amounts. There is a greater need for iodine during puberty, pregnancy, and lactation. The effect of thyroid hormones on both health and personality is marked because they regulate the metabolism of the body. They speed up the pulse, the respiration, the rate at which food is burned, and other body functions.

Perhaps the best known derangement of the thyroid gland is an enlargement called a **simple goiter**. This condition tends to be endemic in regions deficient in iodine. Such regions include the Great Lakes and Pacific Northwest in the United States, the Alps, the Pyrenees, and the Himalayas. As many as 80% of the Chinese men and women working on the Burma Road during World War II showed signs of simple goiter. The soils of Japan have a low iodine content, but the country is goiter free because the people eat much seafood, which is rich in iodine.

Most simple goiters show enlargements of the thyroid gland with little or no effect on general health. Similar glandular enlargments are found in domestic animals in goitrous areas. Individuals in such areas vary in their susceptibility to the development of goiter. The condition is prevented or improved by the addition of iodine-containing foods. It has been largely eliminated in many areas through the use of **iodized table salt**.

Serious conditions resulting from a deficiency of thyroid hormones (**hypothyroidism**) are cretinism and myxedema. **Cretinism** occurs in infants. Causes include faulty anatomic development of the gland, inborn errors of hormone biosynthesis, and a severe endemic iodine deficiency. In cretinism physical and mental development is retarded, and the child is misshapen. The abdomen protrudes. The body temperature is subnormal, and both the pulse and breathing are slow. The face lacks animation. The nose becomes flat. The hands are clumsy. The teeth are of poor quality, and they erupt late. Startling improvement is secured by the administration of thyroid extract. Severe hypothyroidism in youth or adulthood produces a similar condition known as **myxedema** (Fig. 12-2). It is characterized by low basal metabolism, sluggish mentality, thickened skin, and swelling of the face and hands and is treated with thyroid extract.

Hyperthyroidism, or overactivity of the gland, in which an increased amount of thyroxine is released into the blood, is known as Graves' disease or **thyrotoxicosis** (Fig. 12-3). This condition is marked by increased oxida-

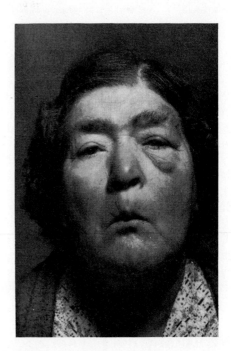

FIG. 12-2 ■ Person with myxedema.

From Schottelius, B.A., and Schottelius, D.D.: Textbook of physiology, ed. 18, St. Louis, 1978, The C.V. Mosby Co.

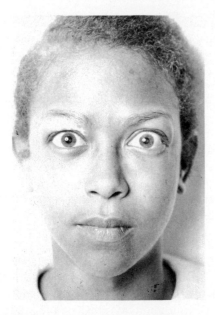

FIG. 12-3 ■ Person with thyrotoxicosis and exophthalmos.

From Schottelius, B.A., and Schottelius, D.D.: Textbook of physiology, ed. 18, St. Louis, 1978, The C.V. Mosby Co.

tion, excessive nervousness, a rapid heartbeat, increased blood pressure, and characteristic bulging of the eyes. A person suffering from such increased metabolism is usually high-strung and irritable. Relief may be given by surgically removing enough of the gland to restore endocrine balance or by prescribing radioactive iodine or certain antithyroid drugs.

Minor deviations in thyroid output occur in both directions with undoubted effects on personality. Sometimes the term "high thyroid" is applied to a thin, alert, excitable, nervous, irritable individual, and "low thyroid" is applied to a person with the opposite characteristics. It is, of course, a mistake to assume that such differences have a single cause.

■■■■■ PARATHYROID GLANDS

The parathyroid glands are four small bodies immediately behind the thyroid. The function of the parathyroids is to maintain the proper ratio of **calcium** and **phosphorus** in the blood. Removal of these glands causes the level of calcium ions in the blood to fall and the level of phosphate ions to increase. In children an insufficient supply of parathyroid hormone interferes with the development of bones. **Hyperparathyroidism** occurs when an excess of parathyroid hormone produces a high blood calcium level. Most of this calcium is withdrawn from the bones, rendering them soft, deformed, and easily broken. Also, calcium salts precipitate in the urine, forming kidney stones. **Hypoparathyroidism** is an insufficient secretion by these glands that leads to greatly increased neuromuscular excitability. Muscular twitchings and tetanic spasms occur. This condition, called **tetany**, usually follows accidental removal of or damage to the glands during thyroidectomy.

■■■■■ ADRENAL GLANDS

The adrenal glands are small flattened bodies lying on the outer, upper extremity of each kidney. They consist of two distinct parts, the **cortex** and the **medulla**, each producing its own characteristic secretion.

The hormones produced by the medulla are **epinephrine** and **norepinephrine**. Stimuli causing the release of these substances include pain, cold, emotions, stress, hemorrhage, lack of oxygen, and low blood sugar. When secreted into the bloodstream, epinephrine causes marked changes in the circulatory system. The rate of heartbeat is quickened, blood pressure is increased, and sugar is released into the bloodstream from reserves in the liver. The pupils dilate. Blood vessels of the skin, mucous membranes, and kidneys constrict, but others (coronary system, skeletal muscles, and lungs) dilate. Digestion is inhibited. There is an increased flow of blood to the muscles. Muscle fatigue is delayed. Epinephrine has been termed the

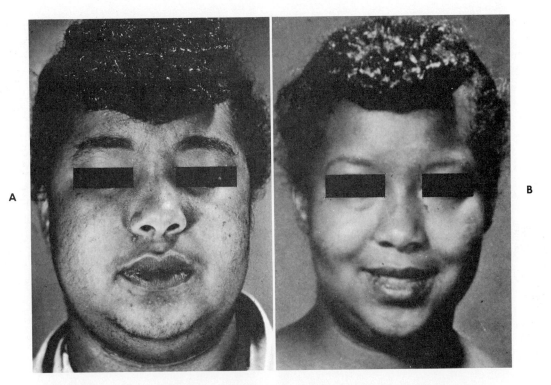

FIG. 12-4 ■ Cushing's syndrome, an endocrine derangement caused by excessive output of hormones by the adrenal cortex. **A,** Preoperative. **B,** Six months after removal of tumor from the adrenal cortex.

Courtesy Dr. William McKendree Jefferies, Highland View Hospital, Cleveland, Ohio.

"emergency hormone," since it brings into play the body processes on which self-preservation depends. The effect of norepinephrine is limited to the constriction of blood vessels.

Only minute quantities of epinephrine are normally present in the blood, the increased output being controlled by nervous excitation. Under the influence of strong emotions, such as fear, anger, joy, or grief, epinephrine is secreted into the bloodstream in increased amounts, and the body is instantly made ready for the performance of unusual physical feats. When these physiologic effects are being produced continually as the result of persistent worry, they are undesirable.

Thomas Addison in 1855 was the first to point out that the secretions of the adrenal cortex are essential to life. He described a severe deficiency that is known as **Addison's disease.** The symptoms include extreme weakness, a lowered metabolic rate, low blood pressure, severe prostration, great susceptibility to fatigue, infections, anesthetics, and anoxia (lack of oxygen), and a bronzelike pigmentation of the skin.

Of the several hormones produced by the adrenal cortex, the best known are **aldosterone** and **cortisol**, which seem capable of preventing certain altered reactions of body cells. Cortisol and its synthetic relatives (collectively referred to as **corticosteroids**) are used in the treatment of rheumatoid arthritis, allergic diseases, and a number of other conditions, including, of course, Addison's disease.

The production of cortical hormones is stimulated by the adrenocorticotropic hormone produced by the pituitary gland and commonly called ACTH. The medicinal administration of ACTH causes the body to increase its own production of cortisol.

An excess of adrenal cortical hormones (namely, cortisol and aldosterone) in the system produces a condition called **Cushing's syndrome**. Blood pressure increases, obesity develops, and hair grows profusely. There is hyperglycemia, bone dissolution, and muscular weakness. The treatment is surgical removal of the gland (Fig. 12-4).

The adrenal glands also produce **androgens** (male hormones) in both sexes. Normally the output is low and of little significance. Hyperactive glands, however, can cause masculinization in females.

■ PITUITARY GLAND

The pituitary gland is about the size of a pea and is located below the brain near the center of the head. It has an **anterior lobe** (anterior pituitary) and a **posterior lobe** (posterior pituitary). Its secretions have such extensive influence on the activity of other endocrine glands that it is sometimes called the "master gland."

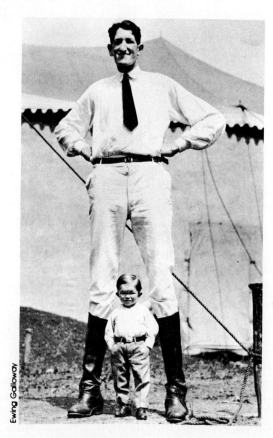

FIG. 12-5 ■ Gigantism and dwarfism.

Secretions of the anterior pituitary are produced in response to **releasing factors** from the brain's hypothalamus. Among the secretions of the anterior pituitary is a **growth hormone** (GH). Overproduction of this hormone in early youth leads to **gigantism** (Fig. 12-5). If secretion is increased after puberty, bones (especially those of the face, hands, and feet) enlarge, and a condition known as **acromegaly** (Fig. 12-6) is induced. Removal or destruction of the anterior lobe in early life leads to physical **dwarfism.** Circus midgets are usually dwarfs. The body proportions are nearly normal, but the size of all structures is greatly reduced. Mental development and function are usually at a normal level.

Other hormones of the anterior pituitary include gonadotropins, prolactin, ACTH, and TSH. **Gonadotropins** stimulate the development and release of ova and the production of female sex hormones. In the male they act on the testes to produce male hormones and influence the development of sperm. **Prolactin** stimulates the activity of the mammary glands following childbirth. The **adrenocorticotropic hormone** (ACTH), mentioned earlier, stimulates the adrenal cortex, and the **thyroid-stimulating hormone** (TSH) stimulates the thyroid gland to produce thyroxine and triiodothyronine.

The posterior pituitary produces the hormones **vasopressin** and **oxytocin**. Oxytocin has a stimulating effect on the muscles of the uterus during childbirth, and it promotes the secretion of milk from the mammary glands. Vasopressin, or antidiuretic hormone (ADH), regulates the amount of water the kidneys remove from the blood. Absence of this controlling factor leads to **diabetes insipidus**, which is marked by great thirst and the passage of a large amount of urine. Treatment centers on administration of ADH.

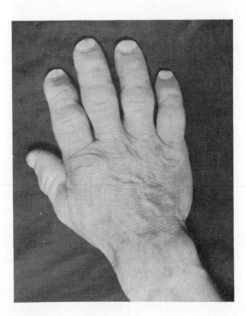

FIG. 12-6 ■ Acromegaly.

From Schottelius, B.A., and Schottelius, D.D.: Textbook of physiology, ed. 18, St. Louis, 1978, The C.V. Mosby Co.

PANCREAS

The pancreas, in addition to its "digestive cells," contains isolated groups of endocrine cells known as the islands of Langerhans. The beta cells of these islands produce **insulin** (L. insula, island), a protein hormone that regulates carbohydrate metabolism, specifically the utilization of glucose. Extensive or complete failure of the islands of Langerhans to secrete insulin causes the disease **diabetes mellitus**, which is characterized by thirst, enhanced appetite, urinary frequency, high blood glucose, weakness, emaciation, and the appearance of sugar in the urine. Untreated diabetes leads to coma and death. The United States Public Health Service estimates that there are about 4 million known case of diabetes in the United States and perhaps nearly as many more undiagnosed cases. Obesity and heredity are predisposing factors. In at least a fourth of the cases there is a family history of diabetes.

The discovery that insulin can be extracted from the pancreas of animals and that it ensures the proper use of glucose made possible the successful treatment of diabetes. In persons in whom the pancreas produces nearly enough insulin, the condition may be controlled by a modification of the diet. Drugs that can be taken orally aid some persons with mild diabetes by apparently stimulating the islands of Langerhans. If the disease is severe, insulin must be injected regularly. The amount needed is influenced by the amount of carbohydrate in the diet and by the amount of exercise the person takes. Exercise decreases the need for insulin by facilitating the burning of blood sugar.

Insulin shock, in which the blood sugar falls drastically below normal, develops when a diabetic person receives too much insulin. A similar condition can develop if the diabetic has too much exercise or too little food. There is an "all gone" feeling, with numbness and tingling of the lips, hands, and feet. Trembling, cold perspiration, muscular contractions, and prostration may follow. The body needs more sugar, and the eating of a lump of sugar or piece of candy or an orange gives prompt relief. Diabetic individuals commonly carry lump sugar or candy for such an emergency. Insulin shock is sometimes produced intentionally by the administration of insulin in the treatment of certain types of mental illness.

Some persons develop disturbances caused by the hyperfunctioning of the islands of Langerhans. The physiologic disturbance is **hypoglycemia** (low blood sugar). The condition may result in faintness, dizziness, sweating, and nervousness when the blood sugar level reaches an unduly low point.

Other cells in the islands of Langerhans, called alpha cells, produce the hormone **glucagon**, whose effect on carbohydrate metabolism is opposite to that of insulin. It has the ability to raise blood sugar and is secreted in response to hypoglycemia. Glucagon is used in the emergency treatment of insulin shock.

PINEAL GLAND

The pineal gland, a tiny white structure (about a tenth of a gram), shaped somewhat like a pine cone and buried nearly in the center of the brain, is, like the thymus, slowly yielding its secrets to the techniques of present-day biochemistry and neurophysiology. In the rat, at least, it now appears that the pineal gland is a neuroendocrine transducer, that is, a gland that converts nervous input into hormonal output. Specifically, the pineal gland manufactures a potent hormone called **melatonin**, which slows the **estrus**, or sex cycle. Moreover, sympathetic bombardment of the gland (as a consequence of impulses relayed from the retina on stimulation by light) inhibits the output of the hormone and thereby accelerates estrus. Thus the current view is that the pineal gland is a true "biologic clock" that regulates sexuality in mammals and, perhaps, the timing of menstrual cycles in humans. Future developments are awaited with enthusiasm.

GONADS

The testes of the male and the ovaries of the female produce spermatozoa and ova, respectively. In addition they act as endocrine glands. Before birth, secretions of these glands help to differentiate male and female sex organs. From birth to puberty the gonads are held in check by the pituitary's growth hormone. Pubertal development is influenced by their secretions (Chapter 13). Changes induced include the development of the breasts and the onset of menses in the female and the growth of a beard and the lowering of the pitch of the voice in the male.

■ Ovaries

The ovaries (in response to pituitary gonadotropins) produce estrogens and progesterone. **Estrogens** accelerate the growth of the accessory sex organs, prepare the uterus for the reception of the fertilized ovum, stimulate the enlargement of the mammary glands, and induce the development of secondary sex characteristics. **Progesterone** is produced by the corpus luteum, which is formed from the follicle from which an ovum has erupted. Progesterone's function is to prepare the membrane lining the uterus for the reception and development of the fertilized ovum. It inhibits the maturation of additional follicles, and thereby ovulation, and prevents menstruation during pregnancy. If the ovum is not fertilized, the corpus luteum undergoes resorption, and menstruation occurs.

When the ovum is fertilized and pregnancy proceeds, the corpus luteum does not degenerate but functions as an endocrine organ for part of the pregnancy, producing both progesterone and estrogens. At childbirth these hormones promptly decrease in the body, thus permitting increase in prolactin, which stimulates milk production.

■ Testes

The testes produce male sex hormones (**androgens**), the most important being **testosterone**. This hormone controls the development of the sex organs and the development and maintenance of the secondary sex characteristics, and it also influences psychosexual behavior and general body metabolism. (The effect of castration on adult animals is seen in the lack of aggressiveness in an ox compared with that of a bull.) There is usually a gradual diminution of sex gland activity rather than an abrupt cessation with advanced age.

THYMUS

The thymus is a flat, elongated gland located behind the sternum. Ordinarily it atrophies between ages 4 and 16 years. It is divided into two pyramid-shaped lobes, which, in turn, are subdivided into numerous lobules. Each lobule displays an outer cortex and an inner medulla. In humans if the sex glands have failed to develop at the age of puberty or have been removed prior to this age, the thymus does not atrophy. The thymus aids in the development of **lymphocytes** (a type of white blood cell) and plays a key role in the body's immunologic system.

PROSTAGLANDINS

The prostaglandins, a family of hormone-like fatty acids present throughout the tissues of the body, are among the most potent of all known biologic materials. Their name derives from the fact that they were first isolated from the prostate gland. Their various effects are numerous: lowering and increasing blood pressure, contracting the uterus, decreasing gastric acidity, relaxing the bronchial tubes, slowing the heart, providing contraception, and so on. Recent work points to the cell membrane as the site of the formation of these agents and also as the site of their basic action. Potential medicinal uses of the prostaglandins include the treatment of high blood pressure, bronchial asthma, stuffy nose, anaphylactic shock, fluid retention, delayed labor, and infertility.

ENKEPHALINS AND ENDORPHINS

Enkephalins and endorphins are recently discovered hormones that have been isolated from the brain and pituitary gland. Although the precise biologic function of these compounds is still uncertain, on an experimental basis (in both humans and animals) they act as potent analgesics in certain types of pain—specifically, pain relieved by morphine and other opiates. Clearly these agents will serve as key tools to unlock the mystery of pain, on the one hand, and its control, on the other.

SELF-TEST

1. __F__ chemical messenger
2. __J__ endocrine glands
3. __N__ simple goiter
4. __A__ adult hypothyroidism
5. __L__ infant hypothyroidism
6. __M__ hyperthyroidism
7. __K__ hypoparathyroidism
8. __B__ hyperparathyroidism
9. __E__ adrenal cortex
10. __H__ adrenal medulla
11. __C__ anterior pituitary
12. __I__ posterior pituitary
13. __G__ beta cells
14. __O__ estrogens
15. __D__ androgens

a. myxedema
b. stones
c. gigantism
d. testes
e. cortisol
f. hormone
g. insulin
h. epinephrine
i. oxytocin
j. "ductless"
k. tetany
l. cretinism
m. thyrotoxicosis
n. iodine
o. ovary

STUDY QUESTIONS

1. What is the basic structural difference between an endocrine gland and an exocrine gland?
2. Hormones are sometimes referred to as "chemical messengers." Does this strike you as an accurate designation?
3. Endocrine dysfunctions and diseases are essentially a matter of "too little" or "too much." What does this mean?
4. "Simple goiter" and "endemic goiter" are synonymous expressions. Explain.

5. Simple goiter has "little or no effect on the general health." Why?
6. What specifically is the purpose of giving thyroid extract to persons with hypothyroidism?
7. What is the purpose of surgery in the treatment of hyperthyroidism?
8. Most cases of hypoparathyroidism are related to thyroidectomy. Why?
9. What is the difference between "tetany" and "tetanus"?
10. What do Addison's disease and Cushing's syndrome have in common?
11. The pituitary gland is sometimes referred to

as the "master gland." Cite examples to support this statement.

12. Gigantism and acromegaly have the same basic cause. What is it?

13. What two pituitary hormones specifically relate to childbirth?

14. Discuss the relationship between stress and the adrenal medulla.

15. Insulin injections (for diabetes mellitus) are certainly a burden. Why not give insulin orally?

CHAPTER 13

The reproductive system

The reproductive system differs fundamentally from the other body systems because its purpose is to ensure survival of the species rather than the individual. But there is a good measure of irony and paradox in this statement because the system obviously necessitates "sex drive," a behavioral force with deep implications for the individual. Stated otherwise, the reproductive system has a unique biologic purpose and colorful psychologic side effects. In short, it is the body system with the most palpable psychosocial ramifications. In the framework of strict biology the basic function of the male reproductive system is to produce and introduce sperm into the female reproductive tract for the purpose of fertilization; the function of the female reproductive system is to produce ova and provide the appropriate environment (within the uterus) for the evolution of the fertilized egg into a new individual.

Male reproductive system

Female reproductive system

Sexual response

Contraception

Disorders and diseases

n the this chapter we shall consider the structure and function of both the male and the female reproductive systems in some detail, together with the highlights of important disorders and diseases that affect them.

MALE REPRODUCTIVE SYSTEM

The reproductive apparatus in the male includes the testes, seminal ducts, seminal vesicles, certain glands, the urethra, and the penis (Fig. 13-1). These structures are discussed in the order named, and in studying them the student should make full use of the accompanying illustrations.

Testes

The testes (sing., testis), the male gonads, are ovoid bodies enclosed in the **scrotum**, a cutaneous pouch suspended from the pubic region. In the fetus, however, they lie within the lower abdominal cavity until about 2 months before birth, when they descend into the scrotum. In the event the testes do not descend and the condition is not corrected, sterility results, for human spermatozoa cannot properly develop or thrive unless their environment is below body temperature, as it is in the scrotum.

The interior of the testis is divided by fibrous partitions into a number of wedge-shaped lobes, each containing one to three **seminiferous tubules**. As shown in Fig. 13-2, these tubules eventually become the ductus epididymis (or **epididymis**). This structure, located on the back of the testis, in turn gives rise to the **ductus deferens**. Also called the **vas deferens**, or **seminal duct**, the ductus deferens ascends the back border of the testis and enters the abdominal cavity, where it travels

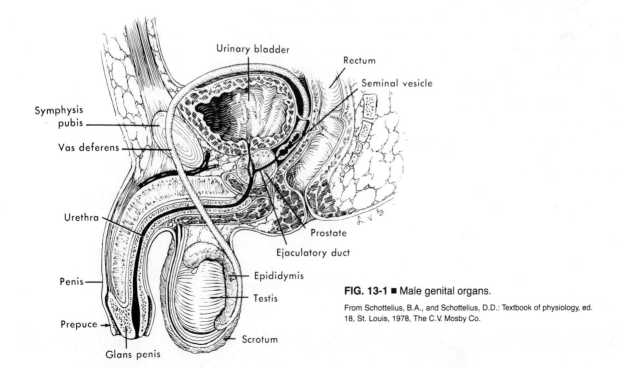

FIG. 13-1 ■ Male genital organs.

From Schottelius, B.A., and Schottelius, D.D.: Textbook of physiology, ed. 18, St. Louis, 1978, The C.V. Mosby Co.

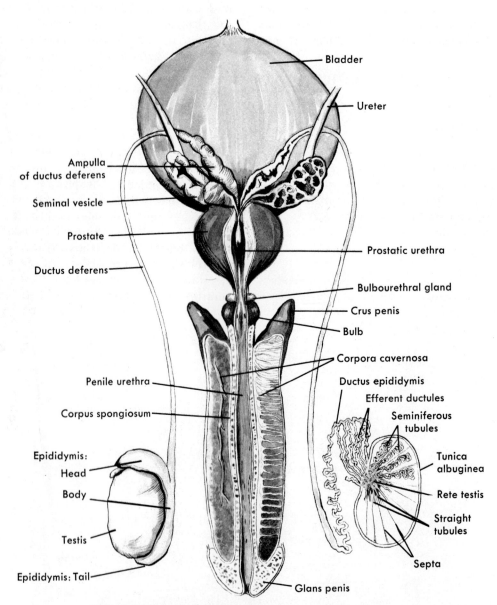

FIG. 13-2 ■ "Exploded" diagram of the male reproductive system.

From DiDio, L.J.A.: Synopsis of anatomy, St. Louis, 1970, The C.V. Mosby Co.

several inches before joining the seminal vesicle.

As discussed in Chapter 12, the testis also serves as an endocrine gland that produces male hormones called **androgens**, the most important of which is **testosterone**. This hormone is essential to male sexual development.

Seminal vesicles

The seminal vesicles are two coiled tubes situated just behind the lower portion of the bladder. Each joins a vas deferens and, in so doing, gives rise to the **ejaculatory duct**, a short tube that passes through the prostate gland to join the prostatic urethra.

Glands

The accessory male glands include the prostate and the bulbourethral (Cowper's glands). The **prostate** is about the size of a walnut and surrounds the neck of the bladder and the urethra. Its median and two lateral lobes are composed partly of glandular matter and partly of muscular fibers, the latter encircling the urethra. The **bulbourethral glands** also lie near the urethra. The prostate and these glands together secrete a thin fluid that enters into the formation of semen.

Urethra

The male urethra is a membranous tube that conveys urine and semen to the surface; it extends from the neck of the bladder to the outside opening and is about 20 cm long. The urethra is divided into three parts on the basis of the structures through which it passes (Fig. 13-1): the prostatic, the membranous, and the cavernous (or penile) portions. About the membranous portion is a band of muscle fibers (**external sphincter**) that remains contracted except during urination and ejaculation.

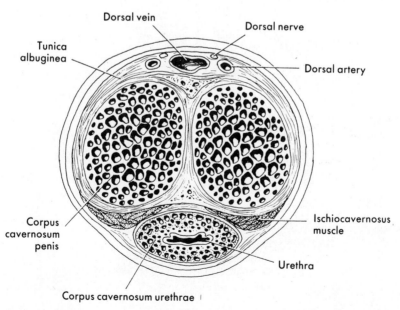

FIG. 13-3 ■ Cross section of penis. Note especially the three columns of spongy tissue.

Modified from Francis, C.C, and Martin, A.H.: Introduction to human anatomy, ed. 7, St. Louis, 1975, The C.V. Mosby Co.

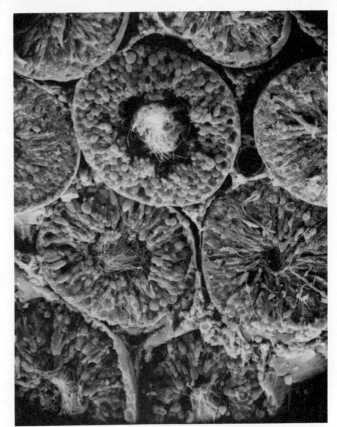

FIG. 13-4 ■ Scanning electron micrograph of seminiferous tubules. Tails of spermatozoa are clearly evident. (×210.)

Courtesy Drs. R.G. Kessel and R. Kardon.

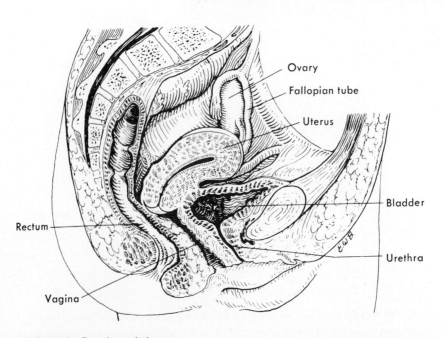

Ovary

Fallopian tube

Uterus

Bladder

Urethra

Rectum

Vagina

FIG. 13-5 ■ Female genital organs.

From Schottelius, B.A., and Schottelius, D.D.: Textbook of physiology, ed. 18, St. Louis, 1978, The C.V. Mosby Co.

◼ Penis

The penis, the male organ of sexual intercourse (coitus), consists of three divisions: the root, the body, and the extremity, or glans penis. The root is attached to the pubic bone by the crura, or extremities, of the corpora cavernosa penis and the corpus cavernosum urethrae (corpus spongiosum penis) (Fig. 13-3). Through the latter passes the urethra. The glans penis is covered with mucous membrane and is ensheathed by the prepuce, or foreskin. The removal of the foreskin is called **circumcision**.

◼ Semen

The collective purpose of the male structures just described is to produce and deliver semen—a whitish fluid composed of sperm cells, or spermatozoa, suspended in the nutrient secretions contributed by the prostate, the seminal vesicles, and the Cowper's glands. The spermatozoa arise in the seminiferous tubules (Fig. 13-4) and are conveyed to the epididymis through the complex system of channels mentioned earlier. Here they assemble, mature, and await discharge. The normal sperm count ranges from 20 million to 200 million per ml of semen.

◼ Intercourse

Sexual union between male and female (at the "mechanical level") amounts to insertion of the erect penis into the vagina, followed by **ejaculation** (the sudden expulsion of semen). Erection results from nerve stimuli that cause the spaces in the spongy, or erectile, penile tissue (corpora cavernosa penis and corpus cavernosum urethrae) to fill with blood and the venous outlets simultaneously to close. In this fashion the erectile tissue is expanded by the increased blood pressure, and the penis takes on an overall length, on the average, of 15 cm. At climax, ejaculation results from the convulsive en masse contraction of the epi-

didymis, seminal ducts, and seminal vesicles, expelling semen through the urethra. The amount of semen ejaculated varies from 3 to 7 ml.

◼◼◼ FEMALE REPRODUCTIVE SYSTEM

The female reproductive system consists of the ovaries, the uterine tubes, the uterus, the vagina, and the vulva (Fig. 13-5).

◼ Ovaries

The ovaries, or female gonads, each about the size and shape of an almond, are located in a shallow depression on the lateral wall of the pelvis (one on each side) and are connected to the back of what is called the **broad ligament** (Fig. 13-6). Another ligament, a fold of peritoneum that passes from the pelvic wall to the ovary, carries blood vessels and nerves.

The ovary is made up of thousands of **ovum-containing follicles** (Fig. 13-7). The fetal ovaries and the ovaries of prepubertal females consist almost entirely of immature follicles, whereas the ovaries of sexually mature females develop graafian (mature) follicles. This process does not occur until the time of puberty because before then the follicle-stimulating hormone (FSH) is not available. Of special interest also is the fact that only the mature graafian follicle can produce hormones and discharge its ovum (egg).

◼ Uterine tubes

The uterine (or **fallopian**) tubes are slender tubes (about 10 cm long) that run from the upper lateral angle of the uterus to the region of the ovary on the same side (Fig. 13-6). They are attached to the broad ligament, and each enlarges into a funnel-shaped mouth called the **infundibulum**. The rim of the latter structure is formed into fringelike extensions called **fimbriae**. To propel along the ova passed into the

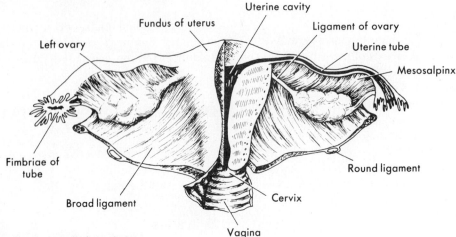

FIG. 13-6 ■ Uterus and allied structures.

Modified from Francis, C.C., and Martin, A.H.: Introduction to human anatomy, ed. 7, St. Louis, 1975, The C.V. Mosby Co.

infundibula, the mucosa of the tubes contain cilia and the walls contain smooth muscle.

■ Uterus

The uterus is the hollow, muscular, pear-shaped organ that houses the embryo and fetus. It is about 7.5 cm long, 5 cm wide, and 2.5 cm thick and has a broad, flattened body above and a narrow, cylindrical part, called the **cervix,** below. The rounded portion that passes above the openings of the fallopian tubes is referred to as the **fundus.** The organ is anchored to the pelvic walls, rectum, and bladder by the broad ligaments and by a number of other ligaments. As shown in Fig. 13-8, the uterine cavity opens into the vagina through the cervical canal. The walls of the uterus are formed of muscle (the **myometrium**), and its lining consists of a very special mucous membrane called the **endometrium.** As we shall soon see, the latter tissue plays a key role in the reproductive process.

■ Vagina

The vagina, the curved, collapsible canal leading from the vulva to the cervix, receives

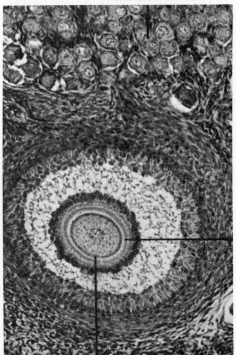

FIG. 13-7 ■ Section of cortex of rat ovary showing ovum within follicle. (×640.)

From Bevelander, G., and Ramaley, J.A.: Essentials of histology, ed. 8, St. Louis, 1979, The C.V. Mosby Co.

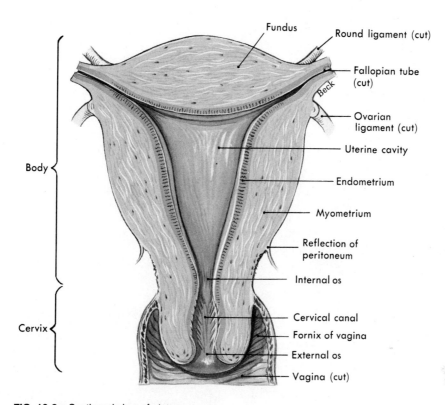

FIG. 13-8 ■ Sectioned view of uterus.

From Anthony, C.P., and Thibodeau, G.A.: Textbook of anatomy and physiology, ed. 10, St. Louis, 1979, The C.V. Mosby Co.

the erect penis during intercourse. It is lined with a mucous membrane thrown into transverse folds, and its walls are composed of smooth muscle. The vagina is about 8 cm long and is capable of great distention. In the virgin the vaginal orifice is partly closed by a fold of mucous membrane called the **hymen**. As a consequence of sexual intercourse and childbirth, this structure in time becomes fragmentary. The condition of the hymen on vaginal examination may have medicolegal significance in some cases of rape.

■ Vulva

The vulva, the region of the external genital organs, consists of the mons pubis, the labia majora, the labia minora, the vestibule, and the clitoris (Fig. 13-9). The **mons pubis**, or mons veneris ("mount of Venus"), is a cushionlike, rounded prominence overlying the symphysis pubis. After the age of puberty, this area becomes covered with hair. The **labia majora** (sing., labium majus) are the two large folds of skin and fatty tissue that extend backward and downward from the mons pubis to within about 2.5 cm of the anal opening. The skin of the labia majora contains hair follicles and sebaceous glands. Inner to and lying under the cover of these structures are the **labia minora** (sing., labium minus), two smaller folds of mucous membrane extending backward from the clitoris. The labia minora do not contain hair follicles but have many glands and blood vessels. The cleft between them leads into the **vestibule**, the slight recess containing the vaginal and urethral orifices. Opening into the vestibule are two ducts from Bartholin's glands,

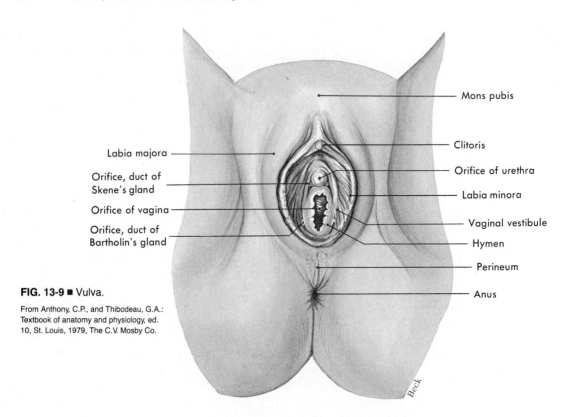

Mons pubis

Clitoris

Orifice of urethra

Labia minora

Vaginal vestibule

Hymen

Perineum

Anus

Labia majora

Orifice, duct of
Skene's gland

Orifice of vagina

Orifice, duct of
Bartholin's gland

FIG. 13-9 ■ Vulva.

From Anthony, C.P., and Thibodeau, G.A.:
Textbook of anatomy and physiology, ed.
10, St. Louis, 1979, The C.V. Mosby Co.

which secrete small amounts of lubricating fluid. The **clitoris**, the small, elongated body situated at the anterior angle of the vulva, corresponds to the penis in the male. It is composed of erectile tissue and becomes hard and erect upon sexual stimulation.

■ Mammary glands

The mammary glands, or breasts, are the milk-secreting organs in the female (Fig. 13-10). They are composed of glandular tissue organized into some 20 lobes, which, in turn, are organized into lobules. The lobes are partitioned by connective tissue, and the whole mass is embedded in a variable but large amount of fatty tissue. At its center the breast is surmounted by the **nipple**—a small, dark, conical structure composed of erectile tissue. The lactiferous (milk) ducts meet here and open to the exterior on its surface. About the nip-

ple is a circular area of pigmented skin known as the **areola**.

Before the age of puberty the mammary glands are composed mostly of connective tissue, but with the onset of puberty the ducts and glandular tissue undergo rapid development. This rapid physiologic activity stems from the abundance of female hormones. Estrogens stimulate development of the duct system, and progesterone stimulates the glands proper. This is especially true during pregnancy, when these hormones reach their highest levels.

Lactation. The secretion of milk by the breasts (lactation) is provoked chiefly by **prolactin**, the lactogenic hormone of the anterior pituitary. It is believed that the sudden drop in the high levels of estrogen and progesterone at the end of pregnancy brings about the release of prolactin. Finally, the act of sucking plays a role by means of **oxytocin**. This hor-

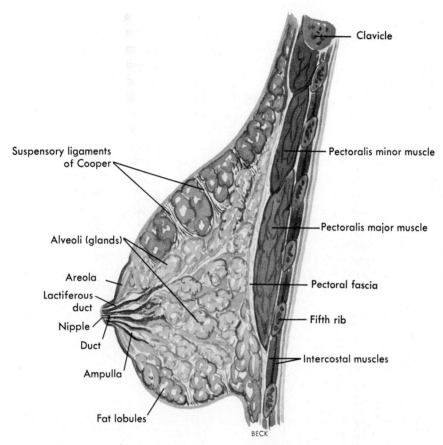

Clavicle

Suspensory ligaments
of Cooper

Pectoralis minor muscle

Pectoralis major muscle

Alveoli (glands)

Areola

Pectoral fascia

Lactiferous
duct

Fifth rib

Nipple

Duct

Intercostal muscles

Ampulla

Fat lobules

BECK

FIG. 13-10 ■ Lateral view of breast (sagittal section).

From Anthony, C.P., and Thibodeau, G.A.: Textbook of anatomy and physiology, ed. 10, St. Louis, 1979, The C.V. Mosby Co.

mone does not increase the production of milk, but it does stimulate its release by contracting the glands and milk ducts.

■ Menstrual cycle

The periodic discharge of blood from the vagina (**menstruation**) is only one phase of a tremendously interesting hormonal time-piece whose mainspring is situated in the anterior pituitary. When a girl reaches the age of 10 to 14 years, the anterior pituitary starts to secrete the **follicle-stimulating hormone** (**FSH**) and the **luteinizing hormone** (**LH**). The follicle-stimulating hormone causes a few of the immature follicles to grow and release estrogens, one of the two major types of female sex hormones (Fig. 13-11). A few days after the release of FSH, the pituitary starts putting out LH, which increases the rate of follicular growth and secretion even more. Finally, one of the follicles becomes so large that it ruptures, expelling its ovum (**ovulation**). When this happens, the follicular cells (still under the influence of LH) increase in size, become fatty and yellow, and thereby become a structure called the **corpus luteum**.

The corpus luteum secretes large quantities of both estrogens and progesterone. Estrogens cause the endometrium to grow in thick-

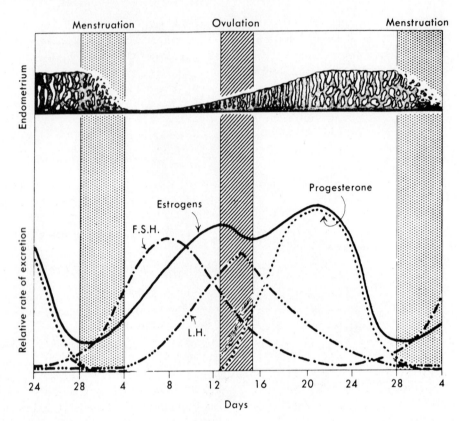

FIG. 13-11 ■ Menstrual cycle in graphic form. *FSH*, Follicle-stimulating hormone; *LH*, luteinizing hormone.

ness (Fig. 13-11), and progesterone enhances endometrial blood flow and nutrient secretion. The purpose of this process, of course, is to provide a suitable environment in which the fertilized ovum can grow.

If fertilization occurs, the developing ovum itself becomes an endocrine gland and releases a gonadotropic hormone that sustains the corpus luteum. Otherwise, the corpus luteum halts its activity, and the output of estrogens and progesterone drops to low levels. As a consequence, the endometrium degenerates and sloughs off into the uterine cavity; the debris, or **menses** (averaging about 60 ml), contains blood, mucus, and dead endometrial cells. While this sloughing process is going on,

the low levels of estrogen and progesterone stimulate the output of FSH and thereby set the stage for a new cycle.

With these facts in mind, the student should carefully study the graphic representation of the cycle presented in Fig. 13-11. In addition to distilling the information already discussed, the illustration gives the arithmetical data for the "statistical woman," that is, a cycle of 28 days, menstruation lasting 4 days, and ovulation occurring on the fourteenth day. Note especially that the cycle begins and ends on the first day the menses appears.

Period of fertility. Since the ovum can be fertilized by a sperm cell only during the 24-hour period after ovulation, and since the sperm cell can live in the vaginal canal usually for no more than 72 hours, it follows that fertilization does not ordinarily occur unless there is intercourse shortly before, during, or shortly after ovulation. Because ovulation in most instances occurs on or about the fourteenth day of a 28-day cycle, the meeting of the ovum and sperm is statistically most likely to occur somewhere around the thirteenth, fourteenth, or fifteenth day. Although many women have cycles as short as 20 days or as long as 40 days, it appears that ovulation still follows a rather definite schedule, that is, 14 days before menstruation. For example, if a woman has regular cycles, say of 33 days' duration, ovulation will occur on or about the nineteenth day (33 − 14 = 19). When the cycles are erratic (for example, 28 days one time, 20 the next, 35 the next, and so on), ovulation cannot be predicted with accuracy.

Menopause. In the average woman at about the age of 47 years, the follicles no longer secrete their hormones in full amounts, and the monthly periods grow irregular and stop. This is termed the **menopause**. Aside from signaling life's advancing years, the menopause is often accompanied by distressing physical and emotional signs and symptoms such as nervousness, headache, "hot flashes," and the like. Since the syndrome is usually benefited by estrogenic therapy, there is good reason to believe that the sudden drop in hormone output is the underlying cause of the menopausal symptoms. Psychosomatic factors undoubtedly play a role, perhaps the major role in many instances.

■ Intercourse

The sexual act is enhanced by the swelling of the erectile tissue about the vaginal opening and the secretion of large quantities of fluid and mucus by the vaginal walls. The tight but distensible and lubricated opening thus provided intensifies the stimulation resulting from the to-and-fro movement of the penis in the vaginal canal. Sensations also arise in the clitoris from the movement relayed through the labia. The climax itself is characterized by a "strong, exotic sensation" and by slow, rhythmic peristalsis-like contractions of the vagina. These effects may serve to hasten along the ejaculated semen into the cervical canal. Although the sexual act is said to reach its highest emotional development when the male and female experience climax at the same time, this is by no means a prerequisite for successful fertilization. Indeed, fertilization is easily accomplished by artificial insemination.

■ SEXUAL RESPONSE

The pioneer studies of Masters and Johnson on the precise physiologic nature of the sexual response indicated that males have only one typical response, whereas females have at least three. Nonetheless, for both sexes a given response was found to consist of four phases: excitement, plateau, orgasm, and resolution. The **excitement phase** is characterized by erection of the penis in the male, and enlargement (in length and diameter) of the vagina and clitoris in the female. The **plateau phase** amounts to an extension of the excitement phase—namely, the penis and testes increase in size in the male, and there is full expansion of two thirds of the vagina in the female; heart rate ranges from 100 to 160 beats per minute in both sexes. The **orgasmic phase** is characterized by ejaculation in the male and by vaginal, uterine, and pelvic contractions in the female. The **resolution phase** is characterized by the rapid loss of vasocongestion (blood engorgement) and penile erection in the male and the gradual loss of pelvic and clitoral vasocongestion in the female; the heart rate returns to about normal in both sexes. Masters and Johnson found that multiple orgasms are rather common in women (sometimes several in rapid succession) but decidedly uncommon in men.

Orgasm in the male, as indicated, is well defined and virtually synonymous with ejaculation. The details of orgasm in the female are still open to debate and speculation. Indeed, Masters and Johnson have theorized that the female orgasm may depend more on the woman's feelings for her partner than actual physical stimulation. At the physiologic level many researchers believe that there are two kinds of orgasm—**clitoral** and **vaginal**—and further that a given woman may experience neither, either, or both. According to Fox and Fox the vaginal orgasm seems to be intensely emotional and always satisfying, whereas the clitoral is somewhat "localized" and not always completely satisfying. Psychologically and philosophically, however, the true orgasm may simply be the tip of the overwhelming feeling of love occasioned by the sexual act.

■ Masturbation

Masturbation is the excitation of the genital organs, usually to orgasm, by means other than sexual intercourse. Although the word comes from the Latin (L. manus, hand + stuprave, to defile), meaning to "defile by hand," it should be noted that masturbation is performed by just about any means, including the use of pillows in males and electric vibrators in females. Masturbation has long been incorrectly associated, in the minds of some people, with perversion and mental illness, and yet it is a sexual activity practiced by the majority of human beings at least sometime in their lives. The naturalness of the act is further underscored by the fact that the subhuman primate engages in self-stimulation of the genitals. The male rhesus monkey masturbates even in the presence of the female.

Researchers say that almost all men and a majority of women masturbate to orgasm at least a few times during their lives. In Kinsey's studies 92% of the men had masturbated to orgasm at least once. Most of the males began between the ages of 13 and 15, whereas

most of the 58% of the females who had masturbated had not started before age 25, 30, or 35. The more recent Hunt Survey gathered much the same information. Interestingly, Kinsey found that the average woman reaches orgasm 95% of the time when masturbating compared to the much lower figure of 73% of the time during intercourse. Furthermore, Masters and Johnson found that masturbation produces the most intense orgasm in women.

■ CONTRACEPTION

The contraception revolution notwithstanding, birth control remains a problem for sexually active couples and is one of the greatest areas of sexual ignorance. The pill, the IUD, and the vasectomy, all hailed in their time as "the answer," have been subjected to agonizing reappraisals. There is still no perfect contraceptive—100% effective, safe, convenient, easily available, inexpensive, reversible, and without distressing side effects. The best that can be said is this: Couples who want to keep sexually active without fear of pregnancy must search for the method of birth control most suitable to their needs. This, of course, brings up such matters as life-style, age, health, and priorities. For example, women who smoke should avoid the pill because smoking tends to enhance side effects, some of which can be dangerous. The contraceptives in current use are described as follows.

■ Oral contraceptives

Oral contraceptives are synthetic female hormones that inhibit ovulation. The regular "pill" contains a **progestin** and an **estrogen**; the so-called minipill contains only a progestin. The pill is 98% to 99% effective, and the minipill is 97% to 99% effective. The minipill has fewer side effects but must be taken every day without fail. (The regular pill has a margin of error.) Possible side effects from the pill include breakthrough bleeding, nausea, breast tenderness, headache, depression, weight changes, changes in libido, cystitis, blood clots, stroke, high blood pressure, and gallbladder disease. Possible minipill side effects include menstrual irregularity, nausea, headache, vaginal discharge, depression, cardiovascular disorders, and ectopic pregnancy.

A promising male contraceptive is a chemical called gossypol. This chemical, extracted from the cotton plant, selectively inhibits an enzyme necessary for normal metabolism in sperm and in sperm-generating cells in the testes. However, gossypol has potential risks, which means that current research involves the development of related agents that are free of extraneous effects.

■ Intrauterine device

The intrauterine device (IUD) is a twist of plastic inserted into the uterus that somehow prevents conception or implantation of the fertilized ovum. Studies show a user effectiveness of 94% to 99%, an effectiveness close to that of the pill. Possible side effects include heavy menstrual flow, cramping, breakthrough bleeding, painful intercourse, skin rashes, perforation of the uterus, ectopic pregnancy, and pelvic infection (that can result in sterility).

■ Diaphragm

The diaphragm is a dome-shaped rubber device with a flexible rim that is inserted into the vagina to cover the cervix and thereby prevent the entrance of sperm into the uterus. Before insertion it must be coated with a spermicide. Needless to say, there can be technical problems with this form of contraception, and not all women can use a diaphragm. Above all, the user must be highly motivated and conscientious. Effectiveness ranges from a low of 80% to a high of 97%. Possible side effects include local irritation and increased susceptibility to bladder infections.

■ Condom

The condom—the most popular contraceptive worldwide—sheathes the erect penis and thereby prevents entrance of sperm into the vagina. User effectiveness ranges from a low of 65% to a high of 97%. The most reliable condoms are of an FDA-tested quality. The only possible side effect is irritation of the penis or vagina.

■ Cervical cap

As its name suggests, the cervical cap is a thimblelike rubber cap that fits snugly over the cervix. Like the diaphragm it blocks sperm from entering the uterus, but unlike the diaphragm it requires little spermicide and, above all, can be worn several days at a time. User effectiveness and possible side effects are still in the statistical mill at the time of this writing.

■ Spermicides

Spermicides are vaginal preparations that kill sperm. They are marketed in a variety of forms: foams, creams, jellies, and suppositories. To be effective they must cover the cervical opening and, equally important, they must be given time to work (about 10 minutes). Furthermore, it must be understood that the effect wears off within an hour or so. Reading the directions on the label is crucial. User effectiveness ranges from a low of about 65% to a high of about 97%. Using a spermicide along with a diaphragm or condom obviously increases protection. Possible side effects are limited to irritation of the vagina or penis.

■ Natural methods

All natural contraceptive methods relate to the fact that a woman is fertile for only a few days in each cycle. Clearly, the trick and challenge is to pinpoint these days. The original natural method of contraception, the **rhythm method**, is based on arithmetic. In order to use this method successfully, the menstrual cycles must be regular. To determine the "period of abstention," 18 days is subtracted from the length of the shortest of the previous 12 cycles and 11 days from the longest. For example, if the woman's cycles vary between 26 and 29 days, the couple must abstain from intercourse from day 8 through day 18 of each cycle.

More dependable natural methods include the basal body temperature (BBT) method, the Billing's (ovulation) method, and the symptothermal method. **The BBT method** is based on the fact that body temperature rises steadily after ovulation. To determine the basal (lowest) body temperature (BBT), a reading is taken first thing every morning before sitting up. When the BBT has risen and has remained elevated for 3 full days, it signals the start of an infertile period lasting until menstruation. **The Billing's method** is based on the fact that vaginal mucus becomes abundant, clear, and slippery as ovulation approaches. Four days after this peak, when the mucus is sticky and thick again, an infertile period begins that runs until menstruation. The **symptothermal method** combines BBT and ovulation with observation of cervical changes (namely, at peak fertility the cervix may rise, soften, and widen). The BBT method has a user effectiveness of 93% to 99% if there is no intercourse before ovulation. The Billing's method and symptothermal method have user ratios of 75% to 98% and 90% to 99%, respectively.

■ Sterilization

Sterilization, the surest way to avoid unwanted pregnancies, is virtually 100% effective. For women it involves blocking off the uterine tubes (**tubal ligation**). In men the operation, called a **vasectomy**, is quite simple. It involves a small incision on each side of the scrotum and the tying off of the vas deferens.

Both operations are difficult to reverse and should not be elected by anyone who expects a reversal at a later date. Authorities agree that sterilization does not affect sexuality—indeed, if anything, sexuality is enhanced because the fear of pregnancy is gone.

■■■ DISORDERS AND DISEASES

Disorders and diseases peculiar to the reproductive (urogenital) system are many and various. Problems in the male include urethritis, inflammation of a testis (orchitis), undescended testes (cryptorchidism), enlargement of the prostate (benign prostatic hypertrophy), cancer of the prostate, and impotence. Gynecologic (female) disorders and diseases include inflammation of the vagina (vaginitis), inflammation of the vulva (vulvitis), menstrual dysfunction, breast cysts, ovarian cysts, breast cancer, uterine cancer, infertility, frigidity, and toxic shock syndrome. Venereal diseases, infections spread by sexual intercourse, are discussed in the next chapter.

■ Infertility

About 10% of married couples encounter infertility. Male infertility may be caused by (1) defective sperm production, (2) obstruction of the seminal tract, or (3) defective delivery of sperm into the vagina. (The sperm count should exceed 20 million per ml of ejaculate.) Female infertility may be caused by (1) a hormonal defect, (2) tubal disorders, or (3) a uterine abnormality. Treatment of infertility obviously depends on the cause, and in many cases the results are gratifying. Recently, drugs that induce ovulation (ovulatory agents) have been introduced to foster fertility. Two such agents are clomiphene citrate (Clomid) and human menopausal gonadotropin (HMG).

In vitro fertilization. Defective uterine tubes, which occur in 1 out of 500 women, often result in sterility. To circumvent the problem, medical research turned to in vitro ("in glass") fertilization, the procedure whereby fertilization is carried out in a Petri dish and the resulting conceptus then implanted into the uterus. It was the perfection of the technique by Doctors Patrick Steptoe and Robert Edwards that, on July 25, 1978, led to the birth in Britain of Louise Brown, the first child conceived in this manner. The technique, in brief, runs as follows: At the time of ovulation a device called a laparoscope is inserted through a small incision in the abdominal wall. Bundles of glass fibers (in the device) carry light into the cavity, while other fibers enable the surgeon to look in, seek out the ripe ovum, and extract it with a suction needle. Once it is removed, the ovum is placed in a dish with a special chemical mixture and then exposed to the husband's sperm. After the fertilized ovum has undergone a few divisions, it is inserted through the cervix and implanted in the endometrium.

■ Impotence and frigidity

Impotence is inability of the male to attain or sustain an erection satisfactory for normal coitus. Possibly half the adult male population experiences transient impotence. Psychic factors are responsible for about 90% of cases. Physical factors include systemic disease, faulty genitals, neurogenic disorders, surgical procedures, and drugs. Interestingly, aging is not an inevitable cause of impotence, even into the eighties.

Frigidity is inability of the female to experience sexual pleasure and satisfaction. Only about 50% of all women experience orgasm during coitus. Psychic factors are responsible for most cases. Physical causes include systemic disease, nervous system disorders, muscular disorders, localized disease, and drugs. Treatment of both impotence and frigidity relate to the underlying cause. Psychic factors call for counseling and psychotherapy.

■ Cancer

Breast cancer is the leading cause of all deaths among women 40 to 44 years of age, and over the past 50 years there has been no great improvement in the mortality rate. For 1982, the estimated number of new cases was 110,000, and the estimated number of deaths was 37,000. The incidence is highest among women of middle age and older, but the American Cancer Society warns that breast self-examination should begin as a monthly health habit at high school age. If breast cancer is discovered in a **localized stage**, modern therapy (surgery, radiation, and chemotherapy) can effect a 5-year survival rate of 85%. Once the malignancy has spread to the lymph nodes, this figure drops to about 56%.

In contrast to the rather dismal figures for breast cancer, cancer of the uterus has dropped 65% over the past 40 years. **Cervical cancer** (which involves the neck of the uterus) is readily detected by the **Pap test** (about 95% accurate) in the **precancerous** condition, a situation that renders treatment about 100% successful. Of great etiologic significance is the considerable body of evidence that implicates the **herpes simplex virus** as the causative agent. Since the virus (specifically type 2 herpes simplex) is transmitted sexually, the American Cancer Society stresses the possibility of cervical cancer in sexually active females.

Endometrial cancer (which involves the body of the uterus) is mainly a malignancy of mature women, especially those in the 50 to 64 year age group. Recent studies suggest an upward trend in this cancer, a trend that most authorities associate with the increased use of estrogens. The Food and Drug Administration has issued a warning to this effect, and physicians are urged to curtail their use. The American Cancer Society holds that the Pap test is ineffective in detecting endometrial cancer and cautions every woman at menopause to have a pelvic examination. Further, those at high risk (women with a history of estrogen therapy, infertility, abnormal uterine bleeding) should also have an endometrial biopsy.

The chief cancer of the male reproductive system is **cancer of the prostate**, which accounts for 10% of all male cancer deaths. The incidence has increased by more than 25% in the past 25 years, but the 5-year survival rate has continued to show steady improvement.

■ Toxic shock syndrome

In 1979 national concern was aroused over what is now called **toxic shock syndrome** (TSS), a mysterious illness that primarily affects young women using tampons during menstral periods. More than 700 cases of the disease were reported, and it was blamed for at least 65 deaths. Because a particular brand of tampon was statistically associated with many cases, that product was withdrawn from the market. Other manufacturers are now supplying warnings on or inside tampon packages to alert the estimated 50 million American women who use tampons to the possible danger. It should be stressed, however, that TSS is a rare disease with, at most, 15 cases per 100,000 menstruating women per year.

Cases of toxic shock syndrome not associated with menstruation account for about 13% of the total reported cases. Among those affected are postsurgical patients, burn patients, women who have just given birth, and patients with boils or abscesses. In a few persons the disease has occurred without any apparent preexisting medical condition.

Toxic shock syndrome is characterized by vomiting, watery diarrhea, and a high fever (over 104° F in most cases). There is a rapid progression to low blood pressure, faintness, and shock, usually accompanied by a sunburnlike rash. Everything from the kidney to the lung and heart can be affected. The acute phase of the disease lasts 3 to 7 days. Most deaths have occurred within a week. The immediate cause has been identified as a toxin released by a certain strain of *Staphylococcus aureus*, a common cause of boils and skin abscesses. Just how tampons are involved is still under investigation, but there is evidence that tampons soaked in blood support bacterial growth. It is possible that tampons (perhaps during insertion) may cause microlacerations that serve as a breeding ground for infection. Treatment of TSS, usually carried out in an intensive care unit, centers on the use of antibiotics and intravenous fluids.

■■■■■ SELF-TEST

1. _C_ male gonad
2. _J_ male hormone
3. _O_ vas deferens
4. _B_ conveys urine and semen
5. _N_ glans penis
6. _I_ corpora cavernosa
7. _L_ female gonad
8. _A_ uterine tube
9. _G_ uterine neck
10. _K_ uterine lining
11. _m_ uterine muscle
12. _D_ vaginal orifice
13. _F_ external female genitals
14. _H_ mammary glands
15. _e_ female hormone

a. infundibulum
b. urethra
c. testis
d. hymen
e. progesterone
f. vulva
g. cervix
h. nipple
i. erection
j. testosterone
k. endometrium
l. ovary
m. myometrium
n. foreskin
o. epididymis

◼◼◼◼ STUDY QUESTIONS

1. The pathway of a sperm cell from its place of origin to ejaculation involves the following structures: ejaculatory duct, ductus deferens, ductus epididymis, prostatic urethra, cavernous urethra, seminiferous tubules, and membranous urethra. From "start to finish," what is the proper order of these structures?

2. The testis, the male gonad, has two primary functions. What are they?

3. The male urethra is about 20 cm long, and the female urethra is about 4 cm long. Why this considerable difference?

4. What is meant by circumcision, and what is its purpose?

5. The body of the penis is composed mainly of the corpora cavernosa penis and the corpus cavernosum urethrae. These structures are often collectively referred to as "erectile tissue." Why?

6. What is the difference between sperm and semen?

7. If an ejaculation measures 6 ml in volume, what is this in terms of a fluid ounce?

8. For any particular ejaculation what two factors determine the number of spermatozoa involved?

9. The ovary, like the testis, has two fundamental functions. What are they?

10. If the average dimensions of the uterus are converted to inches, they are as easy to remember as "1-2-3." Try it and you will see.

11. "Cervix" in Latin means "neck." Does this fit in with the position of the cervix in relation to the uterus?

12. The vagina is "capable of great distention." Can you think of two reasons why this is so?

13. Using the figures cited in the text, determine how the average vagina and average erect penis compare in length? Does this make anatomic sense?

14. Occasionally the hymen completely covers the vaginal orifice (a condition called imperforate hymen). What would be the result of this condition, and what would have to be done?

15. "Labium" (pl., labia) in Latin means "lip." Why is this term used in connection with the vulva?

16. The name "mons pubis" ("pubic mount") underscores its prominence. Why is it so prominent?

17. What part of the vulva corresponds most closely to the male genitals?

18. Hormone levels in the blood rise and fall when the occasion demands. Illustrate this fact using prolactin and oxytocin as examples.

19. Four hormones (at least) are involved in breast development and lactation. What are they?

20. At the end of the menstrual cycle the low blood levels of progesterone and estrogens stimulate the production of FSH and thereby set the stage for a new cycle. This is an example of "negative feedback." Why is it "negative?"

21. The menopause may be as emotional as it is physical. Discuss in detail.

22. Male but not female orgasm is essential to the process of fertilization. Why so?

23. Oral contraceptives prevent ovulation by inhibiting the output of "releasing factors" (by the hypothalamus). Can you explain the mechanism of this action?

24. In a sense saying "no" is a mode of contraception. Do you agree?

25. Other things being equal, which has the greater bearing on infertility—impotence or frigidity?

CHAPTER 14

Pregnancy and childbirth

Pregnancy (gestation) is the period of carrying a developing offspring in the uterus after conception. More precisely it is the period during which the fertilized ovum—a cell about the size of the dot over an "i"—evolves into a new individual. The actual sequence of events is awesomely complex and, in a sense, constitutes the mystery of life. In humans the developing organism is an embryo from about 2 weeks after fertilization to the end of the eighth week; from then until birth the developing offspring is a fetus. The embryonic period is by far the most active—indeed, "explosive"—because it sets the stage for virtually all body systems. Childbirth (labor) is the process by which the fetus is expelled from the uterus through the vagina into the outside world. In the present chapter we will take a close look at pregnancy and childbirth and will consider a number of associated matters, including complications of pregnancy, birth defects, and drug use.

Embryonic development

Pregnancy tests

The expectant mother

Childbirth

Complications of pregnancy

Birth defects and inherited disorders

Drugs in pregnancy

Drugs in nursing mothers

Infant mortality

The charge of semen ejaculated into the vagina usually contains about 500 million sperm (Fig. 14-1). Traveling at a speed of 3 to 4 mm per minute, most will arrive in the upper reaches of the uterine tubes in a little over half an hour. In order for **fertilization** to occur, a sperm must encounter the fresh ovum either here or in the pelvic cavity before the ovum enters the tube. An encounter elsewhere is generally of no avail, for, by the time the ovum reaches the uterus, it has acquired an armor of mucus. As soon as a single sperm enters the ovum, the remaining sperm are "shut out" by some sort of chemical mechanism.

■ EMBRYONIC DEVELOPMENT

Shortly after fertilization the sperm head swells into the **male pronucleus**; the original nucleus of the ovum is the **female pronucleus**. The two nuclei, each containing the haploid number of chromosomes, then fuse into the 46-chromosome **zygote** (Fig. 14-2), the cell destined to become the new individual. In about 24 hours the zygote undergoes the first **cleavage**, and the product continues to divide every 12 to 15 hours thereafter. By the time the fertilized ovum reaches the uterus (3 or 4 days), the segmented mass, now called the **morula**, contains about 25 cells. It is still barely visible to the unaided eye.

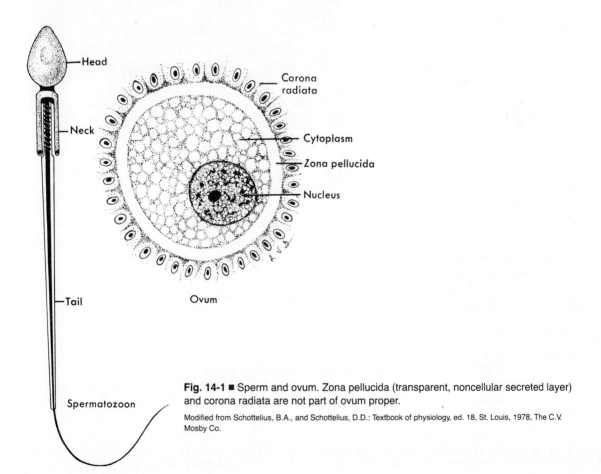

Fig. 14-1 ■ Sperm and ovum. Zona pellucida (transparent, noncellular secreted layer) and corona radiata are not part of ovum proper.

Modified from Schottelius, B.A., and Schottelius, D.D.: Textbook of physiology, ed. 18, St. Louis, 1978, The C.V. Mosby Co.

Columnar epithelium

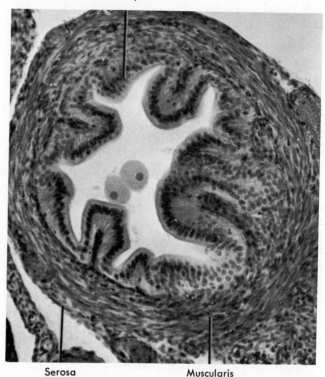

Fig. 14-2 ■ Section of fallopian tube of mouse showing two fertilized eggs (zygotes) in lumen. (×200.)

From Bevelander, G., and Ramaley, J.A.: Essentials of histology, ed. 8, St. Louis, 1979, The C.V. Mosby Co.; courtesy Dr. H. Browning.

Serosa   Muscularis

As growth continues, the new cells arrange themselves in such a way that a cavity forms within the mass, with a cluster of cells (the inner cell mass) projecting into the cavity. This hollow-ball structure is called the **blastocyst**, and the cavity within is the **blastocele**. The cells forming the outer layer of the blastocyst are referred to en masse as the **trophoblast**. The trophoblast secretes enzymes that digest away a tiny bit of the endometrium, and its cells engulf the digested products. In this fashion, the blastocyst situates itself into the uterine wall (implantation) and in the process derives its sustenance.

By the end of 2 weeks the blastocyst is completely embedded within the endometrium, and the trophoblastic cells are rapidly growing and dividing. Soon they and adjacent cells start to form the fetal membranes. The **chorion**, the outer membrane, sends out thou-

sands of microscopic projections (villi) that invade the surrounding mucosa and lay the groundwork for the **placenta**, the cakelike mass within the uterus that will establish communication between mother and offspring by means of the **umbilical cord**.

■ Embryonic disk

While the process just described is taking place, drastic changes are taking place inside the inner cell mass. Two cavities have appeared in the mass, and a new layer of cells (the mesoderm) has grown over the original lining of the blastocele, passing between the two new cavities. The cavity closest to the trophoblast, the **amniotic cavity**, is destined to house the embryo, which has not yet appeared; the outer cavity, the yolk sac, serves no purpose in humans and ultimately degen-

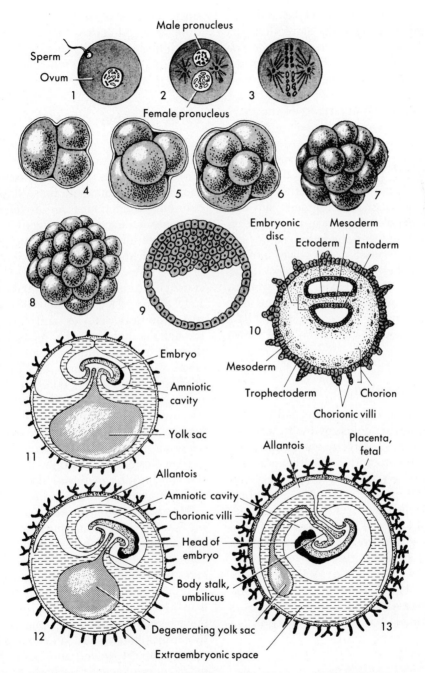

Fig. 14-3 ■ Embryologic highlights of mammalian gestation from time of fertilization, *1*, to development of the fetal placenta, *13*. Stages *8* and *9* are called the morula and the blastocyst, respectively.

Modified from Woodruff, L.L.: Animal biology, New York, 1961, Macmillan, Inc.

erates and disappears. The three-layered plate of cells running between the amniotic cavity and the yolk sac, aptly referred to as the **embryonic disk**, now becomes the crucial area of development, for this is where the embryo is formed.

The **ectoderm**, the outermost of the three layers of the embryonic disk, evolves into the skin, the nervous system, the external sense organs, and the mucous membranes of the mouth and anus; the **mesoderm**, the middle layer, evolves into the connective tissues, muscles, blood vessels, sex organs, and epithelium of the pleura, pericardium, peritoneum, and kidney; and the **entoderm** (or endoderm), the innermost layer, evolves into the epithelium of the pharynx, respiratory tract, gastrointestinal tract, bladder, and urethra. Some idea of how these transformations take place in the early stages can be obtained by a close study of the diagrammatic sections shown in Fig. 14-3.

■ Sex determination

In each human somatic (body) cell 2 of the 46 chromosomes are concerned with sex. Two X chromosomes characterize the female, and an X and a Y chromosome characterize the male. Thus all ova carry an X chromosome, whereas half the sperm cells carry an X chromosome and the other half a Y chromosome. When an X sperm cell fertilizes an ovum, the offspring is a girl; conversely, when a Y sperm cell fertilizes an ovum, the offspring is a boy. Since it is the father who carries the odd chromosome, he should by no means blame the mother in the event the sex of the offspring is not to his liking.

■ Twinning

If two or more ova, instead of the customary one, are released and fertilized simultaneously, **fraternal twins** result. **Identical twins** (Fig. 14-4), on the other hand, result from a single fertilized ovum that has split one or more times into cell masses that develop into separate but identical offspring. In the instance of quintuplets, there are four such divisions before implantation.

■ The placenta

The placenta makes intrauterine life feasible. As shown in Fig. 14-5, this structure is essentially a mass of blood sinuses formed by the placental septa. Into these sinuses extend chorionic projections from the fetal portion of the placenta, each covered with an enormous number of microscopic villi containing blood capillaries. Maternal blood flows into and out of these sinuses by means of a well-channeled system of vessels derived from the uterine wall. Fetal blood is led into the villi through the two **umbilical arteries** and then led back through the **umbilical vein**. As the blood moves through the villi, nutrients are absorbed and waste products are removed. This is largely effected through simple diffusion; that is, since the concentration of oxygen and nutrients is greater on the maternal side of the placental barrier, they diffuse from the mother to the offspring. By the same token, fetal wastes (carbon dioxide, urea, and the like) diffuse from the villi into the maternal blood, from which they are excreted by the kidneys.

Placental hormones. Aside from serving as a food source and purifier, the placenta also secretes hormones, without which pregnancy cannot continue. When fertilization occurs, the **corpus luteum**, which normally degenerates at the end of each menstrual cycle, is maintained by chorionic gonadotropin hormone secreted by the developing ovum (at first by the trophoblast and later by the chorionic membrane). However, after about the fourth month of pregnancy, the chorionic gonadotropin concentration drops to low levels, and the corpus luteum ceases to be stimulated sufficiently to produce the necessary high levels of estrogens and progesterone. At this time

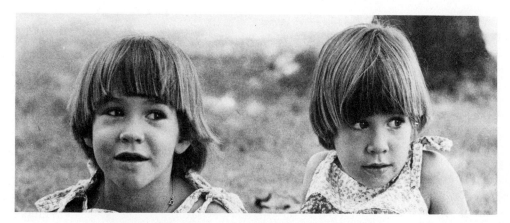

Fig. 14-4 ■ Identical twins illustrate the force of heredity.

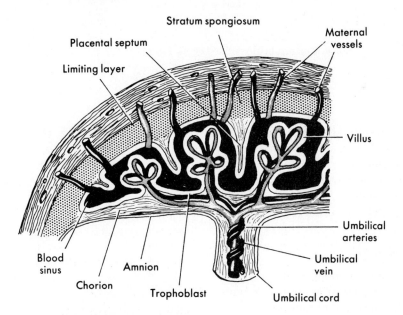

Fig. 14-5 ■ Basic structure of the placenta.

Modified from Guyton, A.C.: Function of the human body, Philadelphia, 1959, W.B. Saunders Co.; after Gray.

the placenta takes over the job and pushes the concentration of these hormones to well over 50 times their peak value during nonpregnancy.

Estrogens and progesterone are especially vital during pregnancy. In brief, estrogens thicken the uterine musculature, greatly en-hance the uterine blood supply, enlarge the breasts, and facilitate embryonic development. Progesterone relaxes the uterine musculature until the time of birth, aids the development of the endometrium, prevents ovulation, and enlarges the breast glands.

A placental estrogen of special diagnostic

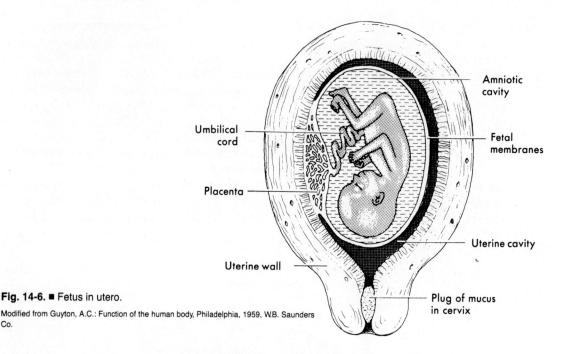

Fig. 14-6. ■ Fetus in utero.

Modified from Guyton, A.C.: Function of the human body, Philadelphia, 1959, W.B. Saunders Co.

significance is **estriol**. The maternal urinary concentrations of estriol increase throughout pregnancy and decrease just before delivery. If estriol levels suddenly fall or do not rise rapidly (during pregnancy), a fetal difficulty should be expected.

■ Fetal membranes

Two membranes surround the fetus: the **amnion** and the **chorion** (Fig. 14-6). The amnion, the innermost membrane, is a thin, transparent tissue that encloses the amniotic cavity; to equalize and cushion the pressures bearing on the fetus, this cavity is filled with a watery liquid called the **amniotic fluid**. The chorion, the thick, outermost membrane, is actually composed of two layers. The portion of the chorionic surface that gives rise to the villi and forms the embryonic and fetal placenta is called the chorion frondosum. The remaining surface, the chorion laeve, is membranous and smooth.

TABLE 14-1

Typical fetal growth pattern*

Age (weeks)	Length (cm)	Weight
8	2.5	2.8 g
12	10	28.0 g
20	25	340.0 g
28	35	1.0 kg
36	45	2.3 kg
40	50	3.2 kg

*The developing organism from about 2 weeks to the end of 8 weeks is called the embryo.

■ Fetal and maternal growth

The fetus (the developing organism from 8 weeks on) utilizes prodigious amounts of nutrients supplied by the mother's blood. It evolves from an average weight of 28 g (1 oz) at 3 months to an average weight of 3.2 kg (7 lb) at the time of birth. The bulk of this terrific increase in weight occurs during the last 3 months of pregnancy (Table 14-1). Infants weighing 2.5 kg or more are considered **mature**; a **premature** infant weighs between 1 and 2.5 kg.

◼◼◼ PREGNANCY TESTS

No woman is indifferent to the possibility of pregnancy, and not uncommonly it is the most important issue she has to face. Clearly, then, the advent of the in-home pregnancy test was of considerable significance. Such tests are ultraprivate, safe, fast, easy to perform, and, above all, virtually 100% accurate. All are based on the presence of **chorionic gonadotropin**, which appears in the urine in a matter of days following conception. As indicated, the test is carried out by adding a few drops of urine to the testing material and reading the result (negative or positive) in a matter of minutes.

◼◼◼ THE EXPECTANT MOTHER

The mother undergoes tremendous change during pregnancy. Her metabolism is accelerated, her tissues hold excess fluid, and last but by no means least, she gains an average of about 20 pounds (fetus, 7 pounds; uterus, 2 pounds; placenta and membranes, 2½ pounds; breasts, 2 pounds; fat and extra fluid, 6½ pounds). If all goes well throughout pregnancy and during delivery, these anatomic and physiologic alterations reverse themselves in an amazingly short period of time. Indeed, there is good reason to believe that a normal pregnancy strengthens the body.

There is every reason for a healthy and safe pregnancy. Safeguards against health dangers are ample for the intelligent woman in good health. It is common practice for the expectant mother to place herself under the care of a physician. If begun early, general medical supervision enables the physician to start treatment in time if anything is wrong. The

physician's examination is very complete. It starts with a health history of any childhood diseases and later illnesses, such as heart trouble, rheumatic fever, diabetes, tuberculosis, or venereal disease. The physician asks about previous pregnancies or miscarriages, examines the heart and lungs, and checks the throat, nose, ears, and teeth for any sign of infection. A blood sample is sent to the laboratory for detailed analysis. Another test made quite routinely is the Pap test to detect cancer of the cervix or uterus. The physician makes effective preparations for proper care at the time of childbirth and gives advice about regular body exercise, adequate rest, and needed adjustments in the life of the family.

The elimination of wastes for the fetus puts an added burden on the mother's kidneys during pregnancy. It is particularly important that the condition of the kidneys be watched, since they must remove all the nitrogenous waste. A urinalysis is made at each visit to the physician to check the functioning of the kidneys.

It sometimes happens that the pelvis is too narrow, making the normal birth of the child difficult or impossible. By careful pelvic measurements it can be determined in advance whether the largest part of the baby, the head, will have sufficient space to pass through the narrowest part of the pelvis. Arrangements may have to be made for birth by **cesarean section,** in which the delivery is made by way of an incision through the abdominal and uterine walls.

It is important to the health of the baby that the mother avoid infectious disease during the first months of pregnancy, particularly in the second month. There is clear evidence that German measles at this time occasionally produces defects in the central nervous system of the infant. Other infections at this stage of pregnancy are suspected of injuring the fetus.

Research studies show a positive correlation between the mother's diet during pregnancy and her health and the health of her new baby. These studies present evidence that a good prenatal diet helps the mother by reducing the incidence of toxemias and other complications; it lowers maternal mortality and makes greater the likelihood that the infant can be breast fed. The benefits of good maternal diet for the baby are better growth, development, and physical condition at birth. Good prenatal diet also appears to reduce the incidence of stillbirths and premature births.

■■■ CHILDBIRTH

The duration of pregnancy averages 280 days from the beginning of the last menstrual period; about 90% of all births occur within a week before or after this figure. The actual birth process is called **labor**, **parturition**, or simply **childbirth**. The physician prepares the expectant mother, especially in the case of the first child, for the procedures to be expected. There is growing interest in so-called **natural childbirth**, in which exercise and psychologic preparations are added to the usual prenatal practices. Needless fears and tensions are eliminated, and the expectant mother approaches the delivery with confidence and enthusiasm, ready to do her part in promoting the birth process.

An examination of professional care at delivery shows that in the United States over 90% of babies are delivered in hospitals under the care of a physician who has at hand such hospital resources as may be needed. Other babies are delivered by **midwives**. These specialists can serve effectively in normal deliveries and know when it may be necessary to call in a physician. Maternal death in childbirth is now extremely rare, only about 3 in 10,000 births. Some women prefer to have babies at home, and many physicians support the idea in normal pregnancies.

The process of childbirth has three stages. The **first stage** begins with weak uterine contractions (labor pains) and ends with the complete relaxation of the cervix of the uterus. The first contractions are 15 to 40 minutes apart and grow gradually stronger and more frequent over a period of about 12 hours for first babies and about 8 hours for subsequent births. The expectant mother can reduce the discomfort somewhat by breathing deeply and relaxing during the contractions. The **second stage** encompasses the passage of the baby through the birth canal, generally lasting from ½ to 2 hours. The amniotic fluid ("sac of water") in which the baby lived in the uterus breaks, and the uterine muscles begin more vigorous contractions. These, aided by strong contractions of the mother's abdominal muscles, move the baby through the birth canal and free it from the body of the mother (Fig. 14-7). The **umbilical cord** is tied off and cut. Since the cord has no nerves, this is not painful to either mother or child. Also, to ensure proper ventilation the physician must suction mucus from the baby's mouth and throat. The baby cries and inflates the lungs for the first time. Then the baby is cleaned and given an identification bracelet or number. The attached portion of the umbilical cord later dries up, leaving the navel (or **umbilicus**). The third stage of childbirth is the expulsion of the **afterbirth**, which consists of the placenta and fetal membranes. This is accompanied by a blood loss of 400 to 500 ml, as a result of the placenta being "torn away" from the uterine wall.

In a few cases the infant moves toward birth with the hips first instead of the head. This is called **breech presentation**. It is somewhat more difficult but can be handled effectively by the experienced obstetrician. Cesarean section is sometimes necessary because the woman's pelvis is too narrow, making the normal birth of the child difficult or impossible. Or the mother may have a heart condition or some other limitation that makes her a poor candidate for the rigors of labor. The section is usually performed about 2 weeks before the expected date of birth. An incision is made in

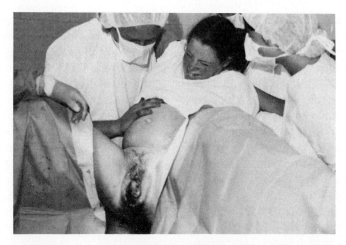

"I started pushing."

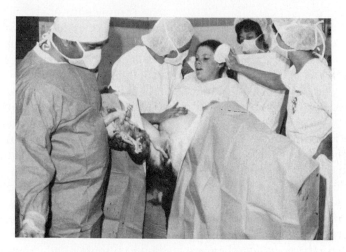

"Stopped pushing and opened my eyes."

Fig. 14-7 ■ The second stage of labor. Expression on mother's face is not a reflection of pain but rather of her strong effort in "pushing."

From Phillips, C.R., and Anzalone, J.T.: Fathering: participation in labor and birth, St. Louis, 1978, The C.V. Mosby Co.

the abdominal wall and in the uterus, permitting the direct delivery of the infant.

Following normal delivery the mother is returned to her own room as soon as possible. The next day she usually walks about the room a little, and she returns home in about 3 days. She may suffer some discomfort for a few days, and the resumption of household responsibilities plus the care of the new baby may be a heavy load. Rest and encouragement are important. After 6 weeks the uterus should be back to normal size. About 80% of nursing mothers do not menstruate for the first few months, although menstruation may return within 6 weeks after childbirth.

Breast feeding is important for the health of the mother as well as the infant. For the first 2 or 3 days the mother's breasts produce **colostrum**, after which they begin to secrete milk. Colostrum is a watery fluid that has a substantial immunizing effect on the infant. Breast feeding not only protects the infant from possible malnutrition or infection but also is emotionally satisfying to both mother and child. The mother sometimes worries that breast feeding may affect her figure, but proper supports will minimize this danger. Appropriate abdominal exercises are also helpful in figure control.

■ Fathering

During pregnancy and birth fathers have tended to be undervalued in our culture and clearly discriminated against. Some hospitals still treat them as excess baggage. But the medical profession and the public in general are starting to rethink the situation, and many hospitals are promoting father participation, inviting him to childbirth preparation classes and accepting him in the delivery room. Indeed, Phillips and Anzalone, a nurse-physician team, have co-authored *Fathering: Participation in Labor and Birth*, in which they attempt to create a new understanding of fathers. They believe that parents should at least be given the option to decide for themselves whether or not they want to share the birth experience—an experience those authors believe will make the couple better human beings.

■ COMPLICATIONS OF PREGNANCY

There are, understandably, a number of possible complications of pregnancy, especially in teenage pregnancies. Among others,

these include certain infections, anemia, trimester bleeding, hyperemesis gravidarum (pernicious nausea and vomiting), eclampsia (coma and/or convulsive seizures), erythroblastosis fetalis (Rh factor incompatibility), ectopic pregnancy (implantation outside the uterine cavity), and spontaneous abortion (miscarriage). By convention, abortion is defined as delivery or loss of the "product of conception" before the twentieth week of pregnancy. About 35% of women bleed or have cramping sometime during the first 20 weeks of pregnancy; about 20% actually abort. Since in 90% of spontaneous abortions the fetus is either absent or grossly malformed, and in an additional 5% it has chromosomal abnormalities, spontaneous abortion may be a natural, purposeful rejection. If a woman has three or more successive pregnancies that end in spontaneous abortion, she is said to have **habitual abortion**.

Other forms of abortion are **missed abortion** and **septic abortion**. Missed abortion occurs when the fetus has died but has been retained in utero for a month or longer. After about 6 weeks the dead fetus syndrome may develop, characterized by possible massive bleeding when delivery finally occurs (usually between 12 and 20 weeks). Septic abortion develops when the uterine contents become infected before, during, or after an abortion. Blood poisoning and shock are possible, and the prognosis is commonly grave. Septic abortions are typically associated with induced abortions done by untrained persons. As a consequence of legalized induced abortion, the septic abortion rate in the United States has fallen dramatically.

■ BIRTH DEFECTS AND INHERITED DISORDERS

Specters of birth defects and inherited disorders can throw a pall over the bright expectations of parents-to-be. The process of genetic counseling, along with new ways of determining whether a fetus is likely to be normal, has taken much of the mystery out of predicting pregnancy outcomes. Through genetic counseling a couple may be told if an inheritable disease or disorder is likely to be carried to an offspring or if a high-risk pregnancy may develop. The medical procedures used for these determinations include removing a sample of fluid from the pregnant uterus, taking sound "pictures" of the fetus and uterus, and examining pelvic structures and the developing fetus by insertion of special medical devices. Fetal abnormalities that may be identified or ruled out through prenatal testing and counseling include sickle cell anemia, Tay-Sachs disease, phenylketonuria (PKU), Down's syndrome (mongolism), hemophilia, thalassemia (a type of anemia), and neural tube defects such as spina bifida.

Genetic counseling can actually start before the couple marries, because knowing that their pairing may result in a child with an inherited disorder can make a difference in the couple's decisions about marriage and childbearing. Some inherited disorders are carried by the mother and passed on almost exclusively to male children. These disorders are known as **X-linked recessive** disorders and include color blindness, hemophilia, and childhood muscular dystrophy. They are called X-linked recessive because they are carried on the X sex chromosome of the mother.

Other inherited disorders, called **autosomal recessive**, are inherited only if both parents carry the gene for the disorder. Even then, the chances are only one in four that each offspring will have the disease. Years ago knowing that such a disease existed in the families of two people planning to marry might have been enough to call off the wedding. But today carrier tests for these genetic disorders often rule out one or both partners as carriers. Three of the more common disorders transmitted in this manner are sickle cell anemia, Tay-Sachs disease, and thalassemia. All three are most commonly found in ethnic or racial

groups whose ancestry can be traced to specific geographic areas. This is understandable because people with similar ancestral backgrounds are more likely to have similar genetic makeups.

Although most of the testing for carriers of genetically transmitted diseases is done through blood analysis, some diseases require other types of testing. An example is cystic fibrosis, one of at least 2000 **inborn errors of metabolism**. Carriers of this disease, which affects one of every 1000 babies born in the United States, can be detected by measuring the amount of salt in perspiration.

Once a high-risk pregnancy occurs, there are several methods of determining whether the offspring will be normal. Amniocentesis, ultrasound, alpha-fetoprotein (AFP) testing, fetoscopy, and placental aspiration can diagnose a host of genetic, chromosomal, and other abnormalities. A diagnosis can ease parents' fears or alert them to the probability of serious birth defects, and it can allow parents the option of terminating pregnancy or of preparing to take both prenatal and postnatal measures to minimize the effect of the abnormality.

Amniocentesis is a procedure usually performed in the obstetrician's office during the fourteenth to eighteenth week of pregnancy. After administering a local anesthetic, the physician inserts a hollow needle into the uterus through the abdominal wall and withdraws a small amount of the amniotic fluid that surrounds the fetus. Nearly all fetal chromosomal abnormalities can be diagnosed in this way. Amniocentesis can also be used to diagnose at least 75 inborn errors of metabolism, to help identify neural tube defects, and to determine sex where there is a risk of X-linked genetic disorder. Women contemplating amniocentesis should be aware that, although considered safe, the procedure is not entirely without risk and should be undertaken only when there is a serious question about the normality of the fetus.

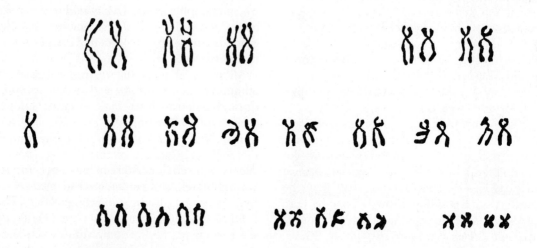

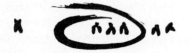

Fig. 14-8 ■ Down's syndrome, with chromosomes arranged in pairs. Note the additional chromosome in the group circled.

From World Health **14**:July-August, 1961.

One of the more common reasons for performing amniocentesis is to rule out Down's syndrome. Down's syndrome children may be severely mentally retarded. They have heart disorders and respiratory problems that often result in death before adulthood. Down's syndrome, or mongolism as it is sometimes called, is a nonhereditary chromosomal abnormality (although there is a rare form of mongolism that is inherited). In Down's syndrome the child has 47 chromosomes, rather than the usual 46. The extra chromosome involves the pair designated chromosome 21—hence the expression **trisomy 21** (Fig. 14-8). Because of the increased risk of Down's syndrome with age, many physicians recommend that all pregnant women over age 35 have amniocentesis performed.

Ultrasonography (or "sonography") is frequently an adjunct of amniocentesis. It does not involve the use of ionizing radiation such as x-rays. In pulse echo sonography high–frequency sound waves are directed into the abdomen of the pregnant woman to produce a picture of the uterus, placenta, and fetus (Fig. 14-9). The procedure produces no discomfort and reduces the necessity of x-ray examination and radioisotope (radioactive tracer) scanning. Ultrasound can be used before amniocentesis, to locate fetal structures, the umbilical cord, and the placenta, and to determine that the fetus is alive. The procedure should not be considered entirely risk free and should be undertaken in pregnancy only when there is a clear medical indication.

The **alpha-fetoprotein** (AFP) **test** helps diagnose neural tube defects by measuring the level of AFP (a normal fetal liver product) in maternal blood and in amniotic fluid. High levels of AFP may indicate the fetus has **anencephaly** (a defective formation of the brain that invariably results in the death of the baby shortly after birth) or **spina bifida** (abnormalities in the spinal column requiring surgical correction after birth and possibly also resulting in paralysis and mental retardation). The

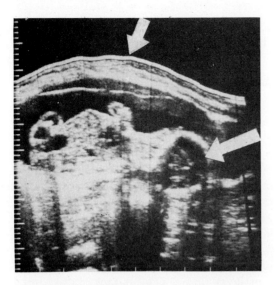

Fig. 14-9 ■ Sonogram of normal pregnancy. *Upper arrow*, Abdominal wall of mother. *Lower arrow*, Fetal brain. Thin white line below abdominal wall is the placenta.

Courtesy Newton-Wellesley Hospital, Newton Lower Falls, Mass.

incidence in the United States of anencephaly and spina bifida is 1 to 2 per 1000 births. However, elevated AFP levels may also indicate multiple pregnancy or fetal death.

Fetoscopy and placental aspiration are more recent techniques used to gain information about the fetus. In **fetoscopy** a small device is inserted through the woman's abdomen, enabling the physician to view the fetus and placenta directly. Before the device is inserted, the positions of the fetus, placenta, and umbilical cord are determined by ultrasound. Small samples of fetal tissue and blood can be obtained by this method. These samples enable physicians to diagnose abnormalities, such as beta-thalassemia and hemophilia, that cannot be diagnosed by testing the amniotic fluid in the womb. In **placental aspiration**, after locating and measuring the thickness of the placenta via ultrasound, the physician inserts a needle into the inner surface of the placenta and aspirates, or draws up by suction, a sample of fetal blood.

Therapeutic abortion often remains the only alternative once an affected individual has been conceived, but neonatal medicine is making great progress in actually treating the fetus. Sometimes the mother is put on a special diet; sometimes she is given corrective drugs; and sometimes the fetus is dealt with directly in the uterus by microsurgical techniques.

■ DRUGS IN PREGNANCY

Drugs taken during pregnancy enter the fetal circulation, and certain ones may cause severe problems, including birth defects. The classic disaster occurred in 1960-1962 with the appearance of 4000 deformed babies in Germany and nearly 1000 in Great Britain—all born to mothers who had taken a sleeping aid called thalidomide. The United States was spared the tragedy because the Food and Drug Administration had not approved the drug for sale. Drugs, chemicals, and infectious agents (such as the rubella virus) that cause birth defects are called **teratogens**. The period of organ formation (organogenesis)—between the third and eighth week—is generally considered the critical period. Drugs taken after this time are not likely to be teratogenic, but they may alter the growth and functioning of normally formed tissues. Drugs causing fetal problems include antineoplastics (cancer drugs), cortisone, radioactive iodine, narcotics, and certain sedatives, analgesics, and antibiotics. A rather special case involves the antibiotic tetracycline. Yellow discoloration of the teeth and faulty enamel occur in children born to mothers given this antibiotic during the latter half of pregnancy.

■ Alcohol

The incidence of alcohol-induced birth defects is now estimated to be one for every 100 women consuming more than one ounce of alcohol daily in early pregnancy. The **fetal al-**

cohol syndrome therefore accounts for the occurrence of approximately one birth defect in every 5000 births in the United States. Affected infants are often of low birth weight, mentally retarded, and may have behavioral, facial, limb, genital, cardiac, or neurologic abnormalities.

The risk and degree of abnormality increases with increased alcohol consumption. According to a Boston City Hospital study of infants born to heavy drinkers (average 10 drinks a day), 29% had congenital defects compared to 14% for moderate drinkers and only 8% among nondrinkers. Furthermore, 71% of infants born to women who consumed more than 10 drinks daily had detectable physical and developmental abnormalities. Safe alcohol consumption levels during pregnancy have yet to be determined. But, in view of the association between high levels of consumption and fetal abnormalities, women who are pregnant or who think they might be should be encouraged to use caution where alcohol is concerned. And women alcoholics, until treated effectively for their addiction, should be encouraged by public information programs and by direct counseling to avoid conception.

■■■■ DRUGS IN NURSING MOTHERS

Most drugs appear in the nursing mother's milk, but the effect on the infant depends on a number of variables, including the type of drug, the amount of milk ingested, and infant tolerance. Drugs that should not be taken by nursing mothers include atropine, anticoagulants, bromides, cathartics (except senna), ergot preparations, iodides, mercurials, narcotics, tetracyclines, and metronidazole (Flagyl). The following drugs are not contraindicated, but the infant should be watched carefully for adverse effects: antibiotics (other than tetracyclines), barbiturates, corticosteroids, diuretics, lithium, nalidixic acid, oral contra-

ceptives, phenytoin, reserpine, aspirin, and sulfonamides (sulfa drugs).

■■■■ INFANT MORTALITY

For 1978 the infant mortality rate was 13.8 per 1000 live births (compared with 162 per 1000 live births in 1900), with the rate for black babies 92% higher than for whites. The greatest single problem associated with infant mortality is low birth weight; nearly two thirds of the infants who die are low in weight at birth. Maternal factors associated with a high risk of low–birth weight babies include age (17 and under, 35 and over), minority status, previous unfavorable pregnancy outcome, low education level, low socioeconomic status, interpregnancy interval less than 6 months, inadequate weight gain during pregnancy, poor nutrition, smoking, misuse of alcohol and drugs, and lack of prenatal care. High-quality early and continuous prenatal, birth, and postnatal care can decrease a newborn's risk of death or handicap from complications of pregnancy, low birth weight, maternal infection from sexually transmitted disease, and developmental problems, both physical and psychologic.

The records of many demonstration projects, both domestic and foreign, amply confirm that dramatic improvements can be made in the indicators of maternal and infant health. For example, the infant mortality rate for American Indians was reduced by 74% between 1955 and 1977, and maternal mortality decreased from 2.2 times the total U.S. rate in 1958 to below the total U.S. rate by 1975-1976. Unfortunately, studies have not generally been designed to yield firmly defensible data on the relative contribution of such programs. However, the evidence indicates that emphasis should be placed on family planning that optimizes the timing of pregnancies, on early identification of pregnancy, and on routine involvement of all pregnant women in prenatal care.

■■■■ SELF-TEST

1. __J__ sperm plus ovum
2. __C__ embryonic disk
3. __L__ X plus Y
4. __A__ X plus X
5. __H__ umbilical cord
6. __O__ fetal membrane
7. __B__ pregnancy test
8. __N__ breast secretion
9. __K__ spontaneous abortion
10. __F__ X-linked disorder
11. __m__ autosomal recessive
12. __E__ Down's syndrome
13. __I__ rubella virus
14. __D__ sonography
15. __G__ AFP test

a. female
b. gonadotropin
c. ectoderm
d. ultrasound
e. trisomy
f. hemophilia
g. anencephaly
h. placenta
i. teratogen
j. fertilization
k. miscarriage
l. male
m. thalassemia
n. colostrum
o. amnion

IUD –
INtRA – UtERa DEViSE

autosomal – body cElls.

■■■■ STUDY QUESTIONS

1. What is the relationship among the terms zygote, embryo, and fetus?
2. What is the relationship between the umbilical cord and the placenta?
3. What is the relationship between the amnion and the amniotic cavity?
4. Normally all ova are identical. The same cannot be said of sperm. Why?
5. Why, precisely, are identical twins "identical"?
6. Quintuplets result from four "splits" of the zygote. By means of a diagram show what happens. (Two diagrams are possible.)
7. What are the chances of fraternal twins being brother and sister?
8. Which is correct, "estrogen" or "estrogens"?
9. Premature infants weigh between 1 and 2.5 kg. Give this weight in pounds.
10. Pregnancy can be detected in a matter of days following conception. How is this possible?
11. A pregnant woman with poor kidney function is potentially at high risk. Specifically, why?
12. What is the origin of the word "cesarean"?
13. Why is the navel also called the umbilicus?
14. In a sense the third stage of labor is an excellent example of the expression "anticlimax." Why so?
15. An excessive loss of blood after childbirth is called postpartum hemorrhage. What would constitute an "excessive loss"?
16. Colostrum and milk provide the newborn with protection against infection. Is this permanent protection? Explain.
17. Breast feeding affords a number of advantages. How many can you name?
18. As a consequence of legalized abortion, septic abortion in the United States has fallen dramatically. Why?
19. A single X-linked recessive gene, such as that of color blindness, manifests itself only in the male. The reason this is true is related to the fact that the Y chromosome is restricted to sex genes. Can a female be color blind? Explain.
20. If one partner of a couple possesses the gene for Tay-Sachs disease, will the offspring have the disease? Explain.
21. Pulse echo sonography is frequently an adjunct to amniocentesis. Why so?
22. Amniocentesis is a key backup tool in genetic counseling. Explain in detail.
23. Teratogen (an agent that produces birth defects) is a word with an interesting origin. What is its literal meaning?
24. What are your personal views on drinking during pregnancy?
25. Of the factors cited in the text that are associated with high infant mortality, which one do you consider the most important?

CHAPTER 15

Sexually transmitted diseases

Sexually transmitted diseases (STDs)—venereal diseases (VD)—are infections grouped together because they spread by transfer of infectious organisms from person to person during sexual contact. Sexually transmitted diseases are major public health problems because they cause enormous human suffering, cost over 1 billion dollars annually, and impose tremendous demands on medical care facilities. Women and children bear an inordinate share of the burden of sexually transmitted disease: sterility, ectopic pregnancy, fetal and infant deaths, birth defects, and mental retardation. Cancer of the cervix may be linked to sexually transmitted herpes virus type 2. Some experts claim that the only way we will control the problem is by developing preventive vaccines, but until that time arrives, the best protection is awareness through public education.

Public health authorities estimate that some 10 million cases of sexually transmitted diseases (STDs) occur annually in the United States, 85% of these in 15 to 30 year olds. Many STDs can be transmitted without sexual contact, although this is not common. For example, scabies or crab lice may be acquired by sleeping in contaminated bedsheets or by engaging in sexual foreplay; syphilis may be transmitted by skin-to-skin contact if the chancre (the primary lesion) is present. A lab technician working with STDs can become accidentally infected through a skin cut, and thousands of babies are born yearly with an STD. Other factors, such as emotional tension, drug use, or pregnancy, can also trigger a genital infection. Herpes infections are found even in celibates.

The dramatic rise in the incidence of STDs relates in large measure to (1) the "new morality" that cropped up in the 1960s and (2) the advent of the contraceptive pill. The discoverers of the pill themselves were among the first to admit this unforseen spin-off—that is, that effective contraception has allowed greater numbers of women to be more sexually active. Other factors behind the STD upsurge include legalized abortion and the emergence of drug-resistant strains of the gonorrhea pathogen, especially those imported during the Vietnam War. Finally, there are all sorts of "incentives" from the movies, television, magazines, and how-to-do-it sex books. The joy of sex is in the air, and, literally, so are its consequences.

PREVENTION

Abstinence and fidelity are the best ways to avoid STDs. The more people with whom a person has intimate contact, the greater the risk of exposure. Though no method is fail-safe, a sexually active person can reduce the chances of getting an STD (1) by not having sex with persons not well known, or with persons potentially infected with an STD; (2) by using a condom or a contraceptive foam, cream, or jelly; (3) by douching after intercourse; (4) by washing exposed areas after contact; (5) by urinating after contact; and (6) by being on the alert for sores, discharges, and other signs of infection. STD education is paramount and, as indicated above, should have two major outcomes: The population in general would adopt actions or modify behavior so as to minimize or prevent infection, and persons who do contact an STD would recognize it and seek proper medical care. Obviously these outcomes depend on a basic understanding of the major STDs, which is the aim of the present chapter.

SPECIFIC STDs

"Venereal disease" (VD) is no longer an adequate expression to describe sexually transmitted diseases, since the term traditionally has been limited to syphilis, gonorrhea, and three relatively rare infections—chancroid, granuloma inguinale, and lymphogranuloma venereum. Today a good two dozen infections are known to be sexually transmissible. Those of major concern, in addition to syphilis and gonorrhea, include trichomoniasis, nongonococcal urethritis, candidiasis, genital herpes, hepatitis B, cytomegalovirus infection, group B streptococcus infection, genital warts, pediculosis pubis, and scabies. The highlights of these infections will be presented. It is important to keep in mind that an infected person may harbor two or more STDs. Trichomoniasis and candidiasis often occur together in women and, in certain populations, syphilis and gonorrhea occur together in both sexes. An individual with gonorrhea, syphilis, scabies, and pediculosis pubis is certainly not a figment of the imagination.

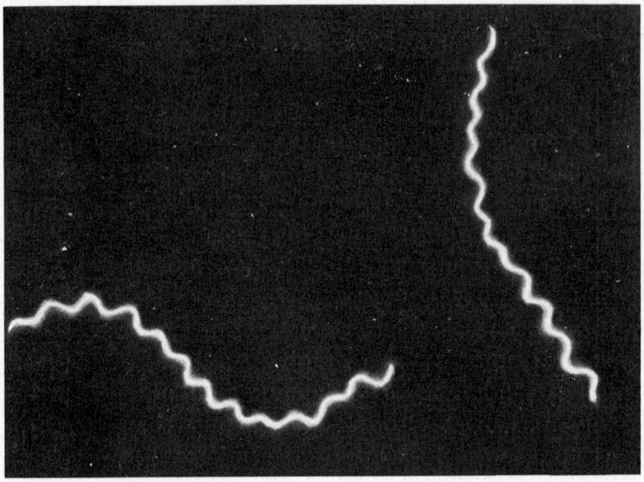

Fig. 15-1 ■ *Treponema pallidum*, the cause of syphilis. (×6000.)

From Kraus, S.J.: JAMA **211**:2141, 1970. Cooyright 1970, American Medical Association.

■ Syphilis

Syphilis ranks third (exceeded only by chickenpox and gonorrhea) among reportable diseases in the United States. An estimated 80,000 to 85,000 new cases occurred in 1980, and about 325,000 untreated cases (including all stages) exist at present. Although much less common than gonorrhea, syphilis is much more dangerous. Untreated, it results in the degradation of mind and body and eventually in death. The causative organism is the bacterial spirochete *Treponema pallidum* (Fig. 15-1). In acquired syphilis the spirochetes typically are passed along by the sexual act, but any form of intimate body contact suffices if it involves the transfer of liquid infectious material. Kissing and abnormal sex practices are recognized modes of transfer, and initial syphilitic lesions on occasion involve the lips, tongue, tonsils, eyelids, breasts, or fingers. Congenital syphilis results when the spirochete is passed from mother to fetus.

Acquired syphilis. After sexual intercourse with an infected person, the **chancre**, the hallmark of **primary syphilis**, appears in about 3 weeks at the portal of entry; the usual sites are the penis, scrotum, vulva, vagina, and cervix. Usually single rather than multiple, the chancre has a firm base and a raised border; it varies from the size of a pinhead to the size of the end of the thumb. The surface appears eroded, and gentle pressure calls forth a watery discharge rather than pus. Another characteristic feature of primary syphilis is the development of swollen regional lymph nodes (buboes). In a month or so the chancre heals, with or without treatment, leaving a pale scar; the buboes, if they occur, may or may not persist.

The passing of the chancre heralds the end of the primary stage of syphilis and the beginning of the **secondary incubation period**, during which time the spirochetes swim about in increasing numbers and set up foci of infection throughout the body. This state continues for weeks or months (about 6 weeks on the average), until one day the victim arrives at the **secondary stage** of infection, the characteristic features of which are a generalized skin eruption and mucous patches. The rash is highly varied and may simulate almost any skin lesion—measles, for instance. The mucous patches are circular, multiple areas of erosion on the membranes of the mouth, throat, genitalia, and rectum. They teem with spirochetes. The rash, patches, and other signs and symptoms last from 6 weeks to 6 months and then disappear with or without treat-

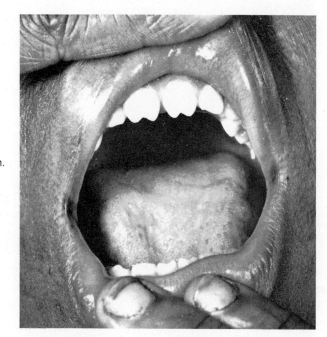

Fig. 15-2 ■ Congenital syphilis. Hutchinson's teeth.

From Wehrle, P.F., and Top, F.H.: Communicable and infectious diseases, ed. 9, St. Louis, 1981, The C.V. Mosby Co.

ment. Then follows the asymptomatic **latent period**, which lasts from a year to a lifetime, depending on the outcome of the continuing battle between the spirochetes and the forces of immunity.

Some one third of afflicted persons eventually develop **tertiary** (late) **syphilis**, the cardinal lesion of which is an inflammatory scarring and weakening of the aorta. Commonly, heart murmurs and heart failures occur. Other cardiovascular possibilities include an outpouching (aneurysm) of the aortic arch and an infected heart muscle. Another major tertiary ramification is neurosyphilis, the most severe form of which is a general semiparalysis arising from a spirochete invasion of the brain. There is considerable microscopic disorder of the cerebral cortex and widespread loss of nerve cells. All this leads to changes in the intellect, memory, mood, and behavior; terminally, there is a dementing psychosis. Finally, about 10% of persons in the third stage of syphilis develop soft, rubbery tumors called **gummas**. The location, number, and effects of

these lesions are varied and, along with the cardiovascular and nervous involvements, make syphilis the great imitator that it is.

Congenital syphilis. The fetus "acquires" syphilis sometime after the fifth month of pregnancy in untreated women, and almost always the result is miscarriage, stillbirth, or a diseased baby. Quite to the contrary, women who become pregnant many years after infection often give birth to normal babies.

Babies born with congenital syphilis are not likely to show evidence of the disease for 3 or 4 weeks, when some sort of skin eruption almost always appears. Other distinguishing marks in the early days are cracking of the lips, enlarged spleen, snuffles, and a peculiar cry. In overall appearance the syphilitic infant is puny, withered, and shriveled and has the face of a little old person. Juvenile lesions appear at an average age of 10 years. The classical feature here is **Hutchinson's triad**: inflammation of the cornea, often resulting in blindness; deafness from auditory nerve damage; and notching of the upper incisors (Fig. 15-2).

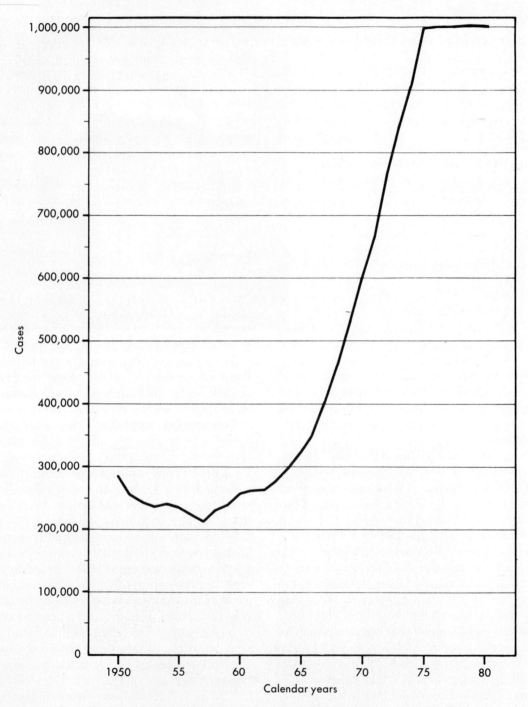

Fig. 15-3 ■ Reported cases of gonorrhea, United States, calendar years 1950-1980.

Centers for Disease Control, Atlanta, Ga.

Additionally, there are considerable and widespread skeletal changes and, not uncommonly, neurosyphilis.

Diagnosis and treatment. To establish whether a chancre is really a chancre or a mucous patch is really a mucous patch, a drop or two of exudate is examined for the presence of spirochetes. Unfortunately, the diagnosis of syphilis is seldom this straightforward because well over three fourths of syphilitic persons seen by doctors are in latency and thus without signs and symptoms. In this situation the diagnosis must be made on a basis of telltale antibodies and blood tests. Useful screening tests are the RPR and VDRL; the most accurate confirmatory procedure is the FTA-ABS test.

Treatment of syphilis centers on the use of penicillin to kill the spirochetes and follow-up blood techniques to monitor the response. Generally, cures are produced in about 90% of early syphilitics receiving one course of treatment and in a substantial proportion of those who must be re-treated. The outlook in late syphilis is from good to excellent when the cardiovascular and nervous systems are not involved. In asymptomatic neurosyphilis where the only sign is a "positive" cerebrospinal fluid, immediate therapy can prevent the development of dangerous complications. Congenital syphilis responds dramatically to penicillin, and complete cures are the rule when the infection is caught early. Afflicted youngsters under age 2 usually are cured in 1 year, and even in late congenital syphilis (12 years or older), the outcome is good, provided there has been no real damage before starting treatment.

■ Gonorrhea

Gonorrhea is the most common STD of universal stature; an estimated 2.5 million new cases occur annually in the United States—a national epidemic (Fig. 15-3). The cause is *Neisseria gonorrhoeae*, a coccal (spherical) shaped bacterium that occurs in pairs; it is commonly referred to as the **gonococcus** (Fig. 15-4). The infected partner infects the nonin-

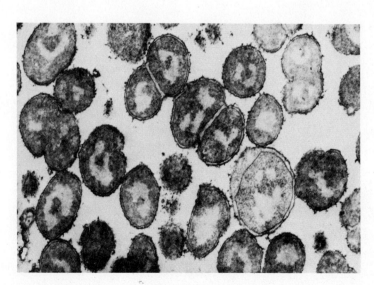

Fig. 15-4 ■ *Neisseria gonorrhoeae*, the cause of gonorrhea, cross section, as seen under the electron microscope. (× 100,000.)

fected partner by introducing the pathogen into the fluid products of the sexual act. The gonococci are massaged and washed into the urethra in a most efficient manner, and, in a matter of days, infection is established. The usual incubation period runs between 3 and 9 days.

In the typical male case the first signs are burning on urination and the appearance of a pus-filled discharge. The urethral orifice is usually inflamed and puffy. The infection works its way upward and backward through the urethra and shortly incites real trouble in the prostate gland (prostatitis) and in the seminal vesicles, the former squeezing the urethra and causing urinary retention and the latter causing fever and pain. Further advancement of the infection into the seminal duct leads to inflammation of the epididymis and testis.

Complications include sterility and inflammation of the joints and heart valves.

In the typical female case the early stages usually do not appear; perhaps 9 out of 10 victims may be completely without initial signs and symptoms. The female becomes a healthy carrier par excellence. When the early phase is evident, however, it begins with painful urination and vaginal discharge. The cervix is involved almost immediately, and, from this location, the infection spreads to the uterine tubes. In untreated cases the tubes get larger and larger and fill with pus; the entire pelvic area eventually gives way to fibrosis, abscesses, and adhesions. This pelvic involvement, referred to as **pelvic inflammatory disease** (PID), is by far the most common and most serious complication in females. Other

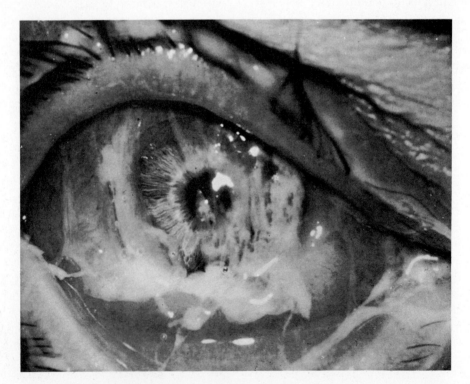

Fig. 15-5 ■ Acute gonococcal conjunctivitis.

From Donaldson, D.D.: Atlas of external diseases of the eye, vol. 1, St. Louis, 1966, The C.V. Mosby Co.

complications are the same as in the male: involvement of the joints and heart valves.

Diagnosis of gonorrhea centers on the isolation of *Neisseria gonorrhoeae*, and treatment amounts to the use of large doses of penicillin or other antibiotics. The result is often dramatic, and "single shot" cures are not uncommon. Untreated gonorrhea is communicable for months and often, especially in females, for years. For the sake of precious time, all contacts should be considered infected and given penicillin or tetracycline at the earliest hour. Expectant mothers known to have gonorrhea should be given appropriate therapy during pregnancy, and, if this is not possible, the newborn should be given penicillin immediately on delivery.

The conjunctiva of the eye affords rich soil for *Neisseria gonorrhoeae* (Fig. 15-5). If unchecked, gonorrheal conjunctivitis can easily result in blindness. Adults may infect their own eyes or someone else's by touching them with contaminated fingers; newborn babies pick up the eye involvement (**ophthalmia neonatorum**) as a consequence of having passed through a birth canal laden with gonococci. Instilling 2 drops of 1% silver nitrate solution into each eye immediately after birth has reduced tremendously the incidence of blindness caused by ophthalmia neonatorum.

■ Trichomoniasis

Trichomoniasis ("trich" or TV) is one of the most common STDs in America. Because 50% of women harbor the pathogen—a protozoan by the name *Trichomonas vaginalis*—and many men become unsuspected carriers, the infection has an estimated incidence of 3 million cases a year. Men and women frequently have asymptomatic infections of the genital tract from this organism. The classic trichomonal vaginitis syndrome consists of a frothy, yellowgreen or white discharge and a red, irritated vaginal wall. Recent studies, however, reveal that these signs are not specific for trichomoniasis and that only a minority of women with this infection will have the classical findings. Severe consequences of this infection have not been documented.

Because trichomoniasis cannot be diagnosed on the basis of signs and symptoms, laboratory tests are essential. The "wet prep" is an inexpensive, quick test in which a sample of vaginal discharge is mixed with a drop of saline solution on a slide and examined microscopically for the presence of the pathogen. Culture methods are more sensitive but are not used routinely because of cost. Metronidazole (Flagyl) is the drug used in the treatment of trichomoniasis, but the drug is contraindicated in pregnant women or lactating mothers. It is about 95% effective. The rate of permanent cure in women can be improved if they and their sexual partners are given metronidazole at the same time.

■ Nongonococcal urethritis (NGU)

Urethritis in males that is not caused by gonorrhea is referred to as **nongonococcal urethritis** (NGU). The incidence of this STD is estimated to be about 2.5 million cases annually. Postgonococcal urethritis (PGU), a variant of NGU, occurs when urethritis recurs after successful treatment for gonorrhea. PGU probably represents coinfection with *Neisseria gonorrhoeae* and some other pathogen. Bacterial microbes associated with NGU (and PGU) include *Chlamydia trachomatis* and possibly *Ureaplasma urealyticum*. The incubation period of this disease is longer (1 to 3 weeks) than that of gonorrhea, and the symptoms are often milder. NGU is diagnosed by excluding gonorrhea. NGU responds to treatment with the antibiotic tetracycline. Persons allergic to tetracycline may take erythromycin. Women with NGU contacts are frequently asymptomatic although they are likely to have cervical infection. NGU may cause pelvic inflammatory disease (PID) and post-partum infections, and it may be transmitted from an infected mother to the newborn (causing conjunctivitis or pneumonia).

■ Genital herpes

Two types of **herpes simplex virus** (HSV) cause skin problems. The common **cold sore** is usually caused by type 1, and type 2 usually infects the genital area. Occasionally type 1 herpes simplex virus can be found in the genital area. Genital infections—**genital herpes**—usually begin 3 to 7 days after exposure. The person may note an area of burning, tingling, or pain on the genitalia; then small, grouped blisters, which ulcerate, appear. Associated with these lesions may be severe pain, swollen lymph nodes, and constitutional symptoms such as fever. When the lesions appear on the cervix or vaginal wall, there are frequently no symptoms. The primary infection usually persists for several weeks, heals spontaneously, then may recur. Recurrent infections are usually milder and shorter than primary infections. However, some persons may have recurrences monthly, which may be disabling. Serious complications are rare in men, but infected women can transmit the infection to the newborn at the time of delivery. Neonatal infection is often fatal or, if the infant survives, may lead to lifelong brain damage. Genital herpes is also associated with cervical cancer, but a cause and effect relationship has not been established.

Genital herpes is highly variable, and the diagnosis can be confirmed only by isolating the virus by tissue culture. For pregnant women who have active lesions at the time of delivery, many experts recommend cesarean section to prevent transmission to the newborn. Estimates of the incidence of genital herpes vary widely, but virtually all who have studied this STD agree that it is a very serious public health problem. Current control strategies beyond careful counseling of pa-

tients have not been developed for this infection. Major research efforts are under way to develop a definitive treatment and to understand more completely the immunologic relationships between the host and the infectious agent. Several new drugs look promising and may eventually prove effective. One such agent, acyclovir (Zovirax), has proved effective when used immediately at the first sign of infection, and the oral form of the drug may prevent recurrences.

■ Cytomegalovirus infection

Cytomegalovirus (CMV) infection is a viral disease occurring congenitally, postnatally, or later in life. It ranges in severity from an asymptomatic infection without consequences to disease manifested by fever, hepatitis, and (in newborns) brain damage, to stillbirth or perinatal death. Twenty-five percent of all serious infant retardation and about 20% of infant cerebral palsy is attributed to congenital infection. The cytomegalovirus is ubiquitous; infected persons may excrete the virus in the urine, saliva, milk, cervical secretions, and semen. Infection may be acquired in utero, during birth, or by contact with infected secretions or excretions at any time thereafter. Clearly, it is an STD of considerable prominence. There is no specific therapy that to date has yielded clear-cut clinical results.

Of special concern and worry is that CMV infection may damage the body's immune system and thereby set the stage for an unusual assortment of exotic disorders—some of them deadly—in homosexual males. Among such diseases are a particularly virulent form of pneumonia (**pneumocystosis**) and a lethal cancer (**Kaposi's sarcoma**) most often found in equatorial Africa. Since homosexual women are not affected, researchers conclude that both diseases are closely linked to the life-style of gay men with many sexual contacts. No effective treatments have been developed. Physicians and gay activists are encouraging homosexuals to practice better hygiene, reduce their sexual contacts, and get the names of those they do have sexual contact with.

■ Hepatitis B

Hepatitis B (**serum hepatitis**) has emerged as an important sexually transmitted disease among homosexual men. Essentially, it is a liver infection caused by hepatitis B virus. Preliminary data from selected homosexual groups indicate that up to 20% to 25% of uninfected men will become infected with hepatitis B virus each year. Studies of selected populations indicate that more than 50% of male homosexuals may have antibodies to hepatitis B virus, indicating past infection. Penile-oral or penile-anal transmission appears to be most common. There is no known effective treatment; most patients recover without treatment. Recently a vaccine against hepatitis B has been developed and evaluated in homosexual men. Vaccination prevented more than 90% of the episodes of hepatitis B. Blood serum from gay volunteers was used in the development of the vaccine.

■ Group B streptococcus infection

Group B streptococcus infection is caused by bacteria named beta-hemolytic streptococci. Most adults do not show symptoms although infection is common, especially in women. About 50% of 12,000 annually infected newborn infants die from the disease, and many survivors suffer damage to the brain, sight, and hearing. The infection is diagnosed by a lab culture from possible infection sites, and it is curable with antibiotics.

■ Candidiasis

Candidiasis is a fungal (yeast) infection caused by the pathogen *Candida albicans*. It is usually limited to the skin and mucous membranes; uncommonly, the infection may become systemic and cause life-threatening infection of the internal organs. Infection of the vulva and vagina (**vulvovaginitis**) is relatively common, especially in pregnancy or in diabetes mellitus, and it appears as a white or yellow discharge with inflammation of the vaginal wall. Itching is intolerable, to say the least. Infection of the glans penis is less common but is often seen in males whose sexual partners had candidal vulvovaginitis. *Candida albicans* is a common inhabitant of the vagina and most of the time is held in check by normal vaginal bacteria. Typically, trouble (vaginitis) arises when the vaginal environment is altered by such factors as pregnancy and diabetes mellitus. Other known factors that affect the vaginal environment include oral contraceptives, hormone therapy, and antibiotics. The detection of candidiasis is made by examining vaginal secretions under a microscope or by taking a culture. Treatment usually consists of oral or vaginal medications containing the antibiotic nystatin. When one sexual partner has recurrent candidiasis, both partners should be treated. The incidence of spreading the disease at birth is quite low, and if it is contracted by the newborn, candidiasis can be easily controlled.

■ Condylomata acuminata

Condylomata acuminata (**genital warts**) are caused by a virus related to the one that causes the common skin wart. The number of cases of the infection per 1000 patient visits to STD clinics (1978-1979) was 37 for men and 24 for women. The incubation period is about 3 months. Typical lesions are white-to-gray and may extend to the surrounding skin of the genital area where they appear as typical warts (Fig. 15-6). The diagnosis is based on the appearance of the lesions. All therapeutic agents are irritants that cause sloughing of the skin containing the virus; therapies do not selectively inactivate the virus. A 20% alcoholic so-

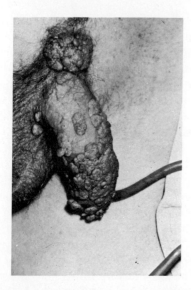

Fig. 15-6 ■ Condylomata acuminata of penis. Note giant wart at penile-abdominal junction.

From Winter, C.C.: Practical urology, St. Louis, 1969, The C.V. Mosby Co.

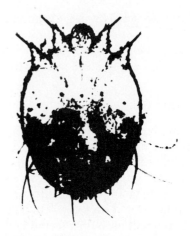

Fig. 15-7 ■ *Sarcoptes scabiei*, the itch mite. (×125.)

Photograph courtesy Reed & Carnrick Pharmaceuticals, Kenilworth, N.J.

lution of podophyllin in benzoin is often highly effective. Podophyllin-resistant lesions are treated with cryosurgery. Efforts to prevent the spread of genital warts are mostly limited to use of a condom until treatment is completed and the warts are gone. Sexual contacts should also be examined to avoid reinfection.

■ Pediculosis pubis

Pediculosis pubis, infestation with pubic lice, is caused by *Pthirus pubis*, the crab louse (p. 145). The number of cases of the infestation per 1000 patient visits to STD clinics (1978-1979) was 37 for men and 24 for women. The crab louse infests the hair of the pubic region and attaches eggs or nits to the hairs. After 1 week the larvae hatch, and in 2 weeks they develop into adult crab lice. The lice attach themselves to the hair base and feed on the blood of the host. Persons become aware of the infection because they see the lice or the eggs or because intense itching develops after 2 to 3 weeks. The diagnosis is confirmed

by identifying typical eggs or lice in the pubic hair. One percent gamma benzene hexachloride (Kwell) applied as a cream, lotion, or shampoo is effective therapy for both lice and the eggs. Killed eggs may remain fixed to a hair until the hair is shed. Clothing and bedding can be decontaminated by thorough washing or dry-cleaning.

■ Scabies

Scabies is a highly contagious infestation caused by *Sarcoptes scabiei* (itch mite) (Fig. 15-7). The number of cases of the infestation per 1000 patient visits to STD clinics (1978-1979) was 11 for men and 5 for women. Among children or in poor living conditions scabies is usually transmitted by nonsexual contact, but sexual transmission makes an important contribution in western society. Initially the gravid female mite burrows into the skin, depositing feces and eggs. The infestation may pass unnoticed for 1 to 3 months when hypersensitivity develops and itchy, red, raised lumps appear; the distribution pattern is shown in Fig. 15-8. The itch is quite noticeable and may become unbearable in warm weather, after a bath, or in bed. The major complica-

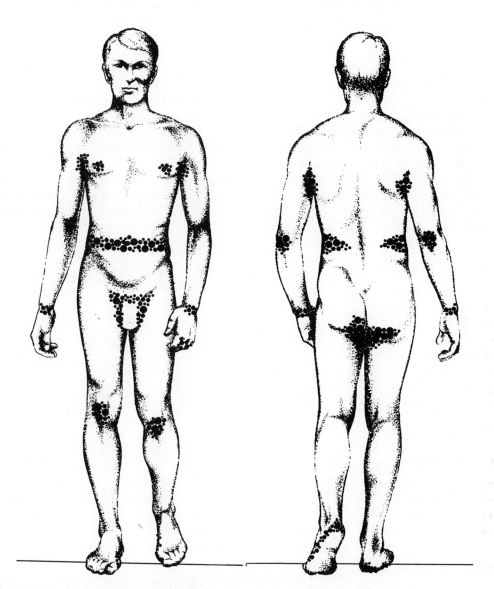

Fig. 15-8 ■ Distribution pattern of scabies.

Courtesy Reed & Carnrick Pharmaceuticals, Kenilworth, N.J.

tion is bacterial infection from scratching. Scabies is treated effectively by applying gamma benzene hexachloride (Kwell) to the skin.

■ Rare STDs

Although reportable by law (in most states), chancroid, granuloma inguinale, and lymphogranuloma venereum are rare compared to the other STDs that have been described. For example, whereas gonorrhea has an incidence of over 400 cases per 100,000 population, chancroid averages about 0.25 cases. **Chancroid** is an acute, localized STD caused by the bacterium *Haemophilus ducreyi*. It is characterized by painful genital ulcers and inflamed in-

guinal (groin) lymph nodes; sulfa drugs usually provide effective treatment. **Granuloma inguinale** is an STD caused by the bacterium *Calymmatobacterium granulomatis*. It is characterized by deep, pus-oozing ulcers of the skin of the external genitals and is successfully treated with streptomycin. **Lymphogranuloma venereum** is an STD caused by a strain of *Chlamydia trachomatis* (another strain of which is responsible for NGU). The infection is characterized by a transient, ulcerative lesion of the genitals followed by inflammation of inguinal lymph nodes and serious local complications. Tetracycline is the drug of choice in the treatment of lymphogranuloma venereum and usually produces satisfactory results.

■ SELF-TEST

1. _B_ primary syphilis
2. _G_ tertiary syphilis
3. _m_ congenital syphilis
4. _K_ female gonorrhea
5. _O_ male gonorrhea
6. _A_ newborn gonorrhea
7. _E_ CMV infection
8. _I_ homosexual transmission
9. _D_ yeast infection
10. _H_ condylomata acuminata
11. _F_ pediculosis pubis
12. _C_ itch mite
13. _J_ *Trichomonas vaginalis*
14. _L_ *Chlamydia trachomatis*
15. _N_ genital herpes

a. ophthalmia neonatorum
b. chancre
c. scabies
d. *Candida albicans*
e. infant cerebral palsy
f. crab louse
g. semiparalysis
h. warts
i. hepatitis B
j. pathogenic protozoan
k. PVD
l. NGU
m. Hutchinson's triad
n. blisters
o. painful urination

■ STUDY QUESTIONS

1. What is the difference, if any, between VD and STD?
2. In your view what are the major factors involved in the tremendous increase in sexually transmitted diseases?
3. As a wit once said, "You have to go out of your way to catch VD." Do you agree?

4. What is the basic distinction between acquired syphilis and congenital syphilis?
5. Syphilis passes through the following "phases" of development: primary stage, secondary stage, tertiary stage, latent period, primary incubation period, and secondary incubation period. Put these in the proper order.

6. By definition, latent syphilis is asymptomatic, that is, without signs and symptoms. How, then, is it diagnosed?

7. Penicillin is generally a magic cure for syphilis, but sometimes it is worthless in the very late stages of the infection. Why?

8. Relative to gonorrhea, the "female is a healthy carrier par excellence." Explain in full.

9. What is the literal meaning of "ophthalmia neonatorum"? What is the usual cause and means of prevention?

10. What is the real proof that a given infection is indeed gonorrhea?

11. Many infectious diseases we get just once and that's it. What about syphilis, gonorrhea, and other STDs?

12. The only sure way to cure trichomoniasis is to treat both sex partners simultaneously. Why?

13. What is the fundamental distinction between NGU and gonorrhea?

14. What, if any, is the connection between the common cold sore and genital herpes?

15. What is the chief danger associated with genital herpes?

16. What is the chief danger associated with cytomegalovirus (CMV) infection?

17. Why is the sexual transmission of hepatitis B mainly associated with homosexual men?

18. The prevention of hepatitis B is unique among the STDs. Why so?

19. Candidiasis usually arises "when the vaginal environment is altered." What does this mean?

20. What, if any, is the relationship between condylomata acuminata and common skin warts?

21. Distinguish between the terms pediculosis, pediculosis capitis, pediculosis corporis, and pediculosis pubis.

22. Is scabies a form of pediculosis? Explain.

23. What is the difference between chancre and chancroid?

24. What do NGU and lymphogranuloma venereum have in common other than the fact that they are both STDs?

25. Soap—just about any kind—is highly bactericidal and virucidal. Discuss the implications of this fact for venereal disease.

CHAPTER 16

The family

The family, to state the obvious, is the basic unit of society. Strong, happy families make a strong, happy society; weak, unhappy families make a weak, unhappy society. Accordingly, those who start the family—the parents—have a grave responsibility. If they are successful, their children and society benefit; if they fail, their children and society suffer. First and foremost, parents are the ultimate teachers in that wittingly and unwittingly they teach by example. Fundamentally, they demonstrate right from wrong, whether it be the right way to brush the teeth or the right way to get along with one's neighbors. All the little things count because taken together they determine the quality of the society in which we find ourselves. In some form or other the family will remain, but as to its future quality, no one can say for sure. There are good signs and there are worrisome signs. What we must do is take stock and then go on to perfect this primordial institution.

The high divorce rate in the United States (one divorce for every two marriages in 1981) has direct implications for the mental and physical health of the nation. Much has been said recently about the weakening of the family by changes resulting from urbanization and industrialization. In agricultural living the extended family, with an uncle or aunt as well as grandparents, carried on some projects in which all members of the family could take a part. Father and son, mother and daughter spent much time together. The family went to church together and depended on it for many social activites.

The small nuclear family in the city of today lives under conditions that have changed the quality and extent of familial relationships. These include the stress of mobility, the loss of contact with nature, and a reduced sense of identification with the community. The changing environments brought about by frequent moves are unfamiliar, and the children may have no idea about what the father or the working mother does during the workday.

Despite many changes the family still remains the basic unit of society and a fundamental source of stabilization for the individual. Marriage affects a great many people. Initially, it involves the two people, then their parents, relatives, and friends, and subsequently their own offspring. It is the beginning of long and far-reaching relationships.

Interestingly, many studies have shown that marriage is associated with good health. One reason may be that marriage can lead to more definitive and regular life-styles and less risk-taking. Persons living together, especially if there are children to care for, tend to be more scrupulous about their own and each other's health care practices—diet (good nutrition), recognition of disease symptoms, and the like are more certain to be considered and noticed than in those who live alone. Another reason could be that seriously unhealthy persons tend to remain unmarried.

■■■ THE MODERN FAMILY

The size of the American family has been steadily decreasing in the past decade. The average household size declined sharply from 3.11 persons in 1970 to 2.75 in 1980. (A **household**, as defined by the Census Bureau, refers to all persons who occupy a housing unit, including related and unrelated persons.) The smaller size of the American family of today is no doubt due in part to the widespread use of contraception. This is especially true of the better educated, more affluent middle class of the population. More couples practice birth control than ever before, and there are more effective methods of contraception.

The planned childless marriage has also contributed to the smaller family size. Today it is no longer taboo to enter into marriage without the idea of procreation in mind. A survey (1980) showed that the majority of young married couples polled felt that refusing to have children was not necessarily selfish and that it was perfectly all right to be married and to choose not to have children. Another survey showed that the majority interviewed believed childless marriages were the happiest.

Turnabouts in family living have occurred that affect traditional roles and arrangements at home and at work. Basic shifts in the stereotyped sex roles of marriage partners have occurred in large measure because of the women's liberation movement and the recognition, thereby, of the equality of women. Since it can no longer be said that "the woman's place is in the home" (since half, or perhaps even more, of American families are composed of working wives and husbands), it is not uncommon for both partners to play a dual role and share responsibilities in the home. Child rearing and housework, for example, today may involve the husband as well as the wife. And of no little importance in an inflationary economy, a working wife's contribution to family finances has become increasingly significant in recent years. By way of contrast, in 1955 the typical husband-wife family contained only one breadwinner, the husband. In that year only 26% of couples were partners in the labor force.

Despite these and other changes and a reduction in religious and moral values, as well as such threatening influences as drug and alcohol addiction and teenage promiscuity, the family remains our basic unit of society. The family is definitely changing, but nonetheless, according to researchers, top priority is still placed on the family and on marriage. Interestingly, young adults are becoming noticeably more conservative in their attitudes toward life-style, and there is an apparent shift toward a reaffirmation of traditional middle-class values. In 1979 the American Research Corporation conducted a survey in which 41% of the women polled said they chose to be mothers and stay at home. One third of the women polled showed a preference for a combination of motherhood and a full-time career. A survey (1978) carried out by the American Council of Life Insurance asked young adults 14 to 25 years of age which of life's goals was the most important to them. Forty-five percent answered, "to develop as an individual"; 34% replied, "to have a happy family life"; 13% answered "to have a fulfilling career"; and 7% responded, "to make a lot of money." The same survey demonstrated that 65% of these persons would like to have the kind of life that provides a good job, a nice family, a home in a pleasant neighborhood, and a role in the community. Furthermore, women's liberation notwithstanding, it seems that women are more likely to support the traditional life-style (73%) than are men (58%).

■■■■ SOCIAL RELATIONS BEFORE MARRIAGE

Prior to the twentieth century social relations between men and women before marriage were carried out largely under chaperoned or strictly supervised circumstances. Today there is usually abundant opportunity for a couple to have as much or as little intimacy as they deem desirable. Young Americans, women in particular, encounter much more freedom than was customary in the past. This freedom presents a great responsibility to young persons to maintain a standard of conduct that will result in a level of happiness for both the present and the future. There is, of course, a very real danger that the young person may be swept off his or her feet by the excitement of the moment. Choices of personal life-style must be made in the context of a society that, in addition to providing an overabundance of freedom, fosters and glamorizes potentially hazardous behavior. The advertising media, movies, television, and pop music, as well as examples set by older adults, bombard young persons almost every hour of the waking day.

The pattern of premarital conduct poses certain problems in a culture in which several years may intervene between sexual maturity and marriage. Often the period stretches from 5 to 10 or more years while young persons complete their schooling and establish their economic independence. During these years adolescents and young adults face social and sexual problems that require decisions based on intelligence and mature judgment. It is the time when these individuals are struggling to establish an acceptable sexual identity—when they are learning what is involved in being a man or woman and knowing how to manage a lasting relationship with someone of the opposite sex. Many young persons during this period find group activity entirely satisfying (Fig. 16-1), perhaps meeting together with one another at the movie theater, coffee house, or local community center. Whether a loner or part of the crowd, the young person eventually will come face to face with the exciting and depressing ups and downs of adolescent love.

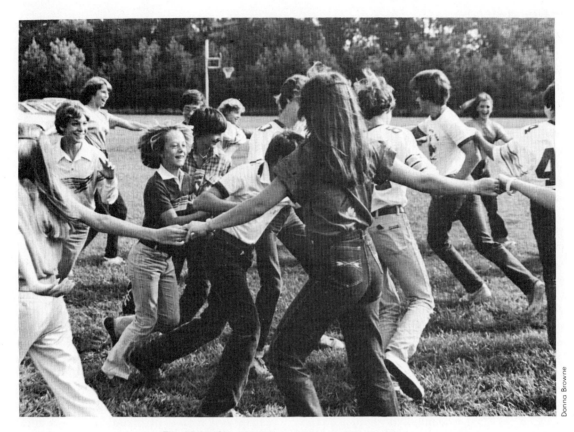

Donna Browne

Fig. 16-1 ■ Group activity promotes social adjustment.

■ Dating

Studies have shown that, contrary to what some believe, dating is not a thing of the past. Despite a large amount of publicity surrounding the changing roles of the sexes, it has been demonstrated by researchers that the traditional practices of dating are here with us now—at least for the time being. According to Winch, the functions of dating include (1) the opportunity for recreation, (2) the provision of status, (3) the development of social graces, (4) the development of one's personality, (5) preparation for selecting a spouse, and (6) the development of qualities needed in marriage as father, mother, husband, wife, and homemaker.

Dates can be made through mutual friends and through social, vocational, and church functions; oftentimes they are initiated through school contacts. Usually, in the beginning, the dating relationship is not serious; rather it is a process whereby the young person may build several or more friendships. In most instances, studies have revealed, initiating the date still remains the man's responsibility, as it was in the past. As a result, men face more pressure in dating than women and therefore experience a higher degree of anxiety. The biggest fear is that of rejection—a fear often severe enough to lead men to counseling. One counselor on a college campus reported that he saw more students because of problems associated with dating than for any other reason.

■ Going steady

Going steady is a relationship that commonly develops from dating when the two young persons find their dates especially enjoyable. Although very popular in high school, going steady can shut off a teenager's social contacts too soon and can interfere later on with a mature selection of a mate. The outcome could very well be an infatuation resulting in an early and unhappy marriage. Going steady in college is more often a marriage-oriented process, but a more mature one.

In going steady the two persons find companionship and the reassurance of having someone to rely on for social activities. Certainly the anxiety involved in dating is absent, and each partner derives a feeling of security and worth. Sometimes, however, the couple removes barriers to sexual activity too soon, granting more freedom than either one is capable of handling, especially if one of the partners is very young and/or lacking in sexual experience. The intensity of this latter situation can result in serious emotional disturbances.

Once they have decided to go steady, the couple should be in agreement about what is involved. The more successful relationships usually develop slowly with real affection, in contrast to those in which one partner manipulates the other out of transient and selfish interest. In general, young men are more inclined to regard going steady as a pleasant, temporary friendship, whereas young women, who, according to the experts, tend to be more marriage and family oriented, may be prone to regard it as the beginning of a permanent relationship.

■ PREMARITAL SEXUAL RELATIONS

In seeking answers to the questions, "What shall I do about sexual relations now?" and "How shall I achieve a happy marriage?" the young adult is likely to find the two questions

closely related. In seeking the behavioral pattern that will provide the greatest long-term satisfaction, the young person faces serious and difficult decisions. Continence and sexual intercourse before marriage are determined in large measure by strong forces related to religion, the acceptance or rejection of a specific code of ethics, the family pattern of thinking in regard to sex, and the individual's interpersonal relationships.

■ Continence and virginity

For some persons continence before marriage contributes to successful mating by making the love element more idealistic and by bringing the highest degree of self-respect to the individuals involved. However, in today's world remaining continent can bring about psychologic and social problems for the young adult, especially the adolescent. Normal young persons often have severe conflicts concerning premarital sex as a result of peer pressure. Peer pressure is considered by many authorities as one of the primary reasons why teenagers become involved in sex. Adolescents' decisions concerning their sex life in large part are based on what their friends are doing. The standards they grow up with will affect their choice—teenage virgins still exist, but their reasons for remaining so may be very different from those of a generation ago. There is no longer much concern about a "bad reputation" among friends, fear of pregnancy, or even worry about adult disapproval. Often teenagers are ashamed to admit they are not ready for sex. And, as we all know, the promotion of sexual precocity as the norm by the media contributes in no small way to the confusion. Add to all this a lack of knowledge of the facts of life and the difficulty and embarrassment many parents experience in discussing sexuality with their children.

Continence and virginity are entirely consistent with physical, mental, and social health, yet, according to statistics, at age 19 only one in five young men in the United States in 1981 was a virgin, and only one in three young women had not lost her virginity. Furthermore, most children had had their first sexual experience by the time they were 16 years old, and approximately 12 million teenagers were sexually active in that same year.

This is not to say, however, that there are not adolescents who demonstrate a high degree of maturity about sex. They are interested in developing meaningful relationships and ask themselves about possible emotional or physical consequences of sexual experimentation. Parents should talk with their children and work to encourage in them wholesome attitudes toward their own sexuality. They should discuss the legal and moral implications of sexual activity and the young person's willingness to accept responsibilities for the well-being of his or her partner as well as the responsibilities of parenthood.

■ Petting

Petting has been defined as "all relations more intimate than kissing but short of actual sexual intercourse." (Once intercourse has taken place, the term "petting" is often replaced by the term "foreplay.") Petting sometimes occurs as a part of casual dates or sometimes results from going steady. It can be "light" or "heavy," but in either case it is sexually arousing and a stimulus for desire rather than a relief from sexual tension. The danger involved is that petting, because of its progressive nature, may push the couple into unexpected and unpremeditated sexual relations.

■ Premarital intercourse

Premarital intercourse (or as some would have it, "promiscuous sex") may be a tender, mutually responsive, passionate communication between two persons who care deeply for one another, or it may be an act performed in haste. If performed in haste, premarital sex

can be harmful and damaging. Severe emotional effects may result as well as anxiety, fear of discovery, and guilt. Longstanding feelings of shame and self-reproach, disillusionment, and a loss of self-respect or respect for one another are not uncommon among very young, immature individuals. The partners may come away from such an unhappy experience with a negative attitude toward sex, possibly lasting for a lifetime.

The specific dangers of premarital sex include pregnancy (Chapter 13) and sexually transmitted diseases (Chapter 15). These consequences increasingly threaten the health and well-being of millions of adolescents and young Americans each year. Statistics tell us that the odds are not in favor of the approximately 1 million teenage girls who become pregnant each year. In addition to being a poor health risk for herself and her baby, the very young mother (under 20 years of age) faces significant social and psychologic adjustments. Abortion (p. 220) also carries a number of potentially serious consequences. If parents and/or their children need information or believe they need help with a sexual problem, they should not hesitate to contact their physician or a local public health agency.

■■■ CHOOSING A MATE

By the time a person reaches a certain level of maturity, the head as well as the heart should be used in choosing a mate, although as we well know, oftentimes just the reverse happens when two persons "fall in love." The college-age adult should have some understanding of personality and the importance of qualities such as sincerity, fairness, friendliness, intelligence, good health, tact, morals, manners, and a sense of humor that are important in a lifetime partner. Physical attractiveness and congeniality are important, as researchers have shown, but certainly they are not the only characteristics to be considered. Not to be ignored are many well-recognized potentially harmful traits that can threaten an enduring friendship and, consequently, a marriage. These include selfishness, arrogance, restlessness, and suspiciousness. Emotional instability should not be overlooked. However, a person is clearly more than a list of characteristics or personality traits; rather, we see and we know the impact of the total being.

THE ENGAGEMENT

Once two persons decide to get married, they often enter the **engagement period**, which may include the presentation of a ring to the woman by the man as a token of affection and faith. The engagement can be a period in which the two persons plan the pattern of their future life together. It can also provide them an opportunity to compare their views on many matters, not the least of which is sex—its relation to love, for example, and the role it should play in marriage. Also, in the engagement period similarities between the two individuals as well as any differences in their interests, attitudes, and beliefs, can be acknowleged. Any conflicting points of view should be discussed openly, and when a difference in religious or racial background is involved, the situation should be explored thoroughly and accepted without reservations. It is important that the couple recognize the potential impact these latter differences might have on their respective families and on society.

The engagement, ideally, should provide time enough for the couple to be as confident as possible that their feelings for each other are genuine and that the relationship is not merely a temporary infatuation. If one partner finds characteristics in the other that are seriously distrubing, it should be kept in mind that it is a rare occasion, indeed, when one person can make over another—serious flaws can seldom be made to disappear. A certain amount of premarital anxiety is understanda-

bly normal. However, the two persons should seek professional counseling if they are unable to reconcile any differences—especially if they cannot communicate openly with each other. Some professionals believe that all engaged couples would profit by counseling in order to get the marriage off to a good start. It could mean the difference between a happy and an unhappy union.

There should be a realistic understanding of what each person's responsibilities will be in the marriage. Important topics that can be discussed and dealt with include, among many others, finances (perhaps the most important), family size, views on child rearing, housekeeping, and living arrangements.

Before the marriage ceremony, it makes for good sense for each partner to have a thorough physical examination, especially so that any indicated physical correction can be made. Premarital blood tests are a requirement in most states and should be made in any case. This is a time, too, for checking genetic factors that may influence the union. From her consultation with the physician, the woman may secure a prescription for contraceptive devices or drugs, which will minimize her fear of pregnancy without restricting her sexual expression.

MARRIAGE

Sooner or later, statistics tell us, most persons make the decision to get married. It has been estimated that 92% of Americans are willing to take the trek down the aisle at least once in their lifetime. People remarry after one, two, or three divorces. Marriage is still considered a viable institution, and although many young people are delaying it, they still support it. In 1980 married couples comprised 60% of all households in the United States, and over 2½ million marriages took place.

Marriage provides many benefits including companionship, parenthood, achievement, sharing, emotional support, economic and legal ties, and aging together. The ideal marriage, it has been said, is "a relationship between best friends whose companionship and common interests make them stronger than they would have been had they not chosen to live their lives together." Age, heredity, education, temperament, parental approval, manners, morals, religion, culture, race, financial and social background, attitudes, common interests, similar work capacities, and emotional maturity all contribute to a happy marriage.

The average age of people entering first marriages in 1981 in the United States was about 25 years for men and 23 years for women. Teenage marriages appear to be declining. State laws set minimum age requirements for teenagers—usually 18 years for both men and women without parental consent. Such laws generally require parental consent if the individual is below a given age, which varies from state to state. Studies have shown that the happiness level increases with the age of the couple at the time of marriage. One causative factor appears to be the changes that take place in value systems between the ages of 16 and 22 years. Divorces occur more frequently in marriages in which either one or both parties were less than 20 years of age when married. The actual ideal age at marriage, however, is determined by the individual situation and not by statistics.

■ Adjustments in marriage

A happy marriage and a contented home, free from frustrations and resentments, can bring great joy to a couple and can contribute immensely to the success of their lives outside the family. In order to achieve these goals, various problems must be faced and solved by every newly wedded couple. If the lines of communication are always kept open, the marriage will be stronger, and the husband and wife will be brought closer together.

Minor irritations are common to every marriage, but they can build up until they become a danger to marital happiness. The couple who can talk about any hurts or grievances promptly, objectively, and with mutual consideration is likely to avoid calamity. Allowing minor problems to recur continuously and meeting them with sarcasm or nagging can lead to serious trouble. "Let not the sun set upon your wrath" is good advice to bear in mind always.

Few problems are unique although they may seem so to a particular couple. Just about every situation has been or will be met by other couples, and there is usually a solution. When great stress arises beyond their ability to cope, the husband and wife should not be reluctant to seek advice from their clergyman or physician. If the problem is severe enough, a qualified counselor can oftentimes save the marriage from ending in the divorce courts.

According to many experts, the major marital problem has to do with finances. How will the husband and wife spend the family income? Is there going to be a budget? How far will they go in making financial commitments? Do both pool their paychecks if both are employed? Money matters can be a serious source of friction that possibly can be avoided if the couple freely discusses the subject before marriage. Indeed, many couples rely on prenuptial agreements or, after the marriage ceremony, written agreements detailing each other's financial responsibilities.

In our society both partners should recognize and come to terms with the ever changing traditional sex roles. The husband must accept the career-bound wife and the fact that she may not be in the home all day long. And, too, the wife often must be willing to support her husband and postpone her own education or career outside the home so that he may finish his education. Changes in the traditional allocation of household responsibilities may be required and will demand the patience and understanding of both husband and wife.

FAMILY PLANNING

One of the most important decisions that every couple must make together has to do with family planning. Factors to be considered should include the health of the mother, the economic ability to provide for the children in early childhood and during their school and college years, the conveniences for rearing children, the career goals of both spouses, and the cultural affiliations of the family. The couple should ask themselves if the joys of parenthood will outweigh the inevitable frustrations of child rearing. Does the couple have the maturity to raise a family? Do they realize (most young people do not) the financial burden? According to the Department of Agriculture, the cost of seeing a child born in 1979 through birth and up to 18 years under the parental roof will total well over $134,000 by 1997. And the real backbreaker—the cost of 4 years of college—is not included. Some important wrong reasons for making the decision in favor of parenthood are (1) the man sees siring a child as the masculine thing to do; (2) the woman sees childbearing as fulfillment of her femaleness; and (3) the couple believes that having a child can save an unhappy, faltering marriage.

Sometimes family planning involves more than the questions of "when" to have a child and "how many" children. For some people the question is "whether." There are couples at high risk of conceiving a child with an inherited disorder. They may wish to consider that risk in deciding whether or not to have children. Other couples decide against having families because child rearing will not fit into their chosen life-style. In order to prevent the birth of unwanted children, one or both members of a couple can use **contraception** to avoid pregnancy temporarily or **sterilization** to prevent pregnancy permanently. (Both topics are discussed in Chapter 13.) When contraception or sterilization is not used, or when it fails, **abortion** may be considered.

There are many sources of information about family planning, and there is help available to everyone, regardless of marital status or ability to pay. As a starter, not to be ignored are the family doctor or clergyman, local board of health, and local hospital, community or church affiliated clinics. Many college campus physicians are willing to provide students with birth control information. Planned Parenthood, one of the most prominent birth control organizations, has about 200 affiliates across the country with clinics to assist in family planning. Local branches may be located by consulting the telephone directory or by writing to the home base in New York City. Other organizations include the National Clergy Consultation Service, Zero Population Growth (ZPG), National Organization for Women (NOW), and Association for Voluntary Sterilization.

Abortion

In 1973 the Supreme Court of the United States in *Roe vs Wade* declared that a woman has a fundamental constitutional right to have an abortion in the first 3 months of pregnancy. Since that time opponents of abortion (estimated at more than 10 million in number) have been seeking a way to undo the decision. The controversial issue, one that involves moral, ethical, religious, and social values, is perhaps the most passionate and intensely felt issue in politics today, emerging in Congress as a matter of prime importance. At the time of this writing the Helms-Hyde bill—the **Human Life Bill**—has been introduced into Congress declaring that the fetus is entitled to the protection that the Fourteenth Amendment extends to all persons and that human life "shall be deemed to exist from conception." The bill would mean that aborting a fetal life could be defined as murder, thereby making the woman and her doctor subject to criminal prosecution. According to some opponents of the bill, it is not only an attack on abortion but on birth control as well, since the legislation could also make illegal any birth control method that is believed to act after conception.

Adding to this volatile issue, the Reagan Administration in 1981 proposed the elimination of federal financing of abortions in cases of rape or incest. Funds for abortion would be available only when a woman's life is in danger. According to the Department of Health and Human Services, it would be up to the individual states to decide whether or not to finance any abortions at all if the proposal is acted on.

One thing that both sides agree on is that abortion can be a difficult issue for both patients and doctors. It is something not taken lightly by women, and the choice to have one is a woman's alone to make and one that is always sad. Doctors are faced with the decision of whether or not they should perform an abortion. Many feel it is a service that violates their own moral code, and therefore they will not participate in it unless, perhaps, it involves the life of the mother.

There are three major methods of terminating a pregnancy—vaginal evacuation, stimulation of uterine contractions, and major surgery. **Vaginal evacuation** is done by either vacuum aspiration (suction) or dilation and curettage (commonly called D & C). Both procedures are limited mainly to first-trimester abortions. **Stimulation of uterine contractions**, the technique of choice for second-trimester abortions, is effected by the infusion of about 200 ml of 20% salt solution into the amniotic cavity. Labor usually starts within 12 to 24 hours after the infusion, and the uterine contents are usually evacuated within 36 hours. Intraamniotic administration of prostaglandin $F_{2\alpha}$ may also be used to stimulate contractions. Major abortion surgery includes **hysterotomy** (incision of the uterus) and **hysterectomy** (removal of the uterus). Hysterectomy

also sterilizes the woman. Both operations can be performed in both the first and second trimesters. Vacuum aspiration has the lowest complication rate, followed in order by D & C, saline infusion, hysterotomy, and hysterectomy. Complication rates are three to four times higher for second-trimester abortions than for first-trimester abortions. As for the psychologic aspects of abortion, the available data show that most women who have induced abortions do not appear to have adjustment problems.

■ Infertility

Some couples (one out of ten) desire children and appear unable to have them. Research in fertility has helped medical science to aid these persons. When sterility (Chapter 13) occurs (in the man, in one third of the cases) and no children have come after a reasonable period of time, the couple should consult their family physician before they become discouraged and assume that they will never be able to have children. Several of the conditions that cause sterility in a man or woman are correctable, and this can be determined by the physician. However, if, after both have had the recommended tests and medical advice, it still appears that no children can be expected, the couple may well give attention to the possibility of adopting a child.

Adoption offers an opportunity of acquiring a ready-made family. Many restrictions have been dropped in recent years that once made adoption difficult. Many single persons are adopting children; and handicapped children, racially mixed children, and children from other countries are being adopted more frequently. There are public and private agencies that provide information and assistance to those interested in adoption. A licensed agency can be found through a state or local department of social services, the United Way, the Regional Adoption Center, and the Child

Welfare League of America. Information can also be obtained from organizations such as the Adoption Opportunities Branch of the United States Children's Bureau and the North American Council on Adoptable Children, both located in Washington, D.C.

■ PARENTING AND CHILD GROWTH AND DEVELOPMENT

The care of the child is an essential supplement to a good heredity. In today's society there is a growing tendency for both parents to take an active role, and thus we have what is referred to as **mothering** and **fathering**—or **parenting**.

■ Parenting

The love and security a newborn baby needs from the moment he or she arrives in the world outside the mother's womb is no less important than the food and shelter the baby receives. And basically this is what parenting is all about. There is an undisputed emotional attachment between mother and child that, according to some psychologists, begins at the moment of birth. (Others say this attachment begins even earlier—when the baby is still in the uterus.) But the father can begin early to participate in many ways, not the least of which is by being supportive of the new mother.

The physical and emotional changes resulting from pregnancy naturally affect the expectant mother directly. But the father-to-be has anxieties and stresses all his own. Certain matters, such as providing additional space at home for the child, selecting care providers and the birth setting, and deciding how to meet the expenses involved, can be shared by both partners. Other concerns, more personal and emotional, may be unexpected. Is the couple ready for additional responsibilities? How much will each partner react in the months ahead? Both parents will experience apprehensions that are natural, especially if it is a

first child, and these feelings will diminish as the practical and emotional adjustments necessary for adapting to the new roles of father and mother are made. A couple can be drawn closer together in learning about the events of pregnancy and the role each will play, and this will reduce some of the apprehensions. They can participate in prenatal classes (perhaps at the local YMCA) and gather information on the physical changes that take place during pregnancy, on fetal growth, and on the process of labor and delivery. Preparation usually lessens the anxiety and uncertainty. Meeting other expectant parents can also help a couple gain self-confidence.

The newborn baby receives communication by touch and sound. Cuddling and a soothing tone of voice provide early love and security. Soon thereafter, visual contact begins to play an important role. The child who feels wanted develops more normally than one who was rejected before birth and continues to be unwanted after birth.

No new parent is an expert. But mother and father will teach the infant the most important lesson in life—how to interact with other humans. And new parents are always amazed by how much knowledge they have gained through observation and experience. Parents are the most important teachers their children will ever have, and even when children start school, the home is still their classroom. Therefore intelligence, preparation, and guidance are all necessary prerequisites for parenting.

However, there is a growing recognition that in many cases young persons today are not well prepared to meet the problems encountered in child rearing. In the past, in the extended family, preparation for parenthood was obtained by observing one's parents and by caring for brothers and sisters at home. But with today's smaller families and more mothers going to work, many adolescents do not have the training opportunities at home that they will need to become effective parents. To combat this situation, especially in light of the increasing numbers of teenage mothers, divorced persons, single parents, and working mothers, many schools are introducing courses in child growth and development and parenting. Hopefully, the more teenagers can learn, the better equipped they will be to make informed decisions about marriage and parenthood and to cope with the stresses of family life.

There are also many youth-serving organizations in nonschool settings conducting a variety of parenthood education projects for teenagers. Some of these are Boys' Clubs of America, Boy Scouts of America, National 4-H Club Foundation of America, Girl Scouts of the U.S.A., National Federation of Settlements and Neighborhood Centers, the Salvation Army, and Save the Children Federation

(Appalachian Program). The federal government supplies information through various agencies, including the Education for Parenthood Program, sponsored by the Children's Bureau of the Department of Health and Human Services.

Specialists in child growth and development agree that the first 5 years are the most important ones in a child's life. From infancy children try to learn about the world inside and outside the home as well as about the world of feelings inside themselves, such as happiness, sadness, anger, fear, and frustration. They manipulate, investigate, imitate, and want to master as much of their environment as they can. To them, learning is a natural and joyful experience. The ability of children to learn many skills in these early years will depend on their stage of development and

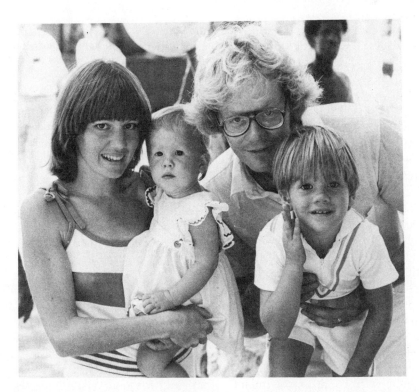

Fig. 16-2 ■ Raising children is basically a human relationship between parents and children.

on the encouragement and opportunities that the parents—the people they love and depend on the most—offer at home and in other surroundings. A responsive and accepting relationship between parents and their children (Fig. 16-2), in which the parents act as guides, teachers, and fellow explorers in a fascinating world, will enhance the children's sense of belonging, sense of responsibility to themselves and others, and their ability to learn and make decisions. These first attitudes learned from the parents will very likely influence the child throughout the rest of his or her life.

Raising children is basically a human relationship between parents and children. There can be no hard-and-fast rules. Parenting styles differ from one family to another and often vary for different children within the same family. However, there are guidelines to help parents develop happy, self-confident, self-disciplined, and healthy children.

■ The infant

Infancy is the first year of a child's life. The chief causes of infant morbidity and mortality are now controlled through intelligent care of the infant and mother. Nevertheless, at no year in life until extreme old age is the death rate so high as during infancy. And within that year the highest death rates occur during the first week and the first month. Prematurity, congenital malformations, acute respiratory diseases, acute gastrointestinal disease, and congenital debility are important causes of infant morbidity and mortality.

Many health hazards of infancy have been removed. For example, ophthalmia neonatorum has been virtually eliminated by treating the eyes at birth with 1% silver nitrate solution. State health departments help to make incubators available for infants born prematurely. Other developments are illustrated by the control of such rare conditions as infant anemia associated with Rh factor and by the

SCHEDULE FOR INFANTS	
Age	**Vaccines**
2 mo	DTP, TOPV
4 mo	DTP, TOPV
6 mo	DTP
15 mo	MMR
18 mo	DTP, TOPV
4-6 yr	DTP, TOPV
14-16 yr	Td (every 10 yr)

SCHEDULE FOR CHILDREN NOT IMMUNIZED IN EARLY INFANCY		
Time interval	**Under 6 yr**	**6 yr and older**
First visit	DTP, TOPV	Td, TOPV
1 mo later	MMR (15 mo or older)	MMR
2 mo	DTP, TOPV	Td, TOPV
4 mo	DTP	
10-16 mo (or preschool)	DTP, TOPV	Td, TOPV
14-16 yr	Td (every 10 yr)	Td (every 10 yr)

DTP — Diphtheria and tetanus toxoids and pertussis vaccine adsorbed
Td — Tetanus and diphtheria toxoids adsorbed (for adult use)
TOPV — Trivalent oral polio vaccine
MMR — Measles, mumps, rubella

● ● ● ●

★ All recommended vaccines must be taken for complete protection. Partial immunization does not ensure against the disease.

★ Any interruption in the schedule does not necessitate starting the series again. Simply complete it.

★ Doctors may vary the schedule in order to meet individual needs.

★ If unsure whether an immunization is needed or not, immunize!

Fig. 16-3 ■ Immunization schedule recommended by the Massachusetts Department of Health.

prevention of mental retardation arising from phenylketonuria and galactosemia.

To ensure good health and development the parents should have the baby examined regularly by a doctor, with monthly visits at first and less frequent visits later. Families who cannot afford visits to a private physician can

FAMILY IMMUNIZATION RECORD

■ Ask your doctor when shots are due.

■ When shots are given, have your doctor enter dates under child's name.

SHOTS FOR ▼	CHILD'S NAME ▶				
● DIPHTHERIA ● TETANUS ● WHOOPING COUGH One immunization (one shot each date) can immunize for all three if doctor recommends.	AT AGE 2 MOS.*				
	2 MOS. LATER				
	2 MOS. LATER				
	12 MOS. LATER				
	BOOSTER 4-6 YRS. OLD				
● POLIO One oral immunization each date.	AT AGE 2 MOS.*				
	2 MOS. LATER				
	2 MOS. LATER				
	12 MOS. LATER				
	BOOSTER 4-6 YRS. OLD				
● MEASLES ● MUMPS ● RUBELLA (German measles) {Triple immunization (one shot for all three). Measles booster at 15 mos. if first immunized before 1 year.	AFTER 1 YEAR OLD				
	AFTER 1 YEAR OLD				
	AFTER 1 YEAR OLD				
	*For children already beyond infancy, don't delay. See your physician and start series now.				

Fig. 16-4 ■ A sample Family Immunization Record.

attend a well-baby clinic or a child health conference located at a hospital or local health center where physicians and nurses work as a team. When they are born, babies have a natural protection from many diseases. But this protection does not last—it wears off anytime during the first 6 to 12 months of life. Protection against infection is crucial and should be provided by **active immunization**. The United States Public Health Service recommends vaccinations for the "Big Seven" infections; most states require these vaccinations for entrance to public school. The Big Seven are **diphtheria**, **pertussis** (commonly known as whooping cough), **poliomyelitis** (polio), **tetanus** (lockjaw), **rubeola** (measles), **rubella** (German measles, three-day measles), and **mumps** (Figs. 16-3 and 16-4). The importance of early immunization should be obvious to all (Table 16-1).

There is less tendency today to force infants into a rigid time schedule of eating, sleeping, and elimination, so long as there is a sound basic plan. Parents ask, "Do we pick the baby up or let him or her cry it out?" Opinions of experts vary as to the answer to this and myriad other questions. Primarily, there is no doubt the infant needs attention and an en-

ronment that provides a feeling of security. Picking up the baby and soothing it can provide the necessary security. Physicians have been known to write prescriptions for TLC ("tender loving care") as well as for medications. As stated earlier, caring for a baby requires intelligence, preparation, and guidance. Books written specifically for parents abound, and local agencies, such as the YWCA, offer programs to help parents cope with some of these problems.

■ The preschool child

The preschool child from 1 to 5 years of age has increased activities that multiply exposure to communicable diseases and opportunities for accidents. Because the child is growing and developing so rapidly, nutritional, emotional, medical, and dental needs change. The parents still need much time to give the child necessary training. It may not be provided by some parents because they do not understand the child's requirements.

Although the mortality rate among children from 1 to 5 years of age is low, continued medical supervision is desirable. A health exami-

■■■■■■■■■■■■ **TABLE 16-1**
The "Big Seven" and the dangers they can impose

Disease	Description	Possible dangers
Polio	A viral disease with three known strains	Permanent paralysis Deformity Death
Diphtheria	A serious bacterial infection	Pneumonia Heart failure Nerve damage Death by suffocation
Pertussis (whooping cough)	A bacterial respiratory tract infection	Pneumonia Brain damage Death
Tetanus (lockjaw)	A noncontagious disease caused by bacteria found in the soil	Muscle spasms Severe nervous system damage Death
Rubeola (measles)	A highly contagious viral disease	Brain damage Mental retardation Pneumonia, respiratory problems Deafness, blindness Death
Rubella (German measles)	A mild viral infection in children, a major tragedy in pregnant women	Miscarriage and stillbirth Severe birth defects including blindness, deafness, and damage to the heart, brain, and other organs
Mumps	An acute viral disease with painful swelling around the jaw and under the ear(s)	Central nervous system damage Deafness Brain damage Kidney inflammation

Data from Massachusetts Department of Public Health, the Massachusetts Hospital Association, and the Massachusetts Medical Society Auxiliary.

nation twice a year by a physician who has had experience in the care of children will enable the parent to learn of any abnormalities that need attention, to know whether the child is growing properly, and to determine whether nutritional needs are being amply met. In most instances deviation from normal in eyesight or in hearing can be most satisfactorily corrected if it is found and treated before the age of 6 years.

A visit to the dentist every 6 months or as often as the dentist deems necessary is important from the time the child is 2 years old. The dentist should watch the growth of the teeth, clean them, and fill cavities. The deciduous teeth are very important in the development of a normal jaw and in aiding the permanent teeth to erupt in proper alignment. It is a mistake to allow deciduous teeth to be neglected because they are only "temporary"

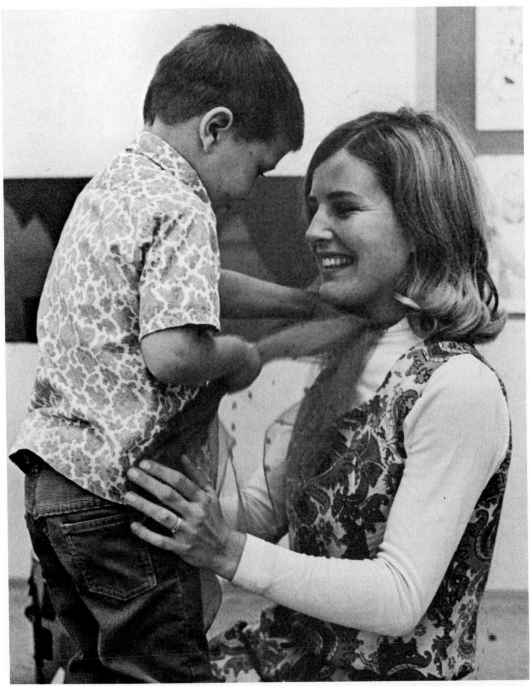

Santa Barbara County Head Start

Fig. 16-5 ■ Proper care is loving care.

From Hendrick, J.: The whole child: new trends in early education, ed.2, St. Louis, 1980, The C.V. mosby Co.

teeth. Brushing the teeth should be started when the child is about 2 years of age. The teeth should be brushed daily with a small, soft brush by the parent until the child is old enough to do it.

Good food habits are important. As the child takes more interest in the world, interest in food often slackens. The toddler is growing less rapidly and may not want or need as much food at 18 months as when he or she was 1 year old. The parents' main aim at this time is to make eating a pleasant experience.

The preschool child needs a well-planned regimen, with attention given to sleep, play, and exercise out-of-doors, as well as to diet. There should be guidance in forming habits of cleanliness and regular elimination. The family physician or public health workers can give help with the problems of child training. **Day care** may be necessary, indeed it is a growing concern in the United States. (This subject will be discussed later on in the chapter.)

Mental health deserves attention. In general parents should remember that pleasant associations help to build desirable habits and that unpleasant associations often lead to antisocial behavior. The judicious use of praise for desirable acts and the withholding of approval or attention for those that are objectionable are most important in child rearing. Children want to obey and accept the guidance of rules. Commands should be sincere, rational, enforced, and consistent. Some of the basic needs of the child are affection, companionship, understanding, a feeling of security provided by a happy home, a kindly parental authority, and a feeling of belonging, which the child gains from participation in the work and play of the family (Fig. 16-5).

■ The school-age child

The period of school age begins with entrance to school, usually at age 5 to 6 years, and lasts until the onset of puberty. Permanent teeth begin to appear, and the body proportions continue to progress. Eriksen referred to this period as "industry versus inferiority"—the child takes pride in undertaking projects and is upset if they do not turn out to be successful. According to Piaget, the concrete operational period of development occurs between 7 and 11 years of age. The child is able to comprehend cause and effect. Perhaps the most outstanding experience of the period is the child's entrance to school—one that can be traumatic or pleasant for both child and parent. The child must adapt to an entirely new sphere of rules and regulations, and the parent must release his or her child into new social realms. Preparation for this release should begin with the preschool child. For example, the parent can help the child to familiarize himself or herself with what school is all about.

■ Pubescence

Pubescence (**puberty, preadolescence**) is the period in which rapid physical changes take place. For example, both boys and girls notice an increased height and weight and the growth of pubic and axillary hair. When **menarche** (beginning of menstrual function) takes place at about 12 to 14 years of age, a girl's gain in height and weight abruptly slows. When spermatogenesis occurs at about age 15, a boy's growth in height slows, but his weight gain often continues as a result of increases in muscle mass. It is essential during this period that both sexes are informed accurately about the physiologic and emotional changes that are taking place.

It is important that the information about what is happening to their bodies be supplied to youngsters before an event takes place. The source can be books, but what they learn may not be nearly so important as being able to talk with a sympathetic adult about physical problems and the way they feel about themselves. Menstruation, for example, can be frightening to a girl if she does not know what it is all about. How this is handled by a parent can also have much to do with the way a girl feels about being a woman. Depending on the attitudes of her parents, she can see menstruation as a "curse" or as an exciting beginning to being grown-up. Much the same holds true for boys—nocturnal emissions (sometimes called "wet dreams") are a worry.

The preadolescent (and the adolescent, for that matter) is concerned that his or her body is changing in visible ways and becoming somewhat unfamiliar. Parents should recognize with tact and sensitivity their child's concern—often unspoken—about physical development or lack of it. This matter seems to cause more pain in the late-developer than to one who matures early. A daughter, anxious to grow up but still possessing a childish figure, can be helped by parents who mention her general good looks and give some time to her choice of clothing. A boy may need to be reassured that his build or physical development is in normal range.

■ Adolescence

Adolescence may be best described as a "process"—a series of rapid, noticeable changes—as well as a period in the young person's life beginning with puberty and ending somewhere between ages 19 and 21. There are no hard and fast rules to tell us when it starts or when it is over. Outward physical and personality changes occur as the youngster grows from a wholly dependent child to an independent adult. A surge of new chemistry, new drives and emotions, begins to race through the child's mind and body. These changes can affect the adolescent's everyday functioning, resulting in highs and lows that swing from cheerfulness through boredom and often down to real depression.

Whether a youngster is overdeveloped or underdeveloped, the diet deserves special attention. What an adolescent eats has a real effect on appearance, growth, and good health; studies show that adolescent nutrition is among the worst in the nation. Adolescents should be encouraged to get at least a couple of balanced meals every day. In this instance it is up to the parent to become informed about the child's dietary needs and encourage the child to eat at home as often as possible.

Adolescence brings new interest in members of the opposite sex and new impulses and desires requiring understanding and guidance. The adolescent's gradual participation in more activities outside the home, at school, church, and clubs, places on community agencies a share of the responsibility to direct new drives into healthful channels.

Adolescents need to know the consequence of sexual relations outside marriage (p. 232), of alcohol and smoking (Chapter 21) and drug abuse (Chapter 22). Young people should be fully informed about both sides of the sexual coin, as well as about the effects of drugs, alcohol, and nicotine. Impulses can be held in check without bringing harm today; restraint can provide a satisfying future life.

Runaway adolescents. For many of the 49 million youth in the nation aged 10 to 21 the adolescent years are traumatic—a time when difficult family- and school-related problems often must be faced. Most young people are able to resolve these problems, but a large number of teenagers (an estimated 730,000 yearly) are unable to cope and try to escape by running away from home. Many of these runaways drift from city to city, sometimes turning to drugs, crime, and prostitution.

State and local social services agencies funded by the Administration for Children, Youth, and Families (ACYF), a branch of the Department of Health and Human Services, provide runaway homeless youth with temporary shelter and follow-up care. In neighborhood centers trained staff and professional consultants of the Youth and Development Bureau of the ACYF try, whenever possible, to reunite runaways with their parents. They try to help young people resolve their family problems and make positive plans for the future. The Bureau also supports the National Runaway Switchboard, a nationwide toll free hot line (800-621-4000) designed to put teenagers in touch with their families and to refer them to local community agencies for needed services. Since 1974, when the hot line was first set up, the volume of calls each month has increased from 500 to many thousands.

■ Sexuality

All parents have a responsibility to prepare their children for family living. Childhood prepares for adulthood, and the best way to prepare for the profession of parenthood is to serve a childhood apprenticeship under wise and loving parents.

Hygienic living in matters relating to sex, as in other phases of life, is encouraged by correct information (as has been said earlier). Sex is not a phase of life separated from all others, nor should be the instruction concerning it. To the 3- or 4-year-old child, answers to questions about what makes the stars twinkle and where he or she came from are of equal interest. The wise parent is candid and unemotional. Sex organs should be referred to by their correct names. Children are sensitive to changes in the tone of voice or facial expression, and parents too often act embarrassed, scold or keep silent, or tell untruths in these situations. As a result the child is made uncomfortable and comes to believe that sex should never be discussed. A truthful answer in each case with facts suited to the child's level of understanding, without information that is neither needed nor understood at this time, will do much to establish healthful attitudes toward life's realities.

Such instruction is entirely or almost entirely a parental responsibility. During this time the child is developing a feeling of security as a member of the family, sharing in the love of the family. The young child plays housekeeping and takes the role of father or mother. A pattern of love and consideration (or lack of consideration) of parents toward each other and toward other members of the family is already being established.

The parent continues to be the person to whom the child most naturally turns for information about reproduction, but soon the school and other outside influences begin to contribute learning experiences. Group instruction from kindergarten through high school, beginning with caring for families of pets and continuing through laboratory courses in biology, provides children with information in physiologic matters. The school contributes to the development of correct social attitudes. But before puberty the child needs more personal information about the changes that he or she is going to experience. Once again, as said earlier, parents are best able to give this instruction. In the event parents are not able for one reason or another, the family physician or an exceptional teacher can provide the instruction (Chapter 27).

■ Day care

As more and more mothers enter the nation's work force, what to do with their children during working hours is perhaps their most worrisome problem. The availability and quality of day care for their children has become an issue of national importance. In some parts of the country there is a shortage of quality day-care facilities for low- and middle-income families.

About 58% of mothers with children 6 to 13 years of age now go to work. Some 41% of women with children under 6 years of age are now in the labor force—the fastest growing group of working mothers. Currently, about

14 million children under 14 are in day-care facilities for 10 or more hours a week. Of these children, some 900,000 are cared for in licensed day-care centers and 300,000 in licensed family day-care homes. The rest receive care in unlicensed day-care homes or are left with relatives and friends.

In licensed day-care centers and licensed day-care homes the quality of care can vary greatly, depending on the effectiveness and enforcement of federal and state regulations. Many unlicensed family day-care homes do not meet even minimum safety, health, and child development standards.

A good day-care center or home should provide the same health, training, and feeding care a parent would give at home. The physical environment should be conducive to a child's fullest social, emotional, creative, physical, and mental development. Finding a situation that meets all these criteria may be difficult, but local civic, social, and religious agencies can provide information on how and where to find out about day care. Other sources include the Day Care and Child Development Council of America (Washington, D.C.), local chapters of the National Organization for Women (NOW), and the Department of Health and Human Services, as well as listings of approved day-care centers from state departments of public welfare, state health departments, or state departments of institutions and agencies.

■ Television

Television has become America's most popular leisure-time activity and an inanimate member of the family. The set is turned on for children the moment they are out of the crib. TV often becomes an inseparable baby-sitter. Researchers have found a low level of parental concern about how much television their children watch and what kinds of programs the children tune in. Parents, according to studies, underestimate the amount of time their offspring spend on TV viewing, and it is estimated by specialists in communications that only about one third of parents control their children's television viewing. Children 2 to 11 years of age, it is further estimated, spend 3½ to 4 hours a day devoted to "the box," and teenagers spend a little over 3 hours daily in front of TV. It has not been determined how much and in what ways watching TV affects children, but some researchers have established one or more of the following results: aggressive behavior in some children, anxiety and insecurity, minority prejudice (as a result of certain programs), and adverse effects on the development of language, imagination, and reading ability. Parents can help to achieve more positive effects by discussing certain programs with their children and by deciding with them which programs are most worthwhile and rewarding to watch and which are not.

■ ALTERNATIVE LIFE-STYLES

According to a study in 1981, only 1 out of 17 families can be described as a nuclear family. And in "The Nation's Families 1960–1980," a report released by the Joint Center for Urban Studies of the Massachusetts Institute of Technology and Harvard University, the comment is made that "however valid it may have been in the 1960's to identify the suburban nuclear life-style as characteristic of the society, it is certainly not valid in the 1980's." According to the latest census data, 10% of the nation's households are headed by women, 2% are headed by men, and 28% are "nonfamily" units with unrelated people living together.

■ Living together

In about a quarter of all United States households persons are living in the same unit as simple arrangements of convenience. These persons have decided that two, sometimes three, four, or more can live in better circumstances than one, if not as cheaply. Some persons find a need for "family" support in the absence of the traditional family. Older persons have discovered shared housing as an alternative to institutional living. In some cases men and women are living together as couples.

■ Cohabitation

No one knows for certain, but it is estimated that about 1½ million unmarried heterosexuals are living together, a number that is rapidly rising. In 1970, for example, there were only an estimated 523,000 cohabitants. Cohabitation is now a part of the American way of life and in many cases proves to be a period of experimentation before the partners move on to a more traditional family life-style, that is, marriage. (Cohabitation sometimes is referred to as "trial marriage.") Many authorities believe that if cohabitation is entered into for all the "right reasons" and not simply as an immature act or act of rebellion or escape, it can provide opportunities for mutual growth for both partners.

Some of the problems encountered by cohabitants are exactly the same as those of married couples. Some problems are very different, such as the slights and discomforts that may come with breaking the rules of society. Furthermore, marriage focuses not only on the present but on the future, as opposed to the focus of the relatively short-lived relationship in cohabitation (an average of 5 years). There is the ever present danger that one or both partners can be hurt emotionally, and if children enter the picture, the arrangement becomes more complex.

When the relationship terminates, attendant complications can lead to great disappointment, hardship, and heartache. It has been said, "You shouldn't have love without a contract." In recent years a contract has been devised to alleviate some of these overwhelming complications. Called a "living together

agreement" (LRA), the contract specifies what is to happen to the couple's mutual property when they break up. Without such an agreement the courts can be drawn into bitter battle as happened in 1976 when the reciprocal property rights of unmarried couples were being tested for the first time (*Marvin vs Marvin*).

Questions can arise other than those concerning the division of material wealth, including the following: Should a divorced person living with a new lover without remarrying receive alimony from a former spouse? How does the insurance company regard "spouse"? What is the answer to discrimination in housing because of the couple's living arrangement? Can a divorced woman be denied custody of her children if she is living unmarried with a man? Can a divorced man be denied visitation rights to his children if he is living unmarried with a woman? Is the man entitled to claim a dependency exemption for the woman he is living with on his income tax return? Can an unmarried cohabitant benefit from the status of "spouse" for purposes of inheritance taxes when the live-in companion dies? Not only do heterosexual couples encounter these and other legal considerations in the various states, but also homosexual cohabitants face many of the same questions.

■ Single-parent families

There are about 5 million single-parent families in the United States as a result of divorce, separation, widowhood, unwed parenthood, and single-parent adoption. Today one out of five, or over 11 million, children are part of these families. Family experts are concerned about the special needs of such families, and, although there is no consistent evidence that single parents per se have more difficulties with their children than do other parents, there may be negative effects on a child's growth and development.

The single parent often feels overwhelmed

by day-to-day problems of managing house-keeping tasks, meeting the needs of the children, and handling financial responsibilities. Added to this is the loneliness felt by the single man or woman. Depending on the age of the children, household chores can be shared by them, day-care centers or baby-sitters can help with the problem of preschool-age children or afterschool supervision, and the children can be taught the importance of money and how to handle it. If the single parent takes time out for adult activities, the resulting relaxation will contribute not only to his or her own health and welfare but also to the happiness of the family.

Sooner or later all single parents must face up to their children's questions as to why they do not have both a father and a mother in the home. The children may worry about the future and feel guilty and perhaps blame themselves for the other parent's absence. To this end, the remaining parent must listen to the children express their feelings and reassure them that these feelings are normal. Above all, the single parent must let the children know in no uncertain terms that they will be loved and cared for.

■ Communal living

In communal living there may be several or many couples sharing the same living accommodations. The commune attracts people of all ages and is a direct response to the social stresses of our times. Ecologic and spiritual reasons are often the basis for this unit of family life.

■■■■ THE SINGLE PERSON

There are many men and women who prefer not to marry, and important as the institution may be, a person should not feel that marriage is the whole of life or that it is a necessity. Indeed, today the unmarried single state is as socially acceptable as the married state. It is not true, as a humorist has suggested, that everyone over 35 years of age is either married or singular. Some of the best services to society have come from single persons whose dominating interest has been a worthwhile cause. Furthermore, celibacy is entirely compatible with health.

It should be pointed out, however, that recent studies indicate that single people who live isolated, friendless lives are at a significantly greater risk of ill health and death than are people with a close network of relatives and friends whom they see often or than are people who actively engage in community activities. In fact, the absence of such social support systems appears to constitute just as strong a risk factor for premature death as do the factors of diet, exercise, and the absence of other more widely recognized attributes of healthy life-style.

The 1979 National Center for Health Statistics survey found that about 6% of the population visited with friends or relatives less frequently than once a month, and men and women were the same in this respect. On the other hand, about 70% of the population visited with close friends or relatives once a week or more frequently. Thus although social isolation is a problem for a small segment of the population, it does not appear to be so for the majority.

■■■■ DIVORCE

Mark Twain said it: "Familiarity breeds contempt—and children." The United States is experiencing an all-time high divorce rate. Over 1 million divorces are granted each year, and over 1 million children end up in single parent families. The greatest number of divorces occur between the first and seventh years of marriage. After this seven-year interval the likelihood of divorce diminishes. Over a third of those marrying are likely to experience one divorce. Half of all marriages of young adults are predicted to end in divorce. Even when divorce is no-fault and by mutual agreement, it is a stressful event, marked by widespread pain identified in no manual of diseases or disorders. Husband, wife, and children share in this pain.

Divorce is usually a 50-50 proposition and, except in the case of alcoholism, mental illness, and desertion, there is no one "cause" that can be pinpointed. There are many interacting forces that can result in the dissolution of a marriage. To begin with, factors that are present in a happy union are usually missing in an unhappy marriage. In the happy partnership the lines of communication and interaction between the two persons are usually wide open, especially as regards finances, sex, and problem solving. As we saw earlier, finances receive top priority as a source of discord between two persons living together. Insofar as the impact of sexual problems is concerned researchers are not in total agreement. Still unresolved is whether sexual dissatisfaction comes about as a result of an unhappy marital situation or whether discord arises in the marriage because of sexual incompatibility.

According to Birchler and Webb, the majority of couples in unhappy marriages make their original problems worse or accumulate new ones because their styles of interaction and problem solving are ineffective, if not destructive. Attempts to change a spouse's behavior through sulking, nagging, complaining, and denying sexual requests simply makes the problem worse.

The marriage in which there is little or no recreational activity between the spouses is heading for trouble. For example, this may occur where one spouse works the night shift and weekends and the other spouse works days. Eventually, they draw so far apart they become virtual strangers.

Some marriages start off with problems because the partners are mismatched. Some marriages break up because of unwanted, unplanned parenthood. Some develop more problems than others because of external events such as unavoidable difficulties with relatives or children or with mental or other forms of illness. For example, one authority reports that couples who decide to keep an autistic child at home rather than in an institution invariably end up in divorce court.

■ Counseling

Before separation or divorce takes place, most researchers agree that the couple should ask themselves, "How can our relations be improved?" Each mate should let the other know more clearly his or her own views on their life together. In other words, the prime need in many troubled marriages is for better communication between the partners.

Help in this regard can be obtained from various reliable sources in addition to reputable marriage counselors. Many churches have family help centers. There are state and county agencies prepared to assist people who need help. Community services may be available in the local area. Some examples of community services agencies are Catholic Social Services, Jewish Family and Children's Bureau, Family Counseling Services, YMCA, YWCA, and Family Service Association of America.

■ Adjustments

People who separate and divorce have two adjustments to make—one to the dissolution of the marriage and another to setting up a new life-style. In the first instance the legal process must be dealt with, that is, property settlement and child custody if children are involved. Setting up a new life-style—becoming single again—can include finding new living accommodations, living on less (or occasionally more) money, getting a job, or applying for welfare. If children are involved, there is an adjustment to be made to single parenthood or to occasional and limited visits with the children. Adapting to a new life-style involves making new friends and forming new heterosexual relationships. Certain feelings must be coped with such as fear, frustration, inadequacy, loneliness, bitterness, anger, regret, disappointment, a sense of failure, depression, relief, guilt, lowered self-esteem, and lowered self-confidence. Personal feelings toward the spouse, such as love, hate, anger, envy, concern, and attachment must be reconciled. There may be possible feelings also of freedom, happiness, and heightened self-esteem that are new and need recognition and acceptance. Divorced persons can find counseling by reliable sources helpful, and often counseling can help the person to avoid repeating the same mistake. Divorced Persons' Program, Self-Help Clubs for Single Parents, and Parents Without Partners, Inc., are a few reliable organizations offering help.

■ Children of divorced parents

Over 1 million children each year share the pain of unhappy marriages, separation, and divorce. An estimated two out of every five children born between 1970 and 1980 will live in a single-parent home for some part of their childhood. There is a growing body of evidence of trauma visited on children by divorce, especially in the first year following the breakup of the marriage. The children face emotional tangles and the stigma attached to the "broken home." In the majority of instances the mother rceives custody, thereby perhaps creating confusion in the children's minds out of a sense of loyalty to both parents. However, today courts are more flexible in making arrangements, and some fathers are being given custody and some mothers are being asked to make support payments for the children. No matter what the basis for disagreement between the former spouses, an arrangement should be made that will work toward the best interests of the children. Almost always, the child's best interests require as much time as possible with both parents,

and for this reason many courts are now considering joint custody.

For children who need help, there are many outside sources available. Some public school systems have support groups for children of divorce. Big Brothers of America, Big Sisters International, and National Youth Courtesy Foundation are but a few organizations on the alert to provide assistance.

■ FAMILY VIOLENCE

Domestic violence is clearly recognized as a serious problem in American families. Approximately 2 million incidents of **spouse abuse** (Chapter 17) occur each year within all social and economic groups. The victims, primarily women, are often severely injured. Each year an estimated 1 million children and youth are victims of **child abuse** (Chapter 17) and neglect. To deal with this serious nationwide problem a National Center on Child Abuse and Neglect was established by Congress in 1974 and set up within the Children's Bureau. The center serves as a focal point for a national effort to identify, prevent, and treat child abuse and neglect.

Incest, or sexual abuse in which the perpetrator and the child-victim are members of the same family, is a highly emotionally charged and socially intolerable form of sexual abuse. For most people incest is the most threatening and difficult form of child sexual abuse to understand and accept. It is also the most difficult form of sexual abuse to detect because incest, by its very nature, tends to remain a family secret. Generalizations about its etiology, effects, and treatment are necessarily tentative because most published research on the subject is based on a small number of cases.

Father-daughter incest and incest involving a father figure are the most commonly reported types; mother-son, mother-daughter, and father-son incest are believed to be more rare. Sexual activity between age peers (brothers and sister, cousins) is probably the most prevalent though least reported type of incest and is not generally considered harmful to the participants (unless it involves the use of power, force, or coercion).

Incest usually has complicated temporary and long-term repercussions. Public disclosure may result in the rejection of the child by both parents, who perceive the child as guilty and a betrayer of the family. The effects of incest also depend on the child's age and level of emotional and intellectual development. Very young children may be less affected by an incestuous relationship than older children, because they may not have incorporated society's concepts of right and wrong and lack awareness of the possible repercussions. If the sexual behavior between adult and child has persisted over a long period of time, if it has involved progressively more intimate incidents, or if the child is old enough to understand the cultural taboo against what has occurred, the effects may be profound.

The pervasive fears of family disruption following disclosure are often well founded. In many communities, particularly those without adequate social service resources, family separation is the only means available to protect the child. The child may be placed in foster care; the father may lose his job or be sentenced to prison; the family's income is jeopardized; the child feels guilty and may be blamed for the breakup of the family; and the family is disgraced in the eyes of the community. The potential for disastrous consequences undoubtedly accounts for much of the resistance to reporting incest. Because offenders usually do not receive any treatment in jail, the father may return to the home, again placing the child and siblings in danger.

Signs of a change from punishment-oriented intervention in incestuous families to intervention with the goal of rehabilitating the family have begun to appear in some communities. This approach, when it is in the best interests of the child, is both hopeful and consonant with the trend toward family rehabilitation as the primary goal in child abuse and neglect intervention. There is an increasing awareness that the wrong kind of intervention can do more harm than good and that the child often does not want to be separated permanently from his or her family. Therefore more sympathetic, sensitive techniques for working with these families developed.

■■■■ SELF-TEST

1. __C__ sexual stimulation
2. __F__ "aging together"
3. __G__ first year of life
4. __I__ menarche
5. __H__ 1 to 5 years of age
6. __J__ 13 to 21 years of age
7. __K__ "trial marriage"
8. __L__ sexual abuse
9. __M__ marriage dissolution
10. __O__ aggressive behavior
11. __B__ virginity
12. __D__ personality trait
13. __E__ "making plans"
14. __A__ family planning
15. __N__ working mother

a. contraceptives
b. continence
c. foreplay
d. congeniality
e. engagement
f. marriage
g. infancy
h. preschooler
i. puberty
j. adolescence
k. cohabitation
l. incest
m. divorce
n. day care
o. television

Kelly

◼◼◼◼◼ STUDY QUESTIONS

1. The text states: "In some form or other the family will remain, but as to its future quality, no one can say for sure." Do you agree? What are your views?

2. A major survey in 1980 showed that the majority of persons interviewed believed childless marriages were the happiest. Does this surprise you? Discuss.

3. Basic shifts in the stereotyped sex roles of marriage partners are due in large measure to the women's liberation movement. Why so?

4. A study in 1979 by the American Research Corporation found that 41% of the women polled said they chose to be mothers and stay at home. Does this surprise you? Discuss.

5. "In stark contrast to the past century, present society provides an overabundance of freedom and fosters and glamorizes potentially hazardous behavior." Elaborate on this statement and provide some examples of "hazardous behavior."

6. Winch cites six functions of dating (p. 215). Do you go along with these? Do you have your own list?

7. One college counselor at a large university reported that he saw more students with problems associated with dating than for any other reason. Does this surprise you? Discuss.

8. Many authorities believe that going steady in high school can shut off a teenager's social contacts too soon and interfere later on with a mature selection of a mate. What are your views?

9. What are your feelings about premarital sexual relations?

10. "The head as well as the heart should be used in choosing a mate" is certainly sound advice. Do you know firsthand of situations where the advice was put to use? Not put to use?

11. In your personal view what is the purpose of the engagement? How long should it be?

12. Do you know firsthand of what one might consider a "perfect marriage"? If you do, how well does it go along with the material presented in the text?

13. Numerous studies show that the major marital problem has to do with finances. Does this surprise you? Discuss.

14. Family planning, in essence, concerns the questions "when," "how many," or indeed, "whether." Discuss each.

15. The major problem in discussing the topic of abortion is that people become so polarized and emotional in their thinking. Logic says that there are obviously pros and cons or "two sides to the story." Discuss in detail your feelings on the subject.

16. Sterilization and the pill are virtually 100% effective as contraceptive measures. Cite the pros and cons for each.

17. Distinguish between hysterotomy and hysterectomy.

18. Infertility can arise from a number of causes in both the male and the female. Cite three for each sex.

19. What are your personal views on adoption?

20. What do you consider the most crucial feature of mothering? Of fathering?

21. Growth and development encompasses infancy, the preschool years, the school-age years, puberty, and adolescence. In your own words characterize each phase by a single sentence.

22. In your personal life what did you find the most difficult problem in early adolescence?

23. What are your personal views on cohabitation?

24. What roles do you think home and school should play in sex education? Be as specific as possible.

25. Do you know firsthand of a marriage that ended in divorce? If you do, how well did the situation agree with the material presented in the text?

CHAPTER 17

Mental and emotional health

Mental and emotional health are essential for the well-being of society in general and of the individual in particular. The other side of the coin—mental illness—clearly is an important psychosocial problem. More people are presently hospitalized for mental illness than for all other diseases combined, and an estimated 1 out of every 10 babies born today will be hospitalized for mental illness at some time during his or her life. On the positive side, though, the past quarter century has witnessed a dramatic drop in the number of patients in mental hospitals, despite an increasing population. This heartening trend is attributed in part to improved treatment (especially the use of tranquilizers and antidepressant drugs) and in part to the current emphasis on returning patients as soon as possible to the community on an outpatient basis. Recent studies show that about half of the patients admitted to hospitals are eventually discharged as improved or recovered, most of those within the first year of entering the hospital. Notwithstanding the common comment that the stresses of modern life are "driving us crazy," the evidence is somewhat to the contrary. The incidence of neurosis is no higher in New York City than in the rural areas of the state, and, what is more, the incidence of psychosis is no higher in developed countries than in a number of primitive societies that have been studied. Other topics directly or indirectly related to mental health and illness include death and dying, suicidal behavior, rape, child abuse, and wife abuse. These too will be considered in the present chapter.

Everyone desires vibrant mental and emotional health that will contribute to achievement, attractive personality, and happiness. What are the characteristics of mental health and how is it achieved? How is successful personality developed? What are the departures from normal emotional health that explain the behavior of some of the persons we meet? What should we know about society's problems in the field of mental illness?

CHARACTERISTICS OF MENTAL HEALTH

Mental health is far more than freedom from mental disease. It means the ability to live comfortably with oneself and others, to understand and accept one's own feelings, to make mature and appropriate (not childish) emotional responses to situations, to be creative, to deal with anxiety and stresses, to endure frustration, to gain satisfaction from constructive achievement, and to use leisure time profitably. Emotionally mature persons are sensitive to the feelings of others and have consideration for them. They have the ability to love and to accept love. They can deal constructively with reality and adapt to change. They are relatively free from symptoms produced by anxieties and tensions. They relate to other people consistently and satisfactorily. Let us consider three broad outstanding qualities from the above statements that are especially characteristic of people who possess a high degree of mental health.

In the first place, well-adjusted persons feel comfortable about themselves. They have self-respect and can live with themselves on pretty good terms most of the time. They have a realistic concept of their capabilities and limitations and have learned to accept any shortcomings they might have. They are willing to exert their capabilities to the maximum along constructive lines. They understand that there are strong and deeply rooted emotions that

should not become overwhelming. Through the years an "emotional maturity" has been approached that is in keeping with ideals of the social structure. Life provides disappointments as well as successes, and both are taken in stride. Well-adjusted people possess that valuable ability of being able to laugh at and not take themselves too seriously.

Another characteristic of mentally healthy persons lies in relationships to other people. They feel comfortable within themselves about others and like people and trust them, and expect the same in return. The cultural differences of other people are respected. Well-adjusted individuals are not overly aggressive in dealing with people nor do they allow others to be overly aggressive with them. They can submerge individuality in order to function as part of a group, and they can assume leadership on occasion. There is a broad sense of responsibility to neighbors and fellow human beings. To possess the friendship and esteem of one's fellows and the love of one's family and to have reasonable assurance of social as well as economic security are important essentials for mental health at all ages.

Finally, mentally healthy persons feel able to meet the usual demands of life. They face their problems, shape their environment when it is possible, and adjust to it when necessary. They do not fear the future but plan ahead, setting realistic goals. They are able to arrive at decisions after having considered the ramifications involved. In summary, mentally healthy people are able to face the problems that confront them and solve these problems satisfactorily.

According to D. L. Farnsworth mental health **is not:**

1. Adjustment under all circumstances. There are many circumstances to which a man should not adjust; otherwise there would be no progress.
2. Freedom from anxiety and tension. Anxiety and tension are often prerequisites and accompani-

ments of creativity and self-preservation, as in war, when anxiety mobilizes the powers for action.

3. Freedom from dissatisfaction. From dissatisfaction progress ensues.
4. Conformity. One criterion of maturity is the ability to stand apart from the crowd when conditions indicate. Mental health is characterized by relative freedom from cultural and personal biases.
5. Constant happiness. In this imperfect world a sensitive, mature person often experiences unhappiness.
6. The absence of personal idiosyncrasies. Many such idiosyncrasies that do not interfere with function enrich the life of the individual and the lives of those who come in contact with him.

No one can have continual peace of mind and complete success, but there are ways to increase mental health and its contribution to happiness. Although it is influenced by our environment, our heredity, and our social relationships, we can, by giving thought and effort to our mental health, largely determine its quality.

■■■■ EMOTIONAL NEEDS

There are certain requirements for mental health in the form of interrelated emotional needs.

Security. From early childhood to old age the individual needs a feeling of reasonable social and financial security. A feeling of insecurity leads to anxiety, timidity, overdependence, and inefficiency. The quest for security, however, needs to be held in balance. Security is relative, and the desire for job security should not be allowed to dominate one's plans so completely as to crowd out the hope of greater achievement. A sound realization of the economics of the family and the individual will be helpful in maintaining financial security.

Independence. We regard freedom and independent action, within the law and within one's responsibilities to society, as a right of the individual as well as an emotional need. We would be unhappy were we denied the right to choose our occupations, our mates, our political party, or our form of worship. We enjoy the proper use of independent action.

Achievement. We are cheered by worthwhile achievement, whether our sense of personal worth is strengthened by our private knowledge that we have done well or whether our success is recognized by others. The small child is praised for desirable behavior. A sincere compliment to a student on an academic, athletic, or other achievement boosts his or her morale. The desire for achievement is a major force in promoting human progress. Sometimes it is so strong as to get out of hand and lead to undesirable or unethical behavior in a child's activities, in student life, in business, or in politics.

Companionship. This is a feeling of acceptance by others, a feeling of belonging and being needed (Fig. 17-1). We enjoy the companionship of our family and our close friends and look forward to reunion with them. Being a wanted and needed member of an athletic, musical, or social group is a happy experience. It is important to build friendships with people we respect and admire. Isolation sometimes produces emotional disturbance among the deaf who are deprived of communication and among communication-deprived refugees. The student does poorly either to be isolated too completely in the interest of studies or to enjoy companionship so much that work is neglected. We sometimes see effects of feeling unwanted on older people or on minority groups.

Love and affection. Mental health is impossible for the individual who cannot give and receive affection. The little child needs to feel parental love. Without it the road toward later maladjustments is set. It is important to express affection within the family. We gain happiness through developing the kind of love

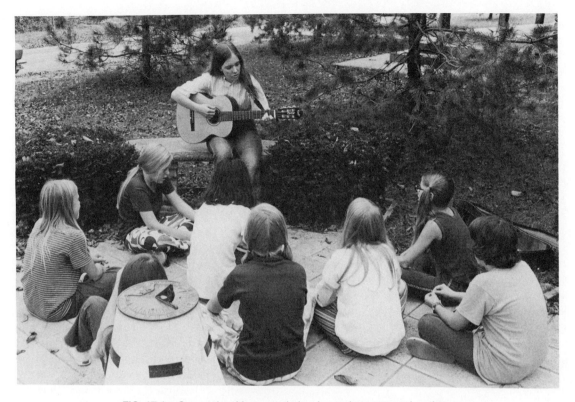

FIG. 17-1 ■ Companionship means belonging and acceptance by others.

that is based on consideration, kindness, tenderness, tolerance, and sympathy.

Self-acceptance. Persons may become emotionally disturbed if they lack self-respect or if they do not accept themselves as worthy and likeable. If unloved and uncared-for as children, if unaccepted by those nearest to them, individuals may find it difficult to accept themselves. As they achieve emotional maturity, individuals recognize their strengths and weaknesses. If there are things that they do not like about themselves but that can be changed (such as lack of courtesy in meeting new acquaintances, for example), they make the needed changes. If there is a defect that can not be changed (lameness, for example), they accept it and adjust to it. They do not make themselves miserable about it.

Variety of experiences. Monotony is deadly. Even the best-liked subject can be pursued for so many continuous hours as to become distasteful. Students should gain a broad, general education before specializing. They should learn to enjoy a variety of recreations and should plan a schedule with a variety of physical and mental activities.

Guidance. People are helped toward desirable and satisfying behavior through appropriate guidance. Emotionally mature parents contribute to desirable emotional and behavioral patterns in their children by setting sound standards of values. Children and young people are entitled to know the standards of behavior set by society. They should not be forced by lack of guidance to experience the distress that comes from failure to comply with society's many demands. Children need guidance and experience in meeting fixed conditions. Most of today's youth have never contended with severe realities of life such as extreme poverty, drought, plague, or economic depression. Many have never faced duties that demand self-discipline.

Time for contemplation. We all need to set aside occasional time for contemplation and planning, for sorting and sifting ideas, for becoming the masters of our schedules instead of allowing the pressures of the moment to make us their slaves.

Faith. Faith in a power or principle greater than ourselves has met an emotional need of humans throughout the ages. A belief in God, in the law of the universe, or in the progress of humanity has given meaning to life and set satisfying goals toward which the individual could move day by day.

■ PROBLEMS OF COLLEGE STUDENTS

For most students, entering college produces a sharp change in their mode of living and in human relations. Many new tensions, pressures, and stresses arise. The established security of the family is left behind, and academic, social, and oftentimes financial security must be sought alone. The degree of independence suddenly increases, and this new freedom should not intoxicate the person to the point of foolish and juvenile behavior. The quest for achievement starts all over again. There is a new setting among peers of differing and conflicting beliefs. New group relations must be formed and new and worthwhile friendships established (Fig. 17-2). A program must be planned that is pointed toward established main objectives but that affords a variety of desirable experiences and acceptable time allotments. The individual is under new authority and finds new guidelines for behavior.

Students' problems, like those of other people, relate to (1) personal characteristics, (2) social relationships, and (3) the demands life makes on the individual. Most problems fit into one of these three categories.

Problems in the first category, **personal characteristics,** include anxieties about physical health. Worries often arise because the student does not have a good work schedule. There may not be enough time for sleep, for recreational activity, for reading, for church, or for cultural interests. The student may always feel hurried and dissatisfied. Perhaps at college there is not time enough to do all the possible interesting and worthwhile things. Time should be allotted first to academic work, health maintenance, and those other things that are of greatest importance; less important activities may have to be postponed.

The second category, **social relationships,** includes the problems of those students who have too few friends or are in too few student activities. Some of these students would be welcomed into more social life, but they withdraw from it because they are timid. Perhaps they "pair up" too completely and lose contact with the group, or they may live socially within a small clique that has unfortunately become "exclusive." There are those, on the other hand, who have too much social life.

In studying the way to make friends, we look for the outstanding characteristics of people who are popular and "wear well." We find they usually seem assured and poised, although not objectionably so. They are friendly and outgoing; they get along well with other people and are genuinely interested in others. They seek opportunities to make and keep new friends. They are fair-minded, not prejudiced. They possess good manners too, which help to smooth the path for their social relationships. They have a realistic sense of their own dependability and personal worth. They are honest, reliable, and sincere. They are usually cheerful and confident, not fearful of the future. They are able to face up to new situations without going to pieces.

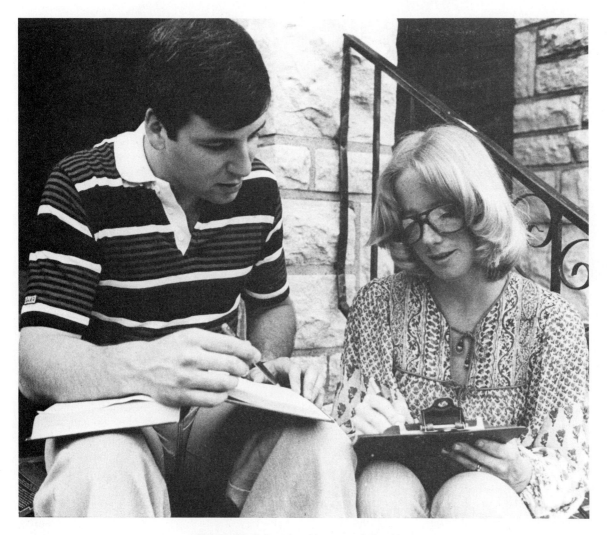

FIG. 17-2 ■ College provides new relationships.

On the other hand, if we consider why the company of certain other persons is unpleasant, we may find that they display irksome and tiresome characteristics. There is the overly sensitive person whose feelings get hurt too easily and who sees slights where none were intended. There is the self-centered individual whose immediate reaction to many situations is, "What's in it for me?" "Where do I come in?" Among the other unpleasant types we may have met are the unstable person, who "blows hot and cold"; the boaster and bore, who constantly expands his or her ego at others' expense; the "spineless" type, who seems so unsure and uncertain when faced with anything new; the prejudiced person, who readily condemns on the basis of inadequate information; and the "whiner," always complaining and never accepting any degree of responsibility for the current plight. We find it difficult to develop a deep friendship with the person who is unreliable and insincere.

College students, like all other adults, have problems in the third category, the **demands of life**. For many there are such problems as insufficient funds, jobs during vacation, dependence on relatives, and part-time work. Obviously these problems have individual, realistic, and often difficult solutions. This is an area in which the advice of parents and student advisors is likely to be helpful.

There are also the problems of students who find the academic requirements dull and uninteresting, distasteful, or almost impossible to meet. They need to consider honestly whether they are working hard enough to get the satisfaction of successful effort or whether perhaps they are embarked on the wrong course.

College students have plenty of hard work and plenty of problems related to personality and mental health. Like other people, they find some of their problems insoluble or only partly soluble. It is clear that effective action, not worry, is the proper prescription. It is also clear that it seems easier to prescribe for others than to treat one's problems objectively.

STEPS IN ACHIEVING MENTAL HEALTH

The late C.E. Turner had a number of suggestions for developing and maintaining mental health. Among others are the following:

1. Develop objectivity toward problems. Learn to accept just criticism without rejecting the person who makes it.
2. Improve skill in dealing with other people. Show appreciation of other members of the family and of the group. Strengthen friendships where problems can be shared. Do not let worries and anxieties cloud contacts with other persons.
3. Face responsibilities. Worrying about them will not drive them away. We have all had the experience of dreading a task and finding it positively exhilarating once we got at it. Avoid spending more time trying to figure out shortcuts than it would take to do the work thor-

oughly. If a decision must be made, get all the facts and then make it. Do not dodge the responsibility.
4. Set appropriate goals. Set short-term and long-term goals in line with your capabilities, neither too easy nor impossibly difficult. Make use of experience.
5. Develop broad interests. In the world of knowledge and in the world of activity and recreation, develop many interests (Fig. 17-3). Many new subjects in college seem dull in the beginning, but the more one learns about them the more interesting they become.
6. Schedule work and then work the schedule. Schedule needed recreation and enough vigorous physical activity to gain a wholesome fatigue.
7. Seek constructive outlets for anger and frustrations. These emotions stimulate the body, through the nervous system, to prepare for fight or flight, neither of which is acceptable in modern society. Vigorous exercise will help adjust the system.
8. Accept limitations that cannot be changed. In the words of Turner: "I have worked with many persons crippled by polio, among whom I have found some of the most cheerful and delightful persons I have ever met. Their mental health was determined not by their misfortune, but by the way they accepted it. In contrast to their attitude was that of a man who had lost his left hand when he was a boy. His parents, instead of helping him to feel that the loss was really unimportant, allowed him to feel that it was a disgrace. He became a lawyer and a judge; but all through college, law school, and professional life he tried to hide the fact that he had lost his hand. He needlessly embarrassed and pained himself."

ADJUSTMENT AND DEFENSE MECHANISMS

What do people do in the presence of strong anxiety, hostility, or fear? We may well examine some of the more common and well-recognized reactions. Some are useful and some are less desirable. Because we are likely to utilize these as escape and defense mecha-

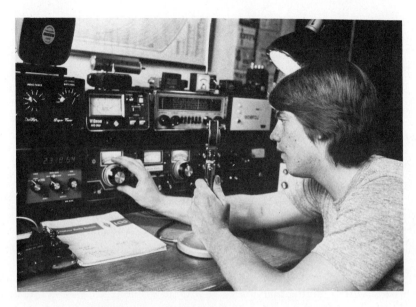

FIG. 17-3 ▪ A good hobby contributes to mental health.

nisms, we should be able to recognize them. They are safety valves when used in moderation but dangerous to achievement and emotional stability when used to excess.

When confronted with an unpleasant task or with anxieties and worries, the individual may practice **withdrawal** from any difficulties by engaging in some more pleasant activity. The student who is behind in studies may forget them by going to a party, watching television, or playing bridge, tennis, or golf. Such escape is sometimes useful as a temporary emotional release, but it does not remove the difficulty.

Sublimation means channeling the energy that might be used for socially unacceptable behavior into acceptable behavior, as when we channel our anger into physical activity or our discontent into creative or socially useful undertakings.

Rationalization occurs when we assume false reasons for our behavior or our failure. We say we failed a subject because we were given excessive assignments, instead of because we lacked effort.

Projection is the shifting of blame to others, as when we justify our wrong behavior because others do the same thing.

Displacement is the transfer of hostile emotions to a person other than the one who caused the reaction, as when a student develops hostility toward an instructor and "takes it out" on a roommate.

Regression is the return to a form of behavior that was satisfactory in an earlier situation, as when a person completely recovered from illness resumes the helplessness of the past weeks to secure attention.

Provocation is a person's intentional stimulation of others toward hostile action in order that his or her own hostility may appear as a reaction, as when one irritates a disliked fellow student until the latter takes the first step in worsening interpersonal relations between the two.

Identification is the gaining of courage or relief from anxiety through attachment to a group, such as one's family or college, or through uncritically adopting the ideas, ways, and values of some admired or famous individual. John may smoke because he identifies with his father.

Denial is the refusal to acknowledge the existence of a threatening situation, as when a student puts out of mind an imminent examination or assumes that it will not be difficult.

◼◼◼◼ PERSONALITY DEVELOPMENT

Why is it that some people possess so many more of the qualities of personality generally considered desirable than do others? What factors go into the building of that much-desired force—the healthy personality?

To the experts in human behavior the word "personality" has a technical meaning. It refers to the total individual and all our reactions—physical attributes, intellectual ability and its development, thoughts, interests, feelings, and hates, loves, joys, and hopes—in fact, all that we are and hope to become. Some of these components, such as the physical ones, are obviously hereditary. Some personality factors appear to be related to constitutional factors. We are strongly influenced by "social heredity," that is, by contact with and imitation of those persons with whom we live.

Perhaps the best way to understand the components of a desirable personality is to consider their chronologic development. Just as there are different stages in physical growth, there are stages in the growth of personality. Each of us passes through common patterns of growing and of aging. We share common physiologic processes, but since heredity and experience vary so extensively, each individual differs from all others. At different phases of biologic growth there are characteristic psychologic problems.

Erik Erikson believed that the **sense of trust** is the keystone in personality development. This starts to form during the baby's first year. Helping this feeling of trust develop is primarily the responsibility of the parents. Except for breathing, the baby at first is totally dependent. The feeling of security grows as the child is cared for and loved.

The need for a sense of trust continues throughout life. Children gradually learn to love and trust their parents. Through this experience they learn to trust others. Feelings of insecurity about parents, on the other hand, are very upsetting to children or to adolescents. If parents fail to respond to the needs of children and to give them love and assurance, they sow distrust and hostility.

In the period from perhaps 1 to 3 years of age the **sense of autonomy** or free choice is developed. The child learns to walk and "gets into everything." The child is testing the world, and testing and exercising newly developed skills. At the same time parental attitudes are a great influence. Too much criticism for destructive or sanitary "accidents" may cause a sense of shame and unworthiness to develop. Too much domination may make the child either defiant or much too submissive. Parental threats to the effect that "I won't love you if you do that" may lead to insecurity and antagonism. Emotions evolve in the emotional climate in which the child lives. The child who is not loved cannot learn to love.

The **sense of initiative** starts to appear about the age of 3 to 5 years. Children begin to act independently and are curious, creative, imaginative, and emotionally close to people. Children in this age group indulge in make-believe grown-up activities.

The **sense of accomplishment** is in the making approximately between 5 and 12 years of age. At the time he or she starts school the individual is the product of earlier experiences that have been developing gradually but continuously. The child is learning to win recognition by producing things, and recognition of accomplishment is important. Criticism is hard to take. Steady attention and perseverance give the satisfaction that comes from completing work. The person in this age group is concerned with relationships between himself or herself and the group; "secret clubs" are evidence of concern with social organizations. Rules are enjoyed; in fact, the conscience seems to be working overtime. Group standards are a tremendous influence, and a sense of personal worth with other children of the same sex and age is tested. Despite all this concern for the group, this individual is by no means ready for emancipation from parents but still turns to them for guidance and security.

Parents do well to set limits of behavior and to enforce wholesome and effective habits of living in home and community. The child learns to adjust to such proper limitations without being unduly disturbed and thus develops the strength of character that makes it easier to recognize and adjust to the more severe limitations imposed by circumstances and by society in later life.

Problems of adolescence, the period from about 12 to 21 years of age, are many and difficult. The period brings confusion and contradictions. The adolescent, now biologically mature and possessing intense emotions and feelings, must find himself or herself all over again. The need for establishing a **sense of identity** ("Who am I, anyway?") is paramount. This sense of identity involves becoming aware of one's own relationship with other people. At this age the drive for independence and emancipation from parental and outside authority is strong. The adolescent must replace this no longer acceptable authority with built-in controls in the form of self-respect, dependability, ambition, and an awareness of the needs of other people.

Pressures within young persons and pressures from their peers, parents, and society in general all demand that they find an answer to this strong drive for independence. On the one hand, adolescents aspire to an idealized maturity. On the other hand, the contemplation of detachment from the family arouses many fears. Aware of their vast inexperience,

they cling to a childhood dependence. Usually they cannot admit their own fears and may complain, sometimes unjustifiably, that it is the parents who will not let them grow up.

It should be pointed out that at this stage of a young person's development parents, too, are faced with parallel problems. They realize that the child should become independent and self-sufficient. They have a great stake in his or her solution of the problems posed by independence, but at the same time they fear the loss of love that will result when the child no longer depends on them. It is helpful for both adolescents and parents to see each other's problems and to make the necessary adaptations.

Young people, in their attempt to develop stability and emotional maturity, often go through a period of rebellion. Growing up and growing away from parents with the retention of filial affection is not easy. Sometimes youths are extremely sensitive to any form of authority and very critical of those in a position of authority. In later adolescence young people engage in endless intellectualization and rationalization about their problems. They may become absorbed in the contemplation of some new or extreme type of social order that purports to offer solutions to social and economic problems. The real reason for these contemplations, however, is their own conflict about fulfilling their needs and desires in the culture in which they find themselves. Their desires and emotions urge them toward decisions quite contrary to those dictated by intelligence or reason.

Another problem encountered at this stage of development is presented by sexual maturity. With our justified belief in education, most young people face years of higher education, followed by the problems attendant on getting established in business or in a profession. There is a long interval in our society between biologic readiness for marriage and the time it is economically feasible. This poses problem of developing a life that is satisfying and at the same time consistent with our ideals.

Problems concerning the choice of vocation are related to this sense of identity. A wise solution to vocational problems is helped by knowing as much as possible about one's own abilities and by setting realistic goals within the opportunities offered by the social structure.

Emotional disturbances in young people may be expressed by antisocial or delinquent behavior. Unpleasant traits and actions may cause the adolescent to be rejected by peer groups at a time when acceptance by the group is vital. As a result of this rejection the adolescent may become antisocial and easy prey for extreme political doctrines or propaganda or may become involved in difficulties with the law.

Actually, adolescents are eager for social acceptance and for the establishment of close friendships with individuals like themselves. They are also eager for the acceptance and approval of those a little older than themselves. They may indulge in "crushes" and hero worship while struggling to work out the problems of identity. They are insecure and uncertain in their relationships with the opposite sex and wonder what to do, what to say, and how to act. Even the most socially successful adolescent is anxious about these things. It is only after individuals have successfully solved the problems posed by the earlier phases of adolescence that they are able to develop a **sense of intimacy** and to become capable of intimate friendship and love for others on a more mature level.

Maturity too presents characteristic problems that challenge mental health. Ideally, the mature individual emerges from the self-absorption of adolescence and expends energies productively on behalf of others—offspring, community, and the broad constructive aspirations of humanity. A broad **parental sense** is developed. Marriage and parenthood offer unique opportunities for personal growth and for the application of principles of mental health. Adjustments are made to factors of social, occupational, economic, and emotional relationships.

FACTORS THAT HELP TO SHAPE PERSONALITY

Although the individual, especially in post-adolescent years, shapes his or her own personality, we must recognize that differences in the mental and emotional behavior of individuals are due in part to differences in physical and "social" heredity. There are physically inherited differences in native intelligence and in many physical characteristics. "Social" inheritance comes from the home, the school, and the community.

Parents may give the child affection, security, and wise guidance. Or they may be ill-tempered, fearful, insecure, or domineering, unreasonable, inconsistent, or actually abusive in varying degrees. Some parents are overprotective. Many are overpermissive. The child's relationships with brothers and sisters help shape the personality. Homes vary in cultural background, religious observance, prejudices, and the graciousness of living. All affect the child's emotional experiences.

For the school-age child the school joins the home in providing the emotional needs (security, independence, achievement, companionship, love, acceptance, variety of experiences, guidance, time for contemplation, and faith) that we have discussed. A well-planned curriculum, well-adjusted teachers, constructive interpersonal relations in work and play, opportunities to achieve success, and special counseling where needed contribute to these needs. It is not possible to have perfect schools, and the existence of severe stress, anxiety, frustration, or violent prejudice lowers mental health and leads toward destructive behavior. Some schools have classes in human relations, in which, through study and discussions, mental health is taught.

Again it is obvious that the mental health of the individual is sharply affected by the nature of the community. Destructive forces in the community are unemployment, low literacy, group prejudices, poverty, lawlessness, and crime. On the other hand, communities that contribute effectively to mental health have adequate employment, churches, schools, law enforcement, health agencies, and mental health services. We recognize the part these forces may have played in shaping the mental health and social attitudes of individuals.

■ Nutritional impact

There is a well-documented correlation between nutrition and childhood development, which in turn has a bearing on personality. Severe malnutrition can have devastating physical and mental effects. Moreover and more insidious, even mild caloric deficiencies in the diet of an infant or pregnant women can prove serious. Recent studies (1981) carried out at Harvard Medical School and the National Institute of Mental Health link minor nutritional problems in early life to the behavioral and social development of youngsters as old as 6 to 8 years. Furthermore, these studies suggest that simply providing calories to undernourished infants and mothers-to-be seems to have a lasting effect on the way the child deals with others and makes use of the environment. Somewhat of a puzzle is the fact that mild-to-moderate malnutrition does not appear to affect higher intellectual and learning abilities significantly. Just why social and emotional characteristics are apparently more vulnerable to nutritional stress than are cognitive (learning) functions is not known, but this fact does seem to indicate something about the development of the brain and central nervous system. Perhaps it is a matter of evolution; that is to say, perhaps emotional and social development are of more recent vintage (than cognitive development) and therefore more vulnerable to stress.

■ STRESS

Many years ago the Canadian physiologist Hans Selye demonstrated that stressful situations—intense cold, intense sound, physical restraints, and the like—caused rats to develop a triad of changes: markedly enlarged adrenal glands, shriveled lymphatic tissue, and bleeding stomach ulcers. These responses always occurred together regardless of the nature of the stressful situation. Accordingly, Selye concluded that they constituted a syndrome and coined the expression **general adaptation syndrome** (GAS). He named the "stressful situation" **stressor** and applied the term **stress** to the state or condition produced by it (a state characterized by GAS).

Selye found that the changes that make up the GAS take place over a period of time in three stages—alarm, resistance, and exhaustion. The **alarm stage** is characterized by an increased output of adrenal hormones (namely, glucocorticoids and norepinephrine) and an enhanced activity of the sympathetic nervous system, all of which arouses the body for "fight or flight." The **resistance** (adaptation) **stage** is characterized by a return to normal—the hormone levels drop, the sympathetic nervous system stops acting up, and there is enhanced resistance to the stressor. In a word, the body "adapts." The **exhaustion stage** develops only when the stress is severe or when it continues over a long period of time. This stage is characterized by the loss of resistance to the stressor and even death of the animal. In applying all this to humans, Selye suggested that most stressors that act on us produce changes corresponding only to the first and second stages. That is, a given stressor—physical or mental—may upset or alarm us, but then we adapt or become accustomed to it. Otherwise, we enter stage three and are in for such troubles as heart irregularity, migraine headaches, or even mental illness. By way of example, high blood pressure and ulcers are much more common among air traffic controllers at large airports than among the general population.

Again, investigators have found that children may fail to grow when they live in an environment that is either physically or psychologically stressful.

No matter what we are doing, we are under a certain amount of physical or mental and/or emotional stress. Ordinarily this is good for us and makes life more interesting. Stress is harmful when it becomes **distress.** Distress is continual stress that causes us constantly to readjust or adapt. Doing something that one does not like to do may prove not only distasteful but also distressful. A rather interesting revelation is the fact that a stressor is not necessarily unpleasant. Indeed, it could actually be a pleasant or happy event. The classic example is a job promotion. In Selye's view what counts is not whether a stress is pleasant or unpleasant but the intensity of the demand it places on us to readjust. A bigger and better job brings or entails more responsibility, and so on. Clearly, an appreciation of stress goes a long way in helping us to understand the difference between mental health and mental illness.

■■■■■ MENTAL ILLNESS

All of us have periods when, to some degree, we feel anxious, depressed, angry, or inadequate in dealing with life's problems. And, accordingly, each of us at times employs some sort of defense mechanism to counter stressful situations. Such a response is certainly understandable—and "normal"—unless it becomes habitual and a way of life. Then the response is considered to be "abnormal" or psychopathologic. Problems of this nature include a variety of disorders in addition to those most people think of as "mental illness." Alcoholism, sexual deviation, suicidal behavior, and insomnia are all forms of psychopathology. Because of this multiplicity, classification systems have been devised to serve as guideposts to mental illness, and the most widely accepted system is the one that groups affected persons according to the behavioral symptoms they display. That is, individuals who behave roughly the same way are given the same label. The major categories under this system are neuroses, psychoses, personality disorders, and psychosomatic disorders. The highlights of each category are discussed below.

■ Neuroses

Neuroses (sing., neurosis) are emotional disorders characterized by loss of joy in living and overuse of defense mechanisms against anxiety. Neurotic individuals can usually get along in society even though their anxiety prevents them from functioning at full capacity. There is a relationship between a neurosis and the stress that preceded it, but in contrast to normal emotional reactions neurotic behavior fails to parallel fluctuations in the individual's situation. By way of example, a severe obsessional or phobic state may be precipitated by bad news but is rarely relieved if the information proves to have been erroneous.

Major forms of neuroses include anxiety, hysterical, obsessive-compulsive, depressive, hypochondriac, and phobic neuroses. **Anxiety neuroses** are marked by exaggerated fear and anxiety reactions that are inappropriately severe and protracted. Normal anxiety usually decreases with repeated exposure to the feared situation, but neurotic anxiety tends to increase and leads to progressive avoidance of and withdrawal from the feared situation and stimuli. Anxiety states are the most prevalent neuroses in highly developed countries.

Hysterical neuroses (conversion reactions) are marked by physical symptoms without underlying organic cause. The symptoms may be sensory (loss of sensation in some body part, blindness or deafness), motor (paralysis of a limb or entire side of the body, speech disturbances, convulsions) or visceral (sneezing, choking, and vague aches and pains).

Obsessive-compulsive neuroses are neuroses marked by recurrent thoughts, feelings, or impulses (obsession) and repetitive acts (compulsion) that the individual recognizes as morbid and to which he or she feels a strong inner resistance. Nonetheless to actually resist their intrusion produces immediate and often overwhelming anxiety.

Depressive neurosis (reactive depression) is a disorder in which long-lasting feelings of dejection arise in response to adverse external circumstances. The precipitating stress may be sudden (such as bereavement, the breakup of a relationship, or a setback in the individual's career), or psychologic pressures may have been exerted over a long time. Neurotic depression differs from episodes of normal sadness in that the individual cannot shake off the feelings of dejection and the effect is disproportionately intense and enduring. The risk of suicide may be considerable in the acute form of the neurosis.

Hypochondria is a neurosis marked by preoccupation with bodily processes and irrational conviction of dysfunction of some region of the body. Heart disease, brain tumor, intestinal obstruction, and venereal disease are common themes. Many hypochondriac individuals take considerable pride in their physique and may have followed athletic pursuits enthusiastically until a relatively advanced age.

Phobias are excessive fears of certain kinds of situations in the absence of real danger, or fears that are totally out of proportion to the amount of danger that a situation may involve. In some cases the choice of the phobic object is purely symbolic; in others it has a close connection with the underlying conflict. Common phobias include fear of high places (acrophobia), fear of closed spaces (claustrophobia), fear of crowds (ochlophobia), fear of animals (zoophobia), and fear of leaving home settings (agoraphobia).

■ Psychoses

Psychoses (sing., psychosis) are mental disorders so deviant from normal that the individual seems to have lost contact with reality. To be psychotic, in laymen's terms is to be insane, crazy, or mad. Some psychoses may be **organic**, that is, associated with some sort of brain damage, but most are **functional** and of unknown cause. Postulated causes relate to heredity, biochemical factors, and psychosocial factors. In some cases it appears that inherited physiologic or biochemical defects are primarily responsible, while in others environmental factors play a key role. It may very well be that an inherited biochemical defect predisposes the individual to a psychotic reaction when under stress. The distinction between organic and functional psychoses is not clear, especially when we consider that general paresis—third state syphilis—was originally classified as functional. Nonetheless, it is practical to distinguish between psychoses of known cause (organic) and those in which genetic-psychosocial factors are assumed to play a major role (functional). Two of the most important and prevalent psychoses (both functional) are manic-depressive illness and schizophrenia.

Manic-depressive illness. Manic-depressive illness is characterized by pathologic mood changes (elation or sadness), spontaneous recoveries and tendencies for the disease to recur. Two genetically independent forms of the illness have now been identified: **bipolar** (cycles of mania and depression) and **unipolar** (recurrent depression). The overall incidence of manic-depressive illness is about 2%. Furthermore, it is twice as common in women as in men and has a high incidence in upper socioeconomic groups. The illness may begin any time from adolescence to old age, but the peak onset is at 30 years of age for bipolar states and 50 years of age for the unipolar states.

In the manic phase a few days' depression

suddenly gives way to a sense of well-being, heightened self-confidence, increased energy, and excessive garrulity. Tactless remarks, inappropriate sexual advances, and paranoid complaints are common features. In the later stages paranoid and grandiose ideas escalate into delusional convictions, and insight is completely lost. The depressive phase is characterized by loss of self-esteem, a feeling of despondency, loss of appetite, diminished libido, slowing of movement and speech, and hypochondria. In severe cases there is depressive delusion—hopelessness, persecution, or bodily decay—and the risk of suicide.

Schizophrenia. Schizophrenia is by far the most common of the psychotic disorders. About half of all neuropsychiatric hospital beds are occupied by patients diagnosed as schizophrenic. The psychosis usually occurs during young adulthood; the peak incidence is between ages 25 and 35. It is found in all cultures, even those remote from the stresses of modern civilization. Of cardinal importance is the fact that schizophrenia occurs with two distinct patterns of onset: "reactive" and "process." The **reactive schizophrenic** has had a fairly adequate social development, and the illness is precipitated by some stress, such as the death of a loved one or loss of a job; the outlook for recovery is good. The **process schizophrenic** has a history of long-term, progressive deterioration in adjustment with but little chance of recovery.

Disturbed thought processes constitute the most fundamental symptom of schizophrenia, and many of the other symptoms—delusions, hallucinations, bizarre behavior, and the like—can be interpreted as manifestations of the schizophrenic's thought process. Withdrawal from the reality of the external world into a private personal world (**autism**) is also highly characteristic. The schizophrenic loses interest in the people and events around him, and in extreme cases the individual may remain silent and immobile for days (**catatonia**) and

may have to be cared for as an infant. The risk of suicide is increased in all stages of schizophrenia, and grotesque violence with self-mutilation (often sexual parts) or murderous attacks may occasionally occur. Matricide, the rarest form of murder, is most often perpetrated by schizophrenics.

■ Personality disorders and sexual deviations

From childhood and throughout their lives, individuals with personality disorders exhibit characteristic patterns of maladjustment in their social, interpersonal, and sexual relationships. In the absence of environmental frustration these persons tend to show little anxiety or emotional symptoms, and they feel that their behavior patterns are "normal" and "right." Actually, taken as a group, personality disorders are pathologic more from society's viewpoint than in terms of the individual's own discomfort or unhappiness. Diagnostic categories of personality disorders include hysterical personality, paranoid personality, obsessive-compulsive personality, schizoid personality, psychopathic personality, and sexual deviations.

Psychopathic personality is the most dangerous personality disorder. Psychopathic (sociopathic) individuals are impulsive, are concerned only with their own needs, and are unable to form close relationships. They tolerate frustration poorly, and opposition is likely to elicit hostility, aggression, or serious violence. Their antisocial behavior shows little insight and, above all, is not associated with remorse or guilt, since these people seem to have a keen capacity for rationalizing and for blaming their behavior on others. In a word the "psychopath" lacks a conscience. Life expectancy is diminished, but among those surviving there is some tendency to stabilization after age 40.

Homosexuality. Since time immemorial researchers of various persuasions have tried to explain homosexuality. A major recent study (1981) of homosexual men and women by the Kinsey Institute for Sex Research found little or no support for most of the traditional theories. In particular the study of nearly 1500 people indicates that the parents' role in a child's sexual orientation has been "grossly exaggerated," as have theories that homosexuality results from a lack of heterosexual opportunities or from traumatic heterosexual experiences. Rather, the Kinsey researchers concluded that a homosexual orientation seems to emerge from a deep-seated predisposition, possibly biologic in origin, that first appears as a failure to conform to society's stereotype of what it means to be a boy or girl. For homosexual men the study showed that "gender nonconformity," which is childhood preference for girls' activities, a dislike of boys' activities, and a feeling that they were not very masculine, was the single most important factor in predicting their eventual sexual orientation. For homosexual women gender nonconformity was the second most important predictive factor, surpassed only by homosexual involvements in adolescence. Nonconformity, however, does not necessarily signal future homosexuality. One fourth of the heterosexual men in the study were nonconforming as youngsters, and only a third of the heterosexual women described themselves as "highly feminine" in childhood. In sum the Kinsey researchers concluded that homosexuality is as deeply ingrained as heterosexuality and that behavioral and social differences between prehomosexual and preheterosexual boys and girls reflect or express rather than cause their eventual sexual preference.

Theories aside, transient homosexual conduct in puberty and adolescence is common, and an estimated 15% of the adult population indulge in both homosexual and heterosexual practices. An estimated 5% of male individuals are exclusively homosexual during their lives. The extent of homosexual behavior in women (**lesbianism**) is not known but could possibly be at about the same level. Facultative homosexuality, frequently exhibited by men confined for long periods with other men, as on board ship or in prison, makes no lasting impression; most resume their usual sexual behavior on release from such environments. Most homosexuals are emotionally stable and conduct relatively normal lives, but studies have shown a higher incidence of alcoholism, neuroses, and suicide among homosexuals than in the general population.

Exclusively homosexual individuals who have never felt any heterosexual attraction consider themselves normal, and one is hard put to dispute this. At the very least they have little or no motivation to change, which means that "treatment" is not only futile but potentially dangerous. However, contrary to what many in the gay society seem to be saying, some homosexuals are strongly motivated to seek help to modify their patterns of adjustment. The best results (in response to behavior techniques and analysis) are achieved in those who have experienced some heterosexual arousal. Frankly bisexual individuals also respond well to therapy. At the psychosocial level, homosexuality deserves understanding and accommodation.

Transsexualism. The transsexual is a person with an overwhelming desire to become a member of the other sex. These persons believe that they are imprisoned within a body that is incompatible with their real sexual identity. Most men of this persuasion regard their genitalia and masculine features with extreme repugnance. Many male transsexuals are adept at acquiring the skills that enable them to adopt a female gender identity; some are satisfied with being given help to achieve a more feminine appearance, together with employment and an identity card that enables them to work and live in society as women. Female hormones are sometimes helpful. The decision to use surgery raises grave social and ethical problems, but some follow-up studies do provide evidence that it may be helpful in well-selected cases.

Female transsexuals are usually the dominant members in lesbian partnerships. Commonly, these persons seek medical help and almost always know exactly what they want—mastectomy, hysterectomy, oophorectomy, and/or male hormones. Sometimes they request an artificial penis (to be fashioned by plastic surgery). Counseling, alterations in social habits, hormones, and/or limited surgery is often helpful. With rare exception, heroic surgery is avoided.

Other sexual deviations. There are, in addition to homosexuality and transsexualism, a number of other sexual deviations. These include transvestism, fetishism, voyeurism, exhibitionism, masochism, and sadism. For the most part these deviations are of minor concern unless they are pronounced, in which case other facets of the personality may suffer. **Transvestism** is the desire to dress in the clothing of the opposite sex. A certain amount of excitement is thus achieved, and public display gives much satisfaction. **Fetishism** is aberrant sexual excitement associated with an inanimate object or body part. For some men and women underclothing, boots, fur, and hair often arouse erotic excitement. **Voyeurism** is gratification from observing the sex organs or sexual acts of others, usually from a secret vantage point. To a degree, of course, this habit is an ingredient of normal sexual curiosity. **Exhibitionism** is the compulsive exposure of the sexual organs in public. Compared with voyeurism, this behavior is a deviation from normal in every sense of the word. **Masochism** is the relatively common aberration in which sexual excitement and satisfaction depend largely on being subjected to abuse or physical pain, whether by oneself or by another. **Sadism** is the association of sexual satisfaction with the infliction of pain on others. Sadists are always potentially dangerous.

■ Psychosomatic disorders

Psychosomatic (psychophysiologic) disorders are physical illnesses in which psychologic factors play a major role. Unlike a neurotic conversion reaction, where no physical cause can be found, a person with a psychosomatic disorder is actually ill. High blood pressure, migraine headaches, skin rashes, ulcers, and asthma are all psychosomatic possibilities. Clearly, just as fatigue or illness can lower one's tolerance for psychologic stress, so emotional stress can lower one's resistance to disease. This is underscored by the fact that psychiatric patients suffer more from physical illnesses of all kinds than do normal persons. It appears that each individual has his own psychosomatic response to stress. For example, the same stressful event may produce high blood pressure in one person and an ulcer in another. All in all, emotional stress can have a significant effect on one's physical health.

■ Therapeutic measures

The treatment of mental illness has developed along two major lines: **somatotherapy** and **psychotherapy**. By somatotherapy we mean treating the body (soma) rather than the mind (psyche). Penicillin has greatly reduced general paresis ("syphilitic psychosis"), and vitamin therapy has just about eliminated the mental disturbances associated with pellagra. The most spectacular somatotherapeutic advances, however, center on the use of psychoactive drugs such as tranquilizers, antidepressants, and lithium. "Minor" tranquilizers, such as diazepam (Valium), are helpful in treating neuroses and psychosomatic disorders, and "major" tranquilizers, such as haloperidol (Haldol), are highly effective in treating schizophrenia. Not only do these drugs reduce agitation and alleviate delusions and hallucinations, but often they decrease the extent of emotional withdrawal and thereby render the patient amenable to psychotherapy (see below). Lithium (as the carbonate or citrate) controls mania (in manic-depressive illness) and prevents mood swings in 75% of cases. Another somatotherapeutic approach is electroconvulsive (electroshock) therapy, which at one time was widely used to treat functional psychoses. Today its use is restricted to severe depression that does not respond to other forms of treatment.

Psychotherapy is the psychologic treatment of mental, emotional, and nervous disorders. The treatment site is a hospital, a community mental health center, or a private clinic or office, and the "therapist" could be a psychiatrist, clinical psychologist, psychiatric social worker, psychiatric nurse, or trained volunteer. For the most part the psychiatrist, who is a physician, is the acknowledged team leader, especially in acute, serious cases. Psychotherapeutic methods and approaches seem to be without number, commonly forming and fading like so many snowflakes. Their absolute value and relative merits are difficult to evaluate because of the problems in defining what is meant by a "cure." Some studies have indicated little or no improvement after psychotherapy, and a few have even reported negative results. In balance it is probably fair to say that proper therapy is of some help most of the time and curative on occasion.

The hallmark of psychotherapy is **psychoanalysis**, which is based on the concepts of Sigmund Freud. This technique uses free association, dream interpretations, and analysis of resistance and transference to investigate mental processes. The therapist—psychoanalyst—in this setting is almost always a psychiatrist. The other modes of psychotherapy stem from the ideas and theories of those who did not go along with Freud and who rejected, especially, his preoccupation with sexual hangups. These other modes include nondirective psychotherapy, behavior modification, group therapy, and cognitive therapy. In actual practice most therapists do not adhere to any one particular method but employ an **eclectic approach**; that is, they select from the various techniques those that they feel are most appropriate for the individual patient. As a matter of fact, a particular method, on close scrutiny, often turns out to be a combination of techniques. Cognitive therapy, for example, combines psychoanalysis with a certain kind of behavior technique.

■ Preventive measures

Maintaining one's mental balance is not unlike maintaining one's desirable weight. Both call for a basic appreciation of the situation and an unrelenting willpower. In the case of excess weight we have eaten too much and/or exercised too little. The solution is to reverse this. In the case of "emotional obesity" it seems reasonable to assume that we have accumulated too much mental energy and that we should release it. One way to do this is through useful work, and another way is through love. Whatever the mechanism or the neural nuts and bolts of the matter may be, this is just about the consensus of the thinkers who have addressed the problem of maintaining mental health. "Mental health," says anthropologist Ashley Montague, "is the ability to love and the ability to work." The master impressionist painter Camille Pissarro was even more specific: "Work is a wonderful regulator of mind and body. I forget all sorrow, grief, bitterness, and I even ignore them altogether in the joy of working." Psychologists Floyd Ruch and Philip Zimbardo look on neuroses as the "loss in the joy of living."

But love and work are not always going to succeed in the prevention of emotional and mental problems, and there comes a time when some of us will need outside help. Indeed, realizing that we need help and seeking it constitute two additional pillars in the prevention of mental illness. No one should ever have any qualms about seeking help—all psychologists agree that it is a healthy sign. Furthermore, problems have a strong tendency to become more severe if untreated—so time is crucial. Today there are all kinds of avenues leading to just the right counselor(s). Information resources include community mental health centers and medical bureaus and the local Department of Mental Health, all listed in the telephone book. And not to be forgotten is one's own physician or clergyman. Practically all colleges have some counseling services available—either through the dean's office, through a separate counseling service, or through the health service. About 10% of our more than 2400 colleges have mental health services that include psychiatrists.

DEATH AND DYING

The dying process is no less complex than life itself. Age, sex, personality, life-style, ethnic background, interpersonal relationships, nature of final illness, and environment are all involved. By way of example, the fact that one person is in early childhood and another in late middle age obviously has a bearing on his or her way of coming to terms with death and dying. Are the last days and hours spent in a sterile clinical setting among strangers or at home among loved ones? And so on. Notwithstanding these many and multileveled variables, the pioneer investigations of Elizabeth Kübler-Ross revealed a similar pattern in the way people respond to the challenges of the dying process. Specifically, Kübler-Ross believes the dying person passes through five stages: denial, anger, bargaining (with God), depression, and acceptance, in this order. Acceptance shows up as an amelioration of depression, but it is not necessarily a happy or blissful state. While many authorities agree that Kübler-Ross's work has been informative, they note that a given person may not exhibit all—or any—of these stages of behavior. In fact, they fear that some dying persons may

become unnecessarily distressed because of lack of "appropriate" behavior in their final days and hours. There is a consensus, though, that dying people do indeed have very special psychologic needs.

■ Hospice

In medieval times the word "hospice" meant an inn, a place where weary travelers could stop to refresh themselves. Today the word has come to mean a way of helping people during the final stage of the journey of life. Because dying persons and their families have special physical, psychologic, spiritual, and practical needs, the specially trained hospice team assists other care providers to meet these needs. Presently there are about 800 hospices in the United States in various stages of development. A forerunner is the Hospice of the Good Shepherd (HGS) in Newton, Massachusetts. The specific goals of HGS are (1) to support both the patient and family so that they can live their lives as fully as possible; (2) to control pain and symptoms that accompany illness; (3) to provide 24-hour coverage, 7 days a week; (4) to develop personalized care plans, which can enable patients to remain at home or in as homelike an environment as possible; and (5) to support family members during the period of bereavement. Services are obtained by referrals from patients, families, physicians, clergy, or other care providers. No referral is accepted without patient and family consent. Hospice services are paid for with a combination of third-party reimbursements, patient fees, grants from public and private organizations and agencies, and donations from individuals.

■ Euthanasia

Those who favor euthanasia ("mercy killing") believe that it is wrong to prolong suffering. Further-more, they say all people should have the right to die with dignity. Surveys of public attitudes toward active and passive euthanasia show that a steadily increasing number of Americans believe there is a right to die. In **active euthanasia** a doctor administers a drug to terminate a patient's life so as to prevent suffering. No place in the world allows this except Uruguay. In Switzerland a doctor can make an overdose of medicine available to a patient who requests it but cannot administer it personally. **Passive euthanasia** is the termination of life-prolonging treatment—colloquially expressed as "pulling the plug." In one form or another, acknowledged or unacknowledged, passive euthanasia has been with us a long time.

The attempt by patients to provide, in advance, informed consent to physicians to terminate care so that the decision would not be left to hospital committees, the courts, or relatives resulted in the so-called **living will**. Since it often becomes appropriate to terminate care only after the patient is in coma or otherwise unable to respond, there are those who feel living wills are the only way for their wishes to be respected. A typical living will may read:

Death is as much a reality as birth, growth, maturity, and old age. If the time comes when I, _____, can no longer take part in decisions for my own future, let this statement stand as an expression of my wishes, while I am still of sound mind.

Other versions of the living will are written as an order, not as a plea. One model provides space for very personal instructions, for example, to administer pain killers, even in amounts that might hasten death. To make the living will binding and to settle legal questions certain states have enacted appropriate legislation. The California Natural Death Act, for example, declares that a death resulting from carrying out a directive (such as a living will) does not constitute suicide. Furthermore, insurance companies are forbidden to invalidate or modify existing life insurance policies if an individual executes such a directive.

An obvious problem in deciding to terminate treatment is establishing when death has actually occurred. Sophisticated medical equipment can keep the heart beating long after the patient has lost the capacity to recover from an illness. In a 1968 landmark case a Richmond, Virginia, jury decided that a patient who had experienced brain death (completely flat waves on an electroencephalogram) was legally dead. In 1981 The President's Commission for the Study of Ethical Problems in Medicine and Biomedical and Behavioral Research urged all 50 states to adopt a simple uniform law defining death. In their view "an individual who has sustained either (1) irreversible cessation of circulation and respiration functions or (2) irreversible cessation of all functions of the entire brain, including the brain, is dead." When officially adopted the statute will be known as the Uniform Determination of Death Act.

■ Bereavement

Bereavement is the process by which a person suffers, sustains, and then recovers from the loss of an essential person. Theorists document five stages: grief, mourning, depression, loneliness, relief, and restitution. Bereavement ceases when the individual is operational again and is able to respond actively to work, recreation, and emotional life. Severe and prolonged symptoms of depression, psychosomatic symptoms (especially gastrointestinal), symptoms resembling those of the deceased person, avoidance of the proscribed rituals, or continual searching and crying at the thought or mention of the deceased may signal the person who has failed to grieve or who is involved in a pathologic situation. The bereaved child is subject to stress from two sources: his or her own immediate response to the loss and the interruption of the usual care necessary for security and proper growth. As a consequence the child sometimes encounters serious problems later in life that typically are related to unresolved feelings surrounding the bereavement. Understanding, appropriate attention, and lots of love will do much to prevent this from happening.

Although it has long been believed that the death of a spouse leads to psychologic distress that might contribute to earlier death and to illness, a recent (1981) Johns Hopkins University study dramatically pointed up for the first time that the impact appears to be more devastating on men. Specifically, men whose spouses have died are much more likely to die, too, in the next several years than men of the same age who are still married. Furthermore, remarriage appears to increase the widowed man's chances of living longer. But the death of a husband has almost no effect on the mortality rate of women, according to this 12-year survey of more than 4000 widowed persons, age 18 and up. The explanation for these findings is obviously a matter of speculation. Constitutional differences in women might make them better able to rebound from the loss. The researchers also suggested that personality characteristics might play a role. Possibly women may have more of a sense of survival.

■ Anatomic gifts

Leaving one's body or its organs to medical science for anatomic study is a practice of long standing. Those who choose to do so certainly serve a worthy cause because the cadaver is obviously an indispensable educational tool in the training of health professionals. In more recent times the cadaver has also become the ultimate resource to repair and replace worn-out parts and organs among the living. The cardinal example, of course, is kidney transplantation (Chapter 7). Other vital "anatomic gifts" in all too short supply include skin, bones, endocrine glands, non-diseased blood, and eye corneas. The fact that corneal transplantation

is such a simple procedure and, above all, that it can give sight to the blind would appear to be something for all of us to think about.

Today more than half of kidney transplants are from cadavers, in many instances from previously healthy subjects who have sustained fatal brain damage but maintain stable cardiovascular and renal functions. The kidneys are removed as quickly as possible and cooled by perfusing with a special solution containing an anticoagulant. If all goes well, donor kidneys can be preserved up to 48 hours prior to transplantation.

The donation of the body or its organs is made quite simple through the Uniform Anatomical Gift Act of 1973. All a person need do is fill out a Uniform Donor Card (Fig. 17-4) available from certain organizations such as the American Kidney Foundation and the National Institutes of Health. Some states allow it to be registered on an automobile driver's license showing that the licensee is a donor. To find a medical institution that has transplant specialists or one that receives entire bodies, the donor should consult a physician or the department of surgery in the nearest medical school or local hospital.

■ SUICIDAL BEHAVIOR

Suicidal behavior includes completed suicide, suicidal attempts, and suicidal ideas. **Completed suicide** includes all the situations in which the circumstances surrounding the death lead to the conclusion that the individual took a positive action with the primary purpose of ending his or her life. This would include what is ordinarily meant when we speak of "suicide" or "committing suicide." **Suicidal attempts** include those situations in which a person performs a life-threatening behavior with the intent of jeopardizing his or her life or giving the appearance of such an intent. **Suicidal ideas** include behaviors that might be directly observed or inferred and that are concerned with or move in the direction

```
┌ ─ ─ ─ ─ ─ ─ ─ ─ ─ ─ ─ ─ ─ ─ ─ ─ ─ ┐
|         UNIFORM DONOR CARD          |
|                                     |
| OF _____ |
|          Print or Type name of donor |
| In the hope that I may help others, I hereby make this anatomical gift, if |
| medically acceptable, to take effect upon my death. The words and marks |
| below indicate my desires         |
| I give   (a) ____ any needed organs or parts |
|          (b) ____ only the following organs or parts |
|                                     |
| _____ |
|        Specify the organ(s) or part(s) |
| for the purposes of transplantation, therapy, medical research |
| or education,                       |
|          (c) ____ my body for anatomical study if needed |
| Limitations or                      |
| special wishes, if any _____ |
└ ─ ─ ─ ─ ─ ─ ─ ─ ─ ─ ─ ─ ─ ─ ─ ─ ─ ┘
```

Signed by the donor and the following two witnesses in the presence of each other:

_____   _____
Signature of Donor   Date of Birth of Donor

_____   _____
Date Signed   City & State

_____   _____
Witness   Witness

This is a legal document under the Uniform Anatomical Gift Act or similar laws.

FIG. 17-4 ■ Uniform Donor Card. Most states require that a donor be at least 18 years of age, and the trend is toward this requirement for all states. Some persons under legal age have probably signed donor cards. Though no law forbids this, an organ can usually be removed from the body of an underage person only with the consent of the next of kin. Filling out a donor card does not mean that your wishes will be followed automatically. Someone must see to it that the donation takes place after death. So tell your wishes to your friends, lawyer, spiritual advisor, doctor, and, above all, to your relatives.

of a possible threat to the individual's life. However, the potentially lethal act is not actually performed.

There are about 200,000 suicide attempts in the United States each year, and about 75,000 are successful. Women make two to three times as many suicide attempts as men, but men are generally more successful in their attempts. Men over 50 years of age are at very high risk. There is a high incidence of suicide among the families of persons who have committed suicide. Professional people appear to have higher than average suicide rates, and among medical specialists the highest rate is among psychiatrists. Suicide is rare among practicing religious groups, particularly Roman Catholics. In comparison with other countries the United States' suicide rate is a somewhat modest 12 per 100,000 people; Sweden's rate is high at about 22 per 100,000 people, and Ireland's is low at about 2 per 100,000.

Of special concern is suicide among teenagers. According to the Surgeon General of the United States, the suicide rate for young people doubled between 1960 and 1980. Suicide now takes more than 5000 young lives annually and ranks as the third leading killer (after accidents and homicides) among young people in the 15- to 24-year age group. As to why young people are killing themselves in greater numbers than ever before, a common theme that seems to cut through all cases is the breakdown of the nuclear family. This is the view of the National Institute of Mental Health. The breakdown can be the result of divorce, both parents working, death, or simply parental self-absorption. Apparently, the parents become so heavily engaged with work or other activities that they neglect to establish any kind of relationship with their children. Thus in a most tragic way teenage suicide underscores the societal potency of the family.

Suicide usually results from multiple and complex motivations. Recognized factors include mental illness (especially depression), social problems (disappointment and loss), personality abnormalities, and physical illness. Often one factor, for example, a disruption in an important relationship, is the final straw. Alcohol also plays a role. An estimated 30% of persons who attempt suicide have been drinking before the act, with about half being intoxicated at the time. This is hardly a surprise when we consider that alcohol itself is a depressant—aggravating the intensity of an existing depression on the one hand and lowering self-control on the other.

We can all help in reducing suicide by being on the alert for changes in mood or behavior of loved ones and friends. And let us not forget total strangers. Statements such as "I can't take it any more" or "I just want to end it all" call for skilled professional help. However, in an emergency virtually anyone can offer emotional support—parents, friends, clergy, police officers, and last but by no means least, bartenders. Many social agencies and lay organizations in large communities offer 24-hour service for those in distress. These suicide prevention centers attempt to identify the potentially suicidal person and to offer help with immediate problems. Above all they keep distressed individuals talking—and as long as you are talking you are still alive.

■■■■ RAPE

Rape is the illicit sexual penetration of any body orifice without consent. Females are the usual victims. It has been a significant enough societal problem to necessitate establishment of **rape crisis centers** across the country composed of supportive personnel available for immediate treatment and counseling. The number of rapes and attempted rapes reported to the police in 1981 was over 82,000 according to Federal Bureau of Investigation statistics. Most rapes are well planned, and over half the attacks involve a weapon (usually a knife). In addition, almost half the rapists are known to their victims. Indeed, in one study about one quarter of the rapists turned out to be a "boyfriend" or "date."

About one half of rape victims exhibit signs of physical trauma. Injury to the vulva and vagina is not unusual; possible medical sequelae include venereal disease and pregnancy. Psychologic stress is typically severe. Anxiety, withdrawal, depression, and a feeling of guilt may all occur. Special care is taken to approach the rape victim with warmth and compassion, and in this regard the female nurse can be especially helpful. Specific treatment calls for the administration of an antibiotic and a contraceptive medication and, if need be, reparative surgery. The married woman's husband is involved early in the support of his wife, and all necessary data are elicited with utmost tact. Since the full psychologic impact cannot be assessed at the time of the emergency, follow-up visits are essential. On occasion long-range problems arise that call for psychiatric intervention.

In a sense there are two kinds of rapists, reported and unreported. Most reported (and sometimes convicted) rapists are young, between the ages of 16 and 24 years; half are white and have previous records of violence (but few of them for sex-related offenses); and most prey on women from their own age group, race, and neighborhood. Unreported rapists are often known to their victims and include acquaintances, friends, bosses, relatives, fathers, and husbands. Indeed, this familiarity accounts in part for the fact that the names of these men do not show up on the police blotter. Rapes of this category are not uncommonly "date rapes"; that is, the man finds the woman differing with his assumption that a date inevitably leads to a sexual encounter.

As to what causes men to commit rape, little is known. In the case of the rapist with a previous record of violence rape could very well be just another manifestation of a disheveled mind. In the case of a teenage rapist it could be a matter of immaturity and not "knowing any better." In the case of the man who rapes his date, it is possible that in his view the woman is merely "playing hard to get." Drugs and alcohol sometimes play a role. In a celebrated case in which three young doctors were convicted of raping a nurse, all three had been drinking. Would they have done such a thing if they had not been drinking?

CHILD ABUSE

According to official estimates a million children are being maltreated by their parents each year in the United States. As many as 200,000 are sexually abused, and probably 200,000 to 300,000 are psychologically abused. The severity of the problem is illustrated by the fact that 3000 children die annually in circumstances suggestive of abuse and neglect. The scars produced by childhood physical and emotional trauma often lead to unhappiness and mental disorders when the child becomes an adult. Numerous studies indicate a definite symptomatic connection between violence prevalent in our society today and the abused, battered children of yesterday.

The average age of the mother who abuses her children is about 26 years, whereas the average age of the father is 30. The lives of the parents frequently are fraught with the problems of divorce, extramarital relations, alcoholism, financial stress, unemployment, poor housing conditions, recurring mental illness, mental retardation, or drug addiction. Studies show that abusing parents are emotionally crippled with a history of unfortunate experiences in their own childhoods. As a child, the typical battering parent was lonely and lacked protection and love. When they become parents, they cannot react normally to the needs of the infant. Longing for care and affection and acceptance, they unreasonably expect the child to meet these needs for them. They see themselves as a child and the child as a small adult capable of nurturing them as their own parents never did (a phenomenon called "role reversal"). When the child is not able to meet such impossible demands, the parents' immaturity and frustrations cause

them to vent their frustrations through violence against the child.

Every state now has a special department or agency to handle reports of child abuse, and a great many private agencies offer various services to abused children and their parents. Above all a suspected case of child abuse must be reported immediately to the proper authorities. Most child abuse treatment programs attempt (1) to prevent separation of parents and child whenever possible, (2) to encourage the attainment of self-care status on the part of the parents, (3) to stimulate the attainment of self-sufficiency for the family, and (4) to prevent further abuse or neglect by removing children from families who show an unwillingness or inability to profit from the treatment.

Interestingly, abusing parents frequently are relieved when reported to authorities. In their own way they are just as sick as the child and now know that they will receive professional assistance. Thus the reporting process tends to improve the family rather than worsen a clearly explosive situation. This is most important to keep in mind because it will encourage us to do the right thing—that is, to report abuse. Stated otherwise, we will be helping the parents as well as the child.

WIFE ABUSE

An estimated 16% of the nation's 47 million married couples have a violent episode at least once a year, and about 4 million husbands and wives have inflicted serious injuries on each other (an event called **spouse abuse**). Although husbands and wives report battering in equal numbers—and kill each other in approximately equal numbers—the researchers report wife abuse ("wife beating") as by far the more serious problem. Well over half of all divorce proceedings include allegations of severe beating by the husband. Furthermore, recent surveys of battered wives found that 35% had been sexually assaulted by their husbands. These assaults have little to do with sex as such but are a continuation of expressions of anger and frustration.

The battering husband, like the rapist, is not easy to characterize, although a number of researchers have provided us with descriptions. The Internal Association of Chiefs of Police, in its training manual, sums up the batterer as "unsuccessful financially, occupationally, and socially." Again, some think the batterer is basically a bully and given to irrational flashes of violent rage. On a more psychosocial level of consideration the Domestic Violence Research Program (at the University of New Hampshire) has gathered a large body of evidence showing that the causes of wife abuse relate to a combination of individual characteristics, cultural patterns, and the or-

ganization of family and society. If we accept this thesis, then the prevention of wife abuse is multidimensional, taking into account the individual, family, and society.

Battered women need close, personal, professional, on-the-spot help. Hospitals around the nation are now establishing services designed to meet the needs of assaulted women, and more should be encouraged to do so. Also crucial is a place to stay. Indeed, experience shows that most battered women would have left home long ago if they had somewhere to go for shelter and advice. Other essential measures include organizations committed to change the sexist structure of the family and society, task forces to expose existing problems, appropriate legal aid, and legislation to define wife abuse as a crime.

■■■ SELF-TEST

1. _C_ childhood development
2. _N_ psychoanalysis
3. _B_ alarm/resistance/exhaustion
4. _J_ hysterical neurosis
5. _L_ depressive neurosis
6. _A_ fear of high places
7. _H_ manic-depressive illness
8. _K_ schizophrenia
9. _I_ lack of conscience
10. _E_ female homosexual
11. _M_ minor tranquilizer
12. _G_ inflicting pain
13. _F_ psychosomatic disorder
14. _D_ mercy killing
15. _O_ general paresis

a. acrophobia
b. stress
c. adolescence
d. euthanasia
e. lesbian *percentage - unknown*
f. ulcer
g. sadism
h. lithium *autonomic nervous system*
i. psychopath *no conscience*
j. deafness
k. catatonia *split personality*
l. bereavement
m. diazepam
n. dreams
o. syphilis

■■■ STUDY QUESTIONS

1. What do you personally consider the most significant attribute of mental health?
2. Mental health is not the absence of personal idiosyncrasies. Cite several examples to support this statement.
3. Do you personally consider faith an essential emotional need?
4. What role does parental guidance play in emotional development?
5. What do you personally consider a major adjustment problem that most college students encounter?
6. Experts agree that a good hobby contributes to mental health. Discuss in detail.

7. The "sense of trust" is said to be the keystone of personality development. Why is trust so basic?

8. There is a well-documented correlation between childhood nutrition and personality. Essentially, it is a "matter of chemistry." Explain.

9. Distinguish between stress and stressor.

10. When does stress enter the pathologic "exhaustion stage"?

11. Cite several examples where good news or a happy event might cause stress.

12. A given stressor does not necessarily cause stress in all persons. Elaborate.

13. Do you think that all of us are a little neurotic? Discuss.

14. What do all neuroses have in common relative to cause?

15. Why are hysterical neuroses also called "conversion reactions"?

16. The fundamental difference between neurosis and psychosis relates to "reality." Elaborate.

17. Neurotic depression (reactive depression) and psychotic depression (manic-depressive illness) are sometimes referred to as "exogenous depression" and "endogenous depression," respectively. Can you account for this practice?

18. What are some phobias other than those cited in the text?

19. The most meaningful and practical classification of schizophrenia relates to the pattern of onset. Why?

20. Do you personally consider homosexuality "abnormal"? Why?

21. Psychoactive drugs have proved spectacularly useful in the management of mental illness. Does this tell us anything about the cause(s) of mental illness?

22. Do you have any firsthand information regarding the value or usefulness of psychotherapy in a particular case?

23. What are your personal views on euthanasia?

24. Is it possible that a "certain type" of person commits suicide? Discuss.

25. In your view what type of person (a) commits rape, (b) abuses a child, (c) abuses a spouse?

CHAPTER 18

Physical fitness

On the average, almost three Americans will suffer a heart attack every minute of the day, adding up to approximately 1½ million each year. Fortunately, during the past decade alone there has been a 25% decline in mortality from coronary artery disease. Among the factors influencing this dramatic decline are changes in life-style that relate to the risk factors associated with coronary artery disease. During the past several years we have witnessed a decrease in smoking among adults, a decrease in cholesterol intake, improvements in the control of high blood pressure, and a growing interest in physical fitness, the subject of the present chapter. Most of the scientific research has found that, compared to physically active people, inactive people have one and a half to two times the risk of having a heart attack. The chance of dying immediately after a heart attack is also three times greater in physically inactive people than in active people. Additionally, those who exercise regularly often lose excess weight and improve muscle strength and stamina. Many also develop an improved self-image, which can lead to further adoption of positive health behavior including that related to smoking and nutrition.

Exercise characteristics

Conditioning exercises

Jogging

Swimming

Recreational activities

Daily activities

Physical fitness can be defined as a positive and dynamic quality of life that is the result of muscular strength, endurance, and circulatory-respiratory efficiency, which interrelate to enhance one's ability to pursue the day's activities with enthusiasm, energy, and alertness (Fig. 18-1). Physically fit persons look better, feel better, and live longer. And the road to physical fitness is well marked—by exercise and sensible eating. Stated otherwise, one does not become physically fit by sitting in overstuffed chairs with one hand on the TV remote control and the other hand in a bag of potato chips. We shall take a look at exercise in this chapter and shall look at eating in the next chapter.

■■■■ EXERCISE CHARACTERISTICS

Exercise means muscular activity, which in turn means the metabolic expenditure of chemical energy. Inasmuch as this energy (measured in calories) comes from the food we eat, it stands to reason that exercise "burns food." An imbalance between what we eat and what we burn obviously results in either a loss or gain in weight. The record is clear that most Americans eat too much and exercise too little. This behavior causes obesity and physical unfitness.

Although exercise is customarily thought of as physical exertion consciously performed to develop or maintain fitness, a more useful understanding of exercise is simply to equate it with any kind of activity. That is, any kind of physical activity uses up calories and contributes to fitness (Table 18-1). The President's Council on Physical Fitness and Sports and the National Athletic Health Institute underscore this point by emphasizing a broad approach to adequate activity and fitness: the synthesis of regular conditioning exercises, recreational activities, and good daily habits. Each of these points will be discussed.

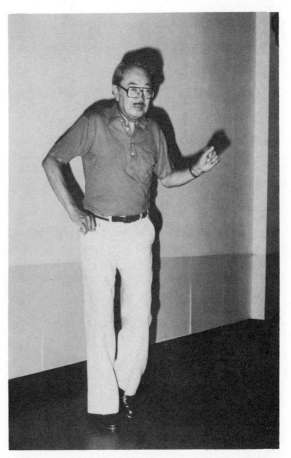

FIG. 18-1 ■ United States Senator (and former college president) S.I. Hayakawa of California tap dancing in his Washington, D.C., office (1981). Senator Hayakawa, a prime example of what it means to be physically fit (at any age!), tap dances routinely for exercise.

■ Aerobic vs anaerobic exercises

Aerobic exercises are the more vigorous types of activity designed to improve organs and systems that help the body process oxygen—the heart, lungs, and blood vessels. These exercises, which include running, (Fig. 18-2), jogging, bicycle riding, and swimming, facilitate breathing, strengthen the heart, open up new blood vessels, and increase endurance. **Anaerobic** exercises include activities of short, intense duration followed by a period

TABLE 18-1

Caloric expenditure by a 150-pound person in various exercises*

Exercise	Calories per hour
Bicycling 6 mph	240
Bicycling 12 mph	410
Cross-country skiing	700
Jogging 5½ mph	660
Jogging 7 mph	920
Jumping rope	750
Running in place	650
Running 10 mph	1280
Swimming 25 yd/min	275
Swimming 50 yd/min	500
Tennis—singles	400
Walking 2 mph	240
Walking 3 mph	320
Walking 4½ mph	440

Adapted from the National Heart, Lung, and Blood Institute.
*A lighter person burns fewer calories; a heavier person burns more calories.

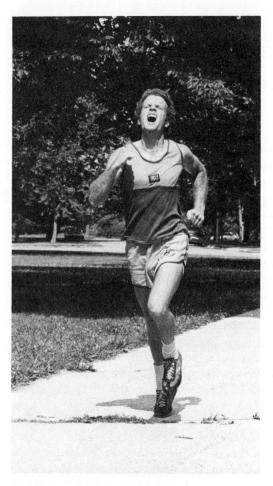

FIG. 18-2 ■ Running, an aerobic exercise, improves organs and systems that help the body process oxygen.

of recovery. Such activities as tennis, handball, and sprinting are examples. These activities require a sudden and high demand on the heart and lungs.

■ Isotonic vs isometric exercises

Isotonic exercises are strength-building exercises that require using muscles through a full range of motion. Examples include weight lifting, push-ups, sit-ups, and pull-ups. This kind of strength-building work is important in maintaining muscle mass, body proportion, and sound posture. **Isometric** exercises are strength-building activities that involve no actual movement. This kind of exercise amounts to pitting muscle groups against one another or against unyielding objects, for example, standing within a doorway and pushing maximally against the jamb on either side. This is usually done for a period of 10 to 15 seconds at maximum effort. Because of the limited movement, isometrics provide little func-

tional strength development and in some cases may limit joint range of motion. Furthermore, isometric exercises may cause dizziness and fainting in some individuals. Isometric exercises are not generally recommended by the President's Council on Physical Fitness and Sports.

■ CONDITIONING EXERCISES

Conditioning exercises are just what the words say—they put us in condition. That is, they not only burn off fat, but what is more, make us trim and strengthen the heart. To achieve success, however, conditioning exercises must be approached with common sense and must be executed conscientiously within the framework of a sound, overall physical fitness program. Such a program, as noted earlier, encompasses recreational activities and good daily habits as well as a conditioning schedule. Persons with health problems such as high blood pressure, heart disease, diabetes, or other chronic or severe illness obviously should check with a doctor before engaging in strenuous exercise. These conditions do not necessarily prevent one from engaging in a physical fitness program, but they do call for some sort of adjustment to meet personal needs and concerns.

The National Athletic Health Institute (NAHI) has devised a straight-forward conditioning program calling for three to four sessions a week of 35 to 45 minutes' duration. The details of a session are set forth in the NAHI's *Exercise Your Right to Live* (Occidental Life Insurance Company of California). In overview, an NAHI session consists of **warm-up**, **flexibility**, **endurance**, and **strength** exercises, in this order, and concludes with a **warm-down** period. The purpose of the warm-up is (1) to loosen and warm the muscles and joints and (2) to increase breathing and heart rate gradually, all in preparation for the more strenuous exercises to follow. Head rotation, trunk rotation, and leg lift are examples. Flexibility exercises are an extension of the warm-up and serve to enhance stretching and, as indicated, body flexibility. Hip stretch, upper trunk stretch, and back arch are examples.

■ Endurance exercises

Endurance exercises are vigorous **aerobic activities** specifically designed to strengthen the cardiovascular system. Examples include jogging, swimming, rowing, jumping rope, and stationary cycling (Figs. 18-3 and 18-4). In the view of most physicians and exercise scientists, physical fitness means cardiovascular fitness. As we know, the heart is a muscular pump, and, accordingly, how well it pumps depends on its muscular strength—strength that comes only from pumping or exercise! A sedentary life provides us with a potentially weak pump; a moderately active life provides us with an adequate pump; a vigorously active life provides us with a strong pump.

In the language of physiology (Chapter 5) a strong heart is characterized by a high **stroke volume** and a low **heart rate**. For example, whereas the average heart rate at rest is usually between 70 and 80 beats per minute, some of the world's top tennis players have rates as low as 30 beats per minute. Other things being equal, a rate of 50 beats per minute or so is a sign of high physical fitness. What all this means is that the heart of a person in good condition gets more rest than the heart of a person in average condition. Within a 24-hour period, for example, a heart with a rate of 80 beats per minute registers about 30,000 times more beats than a heart with a rate of 60 beats per minute. When we put this in the context of weeks, months, and years, the implications are staggering and not a little frightening.

Another possible cardiovascular benefit of endurance exercising relates to the blood itself. Duke University researchers tested healthy adults between ages 25 and 69 who took part in a 10-week physical conditioning program. In a simulated clotting situation, in which researchers inflated a blood pressure cuff around each subject's arm, from which they drew blood, they found an increased level of fibrinolysin following exercise. Since fibrinolysin is a natural clot-dissolving agent, this could well mean added protection against heart attack, stroke, and embolism.

All studies, without exception, show that endurance exercises do what they are supposed to do—provide us with cardiovascular fitness—only when they are vigorous, sus-

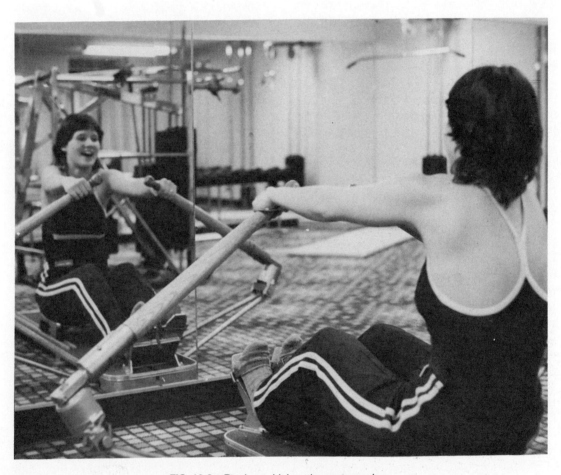

FIG. 18-3 ■ Rowing, a high endurance exercise.

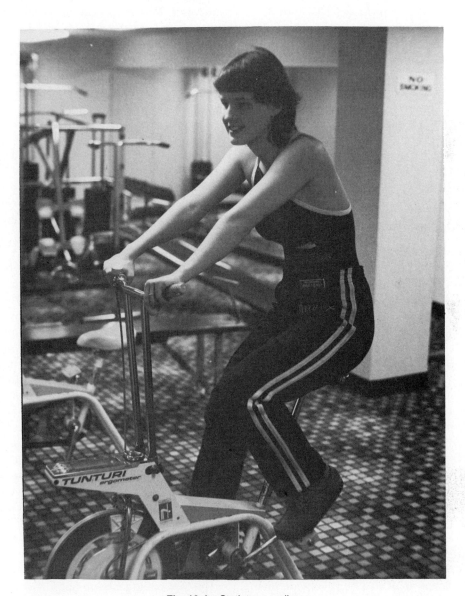

Fig. 18-4 ■ Stationary cycling.

tained, and regular. Vigorous exercise is defined (by the experts) in terms of "target heart rate," which according to the simplest rule of thumb equals 170 minus age. This indicates the approximate maximum pulse rate that strengthens the heart without strain. As another rule of thumb, 15 to 30 minutes of such exercise must be done three or four times a week to assure the desired training effect. And the desired training effect will eventually manifest itself in a lowered resting heart rate. When this begins to happen, one has physiological confirmation of what he or she already feels—namely, a heightened sense of well-being.

■ Strength exercises and warm-down

Strength exercises are designed to improve muscle strength, promote good posture, and contribute to flexibility, coordination, and balance. These can be done through the use of weight-training equipment (under the guidance of a weight coach) or through the use of one's own body. The latter exercises include full push-ups, modified push-ups, full sit-ups, and head and shoulder curl.

The warm-down ("cool-down") period concludes the exercise session and should last for a good 10 minutes. A slow, restful walk usually serves the purpose. This crucial period reduces the intensity of the previous strenuous activity on the one hand and minimizes the chances of dizziness on the other. The abrupt termination of any vigorous or strenuous exercise may cause dizziness and fainting because the circulatory system system is not keeping pace with the body's continuing need for oxygen. Scientists believe that certain other factors may also be involved, such as the "psychology of exhaustion."

■ Clothing

The choice of "conditioning clothing" obviously depends on the type of activity and the weather (Fig. 18-5). Generally, clothes should be reasonably loose and heavy or light enough to protect the body from heat, cold, and wind. Restrictive support garments should be avoided. Plastic or rubberized clothes are dangerous because they do not allow the body to cool itself through the evaporation of sweat. Wearing such clothing during vigorous exercising can result in heat stroke and exhaustion. Most women find it necessary to wear a good bra support, especially while running or jogging. This not only provides general comfort but also prevents soreness and tenderness of the breasts. Finally, the NAHI reminds us not to wear jewelry while exercising. A chain, for example, could catch on something and cause serious injury, especially where exercise machines are involved.

Quality tennis, basketball, or gym shoes are usually suitable for most activities, but running, jogging, and walking call for special shoes. A good running shoe can often spell the difference between running joyfully or having to experience the pain associated with overuse and injury to the foot. A well-constructed shoe, with proper fit, provides proper support for the foot, helps to absorb shock, and protects the foot from being cut or bruised (Fig. 18-6). Proper socks are also important in the prevention of blisters, soreness, and aching feet. The best place to buy proper footwear is at well-established, well-stocked shoe stores. Here, for the most part, one is most likely to get a professional fitting. And that is exactly what is needed for any kind of shoe.

■ Food and water

The old saying about not drinking while "you're playing" has proved to be just another old wives' tale. Indeed, we should always keep a bottle of water handy. Strenuous exercise, especially in the heat, can lead to serious dehydration. Experts say that people exercising or playing hard in hot weather for more than

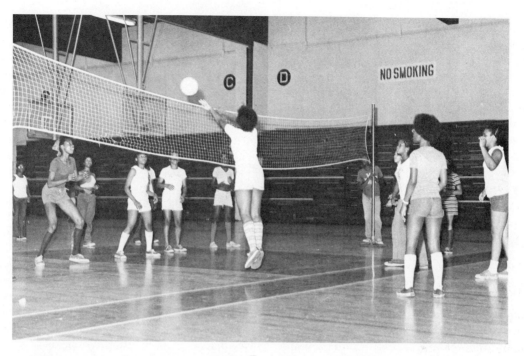

FIG. 18-5 ■ It is a good idea to wear proper clothing for athletic activities.

From Bucher, C.A., and Koenig, C.R.: Methods and materials for secondary school physical education, ed. 6, St. Louis, 1983, The C.V. Mosby Co.

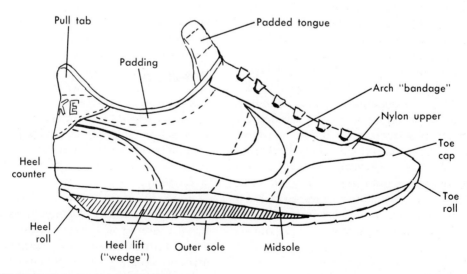

FIG. 18-6 ■ Anatomy of a running shoe.

From Klafs, C.E., and Lyon, M.J.: The female athlete: a coach's guide to conditioning and training, ed. 2, St. Louis, 1978, The C.V. Mosby Co. Artwork by Margaret Miller, Long Beach, Calif.

2 hours should stop for a water break every 15 minutes. This will help maintain the body's proper water balance by replenishing the water lost through perspiration. Warning signals of dehydration can be weakness and/or dizziness. When these symptoms appear, one should stop exercising immediately, take a rest in the shade, and drink a few cups of water.

In regard to food, avoid strenuous exercise for at least 2 hours after a meal. If exercise comes before a meal, the experts say to wait about 20 minutes before eating.

JOGGING

Many people try to make a distinction between jogging and running; others argue that these are just words and that all "joggers" and "runners" are involved in the same activity. The most popular description is that jogging is slower paced and fitness oriented, while running is faster and geared more toward competition. The National Jogging Association (NJA) describes jogging as "a run done at a comfortable pace primarily for exercise and recreation." But whatever the definition, most experts consider jogging as one of the fastest, easiest ways to realize the benefits of aerobic conditioning.

Shoes are crucial. Good jogging shoes have an adequate arch support and a wide heel base. They are flexible and durable, and they are tested for shock absorption, resiliency, and heel resistance. The NJA emphasizes the importance of flexibility exercises before and after jogging and the importance of walking until breathing is back to normal.

How fast one should jog is a key question, and there are several guidelines successful joggers use to find their ideal training pace. Some signals of overexertion are dizziness, tightness in the chest, and nausea. The first important indicator is breathing, which can be checked with the "talk test." If one is out of breath and cannot talk comfortably while jogging, he or she is working too hard and should slow down. Another way to check jogging pace is by means of the target heart rate, which was discussed earlier. This should not be exceeded. To determine heart rate during exercise, the jogger counts the pulse for 6 seconds and adds a zero to the count. If this turns out to be greater than the target heart rate, one should jog more slowly until later on in the schedule when fitness is improved. Since many people have trouble feeling their wrist pulse well enough to count accurately, an alternate way is to press against the carotid artery, easily found just under the angle of the jaw on either side of the neck.

When jogging causes pain and when rest does not help, one should take careful note of where the pain is, what the pain feels like, and when it is most noticeable and least noticeable. Then the person should seek the advice of a licensed health professional in sports medicine. Special evaluations can be done to find out if the feet and legs are vulnerable to problems associated with jogging. Should a problem arise, special therapeutic programs—based on careful evaluations—can be designed to relieve pain, to increase strength and mobility, and to prevent recurrence of the problem.

SWIMMING

If there is such a thing as the "perfect exercise," swimming may come close to it. Swimming can be done by persons of all ages, from 3 to 103 and beyond, who are in almost any physical shape. More people report that they swim regularly for exercise than report that they jog. Many find swimming less boring than jogging because by changing strokes or by doing exercises in the water (Fig. 18-7), they can introduce considerable variety into their activity. Access to an indoor pool can make swimming a pleasurable year-round activity for millions of Americans. Though the annual cost

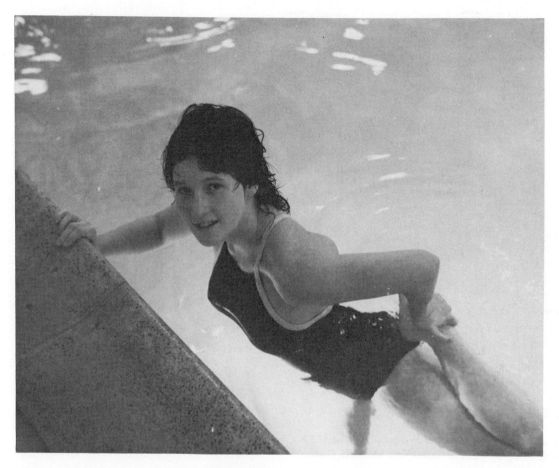

FIG. 18-7 ■ Aqua-exercising.

of pool membership may seem a little high, when one calculates the cost per swim, it is much cheaper than a movie, which exercises only the eye muscles.

Aside from its unique aerobic conditioning effects, swimming has a number of therapeutic attributes. It is often prescribed as the activity of choice for persons with back or joint problems or with injuries incurred as a result of other sports, such as jogging or tennis. Few other exercises strengthen the muscles of the back and abdomen, which help to support the back. The backstroke is especially helpful for those with chronic backaches. Swimming is also

ideal for arthritis. Because the water provides buoyancy, the sport places few mechanical stresses on the body and actually helps to loosen up stiff joints. Swimming is also often recommended for heart patients to improve efficiency of the heart muscle and its ability to withstand the stress of any physical activity. Furthermore, some physicians believe swimming can help counter varicose veins. The explanation is that the improved muscle tone in the legs from swimming massages the leg veins as the legs move, thus helping to avoid venous distention (swollen veins) and varicosities.

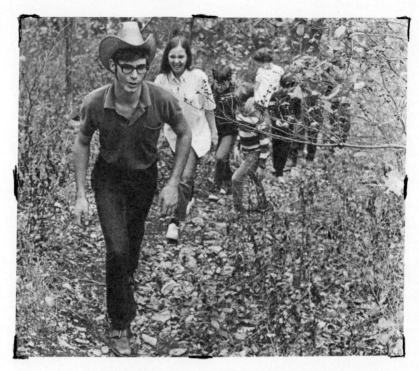

FIG. 18-8 ■ Hiking is an excellent recreational activity.

RECREATIONAL ACTIVITIES

Most people, especially those who wish to lose weight, should supplement their conditioning exercises with recreational activities. Gardening on weekends, bird watching, bowling, golf, hiking (Fig. 18-8), softball, family outings, and the like not only help to burn off calories but also provide relaxation and enjoyment. The experts tell us to avoid highly competitive sports (which not infrequently overpower common sense) and to participate in contact sports only if we are reasonably well trained and conditioned. Such sports can be dangerous.

DAILY ACTIVITIES

To a conditioning program and to recreational activities we should add a little more action each day. Walk to the neighborhood grocery instead of using the car. Park several blocks from the office and walk the rest of the way. Walk up a flight or more of stairs instead of using the elevator; start with a few steps and gradually increase. Stand up to put on and remove stockings and shoes; most people neglect to use their sense of balance. Get off the chair to get what is needed. Bend, stoop, stretch, squat, reach, lift, and carry. These little bits of action, while not taxing, are cumulative in their good effects. A few calories used up by walking, going up steps, bending, or otherwise moving can add up to a fair-sized total in the course of the day. And the contributions these movements make to muscle tone, flexibility, and balance are also significant. Furthermore, walking is the simplest, most basic physical activity, and it is also one of the most beneficial. No matter where it is done, walking has a tonic effect on mind and body. Walking can be a spiritual exercise.

SELF-TEST

1. _G_ aerobic exercise
2. _K_ anaerobic exercise
3. _B_ isotonic exercise
4. _L_ isometric exercise
5. _A_ warm-up exercise
6. _J_ flexibility exercise
7. _N_ stroke volume
8. _M_ heart rate
9. _O_ dissolves clots
10. _I_ "target heart rate"
11. _C_ evaporation of sweat
12. _E_ weakness or dizziness
13. _H_ neck artery
14. _F_ fishing trip
15. _D_ fundamental activity

a. rotation
b. lifting
c. cooling
d. walking
e. dehydration
f. recreation
g. jogging
h. carotid
i. 150 beats/min
j. stretching
k. sprinting
l. pressing
m. 60 beats/min
n. 60 ml/beat
o. fibrinolysin

evaporation – inverse ratio

injection at clot area – heart clot

STUDY QUESTIONS

1. What is your understanding of the expression "physical fitness equals exercise times diet"?
2. Why is it that "exercise burns food"?
3. Aerobic and anaerobic mean (in Greek) "with oxygen" and "without oxygen," respectively. How does this fit in with the application of these terms to exercise?
4. Isometric (in Greek) means the "same length." How does this fit in with the expression "isometric exercise"?
5. What is the basic difference between an endurance exercise and a strength exercise?
6. Why does a weak heart beat at a higher rate than a strong heart?
7. With conditioning exercises does the stroke volume of the heart increase or decrease?
8. Strength exercises alone do not make us physically fit. Why?

9. A sensible diet alone keeps our weight in check but does not make us physically fit. Why?
10. Weight lifting and push-ups are essentially the same kind of exercise. Why so?
11. In order for a given exercise, such as jogging, to pay off in cardiovascular fitness, what three criteria must be adhered to?
12. What is your particular "target heart rate"?
13. In your view or from your experience, what do you consider the ideal endurance (aerobic) exercise?
14. What do you consider the ideal recreational exercise?
15. "Walking can be a spiritual exercise." Elaborate at length.

AVOID WORRY –

CHAPTER 19

Nutrition and the diet

Since we are what we eat, the study of nutrition assumes gigantic and possibly overpowering dimensions. Presently the world's population is growing about 2% per year, while the food supply grows only about 1%. By the year 2000 many authorities believe that the average caloric intake will be just about at the level of starvation. Indeed, in some parts of the world starvation is here right now. Reliable sources estimate that some 50,000 people starve to death each day! Severe deficiency disease is not common in the United States, but nonetheless it can always be found among certain groups, especially infants, the elderly, and those living in extreme poverty. The principal nutritional problem in the United States and other affluent countries is overeating. Stated otherwise, obesity is conspicuously absent during famine. An understanding of nutrition and its health implications is clearly crucial to our physical and psychosocial well-being.

Nutrition is the process of nourishing or being nourished. More particularly it encompasses the interrelated steps by which a living organism assimilates food and uses it for growth and for replacement of tissues. There are all kinds of foods, of course, but all have one thing in common—they contain life-giving chemicals called **nutrients**. In a word, nutrition deals with nutrients. In the present chapter we shall take a good look at all recognized nutrients, the foods with which they are associated, and the diseases and disorders of malnutrition. At the outset, however, we must consider energy—the physical essence of life—and how we measure it: calories for today, joules for tomorrow.

■ ENERGY AND CALORIES

The body, like any machine, needs energy to keep running; the fuel that supplies this energy is called food. Logically, then, the most meaningful way to "quantify food" is in terms of energy, which brings us to one of the more alarming words in the English language, calorie. Actually, there are a number of kinds of calories, but the one of concern to us is the nutritional calorie or **kilocalorie** (kcal). Even nutritionists, however, simply call it "calorie," and for convenience we shall do the same.

The word "calorie" derives from the Latin "calor," meaning heat, which is good to keep in mind because this is the crux of its definition. Specifically, a calorie is the amount of heat (a form of energy) required to raise the temperature of 1 kg of water 1 degree Celsius (C) (Fig. 19-1). By way of example, if the complete combustion of a slice of bread causes the temperature of 1 kg of water to go from 15° C to 110° C, then we say that this particular brand of bread supplies ("contains") 95 calories per slice. In the body a slice of this bread likewise supplies 95 calories, two slices supply 190 calories, and so on. In the International System of Measurement (abbreviated SI) the

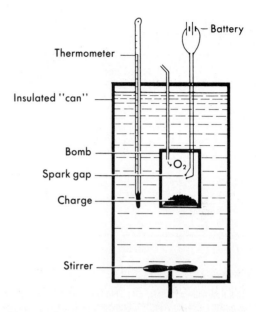

FIG. 19-1 ■ Device (calorimeter) used to measure the caloric content of food. The combustion of the food sample ("charge") causes a rise in the temperature of the water (surrounding the "bomb"), and from this the number of calories supplied by the sample can be easily calculated (see text).

calorie equals 4186 **joules** (J), or 4.186 **kilojoules** (kJ), the joule being the SI unit of energy. Although the joule is the scientifically preferred unit of energy, just when it will replace the calorie in common parlance is anybody's guess. Perhaps by the year 2000 all of us will be "counting our joules."

■ ENERGY AND METABOLISM

Metabolism, we shall recall, is the sum total of all the chemical reactions going on within the body. Metabolic rate refers to the rate at which these reactions are taking place and is expressed in calories per hour. However, because there are so many factors affecting this rate, it is difficult to compare metabolic rates from person to person. For a valid comparison authorities customarily employ what is called the **basal metabolic rate** (BMR), that

TABLE 19-1

Basal metabolic rates

| Age (yr) | Calories per square meter body surface per hour | |
	Male	Female
10-12	51.5	50.0
12-14	50.0	46.5
14-16	46.0	43.0
16-18	43.0	40.0
18-20	41.0	38.0
20-30	39.5	37.0
30-40	39.5	36.5
40-50	38.5	36.0
50-60	37.5	35.0
60-70	36.5	34.0

Modified from Anthony, C.P., and Thibodeau, G.A.: Textbook of anatomy and physiology, ed. 10, St. Louis, 1979, The C.V. Mosby Co.

is, metabolism measured at rest after a 12-hour fast (so-called basal conditions). It represents the minimum amount of energy the body must produce in a given time to keep itself going at the lowest level. This energy is supplied by the conversion of either ingested food or stored food (namely, fatty tissue and liver glycogen). The BMR is calculated as **calories per square meter of body surface area per hour** (Table 19-1) and, for purposes of comparison, is expressed in percent of variation above or below the normal value for a person of the same sex and age. The range usually given as normal is from −10% to +10%. For example, if a 20-year-old woman has a BMR of 40 (that is, 40 calories/m²/hr), this would be expressed as $(40 - 38) \div 38 \times 100$, or +5% (38 being the normal value). In other words, she is well within the normal range. Abnormal BMRs are usually caused by abnormal thyroid activity—up when the thyroid is overactive and down when it is underactive. As we see in Table 19-1 the BMR normally decreases with age and is slightly higher in males than in females.

ENERGY BALANCE

When we say that the body maintains a state of energy balance, we mean that its energy input equals its energy output. Energy input, or intake, per day equals the total calories in the food ingested per day; energy output equals the BMR plus all other activities (expressed in calories). This balance is crucial because it relates to body weight. Body weight remains constant when the body maintains energy balance; body weight increases when energy input exceeds energy output. Body weight decreases when the energy input is less than energy output. Energy input, as noted, derives from food—specifically, carbohydrates, fats, and proteins. Table 19-2 presents the recommended energy (caloric) intake for the general population.

NUTRIENTS

Nutrients are the essential chemical entities contained in food. They are needed to build and maintain body cells, regulate body processes, and supply energy. About 50 nutrients, including water, are needed daily for optimum health. Depending on their metabolic rate and/or molecular structure, nutrients fall into five categories: **carbohydrates**, **fats**, **proteins**, **vitamins**, and **minerals**. Because of the amounts involved, carbohydrates, fats, and proteins are sometimes referred to as **macronutrients**, and vitamins and minerals are referred to as **micronutrients**. The highlights of each each of these categories are presented below.

Carbohydrates

Chemically, carbohydrates contain only carbon (C), hydrogen (H), and oxygen (O), with the ratio of hydrogen to oxygen atoms usually 2:1. For example, sucrose (regular table sugar) has the chemical formula $C_{12}H_{22}O_{11}$. The main

TABLE 19-2

Mean heights and weights and recommended energy intake*

Category	Age (years)	Weight kg	Weight lb	Height cm	Height in	Energy needs (with range) kcal		Energy needs (with range) MJ
Infants	0.0-0.5	6	13	60	24	kg × 115	(95-145)	kg × .48
	0.5-1.0	9	20	71	28	kg × 105	(80-135)	kg × .44
Children	1-3	13	29	90	35	1300	(900-1800)	5.5
	4-6	20	44	112	44	1700	(1300-2300)	7.1
	7-10	28	62	132	52	2400	(1600-3300)	10.1
Males	11-14	45	99	157	62	2700	(2000-3700)	11.3
	15-18	66	145	176	69	2800	(2100-3900)	11.8
	19-22	70	154	177	70	2900	(2500-3300)	12.2
	23-50	70	154	178	70	2700	(2300-3100)	11.3
	51-75	70	154	178	70	2400	(2000-2800)	10.1
	76+	70	154	178	70	2050	(1600-2450)	8.6
Females	11-14	46	101	157	62	2200	(1500-3000)	9.2
	15-18	55	120	163	64	2100	(1200-3000)	8.8
	19-22	55	120	163	64	2100	(1700-2500)	8.8
	23-50	55	120	163	64	2000	(1600-2400)	8.4
	51-75	55	120	163	64	1800	(1400-2200)	7.6
	76+	55	120	163	64	1600	(1200-2000)	6.7
Pregnancy						+300		
Lactation						+500		

From Recommended daily dietary allowances, revised 1980. Food, and Nutrition Board, National Academy of Sciences–National Research Council, Washington, D.C.

*The data in this table have been assembled from the observed median heights and weights of children together with desirable weights for adults for the mean heights of men (70 in) and women (64 in) between the ages of 18 and 34 years as surveyed in the U.S. population (HEW/NCHS data).

The energy allowances for the young adults are for men and women doing light work. The allowances for the two older age groups represent mean energy needs over these age spans, allowing for a 2% decrease in basal (resting) metabolic rate per decade and a reduction in activity of 200 kcal per day for men and women between 51 and 75 years, 500 kcal for men over 75 years, and 400 kcal for women over 75. The customary range of daily energy output is shown for adults in parentheses and is based on a variation in energy needs of ±400 kcal at any age, emphasizing the wide range of energy intakes appropriate for any group of people.

Energy allowances for children through age 18 are based on median energy intakes of children these ages followed in longitudinal growth studies. The values in parentheses are 10th and 90th percentiles of energy intake, to indicate the range of energy consumption among children of these ages.

dietary carbohydrates are **sugars**, **starches**, and indigestible substances collectively referred to as **fiber**. The prime, overall function of carbohydrate in human nutrition is to provide energy, and body tissues require a constant supply. Most authorities believe that we should derive about 58% of our calories from carbo-hydrate—13% as sugar and 45% as "complex carbohydrate" (starches and the like). One gram of carbohydrate supplies 4 calories.

Dietary fiber. The relation of fiber to control of constipation is well established. Water absorption by the fiber softens and increases the volume of the feces, causing the colon to contract and propel its contents faster. Also, there is growing evidence that a high-fiber diet controls the symptoms of diverticulosis. The preventive role of fiber in colorectal cancer has been under investigation by a number of research groups. Although these studies are somewhat inconclusive, they are based on reasonable explanations and have produced a large body of epidemiologic data pointing to such relationships. Scientists have not yet determined how much fiber anyone should eat; that is to say, there is no recommended daily allowance.

A high-fiber diet can cause some distressing side effects, such as a feeling of being "stuffed" or "bloated." Stomach rumblings, usually frowned on in polite society, are caused by changes in the material passing through the intestines. Moreover, large amounts of fiber can impair the body's ability to absorb certain minerals such as iron, copper, and calcium. Experts in nutrition point out that fiber is just one part of a properly balanced diet and that adding it to a poor diet probably will cause more problems than it solves.

■ Fats

Fats are a diverse group of nutrient substances that are insoluble in water and greasy to the touch. Chemically, they contain the same elements as carbohydrates (carbon, hydrogen, and oxygen), but the atoms are "hooked together" in an entirely different fashion. Also the relative hydrogen content is much higher, which explains their greater yield of energy— 9 calories per gram (versus 4 calories per gram for carbohydrates). Fats serve two basic functions in the human body: (1) a primary metabolic function to provide energy, and (2) a secondary mechanical or structural function, for example, to protect vital organs (via fatty tissue).

Saturated vs unsaturated fats. Saturated fats are made up of molecules contain-

ing a maximum number of hydrogen atoms; **unsaturated fats**, such as vegetable oils, are capable of taking on more hydrogen. The important point of this piece of chemistry is that populations like ours with diets high in saturated fats and in cholesterol (a fatlike alcohol) tend to have a higher incidence of atherosclerosis and heart attacks. Eating extra saturated fat and cholesterol will increase blood cholesterol levels in most people. However, there are wide variations. Some people can consume diets high in saturated fats and cholesterol and still keep normal blood cholesterol levels. Other people have high blood cholesterol levels even if they eat low-fat, low-cholesterol diets. There is controversy about what recommendations are appropriate for healthy Americans. The American Heart Association urges us to reduce total fat, saturated fat, and dietary cholesterol in hopes of preventing heart disease. The National Academy of Science, however, recommends that we cut down on our fat and cholesterol intake only in event of a weight problem.

■ Proteins

Proteins contain carbon, nitrogen, hydrogen, and oxygen. Some proteins also contain sulfur, phosphorus, iron, or other mineral elements. The process of digestion converts proteins into chemically simpler compounds called **amino acids**, of which there are 20 or more. Each of the innumerable proteins contains a particular combination of many amino acids in its large and complex molecule. At least eight amino acids must be provided by the proteins of the diet, since the body cannot synthesize them. These are called **essential amino acids**. If they are all present in suitable quantity, the body can form the other amino acids from them. Proteins that contain all the essential amino acids are called **complete proteins**. Animal proteins, such as milk, cheese, meat, fish, poultry, and eggs, are complete

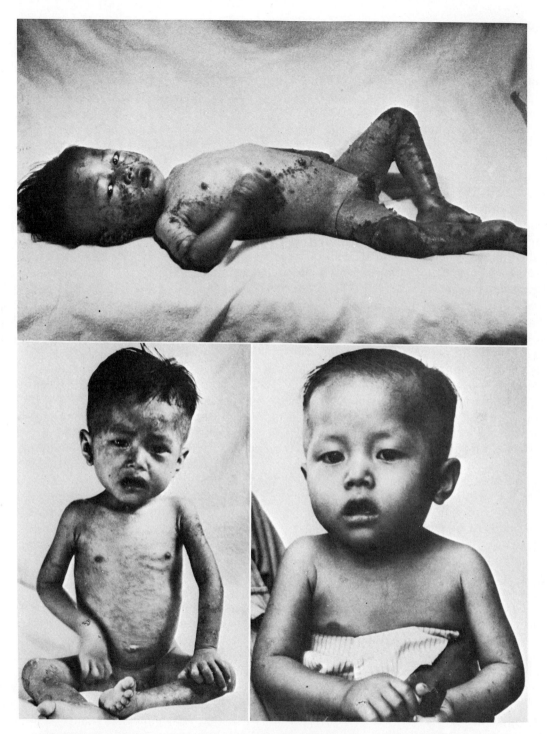

FIG. 19-2 ■ Kwashiorkor and its response to protein. These pictures were taken by the physician who treated the patient. The photograph on top was taken on admission to the hospital; the left photograph, after 4 days; the right photograph, after 1 month.

proteins. Gelatin and the various cereal and vegetable proteins are **incomplete**. All the essential amino acids can be obtained from a combination of vegetable proteins, however. A varied, well-rounded diet contains many proteins so that they supplement one another.

The primary function of dietary protein is the growth and maintenance of tissue. In addition, protein supplies amino acids for other essential nitrogen-containing substances, such as enzymes, hormones, and antibodies. Finally, it has been established that on an average, 58% of the total dietary proteins may be converted to glucose (the body's chief sugar), which is then oxidized ("burned") to supply energy. As a rule of thumb, the daily allowance of protein for the average adult is in the vicinity of 0.8 g per kg of body weight. Thus for a man weighing 70 kg (154 lb) this amounts to about 56 g daily. A total of 75 to 85 g daily is needed during pregnancy and lactation. The requirements for infants and children vary according to growth patterns.

Protein deficiency. Protein deficiencies are either primary or secondary. **Primary deficiencies** stem from a quantitative or qualitative lack of protein in the diet or from increased utilization of protein (for energy) occasioned by a caloric deficiency. **Secondary deficiencies**, on the other hand, are "internal matters"—poor digestion, poor absorption, increased catabolism, excessive loss from the body, or increased requirement.

The classic primary deficiencies are **marasmus** and **kwashiorkor** (Fig. 19-2). Marasmus is a progressive wasting and emaciation, especially in infants, relating to both protein and caloric deficiencies. Kwashiorkor, which occurs in the face of adequate or even excess caloric intake, relates to a lack of most essential amino acids. It is characterized by lethargy, edema, poor skin, decoloration of the hair, and enlargement of the liver. A common cause of death is depletion of potassium. Treatment

centers on the restoration of electrolyte balance and the implementation of a diet based on milk. The treatment of secondary deficiencies involves the giving of protein (for example, transfusions in hemorrhage) and the correction, if possible, of the underlying cause.

■ Vitamins

In 1906 Sir Frederick Hopkins, a British biochemist, proved the existence in normal foods of certain accessory factors essential to the diet, and 5 years later Casimir Funk, believing these factors to be a chemical class called amines, coined the term "vitamine." When further work disclosed that the amino group was not characteristic, Drummond proposed that the "e" be dropped, giving us our present word "vitamin."

Vitamins help to sustain life, promote growth, and maintain health. It is hardly an exaggeration to say that their discovery represents the highest achievement in nutrition. Although the precise mechanisms by which most vitamins work are still not completely understood, biochemists apparently have succeeded in unraveling the essential facts. All known vitamins have been isolated in the pure chemical state and synthesized in the laboratory. By convention they are categorized according to their solubility in fat and water. The **fat-soluble vitamins** include vitamins A, D, K, and E, and the **water-soluble vitamins** include vitamin C and the members of the B-complex group.

Vitamin A. Vitamin A (**retinol**) occurs, as such, only in foods of animal origin (chiefly liver, milk, and eggs); most of what we need comes from beta-carotene, a pigment found in green and yellow vegetables. Vitamin A content is expressed in retinol equivalents (RE). The recommended daily allowances (RDAs) are given in Table 19-3. Deficiencies result not only from inadequate intake of the vitamin or its precursors but also from poor absorption in such conditions as diarrhea and lack of bile. Vitamin A is needed for the proper development of the skin, the bones, and the eyes; the chief signs of deficiency relate to these structures. One of the first signs of vitamin A deficiency is **nyctalopia**, or night blindness. More severe manifestations include ulceration of the cornea, dental defects, and retarded bone growth. It is most important to keep in mind, however, that large amounts of vitamin A are toxic. Recent animal studies show that vitamin A is a cancer inhibitor.

Vitamin D. Vitamin D is unique among vitamins in two respects. It occurs naturally in only a few common foods (in fish oils), and it can be formed in the body by exposure of the skin to ultraviolet rays either from the sun or from a lamp. Vitamin D in the body is predominately associated with calcium and phosphorus; it influences the absorption of these minerals and their deposit in bone tissue. A deficiency results in **rickets** (bone distortion) in infants and children (Fig. 19-3) and in **osteomalacia** (softening of the bones) in adults. On the other hand, excessive intake of vitamin D can be dangerous, producing bone fragility, calcification of various tissues, and kidney stones. The recommended daily allowances are given in Table 19-3. The main food sources of vitamin D are those to which it has been added. Most milk sold today contains 400 IU (international units) per quart. Milk is a "good companion" for vitamin D because it provides calcium and phosphorus as well.

Vitamin E. The term "vitamin E" is applied to four closely related substances called tocopherols, of which alpha-tocopherol is the most abundant and most potent. All are soluble in oil and are absorbed readily from the digestive tract. Vitamin E occurs in wheat germ oil, fresh vegetables, fruits, liver, and muscle. Deficiency states differ considerably in various species. It has been demonstrated without question that vitamin E is essential to the

fertility of male and female rats and mice, but in larger animals and in humans this has yet to be proved. Vitamin E deficiency in rats, guinea pigs, and rabbits results in muscular dystrophy and lesions of the spinal cord. In humans vitamin E helps maintain the natural life of red blood cells and aids the body in utilizing vitamin A and polyunsaturated fats. Other benefits claimed for Vitamin E are still being investigated. Scientists continue to study and evaluate possible relationships to physical exertion, smoking, and air pollution, among others.

Vitamin K. Vitamin K is a fat-soluble vitamin synthesized by intestinal bacteria; an adequate supply is generally assured beyond the first week or so of life. Since the intestinal tract of the newborn is sterile, no vitamin K is produced until a bacterial population develops. Therefore a prophylactic dose of vitamin K is usually given to the newborn soon after delivery. Foods containing vitamin K include green leafy vegetables, tomatoes, egg yolk, and liver. The major function of the vitamin is to stimulate the production (by the liver) of **prothrombin**, an essential agent in the coagulation of blood. A lack of prothrombin results in hemorrhage. No requirement for vitamin K is stated, since a deficiency is unlikely except in certain clinical situations. These include intestinal disease, a lack of bile (which is needed for vitamin K absorption), and prolonged use of antibiotics (which kill off intestinal bacteria).

Vitamin C. By unknown mechanisms vitamin C (**ascorbic acid**) helps maintain the integrity of "intercellular substances" throughout the body; these substances include intercellular cement, tissue fibers, bone matrix, and the dentin of teeth. Vitamin C chemically supports the action of the enzyme that converts folic acid (another vitamin) to its active form (folinic acid), and it facilitates the absorption of iron from food. A severe deficiency of vitamin C results in **scurvy**, a dis-

▰▰▰▰ **TABLE 19-3**

Designed for the maintenance of good nutrition of practically all healthy people in the U.S.A.*

Category	Age (years)	Weight kg	Weight lb	Height cm	Height in	Protein (g)	Calcium (mg)	Phos-phorus (mg)	Mag-nesium (mg)	Iron (mg)	Zinc (mg)	Iodine (μg)
Infants	0.0-0.5	6	13	60	24	kg × 2.2	360	240	50	10	3	40
	0.5-1.0	9	20	71	28	kg × 2.0	540	360	70	15	5	50
Children	1-3	13	29	90	35	23	800	800	150	15	10	70
	4-6	20	44	112	44	30	800	800	200	10	10	90
	7-10	28	62	132	52	34	800	800	250	10	10	120
Males	11-14	45	99	157	62	45	1200	1200	350	18	15	150
	15-18	66	145	176	69	56	1200	1200	400	18	15	150
	19-22	70	154	177	70	56	800	800	350	10	15	150
	23-50	70	154	178	70	56	800	800	350	10	15	150
	51+	70	154	178	70	56	800	800	350	10	15	150
Females	11-14	46	101	157	62	46	1200	1200	300	18	15	150
	15-18	55	120	163	64	46	1200	1200	300	18	15	150
	19-22	55	120	163	64	44	800	800	300	18	15	150
	23-50	55	120	163	64	44	800	800	300	18	15	150
	51+	55	120	163	64	44	800	800	300	10	15	150
Pregnant						+30	+400	+400	+150	†	+5	+25
Lactating						+20	+400	+400	+150	†	+10	+50

From Recommended dietary allowances, revised 1979. Food and Nutrition Board, National Academy of Sciences–National Research Council, Washington, D.C.

*The allowances are intended to provide for individual variations among most normal persons as they live in the United States under usual environmental stresses. Diets should be based on a variety of common foods in order to provide other nutrients for which human requirements have been less well defined. See table for weights and heights by individual year of age.

†The increased requirement during pregnancy cannot be met by the iron content of habitual American diets nor by the existing iron stores of many women; therefore the use of 30-60 mg of supplemental iron is recommended. Iron needs during lactation are not substantially different from those of nonpregnant women, but continued supplementation of the mother for 2-3 months after parturition is advisable in order to replenish stores depleted by pregnancy.

Fat-soluble vitamins			Water-soluble vitamins						
Vitamin A (μg RE)‡	Vitamin D (μg)§	Vitamin E (mg α TE)‖	Vitamin C (mg)	Thiamin (mg)	Riboflavin (mg)	Niacin (mg NE)¶	Vitamin B_6 (mg)	Folacin** (μg)	Vitamin B_{12} (μg)
420	10	3	35	0.3	0.4	6	0.3	30	0.5††
400	10	4	35	0.5	0.6	8	0.6	45	1.5
400	10	5	45	0.7	0.8	9	0.9	100	2.0
500	10	6	45	0.9	1.0	11	1.3	200	2.5
700	10	7	45	1.2	1.4	16	1.6	300	3.0
1000	10	8	50	1.4	1.6	18	1.8	400	3.0
1000	10	10	60	1.4	1.7	18	2.0	400	3.0
1000	7.5	10	60	1.5	1.7	19	2.2	400	3.0
1000	5	10	60	1.4	1.6	18	2.2	400	3.0
1000	5	10	60	1.2	1.4	16	2.2	400	3.0
800	10	8	50	1.1	1.3	15	1.8	400	3.0
800	10	8	60	1.1	1.3	14	2.0	400	3.0
800	7.5	8	60	1.1	1.3	14	2.0	400	3.0
800	5	8	60	1.0	1.2	13	2.0	400	3.0
800	5	8	60	1.0	1.2	13	2.0	400	3.0
+200	+5	+2	+20	+0.4	+0.3	+2	+0.6	+400	+1.0
+400	+5	+3	+40	+0.5	+0.5	+5	+0.5	+100	+1.0

‡Retinol equivalents (RE). 1 Retinol equivalent = 1 μg retinol or 6 μg β carotene.
§As cholecalciferol. 10 μg cholecalciferol = 400 IU vitamin D.
‖ α tocopherol equivalents. 1 mg d-α-tocopherol = 1 α TE.
¶1 NE (niacin equivalent) is equal to 1 mg of niacin or 60 mg of dietary tryptophan.
**The folacin allowances refer to dietary sources as determined by *Lactobacillus casei* assay after treatment with enzymes ("conjugases") to make polyglutamyl forms of the vitamin available to the test organism.
††The RDA for vitamin B_{12} in infants is based on average concentration of the vitamin in human milk. The allowances after weaning are based on energy intake (as recommended by the American Academy of Pediatrics) and consideration of after factors such as intestinal absorption.

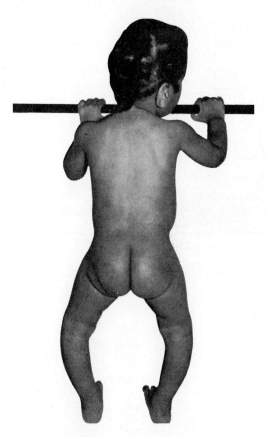

FIG. 19-3 ■ Rickets in young child.

Courtesy Rosa L. Nemire, M.D., and the Upjohn Co., Kalamazoo, Mich.

ease characterized especially by bleeding gums, splotchy hemorrhages beneath the skin, and abnormal formation of bone and teeth. Vitamin C can inhibit the formation of certain carcinogens and may reduce the risk of cancers of the stomach and esophagus. Well-known sources include citrus fruit and tomatoes.

As to whether or not vitamin C prevents the common cold, there is much controversy. Some authorities agree, and others do not. But one thing is for certain: taking excessive amounts of vitamin C can be dangerous. It makes the body more susceptible to kidney stones; it chemically destroys vitamin B_{12} (thereby leading to anemia); and in pregnant women it results in the birth of babies who later develop scurvy because their needs have been inflated in utero. Other reported untoward effects are gastrointestinal upset and diarrhea.

Thiamin. Thiamin (vitamin B_1) occurs in enriched bread, nuts, pork, whole grains, legumes, and liver. Thiamin functions as a key coenzyme in cell respiration; a deficiency leads to general metabolic disturbances. The major signs of deficiency include polyneuritis and enlargement of the heart. When these derangements occur at the same time, the syndrome is called **beriberi**. It is wrong to assume, however, that a thiamin avitaminosis (deficiency) and beriberi are synonymous, because lesser deficiencies lead to a variety of vague and "unimportant" symptoms. Indeed the deficiencies the physician usually sees—and this applies to all the vitamins—are not those depicted by the typical high school or college health text. It is uncommon to find a person with a single avitaminosis; understandably, a poor diet, the usual cause, leads to multiple deficiencies. The recommended daily allowances of thiamin are given in Table 19-3.

Riboflavin. Also known as vitamin B_2, riboflavin is present in milk, liver, yeast, kidneys, eggs, nuts, seafoods, meats, cheese, and green, leafy vegetables. Like thiamin, riboflavin is a key coenzyme in cellular respiration. The chief signs of deficiency include a purplish-red tongue (glossitis), reddening of the lips, fissuring at the angles of the mouth (cheilosis), greasy scaling of the skin, especially of skin folds (seborrheic dermatitis), and extra blood vessels in the cornea of the eye (corneal vascularization). The repercussions of a riboflavin deficiency (ariboflavinosis) in the rat are shown dramatically in Fig. 19-4. The recommended daily allowances are given in Table 19-3.

Niacin. Niacin (nicotinic acid) is a B-complex vitamin present abundantly in rice, bran, liver, yeasts, meat, peanuts, and fish. It

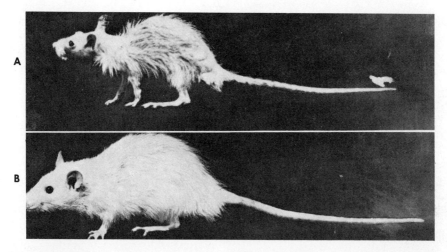

FIG. 19-4 ■ A, White rat with riboflavin deficiency. **B,** Same rat 6 weeks later after being placed on diet rich in riboflavin.

United States Department of Agriculture photograph.

is needed in respiratory reactions and in carbohydrate and protein metabolism. The major signs and symptoms of niacin deficiency relate to the skin, gastrointestinal tract, and nervous system. **Pellagra**, the severe and classic deficiency state, is characterized by skin eruptions and inflammatory redness, diarrhea, and, eventually, mental derangement; it is sometimes a multiple deficiency involving thiamin and riboflavin as well as niacin. The recommended daily allowances of niacin for adults are given in Table 19-3.

Vitamin B$_{12}$ and folic acid. Two members of the B-complex group, vitamin B$_{12}$ (cobalamin) and folic acid (folacin), are required for the formation of tissue. We know this because areas of rapid turnover, such as bone marrow, are the first to reflect a deficiency. Lack of vitamin B$_{12}$, which is usually the result of an inadequate intrinsic factor (needed for absorption), leads to **pernicious anemia**. Lack of folic acid leads to the "nutritional anemias" of infancy and pregnancy and generally retards growth and body development, especially in children. Vitamin B$_{12}$ occurs principally in liver, muscle tissue, milk,

and cheese; folic acid occurs principally in green, leafy vegetables, yeast, soybeans, and wheat. The recommended daily allowances for both vitamins are given in Table 19-3.

Pyridoxine. Pyridoxine (vitamin B$_6$) acts as a coenzyme in the metabolism of certain amino acids. It is present in egg yolk, nuts, whole grains, legumes, kidneys, muscle, liver, and fish. Though the importance of this B-complex vitamin in animals has long been known, its essential role in human nutrition was not appreciated until an unfortunate but nevertheless excusable and instructive incident occurred some years ago. There were widely scattered reports of a nervous syndrome (increased excitability, convulsions, and the like) of unknown origin among infants receiving a commercial milk substitute. An investigation soon demonstrated that the condition resulted from the absence of pyridoxine in the formula. Other deficiency disorders relating to the vitamin are seborrheic dermatitis (dandruff), impaired growth in infants, and vomiting in pregnancy. The recommended daily allowances of pyridoxine are given in Table 19-3.

Pantothenic acid. Pantothenic acid is a B-complex vitamin used by the body in the synthesis of coenzyme A, a cellular agent vital to normal metabolism. Since the vitamin is present in such a wide variety of foods, a deficiency in humans has not yet been described, except in experimental situations. The avitaminosis is characterized by fatigue, malaise, headache, sleep disturbances, colic, vomiting, and impaired muscle coordination. The daily need is believed to be about 10 mg for adults.

■ Minerals

Minerals are the inorganic (noncarbon) elements of food essential to life. Some minerals are needed in relatively large amounts in the diet: calcium, phosphorus, sodium, chloride, potassium, magnesium, and sulfur. "Large" means beyond 150 mg or so. Other minerals, called "trace elements," are needed in much smaller amounts. These are iron, manganese, copper, iodine, zinc, cobalt, fluorine, selenium, and certain other metals (Table 19-3).

Some minerals, such as lead, mercury, and cadmium, are regarded as harmful. Even minerals that the body requires for good health can be harmful if we get too much of them. For example, if all the potassium the body requires in one day is taken in a single, concentrated dose, severe illness can result. Many children under 5 years of age are hospitalized each year because of iron poisoning from accidental ingestion of multiple daily dietary supplements. Some of these children die. Other minerals can cause adverse effects if a person takes as little as twice as much as is required to maintain good health.

Taking too much of one essential mineral may upset the balance and function of other minerals in the body. Excess mineral intake can reduce a person's ability to perform physical tasks and can contribute to health problems such as anemia, bone demineralization and breakage, neurologic disease, and fetal abnormalities. The risks are greatest for very young persons, pregnant or lactating women, the elderly, and those with inadequate diet or chronic disease. There are a number of things we do not know about the function of minerals in the body, particularly the trace elements. It is clear, however, that people who take mineral supplements should not use them in amounts greatly in excess of what the body requires.

Mineral elements have two general body functions: building and regulating. Their building functions affect the skeleton and all soft tissues. Their regulating functions include a wide variety of systems, such as heartbeat, blood clotting, maintenance of the internal pressure of body fluids, nerve responses, and transport of oxygen from the lungs to the tissues.

Calcium. Calcium is present in the body in greater amounts than any other mineral. Almost all of the 2 or 3 pounds present are concentrated in the bones and teeth. Small amounts of calcium help to regulate certain body processes such as the normal behavior of nerves, muscle tone and irritability, and blood clotting. Although growing children and pregnant and lactating women have the highest calcium needs, all people need calcium in their diets throughout life. Milk and milk products are good sources of this mineral. Other good sources are green, leafy vegetables (except spinach and chard), citrus fruits, and dried peas and beans. Meats, grains, and nuts, which are good sources of many other nutrients, do not provide significant amounts of calcium.

Phosphorus. Phosphorus is present with calcium, in almost equal amounts, in the bones and teeth and is an important part of every tissue in the body. It is widely distributed in foods, so a sufficient supply is easily obtained in the diet. Good sources are milk, cheese, meat, poultry, fish, eggs, and whole-grain foods. Vegetables and fruits are generally low in this mineral.

Sodium and chloride. Sodium and chloride (chlorine) are the two elements that combine to form **sodium chloride** (table salt), but each has separate functions in the body. Sodium is found mainly in blood plasma and in the fluids outside the body cells, helping to maintain normal water balance inside and outside the cells. Sodium-rich foods come from animal sources such as meat, fish, poultry, eggs, and milk. Many processed foods, such as ham, bacon, bread, and crackers, have a high sodium content because salt or sodium compounds are added in processing. Chloride is part of hydrochloric acid, which is found in quite high concentration in the gastric juice and is very important in digestion of food in the stomach.

The daily American diet provides a high intake of sodium, much of it added to food as salt. Many authorities believe the intake is much higher than desirable. A reduction of salt in the diet is often prescribed by physicians to lower the sodium intake of persons with high blood pressure, kidney disease, cirrhosis of the liver, and congestive heart disease. A decrease in sodium intake can reduce the retention of water in the system (**edema**), which is typically associated with these health problems. Under conditions of heavy sweating or vomiting, salt intake may need to be increased, but the usual diet provides more than enough to cover losses from normal activities.

Potassium. Potassium is found mainly in the fluid inside the individual body cells. With sodium it helps to regulate fluid balance and volume of fluid in the body. A potassium deficiency is very uncommon in healthy persons but may result from prolonged diarrhea or from diuretics (which cause high urine volume). Deficiency has been associated with extremely inadequate protein diets in children. Potassium is abundant in almost all foods, both plant and animal.

Magnesium. Magnesium is found in all body tissues, but it occurs principally in the bones. It is an essential part of many enzyme systems responsible for energy conversions in the body. A deficiency of magnesium in healthy humans eating a variety of foods is uncommon, but it has been observed in some post-surgical patients, in alcoholics, and in those with certain other diseases.

Sulfur. Sulfur is present in all body tissues and is essential to life. It is related to protein nutrition because it is a component of several important amino acids. It is a part of two vitamins, thiamin and biotin. The complete function of sulfur has not yet been established.

Iron. Iron is an important part of compounds, such as hemoglobin, which are necessary for transporting oxygen to the cells and making use of the oxygen when it arrives. It is widely distributed in the body, mostly in the blood, with relatively large amounts in the liver, spleen, and bone marrow. The only way a significant amount of iron can leave the body is through a loss of blood. This is why people who have periodic blood losses or who are forming more blood have the greatest need for dietary iron. Women of childbearing age, pregnant women, and growing children are most likely to suffer from **iron deficiency anemia** because of their higher needs. Diets that provide enough iron must be carefully selected because only a few foods contain iron in useful amounts. Liver is an excellent source of iron. Other sources are meat products, egg yolk, fish, green, leafy vegetables, peas, beans, dried fruits, whole-grain cereals, and foods prepared from iron-enriched cereal products.

Manganese. Manganese is needed for normal tendon and bone structure and is part of some enzymes. Manganese is abundant in many foods, especially bran, coffee, tea, nuts, peas, and beans. A deficiency in humans is unknown.

Copper. Copper is involved in the storage and release from storage of iron to form hemoglobin for red blood cells. The need for copper is particularly important in the early months of life and, if the intake of the mother is sufficient, infants are born with a store of copper. Copper occurs in most unprocessed foods. Organ meats, shellfish, nuts, and dried legumes are rich sources of this mineral.

Iodine. Iodine is required in extremely small amounts, but the normal functioning of the thyroid gland depends on an adequate supply. With a deficiency of dietary iodine, thyroid enlargement (**goiter**) occurs. Goiter from iodine deficiency (endemic goiter) was common in certain inland areas of the United States, where the soil contains little iodine, until iodized salt was introduced in 1924. The iodization of salt is not mandatory, but, under a 1972 Federal Drug Administration (FDA) regulation, noniodized salt must be labeled with the statement, "This salt does not supply iodine, a necessary nutrient." Foods from the sea are the richest natural sources of iodine.

Zinc. It had been thought that a zinc deficiency did not exist in the United States, but recent studies on the loss of a sense of taste and on delayed wound healing indicate that deficiencies do exist in some persons. Zinc is an important part of the enzymes that, among other functions, transport carbon dioxide (via red blood cells) from the tissues to the lungs where it can be exhaled. Zinc is usually associated with the protein foods. Good sources are meats, fish, egg yolk, and milk. Whole-grain cereals are rich in zinc, but because of the presence of interfering substances, such as phytin, it may not be completely available for absorption.

Cobalt. Cobalt by itself is not essential in the body, but it is a part of vitamin B_{12}, which is an essential nutrient. Vegetarians who do not eat any meat, eggs, or dairy products can become deficient in vitamin B_{12} because it occurs only in trace amounts in plants.

Chromium. Chromium, acting with insu-

lin, is required for glucose utilization. A deficiency can produce a diabetes-like condition. Much remains to be learned about this mineral. Good sources are dried brewer's yeast, whole-grain cereals, and liver.

Selenium. Selenium appears to have a "sparing action" on vitamin E. A variety of problems occur in animals deficient in selenium and vitamin E; most are cured by adding either of these substances to the diet. Selenium's importance to body functioning has been shown in animals, and it is reasonably certain that this element is equally important for humans. The selenium content of foods depends on the amount available to the growing plant or animal.

Fluorine. Fluorine, like iodine, is found in small and varying amounts in water, soil, plants, and animals. Research has proven one benefit and provides strong evidence for a second. Fluoride contributes to solid tooth formation and results in a decrease of dental caries, especially in children. There is also evidence that fluoride helps retain calcium in the bones of older persons. The acceptable level of this mineral in drinking water is only one part per million. In nearly all communities where **fluoridation** of water has been introduced, the incidence of dental caries in children has been reduced by 50% or more.

Other minerals. In recent years the functions of "exotic minerals" in the body have been studied, but, as yet, none has been established as being beneficial for man. Some of these minerals are known to be important to the health of certain plants and animals. Cadmium, lead, and mercury, as noted earlier, are elements that have been found to be harmful and have no demonstrated essential function. Cadmium interferes with the functions of the essential elements of iron, copper, and calcium. Persons exposed to large amounts of cadmium may develop anemia, kidney damage, and, finally, marked bone mineral loss. These effects are less with adequate intake of zinc, iron, copper, calcium, manganese, and ascorbic acid—in other words, a normal diet.

■ Vitamin-mineral supplements

A daily vitamin-mineral supplement in amounts not exceeding U.S. Recommended Daily Allowances (U.S. RDAs) is generally recommended for pregnant and nursing women, heavy drinkers, strict dieters, anyone on prolonged antibiotic therapy, women who take oral contraceptives, and persons who eat a limited variety of foods. Extra iron is often needed by women of childbearing age, especially if they have heavy menstrual bleeding or eat fewer than 1600 calories a day. Persons with intestinal disorders that interfere with absorption of fats may need extra fat-soluble vitamins. Strict vegetarians who eat no animal foods need B_{12} supplements. Persons who take a "one-a-day supplement," however, cannot assume that they have fulfilled their day's micronutrient needs and now can safely consume empty calories or eat haphazardly in place of balanced meals. No supplement currently marketed provides 100% of the U.S. RDAs for all required nutrients. Also, there is a good possibility that natural foods supply essential micronutrients that we do not even know about.

■ FOOD GROUPS

No single food item supplies all the essential nutrients. Milk, for instance, contains very little iron or vitamin C. Clearly, the eating of a variety of foods is good protection against the development of a nutritional deficiency. Variety also reduces the likelihood of being exposed to excessive amounts of contaminants in any single food item. The best way to assure variety and, with it, a well-balanced diet is to select foods each day from each of four major groups: **milk group**, **meat group**, **fruit-vegetable group**, and **grain group** (Fig. 19-5).

■ Milk group

The milk, or dairy, group includes all types of milk used as beverages and in food preparation, all kinds of natural and processed cheese, ice cream and ice milk, yogurt, and foods (such as cream soups and puddings) made with large proportions of milk. The milk group supplies about 75% of the calcium, 40% of the riboflavin, and 22% of the protein available in our nation's food supply. This group also supplies some of almost all other nutrients known to be essential. Children and teenagers need calcium for their developing bones. Pregnant and lactating women need calcium both for themselves and for their babies. Adults need calcium to maintain bone structure. The recommended daily servings of milk (or its equivalent) are as follows: children, three glasses; teenagers, four glasses; adults, two glasses; pregnant women, four glasses; pregnant teenagers, six glasses; and lactating women, four glasses.

■ Meat group

The meat group includes meat (beef, veal, pork, lamb, and wild game), organ meat (such as liver and kidneys), fish and shellfish, poultry, eggs, legumes (such as dry beans, peas, lentils, and peanuts), and nuts. The meat group supplies about 53% of the protein, 53% of the niacin, and 42% of the iron available in our food supply. Because each food of the meat group offers a different combination of nutrients, it is most important to eat a variety of these foods. Lean, red meats are high in B vitamins; dry peas and beans, soybeans, and nuts are high in magnesium; fish and poultry are high in vitamins and minerals and low in calories and fat; and so on. All meat contains cholesterol; egg yolks and organ meats have

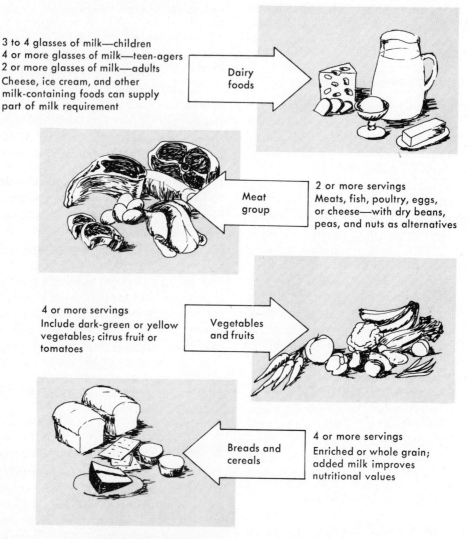

3 to 4 glasses of milk—children
4 or more glasses of milk—teen-agers
2 or more glasses of milk—adults
Cheese, ice cream, and other
milk-containing foods can supply
part of milk requirement

Dairy
foods

Meat
group

2 or more servings
Meats, fish, poultry, eggs,
or cheese—with dry beans,
peas, and nuts as alternatives

4 or more servings
Include dark-green or yellow
vegetables; citrus fruit or
tomatoes

Vegetables
and fruits

Breads and
cereals

4 or more servings
Enriched or whole grain;
added milk improves
nutritional values

FIG. 19-5 ■ Food guide and the four basic food groups.

Courtesy National Dairy Council.

the most. Fish and shellfish, except shrimp, are relatively low in cholesterol.

■ Fruit-vegetable group

The fruit-vegetable group includes all fresh, canned, frozen, and dried fruits and vegetables, except dried beans and peas. The latter are placed in the meat group because of

their high protein content. Corn may be served as a vegetable; corn grits and cornmeal are in the grain group. Fruit and vegetables supply about 90% of the vitamin C and 48% of the vitamin A available in our food supply. This group also supplies a number of vitamins and minerals. Four servings of fruits and vegetables are recommended daily. Since all fruits and vegetables are not equal in nutrients, citrus fruit is recommended daily for vitamin C. This nutrient is not stored in the body, and thus a daily source is necessary. Dark green, leafy, or yellow (orange) vegetables and fruits are recommended three or four times weekly for vitamin A. This vitamin is stored in the body, so a daily intake is not necessary. A serving of cooked fruit or vegetables or juice is ½ cup or a portion ordinarily served, such as a medium apple, banana, or potato or half a medium grapefruit.

■ Grain group

The grain, or "bread-cereal," group includes all grains: barley, buckwheat, corn, oats, rice, rye, and wheat, and the bread, breakfast cereals, grits, and noodle and pasta products made from them. This group supplies about 41% of the thiamin, 27% of the iron, and 15% of the niacin available in our food supply. Grain products supply other essential nutrients also. Four servings of enriched, fortified, or whole-grain foods are recommended daily. Refined white flour needs to have some nutrients restored by enrichment because they are removed in processing. If not enriched, white flour contributes few nutrients in addition to carbohydrate. A serving can be one slice of bread, a pancake, or a small waffle; one half of an English muffin or hamburger roll; 1 cup of ready-to-eat cereal; and ½ cup of cooked cereal, rice, pasta, or noodles. Milk combined with cereals improves the usability of grain proteins for body building and repair. Other examples of grains combined with milk products for high quality include cheese pizza, cheese sandwich, cheese and rice or macaroni casserole, and cheese fondue or soufflé.

■ "Others" group

The National Dairy Council and the United States Department of Agriculture make it very clear that there are indeed a great number of foods not included in the four food groups just described. This, of course, confirms what we already know. For the most part the "others" group provides few nutrients except carbohydrate and fat. These foods complement but do not replace food from the four food groups. Needless to say, they should be eaten or consumed moderately and, in the event of a weight problem, only once in a while or not at all. The "others" group includes butter, margarine, mayonnaise and other salad dressings, molasses, syrup, jam, jelly, candy, desserts, condiments, and the usual beverages: coffee, tea, soft drinks, and alcoholic beverages. Sugar-free carbonated beverages supply virtually no calories, and coffee and tea supply only what we add in the way of sugar and cream. Alcoholic beverages supply calories in the form of ethanol (ethyl alcohol), 1 g of which yields 7 calories.

■ COMBINATION FOODS AND FAST FOODS

Combination foods are prepared from one or more of the food groups described above. Accordingly, they can be exceptionally nutritional. One recipe for meat pie, for example, calls for leftover roast beef (meat group); potatoes, peas, carrots, and onions (fruit-vegetable group); and a crust made from enriched flour (grain group). The most common combination food is undoubtedly the sandwich, or some version thereof. Other things being equal, "chicken salad on rye" with plenty of lettuce is certainly a nutritious combination, cutting across all the major food groups. And the same can be said for **fast foods**, provided that we watch out for the nutritional booby traps. In eating fried fish, for example, we should stick to large pieces of fish rather than tidbits such as clams, shrimp, and oysters, which have far more greasy batter in proportion to "real" food. Condiments, pickles, and potato chips are loaded with salt and certainly should be avoided by those who must watch their sodium intake. A good buy is pizza, which supplies the basic nutrients in approximately the amounts recommended in the dietary goals established by the Senate's Select Committee on Nutrition and Human Needs. A typical slice of pizza has 15% protein, 27% fat, and 58% carbohydrate. Thus either as a snack or as part of a meal, pizza is a reasonably well-balanced food.

FORTIFIED FOODS

It is now standard practice to **fortify** certain foods with additional micronutrients, a practice that has certainly eliminated or drastically reduced a number of deficiency diseases, including endemic goiter, scurvy, and pellagra. Examples of fortification include the addition of iodine to salt ("iodized salt"), vitamin C to fruit juices, vitamin D to milk, vitamin A to margarine, and B-complex vitamins and iron to cereal products. However, indiscriminate fortification of food products for the purpose of generating impressive figures to put on nutrition labels does little to improve public health. Overfortification can encourage careless eating habits and, since some nutrients are toxic in excess amounts, it may even be directly harmful to health. Fortunately, many manufacturers realize this. The nutrition policies of Kraft, Oscar Mayer, Kellogg, General Mills, and many other companies include statements that nutrient additions will be made only when appropriate.

FATTY FOODS

Populations with diets high in fats and cholesterol tend to record high blood cholesterol levels. Persons within these populations usually are at higher risk of having heart attacks. Also, fatty foods appear to increase the risk of breast cancer and digestive system cancers. Extra saturated fat and cholesterol increase blood cholesterol levels in most people. However, there are wide variations among us because of heredity and the way each person's

body uses cholesterol. Some people can consume diets high in saturated fats and cholesterol and still keep normal blood cholesterol levels. Other people, unfortunately, have high levels even if they eat low-fat, low-cholesterol diets. As noted previously, there is some controversy about what recommendations are appropriate for the general population. The American Heart Association tells us to cut down on our current intake of total fat, saturated fat, and cholesterol, advice that should be followed especially by those who have high blood pressure or heart problems or are overweight. This recommendation is not meant to prohibit the use of any specific food item or to prevent anyone from eating a variety of foods. For example, eggs and organ meats (such as liver) do indeed contain cholesterol, but they also, as we know, contain many essential vitamins and minerals, as well as proteins. Such items can be eaten in moderation, as long as the overall cholesterol intake is not excessive. To avoid too much fat, saturated fat, and cholesterol, the U.S. Department of Agriculture suggests that we (1) choose lean meat, fish, poultry, dry beans, and peas as our sources of protein; (2) moderate our use of eggs and organ meats; (3) limit our intake of butter, cream, hydrogenated margarines, shortenings, coconut oil, and foods made from such products; (4) trim excess fat off meats; (5) broil, bake, or boil rather than fry; and (6) read labels carefully to determine both amounts and types of fat contained in foods.

SALTY FOODS

The Food and Nutrition Board of the National Academy of Sciences considers a sodium intake of 1000 to 3000 mg per day safe and adequate for healthy adults. But the typical American consumes 10 to 20 times that amount (almost all as salt), much of it "hidden" in the processed foods that constitute more than half of what we eat. By way of example, a cup of chicken noodle soup contains well over 1000 mg of salt. (A list of foods high in sodium can be found in the box below.)

An excessive sodium intake poses a health hazard to some 60 million Americans who develop high blood pressure after years of consuming a high-sodium diet. In Japan, where salt consumption is the highest in the world, high blood pressure is the leading cause of death. The source of all this salt is soy and other salty sauces and pickled and smoked foods. In societies where salt is infrequently consumed, high blood pressure is virtually nonexistent. If people with high blood pressure severely restrict their sodium intake, their blood pressure will usually fall. At present there is no good way to predict who will develop high blood pressure, though certain groups, such as blacks, have a higher incidence. Low-sodium diets might help some people avoid high blood pressure if they could be identified before developing the condition.

Since most of us consume more sodium than is needed, most authorities believe we should reduce our intake. Helpful hints include (1) learning to enjoy the unsalted flavors of foods; (2) cooking with very small amounts of added salt; (3) adding little or no salt to food at the table; (4) limiting intake of salty foods such as potato chips, pretzels, salted nuts, condiments, cheese, pickled foods, and cured meats; and (5) reading food labels carefully to determine the amounts of sodium in processed foods and snack items. As a final reminder, 1 teaspoon of salt contains 2000 mg of sodium. (A low-sodium diet is 3000 mg or less.)

■■■■ HEALTH FOODS

Advocates of "health," "organic," and "natural" foods—terms for which there is little agreement concerning exact definition—frequently proclaim that such products are safer

Foods high in sodium (250 mg and up per serving)

anchovies	cottage cheese	pickles
bacon	crab, canned	popcorn, salted
barbecue sauce	fish, smoked	potato chips
beans, canned with tomato	flour, self-rising	pretzels
sauce	frankfurters	relish
beef, chipped (dried)	gingerbread	salmon, canned
beef, corned	greens, kale, beet	salt, celery, garlic, onion,
biscuit mix	ham	seasoning, table
biscuits, baking powder	herring, canned	salt pork
bouillon	horseradish	sardines
butter, salted	lobster	sauerkraut, canned
buttermilk	margarine, salted	sausage
catsup	meat extracts	scallops
caviar	meat sauces	shellfish
celery	meat tenderizers	shrimp
cheese, pasteurized	meats, smoked and	soups, canned
processed	salted	soy sauce
cheese, swiss	mushrooms, canned	spinach
chili sauce	mustard	tomato juice, salted
codfish, salted	nuts, salted	tuna, canned in oil
cold cuts	olives	waffles
cookies, commercial	pastrami	Worcestershire sauce

and more nutritious than conventionally grown and marketed foods. Although most of these claims are not supported by scientific evidence, it is difficult for the public to evaluate fact from fancy, particularly in regard to the use of the term "natural" for everything from whole grain flour or bread to potato chips. Suggestions that certain health foods or diets prevent or cure disease or provide other special health benefits are, for the most part, folklore, and sometimes they are downright fabrication. If the label on a food product makes false or misleading claims, the Federal Drug Administration (FDA) can take action on the grounds that the product is mislabeled or misbranded. If false claims are made in advertisements or in other material directly promoting the product, the Federal Trade Commission may be able to take action. But labeling and promotion of fad foods or diets often do not make any direct claim that can be proved false. Instead they refer to a book, a pamphlet, a speech, or a magazine article that has praised the product. Thus these indirect promotions receive protection of the First Amendment.

Scientific rebuttal of food and nutrition myths published and perpetuated in faddist literature often is futile. As one leading nutritionist put it, "Americans love hogwash." And it is expensive hogwash. A recent survey by the U.S. Department of Agriculture found that the cost at the supermarket can run twice as much for health foods as for regular foods. The price for comparable foods, and sometimes even for the same food, rises steadily from the regular supermarket shelf to the health food section of the supermarket to the health food store. Expanded health food sections in some major food stores demonstrate the popularity of these items. Presently, annual retail sales average about 3 billion dollars, a mind-boggling statistic when one considers that more people than ever are going to school and supposedly getting an education.

Finally, some health foods are dangerous, and paradoxically so. Many people are lured to health foods in the belief that since they are "natural," they are ipso facto safer than conventional foods. This is upside-down thinking because hundreds of toxicants are known to occur naturally in foods, toxicants that for the most part are screened out or removed in "processed foods." For example, **aflatoxin**, a potent carcinogen, grows naturally (under certain conditions) on corn, peanuts, and other grains. The FDA monitors foods for aflatoxin and has established safe minimum levels in some foods, such as peanut butter and milk. But there is no way the FDA or anyone can assure that all foods are entirely free of such naturally occurring poisons. Lead, arsenic, and cadmium—highly dangerous metals—occur naturally at very low levels in many foods. In extracts and concentrates, however, these levels are greatly increased. Bulk bone meal, for example, a health food staple, may contain dangerous levels of lead, and a number of poisonings have been reported, all in persons who wanted to improve their health with "high calcium." Herb teas, much favored by health food advocates, contain a galaxy of drug constituents. Sassafras root was found to contain safrole, which produces liver cancer in rats, and the sale of sassafras teas was banned by the FDA in 1976 for that reason. And there are many, many other health food stories of this nature. P.T. Barnum, the great American showman, summed it up over a century ago: "There's a sucker born every minute."

◼◼◼ NUTRITION LABELING

Except for foods "beyond the law" (health foods, organic foods, and their ilk) almost all processed, packaged foods provide nutritional information on the label. Such labeling is mandatory for (1) all foods to which nutrients have been added and (2) foods for which a nutrient claim is made on the label or in advertising. At the top of the panel of the typical food label are the words "Nutrition Information Per Serving," followed by the size of an

```
┌─────────────────────────────────────────┐
│           CHEDDAR CHEESE                 │
│         NUTRITION INFORMATION            │
│             (per serving)                │
│      Serving size = 1 slice (1 oz)       │
│      Servings per container = 16         │
│                                          │
│  CALORIES . . . . . . . . . 120          │
│  PROTEIN . . . . . . . . . . 7 gm        │
│  CARBOHYDRATE . . 1 gm                    │
│  FAT . . . . . . . . . . . . 10 gm        │
│                                          │
│   PERCENTAGE OF U.S. RECOMMENDED DAILY   │
│          ALLOWANCES (U.S. RDA)           │
│                                          │
│  PROTEIN . . . . . . . 15   NIACIN . . . . . . . . . . . . . 0 │
│  VITAMIN A . . . . . . . 4   CALCIUM . . . . . . . . . . 20 │
│  VITAMIN C . . . . . . . 0   IRON . . . . . . . . . . . . . 0 │
│  THIAMINE (B₁) . . . . . 0                │
│  RIBOFLAVIN (B₂) . . . . 6                │
└─────────────────────────────────────────┘
```

FIG. 19-6 ■ Example of food labeling.

average serving and the number of servings per container (Fig. 19-6). **Calories per serving** are given next, followed by protein, carbohydrate, and fat in **grams per serving**. Next appears information about protein, vitamin A, vitamin C, thiamin (B_1), riboflavin (B_2), niacin, calcium, and iron. Amounts of these nutrients are expressed as **percentages** of the U.S. Recommended Daily Allowances (U.S. RDAs) per serving. The U.S. RDAs most commonly given are for adults and for children 4 or more years of age. Special U.S. RDAs are used on baby foods and other products intended for small children. Not all foods contain the seven micronutrients cited. In fact, some foods contain only one or two. If a food contains less than 2% of the U.S. RDAs per serving of a vitamin or mineral, the label shows a zero or an asterisk for that nutrient. (An asterisk and explanation appear at the bottom of the label.)

There are 12 additional micronutrients that may be listed on the label but are not required by the FDA. These are vitamin D, vitamin E, vitamin B_6, folic acid (folacin), vitamin B_{12}, biotin, pantothenic acid, phosphorus, iodine, magnesium, zinc, and copper. They must be listed, however, when added to a food. Other information often given on the label but currently not required includes cholesterol, fat, and sodium. Cholesterol and sodium are given

in milligrams per 100 grams of the product. Fat is given in percent of total calories in one serving of the product, and sometimes stated is how much of the fat is **saturated** and how much **polyunsaturated**. When cholesterol content and fat content are both given (in the manner indicated), the label must carry the following statement: "Information on fat and/or cholesterol content is provided for individuals who, on the advice of a physician, are modifying their dietary intake of fat and/or cholesterol."

■ FOOD ADDITIVES

By broadest definition, a **food additive** is any substance that becomes part of a food product when added either directly or indirectly. An estimated 3000 substances are intentionally added to foods to produce a desired effect, and an estimated 10,000 other compounds or combinations of compounds find their way into various foods during processing, packaging, or storage. Examples of these unintentional additives include traces of pesticides used to treat crops, drugs fed to animals, and chemical agents that diffuse into food from packaging materials. An additive is intentionally used in food for one or more of four purposes: (1) to improve nutritional value (see fortified foods above), (2) to maintain freshness, (3) to help in processing or preparation, and (4) to make food look and taste better. By far the most widely used additives are sugar, salt, and corn syrup. These three, plus such other substances as citric acid, baking soda, vegetable colors, mustard, and pepper, account, according to the FDA, for about 98%, by weight, of all food additives used in this country.

Although the Food, Drug, and Cosmetic Act of 1938 gave the federal government authority to remove adulterated foods from the market, it was not until the Food Additives Amendment was enacted in 1958 and the Color Additive Amendments in 1960 that we had federal laws specifically regulating food additives. In actual practice, however, scientists do not always agree on the safety of a given additive, and often the situation becomes political. For instance, do we or do we not ban saccharin? Commonly, the consumer becomes confused and feels somewhat helpless in exerting any control over what goes into his or her food. But this need not be. Indeed, the FDA believes that the consumer wields the greatest power and control of all—the power of the marketplace. The FDA admonishes us to read the labels to find out what is in the foods we buy, to make our views known to the manufacturers and our representatives in Congress, and to exercise our right to choose.

MALNUTRITION

Malnutrition literally means "bad nutrition." Commonly it refers to conditions, symptoms, and diseases resulting from a deficiency of one or more essential nutrients. It may be classified as primary or secondary, depending on the cause of the deficiency. **Primary deficiency** is caused by an inadequate intake of nutrients. The underprivileged, preschool children, and pregnant and lactating women are particularly vulnerable. High nutrient requirements, early weaning, parental ignorance of proper postweaning nutrition and hygiene, and poverty combine to make the first years of life the most susceptible. **Secondary deficiency** results from failure to absorb or utilize nutrients. Such failure may be due to gastrointestinal disease, impaired endocrine dysfunction, inborn errors of metabolism, severe infection, or degenerative diseases. Specific diseases caused by deficiency malnutrition include kwashiorkor, marasmus, beriberi, pellagra, pernicious anemia, scurvy, rickets, tetany, osteomalacia, endemic goiter, and iron deficiency anemia. All of these have been discussed or touched upon previously. A rather special deficiency disease, anorexia nervosa, will be discussed shortly.

Another kind of malnutrition is not related to nutrient deficiency but rather to excessive amounts of the wrong kind of food—specifically, diets imbalanced in the direction of too many calories and too much fat, sugar, and salt. This form of malnutrition seems to be the principal nutritional problem in the United States. Diseases associated with imbalanced nutrition include heart disease, high blood pressure, diabetes mellitus, dental caries, and, of course, obesity. Except for obesity, all of these conditions have been discussed or touched on before. We shall explore obesity in some detail in the following section.

OBESITY

Weight control is an ever-increasing topic of concern and discussion. And well that it should be because 35% of persons over 40 years of age have weight problems serious enough to threaten health, and up to 40% of school-age children are estimated to be overweight. Girls usually have more of a problem than boys, whose hormones encourage muscle development. Since adolescence is the last opportunity the body has to acquire new fat cells, excessive weight gain during the teenage years can set the stage for a lifetime battle against the bulge. Obesity (being overweight) increases the risk of a number of diseases including hypertension, atherosclerosis, gallbladder disease, kidney disease, gout, and arthritis. It complicates surgery, pregnancy, emphysema, bronchitis, and asthma. All in all, obesity reduces life expectancy.

Obesity is characterized by excessive accumulations of body fat. The ideal percentage of body fat is said to be between 10% and 15% for men and between 15% and 20% for women. Athletes of either sex often have lower values. A diagnosis of obesity is usually made when body weight exceeds 20% of the standard weight given in height-weight tables (Table 19-4). Some authorities have reservations about

TABLE 19-4

Desirable weights for men and women age 25 and over

Height (with shoes)		Small frame	Medium frame	Large frame	Height (with shoes)		Small frame	Medium frame	Large frame
Feet	Inches				Feet	Inches			
Men*					Women†				
5	2	112-120	118-129	126-141	4	10	92- 98	96-107	104-119
5	3	115-123	121-133	129-144	4	11	94-101	98-110	106-122
5	4	118-126	124-136	132-148	5	0	96-104	101-113	109-125
5	5	121-129	127-139	135-152	5	1	99-107	104-116	112-128
5	6	124-133	130-143	138-156	5	2	102-110	107-119	115-131
5	7	128-137	134-147	142-161	5	3	105-113	110-122	118-134
5	8	132-141	138-152	147-166					
5	4	108-116	113-126	121-138					
5	9	136-145	142-156	151-170	5	5	111-119	116-130	125-142
5	10	140-150	146-160	155-174	5	6	114-123	120-135	129-146
5	11	144-154	150-165	159-179	5	7	118-127	124-139	133-150
6	0	148-158	154-170	164-184	5	8	122-131	128-143	137-154
6	1	152-162	158-175	168-189	5	9	126-135	132-147	141-158
6	2	156-167	162-180	173-194	5	10	130-140	136-151	145-163
6	3	160-171	167-185	178-199	5	11	134-144	140-155	149-168
6	4	164-175	172-190	182-204	6	0	138-148	144-159	153-173

Courtesy Metropolitan Life Insurance Company.
*Weights in pounds (in indoor clothing; for nude weight deduct 5 to 7 pounds).
†Weights in pounds (in indoor clothing; for nude weight deduct 2 to 4 pounds).

such tables because total body weight is not necessarily a reflection of body fat; that is to say, total body weight does not take into account the ratio of fat to lean body mass (muscle). A direct (but not infallible) estimate of body fat is the **pinch test**. Approximately half of the body fat is located between the skin and underlying muscle, and at some locations on the body (for example, the back of the upper arm) a fold of skin and fat can be lifted free (pinched) and measured. The average skinfold thickness of the right triceps (Fig. 19-7) is 15 mm for men and 25 mm for women. A person with a skinfold thickness considerably greater than 30 mm is usually what we call obese. And then, of course, there is the mirror test: if you don't like what you see in the nude, you're probably overweight!

■ Cause and treatment

The basic, immediate cause of obesity is a **positive caloric balance**. This results when the average caloric intake exceeds energy expenditure. A surplus intake of only 100 calories per day results in a year's weight gain of approximately 10 pounds! This surplus, whether in the form of fat, carbohydrate, or protein, is converted into fat and stored in the body's energy-storage depots. To say that obesity results from overeating is a reasonable statement provided it is put in the proper context; that is, we put on weight when we overeat in relation to our needs. Some people gain weight on a food intake that would amount to a reducing diet for others. Numerous investigators report that obese persons consume fewer calories than nonobese people.

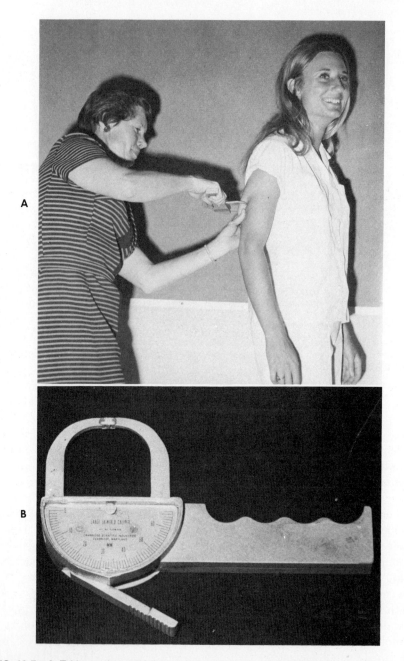

FIG. 19-7 ■ A, Taking a triceps skinfold measure. **B,** Lange skinfold calipers.

From Klafs, C.E., and Lyon, M.J.: The female athlete: a coach's guide to conditioning and training, ed. 2, St. Louis, 1978, The C.V. Mosby Co.

Part of the secret may be that people who tend to stay thin have proportionately more **brown adipose tissue** ("brown fat"), a type of tissue that literally burns excess fat. In babies brown fat seems to act like an auxilliary furnace to help keep them warm.

Unfortunately, obesity is much more than a matter of positive caloric imbalance. Actually it is one of the most baffling problems known to medicine. Factors associated with this infamous imbalance may relate to heredity, growth and development, metabolic defects, brain damage, endocrine disturbances, socioeconomic status, ethnic group membership, religion, or emotional disorders. For example, half the people seeing doctors for obesity treatment exhibit tension, anxiety, frustration, insecurity, depression, loneliness, or plain boredom. In other words, they eat to overcome these problems. Accordingly, weight control entails several approaches, but most important is dieting and exercise. Backup measures include psychotherapy, behavior modification, self-help organizations such as TOPS (Take Off Pounds Sensibly), and commercial organizations such as Weight Watchers. Drastic methods include starvation and surgery (intestinal bypass surgery and gastric reduction). And then, of course, there are the perennial weight-loss gimmicks and gadgets and fad diets, all of which are at best worthless. Some are downright dangerous. Drugs that stimulate brown fat activity are currently under investigation, and these may possibly prove of value.

Dieting. For moderately overweight persons a sensible reducing diet (along with regular exercise) can solve the problem and solve it for good. Success depends on genuine willpower—"mind over calorie"—and common sense. Willpower stems from high self-esteem; that is, if we are horrified by what we see in the mirror (sans clothing), we will do something about it and stay on the diet. Common sense will enable us to identify nutritional

nonsense and laugh at it. There is no magic reducing diet except the one that ensures a **negative caloric imbalance** within a framework of sound nutrition. Persons who are gravely obese need special help in addition to what has just been said, and by all means they should see a physician.

A reducing diet, by definition, is one that ensures a negative caloric imbalance. Unless prescribed by a physician, it should not be below 1200 calories per day. The aim is to lose weight gradually, about 1 or 2 pounds per week; reducing at a faster rate could mean destruction of muscles and organs as well as fat. This is why crash diets are dangerous. Food selection is crucial because with a reduced intake we run the risk of not getting the required nutrients. Selections must be made from the four basic food groups, with special emphasis on items high in quality and low in calories (Table 19-5). Fats and carbohydrates should be kept at a minimum, and junk foods and alcoholic drinks should be reserved for special occasions. In summary, a sensible reducing diet gradually melts away fat but not at the expense of malnutrition. Furthermore, it should be appreciated that once weight control has been achieved, the reducing diet

■■■■■■■■■■ **TABLE 19-5**
Examples of 100-calorie portions

Food	Approximate amount
Banana	1 medium-sized
Bread	1½ medium-sized slices
Butter	1 tablespoon
Cheese, American	1-inch cube
Lettuce	30 large leaves
Mayonnaise	1 tablespoon
Meat, lean	1 small serving
Orange	1 large
Potato, white	1 medium-sized
Sugar	2 tablespoons

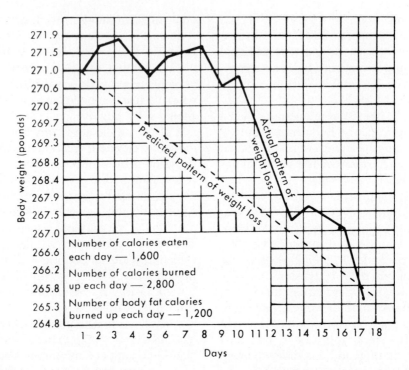

FIG. 19-8 ■ Changes in body weight of overweight person on a reducing diet. Progress chart shows how much body weight can fluctuate as a result of water retention even though daily caloric intake remains constant. This dieter accumulated water for 10 days while losing fat and then showed a rapid weight loss as water was eliminated.

Courtesy Pennwalt Prescription Products Division, Pennwalt Corp., Rochester, N.Y.

is no longer a reducing diet; it becomes a **maintenance diet**, one that will do much to ensure good health for a lifetime.

A reducing diet in action is shown in Fig. 19-8. Note how much body weight can fluctuate as a result of water retention even though daily caloric intake remains constant. This particular dieter accumulated water for 10 days while losing fat (a natural metabolic response) and then showed a rapid weight loss as water was finally eliminated. This is most important to keep in mind because one may very well wonder what's going on and get discouraged. But ultimately the laws of physics prevail and body weight drops, in this case about 6 pounds in 2½ weeks. This loss, incidentally, very closely mirrors the theoretical value. An interesting and helpful fact to remember is that

1 pound of fat contains (yields) 3500 calories. Thus to lose 1 pound a week a reducing diet would have to ensure a negative caloric imbalance of 500 calories daily.

Exercise. Inasmuch as most persons put on weight because they eat too much and exercise too little, it stands to reason that weight control centers on dieting (which we have already explored) and regular exercise. Unfortunately there is a popular belief that one must exercise a tremendous amount to lose a small amount of weight. And, in one way of looking at it, this is true. To lose 1 pound, for example, a person has to walk about 35 miles! This is very discouraging, but clearly the statement is out of context. We don't have to walk 35 miles all at once. Indeed, walking ½ mile every day, which is not a long walk by

TABLE 19-6

Energy expenditures for various activities

Activity	Calories/lb/hr
Sleeping	0.4
Sitting	0.7
Dressing and undressing	0.8
Driving automobile	0.9
Standing	0.9
Typing	0.9
Household tasks, cleaning, dusting, etc.	1.2
Walking (3 mph)	1.8
Bicycling (10 mph)	3.0
Tennis (fast game)	3.5
Swimming (45 yds/min)	3.5
Dancing (fast)	3.9
Squash, handball, raquetball	4.2
Rowing at top speed	7.6
Jogging-running (12 mph)	7.8

any means, will expend in a year's time 36,500 calories and thereby do away with about 10 pounds of fat. Another mistaken idea is that any weight loss achieved by exercise is offset by an increase in appetite and calorie consumption. Studies with experimental animals show that this is not true. Actually, when normally sedentary animals were required to exercise, they ate less food. Only strenuous regular exercise causes people to eat more, and in such instances this increase is appropriate to the increased everyday expenditure. Moreover, recent data show that strenuous exercise increases the BMR for about 6 hours following the bout of exercise, which amounts to a further loss of fat.

Exercise, like the diet, must be regular and sensible. Also, one should consult a physician before beginning any program that involves vigorous or strenuous exercise. This is especially important for those over the age of 35. The experts tell us to increase exercise gradually; for instance, in a walking-jogging program this means all walking for a few weeks, then alternating jogging with walking, very

gradually increasing the amount of jogging. Regardless of the type of exercise, if pain develops or breathing becomes difficult, we should stop. A pulse rate exceeding "200 beats per minute minus age" is another sign to stop. By all means let us never make the mistake of thinking that exercise has to be drastic or "way out." Everyday opportunities can play a significant role in the overall exercise program (Table 19-6). For example, we can take the stairs instead of the elevator; push the lawnmower; rake the leaves; weed the garden; walk instead of driving; walk the dog; stretch, flex, and bend in doing daily chores; and so on.

ANOREXIA NERVOSA

Anorexia nervosa occurs most commonly during adolescence, especially in girls, and is characterized by rapid weight loss, which may begin with extreme dieting in a youngster who is overly concerned about obesity. The essential disturbance is not true anorexia (loss of appetite); rather there is a distorted concept of body image and abhorrence of obesity. Excessive eating followed by induced vomiting is common. The condition may be mild, but usually it is severe and chronic and may result in death. Optimally, care of the teenager with anorexia nervosa is managed jointly by a physician who directs the weight gain and a psychiatrist who deals with the underlying disturbance.

BULIMIA

Bulimia (Gk. boulimia, "ox hunger") is a binge-and-purge behavior that has become a daily affair for growing numbers of young women, threatening their health and interfering with their daily lives. For some the disorder has evolved into a $100-a-day food habit that has forced them into bankruptcy, stealing, and prostitution. Victims may consume up to 60,000 calories in an hour or two, then induce vomiting to prevent obesity, and may repeat the behavior as often as four times a day. Others take big doses of laxatives to prevent their bodies from retaining the enormous amounts of food they consume. The typical bulimic is an unmarried white woman (only about 5% are men) from the middle and upper classes who has some college education. Most are of normal weight and started the binge-and-purge behavior at about age 18 after completion of a diet. Furthermore, bulimics are upwardly mobile, achievement-oriented perfectionists who, despite their accomplishments, have little self-esteem and measure their worth through the eyes of others. Indeed, some authorities see the eating disorder in part as growing out of the stress of trying to be perfect. Aside from creating an abnormal social and working life, bulimia can result in potentially serious and possibly fatal medical complications. Commonly, victims develop severe tooth decay, sore throat, esophageal inflammation, liver damage, and, somewhat paradoxically, malnutrition. Life-threatening complications include stomach rupture and fluid and electrolyte disturbances. The approach to treatment is interdisciplinary and includes psychotherapy, nutrition, social work, and dentistry. Group therapy is often helpful because many bulimics generally feel isolated and alienated.

▬▬▬ SELF-TEST

1. _E_ 4.186 kJ
2. _I_ cal/m²/hr
3. _J_ carbohydrate
4. _A_ fat
5. _G_ protein
6. _N_ cholesterol
7. _B_ vitamin A
8. _L_ vitamin D
9. _O_ vitamin C
10. _D_ niacin
11. _K_ vitamin B$_{12}$
12. _M_ iodine
13. _H_ fluoride
14. _F_ sodium
15. _C_ obesity

a. 9 calories/g
b. nyctalopia
c. caloric imbalance
d. pellagra
e. kilocalorie
f. hypertension
g. amino acids
h. dental caries
i. BMR
j. $C_6H_{12}O_6$
k. anemia
l. rickets
m. goiter
n. atherosclerosis
o. scurvy

[Handwritten notes:]

KCALORIES: 15 × Body Weight —
1/10 of body wght — blood
cal. — CALORIE

B MK —
BASEBALL —
Metallic —
Rythm —

$C_6H_{12}O_6$ photosynthesis —
$CO_2 + H_2O \longrightarrow$ Chlorophyll —
sunlight —

▬▬▬ STUDY QUESTIONS

1. One ounce of Kellog's Bran Buds yields 70 calories. What is this amount of energy in terms of joules (J)? In kilojoules (kJ)?
2. If a young man 19 years of age has a BMR of 31 calories/m²/hr, how would this compare with the normal value (on a basis of percent)?
3. When our caloric intake exceeds caloric output, does this mean that we have taken in more calories or more food? Explain.
4. What is the number of calories in 1 ounce of sugar?
5. What is the number of calories in 1 ounce of fat?
6. Dietary fiber does not supply calories. Why?
7. To say that some fats are "saturated" and others are "unsaturated" is a matter of basic chemistry. Explain.

8. Our protein intake should relate to quality as well as quantity. Explain and give examples.
9. The tissues of the human body contain carbohydrate, fats, and proteins (chiefly as muscle). During starvation, which of the three is the last to be consumed?
10. Relatively speaking, protein is said to be the only "complete food." Why?
11. Why are vitamins and minerals sometimes referred to as "micronutrients?"
12. In the judgment of recognized nutritional authorities the consumption of vitamins beyond what we need is unnecessary and sometimes dangerous. What are your thoughts?
13. A person with pernicious anemia will eventually die unless treated with vitamin B_{12}. Thus it really is a "wonder drug." Commonly, vitamin B_{12} shots (which are quite expensive) are prescribed by doctors for some sort of "pick me up," especially in the elderly. In view of the fact that the use of vitamin B_{12} for this purpose is not be be found in any standard medical text, how do you account for the practice?
14. Aside from vitamin D, what other nutrients are essential in the treatment of rickets?
15. What "precautionary measures" should be observed in the cooking of vegetables?

16. What are your views on vitamin supplements?
17. Why is iron deficiency anemia so common?
18. Endemic goiter is pretty much a thing of the past. Why?
19. The people who are against fluoridation usually cite the fact that fluoride (fluorine) is poisonous. What, if any, is the fallacy in this reasoning?
20. Think up or invent five good sandwiches that would represent the four major food groups.
21. Specifically, what fast foods do you consider a good nutritious buy and why?
22. Are the terms "salt" and "sodium" synonymous? Explain.
23. By rule of thumb our caloric daily needs equal about 15 times our desirable weight. On this basis what are your caloric needs?
24. The laws of science and common sense tell us that there is no way to lose weight (for good!) unless we change our eating habits in general and create a negative caloric imbalance in particular. How, then, do you account for the perennial diet books that hit the best seller list?
✳ If a friend of yours seriously wanted to lose weight, what would be your advice (in 25 words or less)?

(handwritten notes)

(Fluorine — water)

J — joules

```
 120
  15
 ────
 600
 120
 ────
1260
```

✳ Exercise —
✳ Physician —

1st — recognize they have a problem. —

CHAPTER 20

Dental health

Tooth decay is the most common chronic disease of the human species. It causes not only lots of suffering but a substantial economic burden as well. While only 40% of the population seeks dental care, spending about 2 billion dollars each year, 98% of the population requires such care. The United States Public Health Service estimates that if all cavities that develop each year could be treated, the annual cost would reach about 10 billion dollars. The great tragedy in all of this, of course, is that tooth decay is one of the most preventable diseases and perhaps the best example of the old axiom "an ounce of prevention is worth a pound of cure." Furthermore, in the words of the American Dental Association, "Happiness is a Healthy Mouth."

Dentition and tooth structure

Tooth decay and gum disease

Trench mouth

Malocclusion

Erosion and abrasion

Loss of teeth

Tooth injuries

Impaction

Halitosis

Pregnancy and dental health

Oral cancer

The teeth are designed to perform specific functions, the most important of which is chewing food (**mastication**) in preparation for swallowing and digestion. Teeth are necessary for clear and normal speech and also help shape the face. As for their influence on appearance and self-esteem, Fig. 20-1 says it all.

■ DENTITION AND TOOTH STRUCTURE

Dentition refers to the type, number, and arrangement of teeth. There are, of course, two sets of teeth, **primary** (deciduous) and **permanent**. The primary teeth (20 in number) begin erupting at about 6 months of age (Fig. 20-2). These teeth play a key role in the development of the future dentition because they hold space in the jaw for the final position of the permanent teeth that will later replace them. The early loss of any primary tooth could cause the irregular positioning of permanent teeth. The latter (32 in number) begin erupting at about 6 years of age (Fig. 20-3). As shown in the illustrations, the teeth are divided into four groups or types: incisors, canines, premolars, and molars. The **incisors**, with their sharp, chisel-shaped crowns, are the cutting teeth. The aptly named **canines** (cuspids), with their sharp, pointed crowns, are used in tearing; the **premolars** (bicuspids) and **molars** (tricuspids) are the grinders. Whereas the incisors and canines each have a single root, the molars have two or three. The premolars usually have a single root.

The basic anatomy of a tooth is shown in Fig. 20-4. The **crown**, or the portion above the gum, is coated with **enamel**, the hardest substance in the body. Beneath this, and making up the bulk of the tooth, is the **dentin**, a dense, yellow-white, hard, striated material. Within the dentin is the **pulp cavity**, which contains connective tissue, nerve endings, and blood vessels. The **root**, or the portion of the tooth below the **gingiva** (gum), is anchored to the socket of the jawbone by the **periodontal membrane**. The **cementum** is a layer of modified bone forming a sheath for the root.

■ TOOTH DECAY AND GUM DISEASE

Tooth decay, or **dental caries**, is an ongoing process. It begins with **plaque**, the sticky, colorless layer of harmful bacteria that is constantly forming on the teeth. Certain bacteria in plaque act on sugars in the diet (especially sucrose, or ordinary table sugar) to form acids. Each time acid is produced it attacks the enamel for about 20 minutes. After repeated attacks the enamel is broken down and becomes decayed, a process that eventually progresses toward the center of the tooth (Fig. 20-5). If decay is not arrested (by means of a filling) and it reaches the pulp, an abscess forms at the end of the root. When this happens, the tooth becomes painful and will require **endodontic** (root canal) treatment. Without treatment, the tooth will have to be removed.

Gum, or **periodontal**, disease is the most common cause of tooth loss in adults, although it can occur in children as young as 5 or 6 years of age. It attacks and destroys the gums and bone that surround and support the teeth. The disease is usually painless and progresses slowly for many years. But most significant, like tooth decay, it is caused by **plaque**. The most common type of periodontal disease develops in two stages. The first stage, called **gingivitis**, is characterized by red, swollen gums that bleed easily when the teeth are brushed. In the second stage, called **periodontitis** (formerly pyorrhea), the gums begin to pull away from the plaque irritants, creating pockets between the teeth, and these pockets become filled with **calculus** (tartar) and more plaque. Eventually, plaque destroys the supporting bone and the ligaments that connect the root to the bone. Teeth may then be-

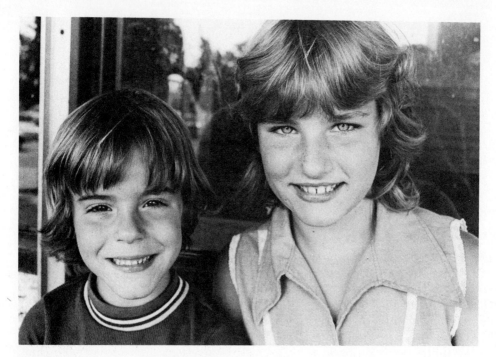

Fig. 20-1 ■ The first and second set of teeth.

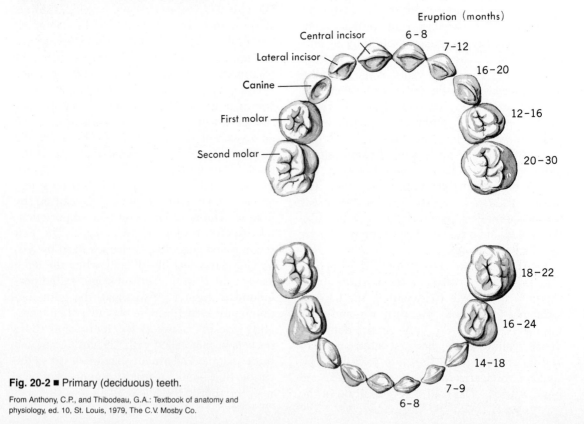

Eruption (months)

Central incisor — 6 – 8

Lateral incisor — 7 – 12

Canine — 16 – 20

First molar — 12 – 16

Second molar — 20 – 30

18 – 22

16 – 24

14 – 18

7 – 9

6 – 8

Fig. 20-2 ■ Primary (deciduous) teeth.

From Anthony, C.P., and Thibodeau, G.A.: Textbook of anatomy and physiology, ed. 10, St. Louis, 1979, The C.V. Mosby Co.

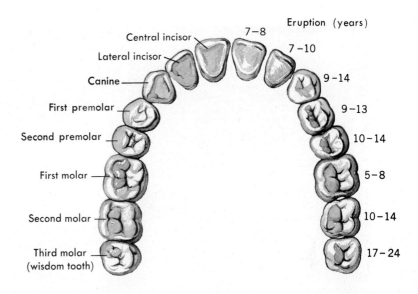

Eruption (years)

Central incisor — 7-8

Lateral incisor — 7-10

Canine — 9-14

First premolar — 9-13

Second premolar — 10-14

First molar — 5-8

Second molar — 10-14

Third molar (wisdom tooth) — 17-24

Fig. 20-3 ■ Permanent teeth.

From Anthony, C.P., and Thibodeau, G.A.: Textbook of anatomy and physiology, ed. 10, St. Louis, 1979, The C.V. Mosby Co.

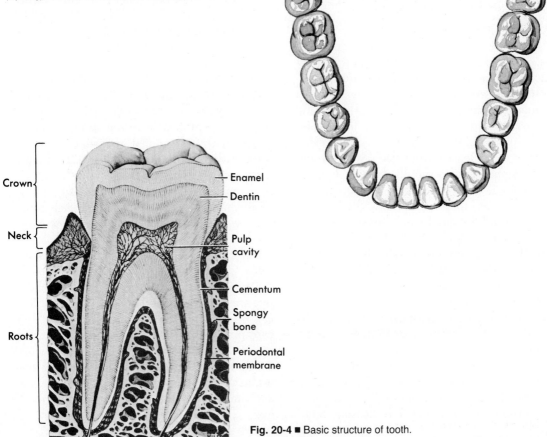

Crown {

Enamel

Dentin

Neck {

Pulp cavity

Roots {

Cementum

Spongy bone

Periodontal membrane

Fig. 20-4 ■ Basic structure of tooth.

Courtesy American Dental Association.

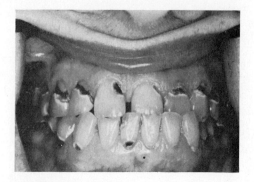

Fig. 20-5 ■ Rampant caries.

From Kerr, D.A., Ash, M.M., Jr., and Millard, H.D.: Oral diagnosis, ed. 6, St. Louis, 1983, The C.V. Mosby Co.

come loose, and they either fall out or must be removed.

■ Preventive measures

There are four sound ways to prevent tooth decay and gum disease: plaque removal, fluoride, diet, and regular dental checkups.

Plaque removal. Plaque removal centers on toothbrushing and flossing. Toothbrushing removes plaque from the outer, inner, and biting surfaces of the teeth. Adults should clean their teeth at least once a day; children and decay-prone persons should clean their teeth more often, especially after meals. Parents should clean their children's teeth until brushing and flossing techniques can be mastered by the children themselves. The brush should have a straight handle, flat brushing surface, and soft bristles. It should be able to reach all teeth. Furthermore, a toothbrush should be replaced every 3 to 4 months. The recommended basic brushing technique calls for placing the brush at a 45-degree angle against the gum line and moving it back and forth with short strokes, using a gentle, scrubbing motion. Flossing removes plaque from between the teeth and under the gum line. The proper or most efficient flossing tech-

nique is related to individual needs and, accordingly, should be demonstrated by the dentist or hygienist.

Fluoride. Fluoride is a mineral nutrient that unites with enamel to make the tooth more resistant to decay. It is most effective when multiple methods of application, as recommended by the dentist, are used during the time the teeth are erupting and forming. The single most effective method of adding fluoride is to drink water that has been **fluoridated.** Benefits are lifelong and are very evident during childhood. Of children who drink fluoridated water from birth, 20% can reach the teenage years without decay. Other methods include the use of tablets or liquid and the professional application of gels and solutions. Fluoride toothpastes and rinses also help reduce decay when used regularly. Products proved effective carry the seal of acceptance of the Council on Dental Therapeutics of the American Dental Association.

Diet. A balanced diet assists the teeth and gums to resist infection. Sugary foods and drinks, especially between-meal snacks, encourage decay beacuse they supply bacterial plaque with the raw material (sucrose) to produce acid. The problem is not just the amount of sugar but also such factors as how often it is eaten and the length of time sugar stays in the mouth. Soft, sticky, sugar-rich foods, such as raisins and caramels, are the worst offenders. For persons who must snack, the safest items are cheese, fresh vegetables, and nuts.

Dental checkups. Regular dental checkups are crucial. Dental diseases and problems can be detected and treated early, and home care practices can be reinforced. X-ray examination should be performed as often as necessary to assist in the detection of decay, malocclusion, bone loss from periodontal disease, and many other conditions not visible to the eye.

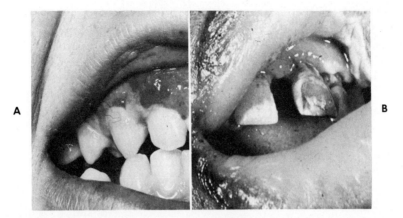

Fig. 20-6 ■ Trench mouth. **A,** Early stage. **B,** Late stage with marked destruction of tissue.

From Bhaskar, S.N.: Synopsis of oral pathology, ed. 6, St. Louis, 1981, The C.V. Mosby Co.

■■■TRENCH MOUTH

Trench mouth is a noncontagious infection characterized by necrosis ("tissue death") and microbial invasion of the gums. The proper dental designation for this potentially serious condition is **acute necrotizing ulcerative gingivitis** (ANUG). Poor oral hygiene, physical or emotional stress, nutritional deficiencies, anemia, debilitating diseases, insufficient rest, and heavy smoking are considered predisposing factors. The onset, usually abrupt, may be accompanied by malaise and fever. The chief symptoms include painful bleeding, ulcerated gums, salivation, and bad breath (Fig. 20-6). Swallowing and talking may be painful, and the regional lymph nodes are often enlarged. Rarely, ulcers appear on the sides of the mouth, throat, and tonsils. Immediate treatment entails removing necrotic debris (debridement) and rinsing the mouth with a 3% hydrogen peroxide solution. Analgesics may be needed to control pain resulting from debridement, and antibiotics may be needed if high fever is present. Gum irritants, such as smoking and spicy foods, are to be avoided. Above all, the underlying cause—poor oral hygiene, poor diet, and so on—must be identified and corrected.

■■■MALOCCLUSION

Malocclusion means that the teeth do not fit together properly when the jaws are closed. It is caused by harmful oral habits, early loss of teeth, dental disease, dental injury, or the abnormal relationship between teeth and jaw size. Untreated malocclusion can affect both dental and general health. Specifically, maloccluded teeth are more difficult to clean, cause facial deformities, and often interfere with proper chewing and speech. Finally, malocclusion can result in emotional problems in some people.

■■■EROSION AND ABRASION

Erosion is the process whereby tooth structure is **decalcified**, usually at the gum line. The cause is unknown, but one contributing factor may be dietary acid, especially excessive consumption of citrus fruits, juices, and carbonated beverages. Abrasion is the wearing away of tooth structures by mechanical forces: prying open bobby pins with the teeth, holding objects between the teeth (such as a pipe or nails), and improper brushing. These are bad habits and should be avoided.

LOSS OF TEETH

The loss of one or more teeth calls for replacement. Otherwise the remaining teeth drift out of position, creating stress and possibly causing injury to supporting tissues. A partial denture (bridge) replaces one or more teeth; a complete denture replaces all the teeth. Dentures call for regular dental visits to assure proper fit and comfort. Home adjustment and repairs can prove dangerous because of possible harm to the mouth.

TOOTH INJURIES

If a tooth is bumped or injured in any way, a dentist should be consulted. Often a baby tooth that has been knocked out can be saved; that is, the dentist replants the tooth in the child's jaw. Under favorable conditions the tooth reattaches to the jaw and will function again. Speed is important. The child—and the tooth—are taken to the dentist immediately. The tooth should not be cleaned but wrapped in a wet cloth or placed in water.

IMPACTION

Dental impaction is the condition in which a tooth is embedded in the jaw, so that its eruption is prevented, or is locked in position by bone, restoration, or surfaces of adjacent teeth, preventing either its normal occlusion or its routine removal. Impacted molars (**wisdom teeth**), particularly third molars, can be painful and may cause adjacent soft tissue inflammation, which can progress to serious infection. Such teeth call for immediate attention and removal.

HALITOSIS

Halitosis, or bad breath (L. halitus, breath or exhalation), is usually due to plaque, periodontal disease, advanced tooth decay, or combinations thereof. Sometimes just the removal of plaque and tartar plus proper daily toothbrushing and flossing may be enough to eliminate the problem. Nondental causes of halitosis include infection of the nasal passages or throat, diabetes mellitus, and lung cancer.

PREGNANCY AND DENTAL HEALTH

Proper nutrition and attention to increased dietary needs during pregnancy will provide a woman with the correct amounts of nutrients required by her and the developing child. Teeth begin forming about the sixth to the eighth week of prenatal life and calcify during the fourth to the sixth month. This dental development can be affected significantly by mineral and vitamin deficiencies. Many women associate pregnancy with increased tooth decay and gingivitis, but both conditions can be avoided by proper dental care and diet.

ORAL CANCER

Most oral cancers begin as early changes in the oral cavity. Excessive use of alcohol and tobacco in any form are recognized contributing factors. Signs of possible cancer include a red sore on the lips, gums, or inside of the mouth that does not heal in 2 to 3 weeks; white, scaly patches inside the mouth or on the lips; swelling or lumps in the mouth or on the lip or tongue; numbness or pain in the mouth without cause; bleeding in the mouth without cause. Often these signs are painless at first and go unnoticed, which is another excellent reason for regular dental checkups. Once again the old axiom applies: Early detection makes successful treatment possible.

■■■■ **SELF-TEST**

1. __L__ primary teeth
2. __N__ permanent teeth
3. __b__ chewing of food
4. __M__ cutting teeth
5. __O__ grinding teeth
6. __C__ crown of tooth
7. __K__ bad breath
8. __I__ pulp cavity
9. __A__ irritated gums
10. __G__ jawbone socket
11. __D__ dental caries
12. __F__ bacterial layer
13. __H__ dental calculus
14. __J__ drinking water
15. __E__ tooth erosion

a. gingivitis
b. mastication
c. enamel
d. decay
e. decalcification
f. plaque
g. root
h. tartar
i. nerves
j. fluoridation
k. halitosis
l. 20
m. incisors
n. 32
o. molars

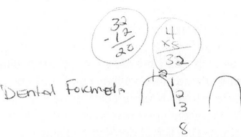

Dental Formula

■■■■ **STUDY QUESTIONS**

1. The fact that tooth decay is the most common chronic disease of the human species is a rather startling statistic, especially when we consider that many health texts (at the college level) devote little or no space to the subject. What, in your view, is the reason for this disinterest?

2. Tooth decay is said to be one of the most preventable diseases. Why is this true?

3. According to the American Dental Association, "Happiness is a Healthy Mouth." What are your views on this statement?

4. In your opinion what role does vanity play in dental health?

5. Since time immemorial the makers of oral products have stressed the social implications of halitosis. From your experience would you say they overstate the problem or hit the nail squarely on the head?

6. Based on your reading of the text, how often would you recommend brushing the teeth, and when?

7. History shows that fluoridation is probably one of the most outstanding and effective public health measures of the present century. How, then, do you explain the fact that certain groups are against fluoridation, to the extent that certain areas of the country are without its benefits?

8. In your own words state the events leading to tooth decay.

9. What is meant by endodontic treatment?

10. What is the difference between gingivitis and periodontitis?

11. In relation to dental health, what single dietary item do you consider the most dangerous? CANDY —

12. What dietary minerals are essential for the proper growth and development of the teeth?

13. Acute necrotizing ulcerative gingivitis (ANUG) is known by several other names. Give two.

14. What is the relationship between the primary teeth and malocclusion?

15. Pregnancy is a "threat" to the dental health of both the mother and the fetus. Specifically, why?

CHAPTER 21

Alcohol and tobacco

Alcohol and tobacco are clearly recognized health hazards, and in immoderate amounts they can usually be relied on to shorten one's life. Nowhere else is the maxim "everything in moderation" underscored in a more dramatic fashion than in the practice of drinking and smoking. There are an estimated 10 million alcoholics in the United States, and alcohol abuse is the number one drug problem of American teenagers and children. Alcohol not only can kill the people who drink it excessively, but also it can endanger the lives of others who come into contact with heavy drinkers. According to the National Council on Alcoholism, half the deaths in car accidents, half the homicides, and one fourth of the suicides are related to alcohol. As for smoking, it kills directly by causing cancer and heart attacks and indirectly by means of fire. In the words of the World Health Organization, "Smoking-related diseases are such important causes of disability and premature death in developed countries that the control of cigarette smoking could do more to improve health and prolong life in these countries than any single action in the whole field of preventive medicine."

Alcohol and tobacco are both drugs. The reason they are dealt with here in a special chapter (and not in Chapter 22 on drug abuse) is mainly because they are household drugs, just like aspirin and caffeine. But they are, as noted in the Overview, potentially hazardous and the most abused of all chemical substances in our environment. What follows are the highlights of these two substances in their various medical and psychosocial ramifications.

▬ ALCOHOL

The use of alcoholic beverages began very early in human history. Egyptian writings of 3000 years ago urged temperance, and the Old Testament and the writings of the Greeks, Romans, Chinese, Japanese, and Indians denounced excessive drinking. In American Colonial history drinking was accepted, but drunkenness was punished by fines, whippings, and confinement in the stocks. The early temperance movement was an appeal for moderation that permitted beer and wine but urged abstinence from distilled spirits.

About 1840 the "total abstinence" movement got underway, culminating in the passage of the Eighteenth Amendment to the Constitution, which prohibited the manufacture and sale of all alcoholic beverages. National prohibition lasted from 1920 to 1933, when it was abandoned because of the bootlegging of illicit liquor and the crime, corruption, and violence related to it. Once more the moderate use of alcoholic beverages has become socially acceptable, although there are those who still feel that total abstinence is desirable.

▪ Chemistry

Alcohol, the active ingredient in wine, beer, hard liquor, and the like, is a natural sub-

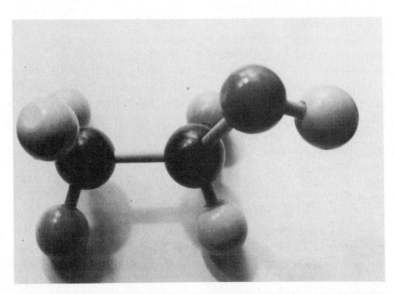

Fig. 21-1 ▪ Chemical model of ethyl alcohol (ethanol), which has the formula C_2H_5OH. The two darkest balls are carbon atoms; the oxygen atom is the darker atom attached to the carbon on the right; all other balls are hydrogen atoms.

TABLE 21-1

Percent alcohol of alcoholic beverages*

Beverage	Alcoholic content
Beer or ale	4% to 5%
Table wines and champagne	11% to 13%
Vermouth	16% to 19%
Dessert wines	19% to 20%
Liqueurs	23% to 46%
Distilled spirits	40% to 50%

*Tables wines refer to dry white or red wine; dessert wines include sweet wines such as port and sherry; liqueurs include sweet, syrupy drinks such as Amaretto, Drambuie, Irish Mist, Grand Marnier, and fruit brandies; distilled spirits ("hard liquors") include whiskey, gin, vodka, rum, and brandy.

stance formed by the reaction of fermenting sugar with yeast. There are hundreds of alcohols known to chemistry, but the kind in all alcoholic beverages is **ethyl alcohol** (Fig. 21-1). For convenience we shall refer to ethyl alcohol simply as "alcohol." Pure (absolute) alcohol is a colorless, light, volatile, flammable liquid with a somewhat stinging taste. The various alcoholic beverages are produced by using different sources of sugar for fermentation. For instance, beer is made from germinated or malted barley, wine from grapes or berries, whiskey from malted grains, and rum from molasses. Hard liquor—namely, whiskey, gin, vodka, and rum—is made by **distillation**, which further concentrates the alcohol resulting from fermentation.

Alcohol strengths of typical alcoholic beverages are presented in Table 21-1. The same alcoholic content, about ½ fluid ounce of pure alcohol, is found in a 12-ounce can of beer, a 5-ounce glass of table wine, and a cocktail containing a jigger or 1½ ounces of 86-proof liquor ("proof" being double the percent of alcohol). In energy potential 1 fluid ounce of pure alcohol supplies about 200 calories of heat.

■ Physiologic action

Unlike other "food," alcohol does not have to be digested. When you drink an alcoholic beverage, 20% of the alcohol in it is normally absorbed immediately into the bloodstream through the stomach walls. The other 80% enters the bloodstream almost as fast after being quickly processed through the small intestine. After it is consumed, alcohol eventually can be found in all tissues, organs, and fluids of the body. Alcohol immediately acts on the brain's central control areas to slow down or depress brain activity.

A low level of alcohol in the blood, such as would result from sipping one drink (for example, a 12-ounce can of beer), has a mild tranquilizing effect on most people. Although basically a **sedative**, alcohol seems to act temporarily as a stimulant for many after they first start drinking. This is because alcohol's initial effects are on those parts of the brain affecting learned behavior patterns such as self-control. After a drink or two, this learned behavior may be altered, making one lose his or her inhibitions, talk more freely, or feel like "the life of the party." On the other hand, one may feel aggressive or depressed.

Higher levels of alcohol in the blood depress the brain activity to the point that memory, as well as muscle coordination and balance, may be temporarily impaired. Still larger intake within a relatively short period of time depresses deeper parts of the brain, severely affecting judgment and dulling the senses. If steady drinking continues, alcohol anesthetizes the deepest levels of the brain and can cause coma or death by depressing heart function and breathing (Fig. 21-2).

As with any drug, the effects of alcohol are modified by several factors, including tolerance, kind of drink, speed of drinking, stomach contents, and body weight. **Tolerance** to alcohol develops with use and, other things being equal, it is the most important factor involved in the impact of a given dose of al-

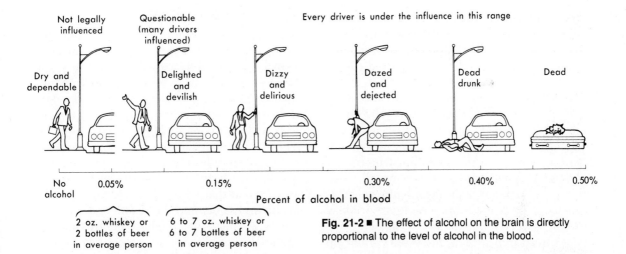

Fig. 21-2 ■ The effect of alcohol on the brain is directly proportional to the level of alcohol in the blood.

cohol. For persons accustomed to its use, a shot of whiskey barely produces a cerebral response; for persons not accustomed to its use, the effects are typically pronounced, sometimes to the point of inebriation. A classic study using a variety of simple visual and motor tests showed disruptions of performance at an average **blood alcohol level** (BAL) of 0.05% in abstainers, 0.07% in moderate drinkers, and 0.1% in heavy drinkers. Stated otherwise, a higher level of alcohol in the blood is necessary to impair the performance of a chronic heavy drinker than to impair a moderate drinker's performance.

The speed of drinking relates to the fact that it takes about 1 hour to burn up ¼ ounce of pure alcohol. This is the amount of alcohol contained in an average highball, can of beer, or glass of table wine. Thus if we sip such a drink slowly and do not have more than one every 2 hours, our consumption does not outpace the body's metabolic machinery. On the other hand, gulping drinks leads to high levels of alcohol in the blood and to consequent depression.

The kind of drink is of concern because some drinks are obviously stronger than others. The alcohol in wine and beer is more dilute and therefore absorbed somewhat more slowly into the bloodstream than alcohol from hard liquor or distilled spirits. Diluting the latter with water helps to slow down absorption, but mixing with carbonated beverages can increase the rate of absorption. In addition to the question of the kind of drink is the matter of whether the stomach is full or empty. Eating, especially before drinking but also while drinking, slows down alcohol's rate of absorption into the bloodstream and produces a more even response to alcohol.

Body weight plays a significant role in the effects of alcohol, a fact not generally appreciated. Alcohol is quickly distributed uniformly within the circulatory system and body fluids. Therefore, if the same amount is drunk by a 120-pound person and a 180-pound person, the alcohol is more concentrated in the lighter individual and, other things being equal, more intoxicating to that person.

■ Drunkenness and hangover

Drunkenness (inebriation) is characterized by a temporary loss of control over physical and mental powers caused by excessive alcohol intake. Symptoms vary, but they can include impaired vision, distorted depth perception, thick speech, and bad coordination. The ability to solve problems is reduced, emotion and mood become unpredictable, memory is impaired, and judgment becomes poor. In most states a person is considered legally drunk when he or she has a 0.10% **blood alcohol level** (BAL). Such a situation generally results when a person weighing 160 pounds has had about four drinks within 1 hour after eating. As noted earlier, a person will reach this stage with fewer drinks if body weight is less than 160 pounds and with more drinks if weight exceeds this figure. Contrary to a widespread impression, one cannot sober up by such devices as drinking black coffee, taking a cold shower, or breathing oxygen. Once alcohol is in the bloodstream, nothing can be done about its effects except to wait until it is metabolized. As noted earlier, the body burns up alcohol at a rate of about ¼ ounce of pure alcohol per hour.

A **hangover** is the body's reaction to excessive drinking. The associated miseries of nausea, gastritis, anxiety, and headache vary from case to case, but there is always extreme fatigue. No scientific evidence supports the curative claims for coffee, raw eggs, oysters, chili peppers, steak sauce, tomato juice, vitamins, or the proverbial "hair of the dog." The experts recommend aspirin, solid food, and rest. The real answer to hangover, of course, is to avoid excessive drinking and drunkenness. Helpful hints include sipping slowly, putting food in the stomach, and paying close attention to one's response to the effects of alcohol. Just an inkling that one is getting close to a potentially sorry state of affairs is the signal to stop.

■ Alcoholism

Alcoholism is marked by dependence on alcohol and loss of control over one's drinking. This loss of control may develop almost im-

perceptibly over a long period, or it may manifest itself almost from the start of a person's drinking. Determination of whether an individual is an alcoholic cannot be made from estimates of how much he or she is drinking. Such estimates seldom are accurate. The crucial issue, experts agree, is how alcohol is affecting the individual's life. A person must be considered an alcoholic if he or she continues to use alcohol despite the knowledge that its use is contributing to problems at home and at work and that he or she is risking personal health and safety and the health and safety of others. Though we might tend to think of "typical" alcoholic people as skid row inhabitants, only about 3% of alcoholic Americans are in that category. Actually, alcoholics come from all walks of life. Indeed, alcoholism is a problem among the clergy, and an estimated 25% of physicians have drinking problems. Most alcoholics are employed, and most have families; they are much like their neighbors and fellow citizens. Alcoholism strikes men and women about equally.

Damage to the liver, heart, and brain is the principal risk of alcoholism. The liver disease known as **cirrhosis**, which is significantly related to alcohol abuse and can lead to death, has been rising rapidly in the past two decades. Damage to the heart includes disturbances in heart pumping action and rhythm abnormalities, which can be life threatening. In the brain the first detectable changes are in abstract thinking. As the disease progresses, brain damage may be severe, with seizures and "blackouts," that is, periods of activity that the individual cannot recall. Continued excessive use of alcohol can result in permanent brain damage. Women run an additional risk. Heavy alcohol intake by a pregnant woman has been shown to result in mental retardation and other birth defects in her infant (**fetal alcohol syndrome**). Furthermore, several studies have identified maternal alcoholism as a possible contributor to

sudden infant death syndrome, in which, for no clear reason, an infant mysteriously dies while sleeping. The Surgeon General's office in 1981 urged total avoidance of alcohol not only by women who are pregnant but also by those who are planning to become pregnant.

Withdrawal. The physical dependence (addiction) with prolonged heavy use of alcohol is best seen when alcohol intake is stopped. The **withdrawal syndrome** that develops is medically more severe and more likely to cause death than withdrawal from narcotic drugs. A continuum of symptoms and signs starts 24 to 48 hours after cessation of intake, although this may not occur until 3 weeks after withdrawal or can start during a period of high alcohol intake. A mild withdrawal syndrome includes tremor, weakness, sweating, exaggerated reflexes, and gastrointestinal symptoms. A severe withdrawal syndrome, or **delirium tremens** (DTs), begins with anxiety attacks, increasing confusion, poor sleep, marked sweating, and a profound depression. Fleeting hallucinations and nocturnal illusions that arouse fear and restlessness may occur. Visual hallucinations involving animals ("pink elephants") are frequent and often incite terror. Vestibular (balance) disturbances may cause the person to believe that the floor is moving, walls are falling, or the room is rotating. Some victims may suffer grand mal epilepsy. The mortality of delirium tremens runs as high as 15%. However, the course is usually self-limited, terminating in a long sleep. The acute period lasts from 2 to 10 days but can be more prolonged in severe withdrawal syndromes.

Treatment and prevention. The first phase of treatment of an alcoholic consists of immediate withdrawal of alcohol. The delirious state that may accompany withdrawal (just described) is managed with tranquilizers, intravenous fluids, and large doses of vitamin C and B-complex vitamins, particularly thiamin. After correction of any nutritional deficiencies associated with excessive alcohol in-

take, the alcoholic's behavior must be changed to stop the cycles of drunkenness and sobriety. Maintaining sobriety once it has been established is difficult because such a person has as fixed a pattern of social habits as he or she does of drinking. The alcoholic has to be warned that after a few weeks (following recovery from the last bout) he or she is likely to drink in a controlled manner for a few days or, rarely, even for a few weeks, but inevitably will repeat the pattern and again become ill. Various types of psychotherapy have been recommended for alcoholism. Group therapy may be helpful, but psychoanalysis is generally considered less useful. Aversive therapy of various forms has been used, most notably a daily dose of disulfiram (Antabuse), a drug that makes one violently sick if alcohol is consumed. Small daily doses of a tranquilizer may help assuage the craving for alcohol in some individuals. The drug appears to be a substitute for alcohol, and the benefit ceases when it is discontinued.

Help for alcoholics is now widespread. Such help can be provided by a physician or clergyman, a local welfare agency, a clinic, a social worker, a psychologist or psychiatrist, a general hospital or psychiatric hospital, an alcoholism treatment center, or the local chapter of Alcoholics Anonymous (AA). Alcoholics Anonymous is probably the best known source of help for alcoholic persons. This organization is a self-help group in which members help each other in a type of group therapy setting that utilizes mutual experience for mutual support. Additionally, **industrial rehabilitation** programs for the alcoholic worker are offered by a growing number of business organizations. The possibility of losing one's job is a strong motivation to seek treatment. With guidance and treatment, many good workers are able to stop drinking, keep their jobs, and lead more productive and satisfying lives. Recovery rates in industry range from 60% to 80%.

Therapy groups for the families of alcoholics include Al-Anon and Alateen. They meet to help themselves and each other and to learn how to cope with the troubles brought about by another person's drinking. And perhaps above all they learn that alcoholism is a terrible illness demanding treatment and understanding. Those who are interested can find the location of the nearest Al-Anon and Alateen group meetings by looking up Alcoholics Anonymous in the telephone book.

The National Institute on Alcohol Abuse and Alcoholism reminds us that problem drinking and alcoholism can never be controlled solely by treating people. The long-range goal must be prevention. And this requires education—at home, in our schools, and in our communities—to develop the nation's habits of moderation in the use of alcoholic beverages and to encourage respect for those who choose to abstain. One immediate step that we as individuals can take toward preventing alcoholism in our own social circles is assuming the responsibilities that we as hosts and hostesses have to our friends. At dinner parties and social gatherings food should be served both before and with drinks. Moreover, other beverages should be made available. Indeed, "close the bar" an hour or so before you plan to break up the party and serve coffee and a tempting dessert.

■■■■ TOBACCO

Tobacco is the dried, processed leaves of the plant *Nicotiana tabacum*. On this continent tobacco has been used for over 400 years, but cigarette smoking came with the twentieth century. In 1900 the annual per capita consumption of cigarettes was 54; today it is about 4000. During this period the per capita consumption of cigars has declined from 122 to 66, that of pipe tobacco from 1¾ pounds to ½ pound, and that of chewing tobacco from 4½ pounds to ½ pound.

■ Chemistry

Tobacco smoke is a mixture of gases and minute droplets of tar; nearly 1000 components of tobacco smoke have been identified. Some components are filtered off as the smoke is drawn through the unburned tobacco, but they are redistilled as the burning ember advances, and the smoke in each successive puff becomes more concentrated. Since cigarette smoke is less irritating than pipe or cigar smoke, it is more likely to be inhaled. Consequently, cigarette smoke is by far the major problem.

The components of tobacco smoke of medical importance fall into four main groups: nicotine, carcinogens, irritants, and toxic gases. **Nicotine** chiefly affects the nervous system and is probably responsible for a smoker's dependence on cigarettes. The effects are pharmacologically complex and include stimulation or sedation, depending on the dose and on the smoker's physical and psychologic state. Other effects on the nervous system, noted only in the first use of tobacco (the "first cigarette"), include headache, dizziness, and nausea. Indirectly, nicotine speeds up the heart and increases blood pressure by causing the adrenal glands to release epinephrine. **Carcinogens**, present in the tar, initiate cancer formation. So-called cocarcinogens accelerate the production of cancer by other chemicals. **Irritants**, as the term implies, irritate the tissues in general and the respiratory passageways in particular. The result is coughing, wheezing, and excess mucus. **Toxic gases** include hydrocyanic acid, hydrogen sulfide and, most especially, **carbon monoxide**. The latter combines with hemoglobin (in the red blood cells) to form carboxyhemoglobin and in so doing prevents the hemoglobin from reacting with and transporting oxygen to the tissues. The average carboxyhemoglobin level in persons smoking a pack of cigarettes a day is about 5%, compared to less than 1% in nonsmokers.

■ Risks of smoking

Smoking cigarettes is likely to shorten one's life. The damage is dose related, with the number of years of reduced life expectancy proportional to the amount of smoking and years of smoking. A 25-year-old person who smokes two packs of cigarettes a day can expect to live 8.3 years less than a nonsmoking contemporary. The chances of a heavy cigarette smoker dying during his or her prime are almost twice as great as a nonsmoker's chances. Smoking directly causes or contributes to the three main causes of American deaths: heart disease, cancer, and accidents.

Cigarettes are deemed responsible for about a quarter of the deaths from heart attack. Along with high blood pressure and high cholesterol, smoking is a main factor in premature death and chronic disability caused by coronary heart disease. Also the carbon monoxide in cigarette smoke may replace oxygen in as many as 12% of a smoker's red blood cells, impairing oxygen delivery to the tissues.

A third of cancer deaths are caused at least in part by smoking, sometimes in concert with occupational exposure to noxious substances such as asbestos, uranium, and dyes. Cigarette smoke contains a number of known cancer-causing agents (carcinogens), including radioactive elements; a major part of a smoker's total radiation exposure comes from cigarettes, which may result in 40 times the recommended maximum annual exposure. Smoking is by far the main cause of the nation's leading cancer killer, lung cancer, which is fatal to 90% of its victims. As girls and women have taken up smoking with a vengeance, their once low risk of lung cancer has risen dramatically, so the disease may soon surpass breast cancer as the leading cancer killer of American women. Other cancers to which smoking makes an important contribution are the nearly always fatal cancers of the esophagus and pancreas as well as the disabling cancers of the larynx, mouth, and bladder.

Cigarettes account for about 70% of the cases of life-limiting chronic bronchitis and emphysema. Lung damage occurs even in young smokers. Smoking has also been linked to peptic ulcer, earlier onset of menopause, hearing loss in older men, sleep problems, impaired athletic performance, excessive numbers of red cells, and malignant (life-threatening) hypertension. Furthermore, smoking adversely affects the action of several important drugs, including tranquilizers and analgesics (pain killers).

And then there is the problem of "passive smokers," for example, the unborn child, who is the most vulnerable. Smoking during pregnancy reduces the oxygen supply to the fetus and increases the risk of stillbirth, low birth weight, and death shortly after birth. It may also impair the physical and social development of surviving offspring. The children of smoking parents have poorer lung function and a higher incidence of wheezing and respiratory infection, including life-threatening pneumonia. Other risks of passive smoking are well established. In addition to general discomfort and allergic reactions, significantly reduced lung function has been shown to occur in those who work near smokers. Nonsmokers inhaling the air in a smoke-filled room can develop high levels of carbon monoxide in their blood, which can interfere with heart function and cause angina pains.

Apart from health considerations but no less important, smoking causes more fatal fires than any other source of combustion, resulting in about 2500 deaths a year. At least 25,000 people are injured, and over $300,000 in property is annually lost as a result of fires caused by smoking.

■ Stopping the habit

Well over 30 million Americans have taken the risks of smoking to heart and have "kicked the habit." Some 55 million continue to puff away, but a 1981 survey showed that a good 45 million of these people would like to quit. And it is never too late. Although those who quit before age 40 benefit most, the risk of death and disability from smoking declines at any point that one quits. Contrary to what some believe, so-called stress-related deaths do not increase among former smokers. The risk of heart attack among men under 65 is reduced by 25% if they stop smoking. The risk starts dropping within a year after quitting and after 10 years reaches the level of those who never smoked! Moreover, there are a number of immediate benefits of quitting: enhanced stamina, improved sleep, fewer headaches and stomachaches, and keener senses of taste and smell. Smoker's cough takes a while longer but, after a few years, it too will disappear.

Many people stop smoking entirely, all at once. Others manage first by cutting down or switching to low-nicotine, low-tar cigarettes. A recent report by the Surgeon General, however, has found that smoking "safer cigarettes" decreases a smoker's chances of developing lung cancer by only a minor extent. It also found little firm evidence that these cigarettes can reduce the incidence of cardiovascular diseases, emphysema, bronchitis, complications of pregnancy, and other disorders linked to smoking. Furthermore, the report goes on to say that even the small benefit derived from such cigarettes is lost if smokers consume more cigarettes or inhale more deeply after switching. Other strategies smokers use to quit range from special chewing gums and "countdown filters" to hypnosis and group therapy. Clearly, different strategies work for different smokers; the trick is to find the one that best suits individual needs and personality.

Local American Cancer Society units offer free Quit Smoking Clinics in many communities as part of a stepped-up national campaign to provide help to people who want to quit. A typical clinic consists of eight sessions over a 2-week period under the guidance of a trained group leader. Other available programs of established value include Freedom From Smoking, Stop Smoking Systems, Quit Smoking, and SmokeEnders.

■■■■ SELF-TEST

1. __O__ nicotine
2. __L__ carcinogens
3. __K__ ethanol
4. __M__ fermentation
5. __D__ 43% alcohol
6. __I__ wine
7. __A__ beer
8. __B__ whiskey
9. __N__ drunkenness
10. __J__ BAL
11. __H__ addiction
12. __G__ cirrhosis
13. __E__ withdrawal
14. __F__ aversive therapy
15. __C__ hemoglobin

a. malted barley
b. distillation
c. carbon monoxide
d. 86 proof
e. delirium tremens
f. disulfiram
g. liver disease
h. physical dependence
i. grapes
j. blood alcohol level
k. ethyl alcohol
l. tobacco tar
m. sugar plus yeast
n. inebriation
o. smoker's dependence

STUDY QUESTIONS

1. What do all alcoholic beverages have in common chemically?
2. What is meant by the expression "absolute alcohol"?
3. Briefly, what is the process of fermentation?
4. Briefly, what is the process of distillation?
5. As it applies to alcoholic beverages, what is the meaning of "proof"? Give an example.
6. Assuming that a certain brand of beer contains 5% alcohol, how much pure alcohol is consumed in the drinking of two 12-ounce cans?
7. How many ounces of pure alcohol are contained in 2 jiggers of 80-proof bourbon?
8. In regard to the above question, how many calories are involved?
9. Pharmacologically, alcohol is a sedative, and yet most people tend to characterize it as a "stimulant." Discuss.
10. Although two persons might have the same BAL (blood alcohol level), it is quite possible that one could be inebriated and the other "sober as a judge." Discuss in detail.
11. Mention as many factors as you can possibly think of that have a bearing on the way a person responds to alcohol.
12. Once alcohol is in the bloodstream, "nothing can be done about its effects except to wait until it is metabolized." What does this mean?
13. How long does it take for 2 ounces of pure alcohol to disappear from the bloodstream?
14. The text states (p. 318) that "the determination of whether an individual is an alcoholic cannot be made from estimates of how much he or she is drinking." Discuss fully and be sure to incorporate your own views.
15. Quite obviously the vast majority of people who drink alcoholic beverages do not become alcoholics. What, then, can be said about the ones who do? Do you have a theory?
16. What are the major medical risks of alcoholism?
17. What are your views on drinking during pregnancy?
18. What is the relationship between physical dependence (addiction) and the "withdrawal syndrome"?
19. What do you consider the best approach to the prevention of alcoholism?
20. Medically speaking, "smoking" is just about synonymous with cigarettes. Why cigarettes?
21. What are the major physiologic effects of nicotine?
22. Although they may not realize it, heavy smokers suffer from a lack of oxygen. Specifically, why?
23. What are the major medical risks of smoking?
24. Lung cancer in women is on the rise. Why?
25. What are your personal views on smoking?

CHAPTER 22

Drug abuse

Drug abuse involves psychoactive ("mind-altering") chemical agents and the people who use them. Alcohol, the number one abused drug, was discussed in the previous chapter. In the present chapter we shall take a look at "pot," "uppers," "downers," and other abused substances, both legal and illegal. The use and abuse of psychoactive drugs has been continuous throughout recorded history and, directly or indirectly, society is the victim. Such drugs destroy health, crush family life, generate crime and violence, and kill innocent people. These are well-known facts. What may not be so well known and appreciated is the tremendous economic burden, both in terms of cost and waste. Drug abuse makes nonproductive citizens out of productive people, strains medical facilities, and increases the cost of running society, especially the jails, prisons, and police forces. Moreover, according to recent figures compiled by the National Institute on Drug Abuse, Americans spend 20 billion dollars a year on marijuana alone. In summary, society has a grave problem, and it is now quite clear that the only solution resides in a real understanding of the problem, that is, in education and family guidance. Other preventive measures can certainly help, but they are clearly not central to the issue.

A drug is any chemical substance that produces physical, mental, emotional, or behavioral changes in the user. Drug effects depend on many variables, including the amount of drug taken, how often it is taken, the way it is taken, and other drugs used at the same time. Also, body weight, set (personality, mood, expectation), and setting of use (environment) help determine how a drug affects a person.

Drug abuse (Fig. 22-1) is the use of a drug for other than medicinal purposes, which results in the impaired physical, mental, emotional, or social well-being of the user. **Drug misuse** is the unintentional or inappropriate use of prescription or over-the-counter drugs, with similar results. Multiple drug abuse is common. People who abuse one drug are likely to abuse other drugs, either by taking a variety of them all at once or at different times. Multiple drug abuse means multiple risk. For example, mixing alcohol with sleeping pills, sedatives, or tranquilizers is especially dangerous.

■■■ CHARACTERISTICS OF DRUG ABUSE

Drug abuse is the excessive or persistent taking of a drug without regard for accepted medical practice. Most often the drug is obtained illegally. Drug abuse commonly leads to **drug dependence**, a condition in which the user has a compelling desire to continue taking the drug either to experience its effects or to avoid the discomfort of its absence. On the recommendation of the World Health Organization, the expression "drug dependence" encompasses "drug habituation" and "drug addiction."

Drug habituation, or **psychologic dependence**, occurs when a person has taken a drug

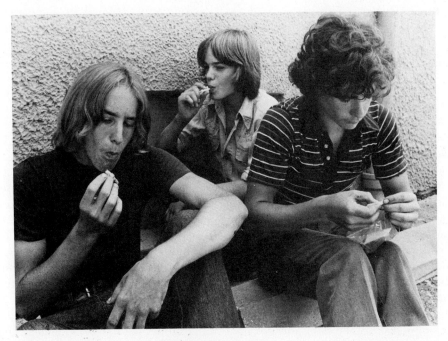

Fig. 22-1 ■ Drug abuse.

regularly because of its pleasing effect and has become so used to having it that the person does not feel comfortable or happy without it. Giving up the habit is a matter of will power. The bodily functions are not upset when the use of the drug is discontinued. The individual may be very uncomfortable, but the problem is psychologic or emotional rather than physical.

Drug addiction, or **physical dependence**, may be defined as the continuing, uncontrolled, compulsive use of a drug, not only to induce intoxication but also to avoid the tortures of its withdrawal. An altered state of body physiology is thus established, and when the drug is withdrawn, distressing symptoms appear. These are associated with the malfunctioning that has been established. Common withdrawal symptoms include discomfort, restlessness, vomiting, diarrhea, aching muscles, slight fever, and elevated blood pressure. The severe discomfort of going without the drug drives the patient back to it. In many cases **tolerance** develops. This is the need to take larger and larger doses to produce a given effect. All drugs discussed here produce psychologic dependence, and the narcotics and sedatives produce physical dependence also.

Individual differences in reaction to specific drugs must be recognized. These differences may appear the first time a drug is used, as when a person has a "bad trip" on LSD. Actually, this applies to all kinds of agents. For example, some persons are violently poisoned by the slightest contact with poison ivy or poison oak, whereas others may handle the leaves of the plant with no harmful results. Also, differences may relate to the individual's potential for addiction. For example, although two persons begin using alcohol in the same way, one of them may never develop any appreciable interest in drinking, whereas the other becomes an alcoholic in spite of his or her best

efforts to escape. No chemical or physiologic explanation for these differences has been found.

Drug abuse provides, in varying degrees, departures from reality with specific changes in health and personality. And in addition to these specific changes it spreads hepatitis and other communicable diseases when unclean needles are used in common to inject the drugs. Drug abuse also boosts the accident and crime rates.

In the interest of convenience, abused drugs are categorized pharmacologically, that is, on the basis of their principal effects on the body. Recognized categories, or classes, include narcotics, sedatives, tranquilizers, hallucinogens, and stimulants.

◼◼◼ NARCOTICS

Opium has been a source of narcotics for thousands of years. It is a sticky resin from the capsule of the plant *Papaver somniferum* (the opium poppy). **Morphine** and **codeine** are extracted from it. **Heroin**, or diacetylmorphine, is a derivative of morphine and three times more potent than morphine. These substances relieve pain and reduce hunger, thirst, sexual urges, and fear. Opium smoking has long been a common form of drug abuse in the East, but this abuse has never been extensive in the West. Morphine and codeine are widely used medically. Persons using these drugs develop tolerance, along with psychologic and physical dependence. In the United States heroin, the opiate most widely subject to abuse, is sniffed, injected under the skin, or injected directly into a vein. It produces a transient euphoria with a sense of relaxation. The duration of the "high" is from 1 to 6 hours. Overdose is common and sometimes lethal.

Narcotic addiction is marked by anemia, pallor, sleepiness, and loss of both weight and appetite. Once the individual is "hooked," he or she is in dire fear of the withdrawal symptoms, which begin about 8 hours after abstinence. The withdrawal syndrome is characterized by perspiration, tearing of the eyes, aching bones and muscles, nausea, vomiting, and diarrhea.

The addict may need to spend hundreds of dollars a day for heroin, and crime is often the only source of this amount of money. Addicts turn to robbery and burglary. Women commonly turn to prostitution. Treatment in a hospital or rehabilitation center is desirable, and in some states addicts are sent to hospitals rather than to jails when they are arrested for possession of the drug. Treatment may consist of psychiatric therapy with guidance and group sessions. It may include drug therapy, namely, substituting the synthetic narcotic methadone for the more addicting heroin. Methadone programs are being viewed with some caution, however, and only time will tell how effective they really are.

◼◼◼ SEDATIVES AND HYPNOTICS

Sedatives calm and allay excitement, and hypnotics induce sleep. Commonly, they are one and the same drug at different dosages. By convention they are categorized as **barbiturates** ("downers"), such as secobarbital (Seconal), and **nonbarbiturates**, such as methaqualone (Quaalude). The barbiturates are the most subject to abuse. Indeed, they are second only to carbon monoxide as the cause of fatal poisoning.

Barbiturates are derivatives of barbituric acid—hence their name. The most commonly abused are the short-acting barbiturates (pentobarbital, secobarbital, and amobarbital). Phenobarbital and other long-acting barbiturates are not frequently abused because they do not act quickly enough. At the outset barbiturates produce relaxation, lassitude, and a reduction in tension. In greater amounts they produce a state very similar to alcoholic intoxication. The abuser may become confused, irritable, depressed, and emotionally erratic. Suicide by overdose, either intentional or unintentional, may occur. The ingestion of barbiturates and alcohol at the same time is especially dangerous and can be fatal. Not uncommonly, the abuse of sedatives may develop from prolonged therapeutic use under medical prescription. The abuser then purchases the drug on the black market to avoid reality and to gain relief from tensions and anxieties. Often the abuser becomes addicted before he or she knows it. As tolerance increases and physical and psychologic dependence develop, the abuser usually becomes careless of his appearance. Judgment and ability to concentrate are seriously impaired, and job loss is common. A paradoxic reaction in some abusers after tolerance has developed is that the drug then produces a reaction of excitation and is taken for exhilaration.

Complete withdrawal is accompanied by serious symptoms of nervousness, anxiety, headache, dizziness, vomiting, low blood pressure and sometimes convulsions, disorientation, and delirium. Abrupt withdrawal can be fatal. In treatment, therefore, withdrawal must be accomplished slowly and carefully under medical supervision and preferably in a hospital.

◼◼◼ TRANQUILIZERS

Tranquilizers are agents that act on the emotional state, quieting or calming the person without affecting clarity or consciousness. So-called **minor tranquilizers**, such as diazepam (Valium), are used in the treatment of anxiety and tension or psychoneurosis; so-called **major tranquilizers**, such as chlorpromazine (Thorazine), are used to reduce psychotic symptoms. Many authorities believe that the primary factor underlying the decline in mental hospital populations in the United States can be identified as the introduction of tranquilizers into treatment programs in 1954 and 1955. The statistics are actually startling. For example, in 1955 the number of resident patients in state and local government mental hospitals in the United States was 559,000, and in 1976 the figure had dropped to 171,000. This is the good news. The bad news is that minor tranquilizers, notably Valium, enjoy wide casual street and home use. Indeed, it is possible that more people misuse and abuse Valium for longer periods than most other drugs. There may be withdrawal symptoms. An abrupt withdrawal of the drug may result in seizures.

■■■ HALLUCINOGENS

Many drugs produce hallucinations. Those of chief concern include LSD (**lysergic acid diethylamide**); **marijuana** (from the hemp plant *Cannabis sativa*); **mescaline** (from the peyote cactus that grows in Mexico and the Rio Grande Valley); **psilocybin** (from the Mexican sacred mushroom, *Psilocybe mexicana*); and DMT (dimethyltryptamine), which is closely related chemically to psilocybin. These agents are also called **psychedelic** ("mind expanding") because of the sensations they produce, but there is no evidence that they improve creative endeavor. Although phencyclidine ("angel dust") and various chemical inhalants are not true hallucinogens, they may produce hallucinations in some abusers. For this reason they are here included in the psychedelic category. Actually, they are somewhat in a class by themselves.

■ LSD

LSD was synthesized by Stoll and Hofmann in 1938. In 1943 a pinch of the drug was accidentally ingested by Hofmann, and he reported the weird sensations produced. The abuse of the drug became apparent in the early 1960s, and by 1965 a stream of patients began to make their way to hospitals. Aldous Huxley and Timothy Leary had published papers expressing their hopes that these drugs would prove "consciousness expanding." Their hopes have been been borne out, but unfortunately they did stimulate the self-administration of the drug.

LSD is highly potent, odorless, colorless, and tasteless. It is most often taken by ingestion in capsules or tablets or in saturated sugar cubes. An LSD "trip" usually lasts about 12 hours. Within 20 to 60 minutes after the drug is taken, the heart rate increases, the pupils dilate, and perceptions become distorted. Colors become more vivid and sounds become more exciting. The sense of time is lost. There may be uncontrolled laughing or crying. Tactile sensations become distorted, and the mood changes toward exhilaration or depression. The "trip" may be either pleasant or harrowing. Sometimes there is depersonalization and an intense feeling of losing one's mind. Sometimes there is panic.

There may be quite complete departure from reality. One youth was killed on the freeway, convinced that he was invisible. Another believed that he could fly and jumped out of a window to his death. A young man in Brooklyn murdered his mother-in-law for no reason that he could remember when he "sobered up."

Serious aftereffects include impairment of judgment, severe depression lasting several months, and cessation of all constructive efforts. Periods of extended psychosis have followed a single exposure, and hallucinations have reappeared without further ingestion of the drug. Evidence of chromosome damage and consequent birth defects is accumulating. There is no physical dependence, but psychologic dependence is strong, and tolerance

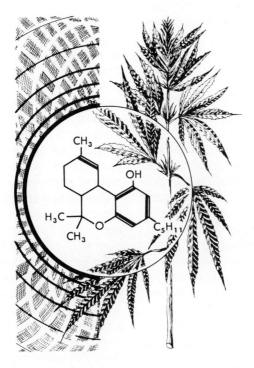

Fig. 22-2 ■ Marijuana and the chemical structure of its active constituent (THC).

builds up quickly. Withdrawal should be carried out under medical care.

■ Marijuana

Marijuana ("pot," "grass," "weed") comes from a plant with the botanical name *Cannabis sativa*, which grows wild and is cultivated in many parts of the world. Containing over 400 chemicals, this plant has the ability to intoxicate its users, primarily because of the psychoactive or mind-altering ingredient called **delta-9-tetrahydrocannabinol** (Fig. 22-2), or THC. It is the THC content, found in various concentrations in different parts of the plant, that determines the potency. And the THC content is controlled by plant strain, climate, soil conditions, and harvesting. Typically, the marijuana used in cigarettes ("joints," "sticks")

is made from dried particles of the whole plant except the main stem and roots. In 1975 the average confiscated sample of marijuana contained 0.4% THC; in 1980 the average THC content was about 4%—a tenfold increase. Sinsemilla, a cultivated form of marijuana that is becoming more frequently available in this country, may contain 7% THC.

Hashish ("hash") is a green, dark brown, or black resinous exudate of *Cannabis sativa*. In the past hashish, which averages about 2% THC, contained more THC than marijuana. However, because of the increased potency of the marijuana on the streets, it is now frequently stronger than hashish. Hash oil is the concentrated extract of hashish. It may contain up to 30% THC, many times the amount found in marijuana. Hash oil is a tarlike substance usually smoked in small amounts in tobacco or marijuana cigarettes or in small glass pipes.

Euphoria and relaxation are commonly reported as the result of smoking moderate amounts of marijuana. Physically, users experience an increase in heart and pulse rate, a reddening of the eyes, a dryness in the mouth and throat, a mild decrease in body temperature, and, on occasion, a sudden appetite. High doses may result in image distortion and hallucinations. Many users claim that marijuana enhances hearing, vision, and skin sensitivity, but these reports have not been confirmed by researchers. Confusion of identity may occur. Panic reactions also occur sometimes, especially when the user is a novice.

Even when other effects are unnoticeable, reaction time, learning, perception, motor incoordination, and attention in task performance are decreased, making smokers a danger to themselves and others (especially when driving). Impaired memory and altered sense of time may be long-term effects along with lung damage and other body changes that might occur; adverse effects on babies born to mothers who smoked marijuana during pregnancy have also been noted. Psychologic dependence can develop. Additionally, a very real danger in marijuana use is its possible interference with growing up. Scientists believe that the drug may interfere with the development of adequate social skills and may encourage a kind of psychologic escapism. Young people need to learn how to make decisions, to handle success, to cope with failure, and to form their own beliefs and values. By providing an escape from "growing pains," this drug can prevent young people from learning to become mature, independent, and responsible.

Decriminalization.   Decriminalization refers to the process of reducing the penalty, which in some states is imprisonment, for possession of small amounts of marijuana. Many feel that, while marijuana use should be discouraged, imprisonment is too harsh, especially for young users. Many states have already changed their laws, making possession of small amounts for personal use a misdemeanor and requiring civil fines, mandatory drug education programs, or involvement in public service instead of prison. Laws remain harsh for dealers of marijuana. As punishment for personal possession decreases, punishment for selling marijuana has increased in every state.

Medical uses.   Like any drug, marijuana has the potential to do either harm or good, depending on how it is used. So far the balance seems tipped toward the harm it does. But the ultimate answer is still locked up in marijuana's complex, largely unknown chemistry. Thousands of cancer patients use THC to relieve the violent nausea and vomiting that accompany chemotherapy. Glaucoma victims smoke joints to ease intraocular pressure. The plant is also being studied as a possible aid to people stricken with epilepsy, acute migraine, or multiple sclerosis. Recognizing its promise, the Food and Drug Administration has classified THC as a Class C drug, one with clinical applications. As of 1981, twenty-seven states had approved the distribution of THC for medical purposes, and one drug company had applied for a license to market it in capsule form. Laboratories that manufacture the pills and researchers who want to test raw marijuana get their supplies not from street peddlers but from a crop grown under government supervision at the University of Mississippi.

■ Phencyclidine

Phencyclidine (PCP) was developed as a surgical anesthetic for humans in the late 1950s. Because of its unusual and unpleasant side effects in human patients (delirium, extreme excitement, and visual disturbances)

PCP was soon restricted to its only current legal use as a veterinary anesthetic and tranquilizer. Nearly all PCP in today's drug culture is made illicitly, since it is easily synthesized in bootleg laboratories. Street PCP comes in various forms: as the powdered "angel dust," as tablets, as crystals, and in pills named "hogs" or "Pea Ce Pills." Smoking the dust, usually mixed with marijuana, parsley, and mint leaves, has become the preferred method of PCP use. The smoker can control the drug's effects better than the pilltaker can.

The reactions to PCP are singularly unpredictable. Most users report that their first experience was a pleasant one. "I feel wired," "I feel powerful," "I feel superior," are typical testimonies. But there are plenty of bad trips. According to one researcher, PCP can make Grimm's fairy-tale characters come to life. Parents, nurses, and doctors appear as monsters or witches, and police cars take on the form of dragons. Psychotic reactions mimic those of the paranoid schizophrenic and include hallucinatory voices and combative or self-destructive impulses. The drug can also give users a distorted sense of their own bodies; people often feel their arms or legs are growing or shriveling. Acute toxic reactions can last up to a week after a single dose, and the mental effects can linger for more than a month, often recurring in sudden episodes while the victim is apparently recovering. Taken in larger doses, PCP can induce seizures, coma, and death.

■ Inhalants

Inhalants are a group of diverse volatile substances people do not normally think of as drugs. The number of such substances is almost endless: model airplane glue, spray paint, gasoline, alcohol, cleaning fluid, nail polish, paint thinner, lighter fluid, hair spray, and just about anything else in an aerosol can. These legal substances, most of which are found in everyday household products, are abused by sniffing or inhaling. The desired effect is a euphoric high with mild hallucinations. During and shortly after inhalant use, the sniffer usually exhibits motor incoordination, inability to think and act clearly, and sometimes abusive and violent behavior. Abuse is on the rise among young people, especially between the ages of 7 and 17, no doubt in part because inhalants are readily available and inexpensive.

By and large inhalants are poisonous and very dangerous. Much of their intoxicating effect comes from cutting off oxygen to the brain or affecting the heart or lungs. Risk of death by suffocation increases when users sniff concentrated spray fumes from a paper or plastic bag. Most deaths, however, have been associated with the propellants used in aerosol sprays. Studies of long-term users of sprays and inhalants have disclosed bone marrow damage, kidney damage, drastic weight loss, and impairment of vision and memory. Fortunately, these serious dysfunctions cease when sniffing stops.

■■■ STIMULANTS

Stimulants are a class of drugs that stimulate the central nervous system. They usually relieve drowsiness and disguise the effects of fatigue and exhaustion. The stronger stimulants typically produce euphoria. Stimulants of chief concern and interest are the amphetamines, cocaine, and caffeine.

■ Amphetamines

Amphetamines, or "uppers" (for example, Benzedrine, Dexedrine, and Methedrine), are prescribed by physicians for minimal brain damage and narcolepsy. Their use in weight control is considered "bad medicine," and some states make it illegal for a physician to prescribe amphetamines for this purpose. These drugs speed up the action of the central nervous system, in contrast with barbiturates, which slow it down. The initial effect is to make the patient feel more alert and less tired. Larger amounts cause excitability, restlessness, unclear speech, tremor of the hands, euphoria or dysphoria, and insomnia. An acute psychosis sometimes develops.

Amphetamines are not legally available without a prescription, but they are available on the street and elsewhere. They are sometimes taken intravenously by serious users. More often they are taken orally. Some people take them for "kicks" and others in the mistaken belief that they increase efficiency. The American Medical Association has this to say on the subject:

Controlled studies have shown that amphetamines can drive trained athletes to increased performance in individual events involving strength and endurance. However, it has also been shown that this practice can, by artificially pushing the athlete beyond his normal endurance level, be harmful or even fatal. Using amphetamines for this purpose also violates principles of sportsmanship, and has been condemned by the American Medical Association and major amateur sports associations. . . .

It should be emphasized that amphetamines are not a magic source of extra mental or physical energy; they serve only to push the user to a greater expenditure of his own resources, sometimes to a hazardous point of fatigue that is often not recognized. Automobile or truck drivers, with or without amphetamines, who continue beyond their usual mental and physical capabilities risk their lives and the lives of others. Students who resort to the use of stimulants for all-night "cram" study sessions are not following sound educational practices and may find that although stimulants increase volubility during examinations, there is a concurrent loss of accuracy.*

---

*From J.A.M.A. **107**:1023, 1966.

Psychologic dependence is brought on rather easily. Tolerance develops and the dosage increases to high levels. The abuser is irritable, unreliable, and unstable, often with emotional deterioration. Abrupt withdrawal leaves the individual tired, sleepless, depressed, and in some cases potentially suicidal or homicidal.

■ Cocaine

Cocaine is a potent stimulant derived from the leaves of the South American tree, *Erythroxylon coca* (not related to the cacao tree from which cocoa and chocolate are derived). The Indians of the high plateau chew the leaves and get enough of the drug to still the pangs of hunger and help them forget fatigue. Cocaine, used medically as a local anesthetic, has a long and continuing history of being abused. It is used, often with heroin, to reduce the sense of fatigue and produce excitement and euphoria. The powder is sniffed, or it is dissolved and injected into a vein. Interestingly, cocaine does not produce physical dependence or tolerance. Withdrawal, however, leaves the subject deeply depressed.

Although infrequent and low-dosage use of cocaine produces few risks, regular or high-dosage use can have quite different results. Repeated inhalation often results in nostril and nasal mucous membrane irritation. Injection with nonsterile equipment can cause hepatitis or other infections. Some regular users experience restlessness, anxiety, irritability, and paranoia while on cocaine. Cocaine psychosis, characterized by hallucinations and paranoid fears, has been reported in heavy users who inject the drug. Cocaine is highly toxic. Overdose deaths from injected, oral, and snorted cocaine have occurred, a result of seizures followed by respiratory arrest and coma. Cardiac arrest sometimes occurs.

TABLE 22-1

Common sources of caffeine

Coffee (6 oz)	
Automatic drip	181 mg
Automatic perk	125 mg
Instant regular	54 mg
Decaffeinated	2 mg
Tea (6 oz) loose or bag	
One-minute brew	20 mg
Three-minute brew	35 mg
Soft drinks (12 oz)	
Mountain Dew	54 mg
Mello Yellow	51 mg
Dr. Pepper	38 mg
Pepsi Cola	38 mg
Diet Pepsi	34 mg
Coca Cola	33 mg
Tab	32 mg
RC Cola	26 mg
Fresca	0 mg
Hires Root Beer	0 mg
Sprite	0 mg
7-Up	0 mg
Cocoa (6 oz) from mix	10 mg
Chocolate	
Baking chocolate (1 oz)	45 mg
Milk chocolate candy (2 oz)	12 mg
Drugs	
Dexatrim capsules (Thompson)	200 mg/capsule
No-Doz tablets (Bristol-Meyers)	100 mg/tablet
Anacin (Whitehall)	32.5 mg/tablet
Midol (Glenbrook)	32.4 mg/tablet
Coricidin (Shering)	30 mg/tablet

Approximate values compiled from standard sources.

■ Caffeine

Caffeine is a naturally occuring stimulant that is found in the leaves, seeds, and fruit of more than 65 species of plants growing in all parts of the world. Coffee has been the greatest source of caffeine in the American diet since the Boston Tea Party more than 200 years ago. Tea, soft drinks, and cocoa follow coffee in order of popularity as food sources of caffeine (Table 22-1). In addition to the diet, an estimated 2000 over-the-counter drugs contain caffeine, including such popular products as Anacin, Excedrin, Midol, No-Doz, and Cope. Many prescription drugs contain caffeine, including Cafergot and Migral, used to treat migraine headaches, and Fiorinal, Darvon Compound, and Empirin Compound with Codeine, used as pain relievers.

Caffeine stimulates the central nervous system. It can help people stay awake, and it seems to reduce boredom created by dull or repetitive tasks. Caffeine appears to increase the body's muscle strength and the amount of time a person can perform physically exhausting work. It can also relieve certain types of headache by constricting the blood vessels and reducing muscle tension. On the negative side, many regular users of caffeine are dependent on its stimulant effects. Regular caffeine consumption equivalent to more than 4 cups of coffee per day can produce a form of dependence. If regular users abstain from caffeinated beverages for a day or two, many experience withdrawal symptoms, such as headaches, irritability, restlessness, or fatigue. But most disturbing is the revelation that caffeine may cause birth defects. Test results in mice, rats, chickens, and rabbits indicate that high doses of caffeine can cause birth defects, such as missing digits and cleft palates. Caffeine was also shown to increase premature births, spontaneous abortions, and stillbirths in the animals studied. Although more evidence is needed before final conclusions can be drawn, these animal test results suggest that pregnant women should be cautioned about their caffeine consumption. The Federal Drug Administration believes that pregnant women should be alert to products that have caffeine in them and should use them sparingly or avoid them altogether.

■ DRUG ABUSE PREVENTION

Drug abuse presents a serious problem to the citizens of any country. Millions of drug abusers not only are withdrawn from productive activities but also add to the national cost of medical care, to the disruption of families, and to the load of physical and mental suffering. What attitudes shall society take? Shall it say: "This is a free country; do what you like. Never mind your responsibility to society. When you become an addict, we will make you a ward of the state while you are under treatment or for life if you do not return to normal health"? Or should it say: "The abuse of drugs is destructive and antisocial. The possession, sale, and use of certain drugs is a crime, and the addict or habitual user will be treated as a criminal, either sick or well"?

In practice neither extreme is followed. The United States and most other advanced countries have made the unrestricted sale, the possession, and the use of specified dangerous drugs illegal. The passage of the Harrison Narcotic Act in 1914 was followed by a sharp reduction in drug abuse. Prior to this act, one person in 400 was dependent on an opiate. By the late 1930s the proportion was reduced to one in 4000. There was further legislation in 1937 and 1951, followed by the enactment of the Drug Abuse Control Amendments in 1965. The Comprehensive Drug Abuse Prevention and Control Act of 1970 established the Drug Enforcement Administration. This law and its subsequent amendments guide the federal regulation of dangerous drugs. They limit the manufacture, sale, and distribution of controlled drugs and the refilling of prescriptions, specifying criminal penalties for violations. Various state laws on drug control have also been passed.

There is no one answer to drug abuse. Authorities do, however, have some ideas about prevention that can be put to use. For example, one suggestion has been to help people develop strong personal values that will reduce the chances they will hurt themselves or others by abusing drugs. Drug abuse is not confined to youth, but if young people between the ages of 7 and 20 years can be prevented from abusing drugs, they are less likely to have serious drug problems when they grow older.

As parents we can raise our children to be thinking, caring adults who weigh the consequences of their actions and make sound decisions about drug use. We should set reasonable but firm limits to our children's behavior and teach them responsibility for their actions. **As persons who work with youth** (teachers, recreation workers, scout leaders) we can guide young people and help them make the difficult choices they face as they grow up. We should try to help them understand society's restrictions and avoid what is considered unacceptable behavior for the common good. **As citizens** we can get the community to offer activities that help young people develop without the need for drugs. Satisfying alternatives to experimentation with drugs are keys to drug abuse prevention. **As friends** we can be good listeners when our friends are in trouble. We should try to provide accurate and helpful information about drugs and their often dangerous effects.

It is not easy to be a good parent, to start a community program, or to be a real friend. And there are many social pressures affecting youth over which parents have no control. But parents can help young people discover their human potential and realize they need not turn to drugs for excitement or to solve their problems. The National Institute on Drug Abuse sponsors a National Drug Abuse Prevention Campaign designed to encourage people to become involved in prevention activities. The campaign has produced pamphlets, posters, and a community action manual, all obtainable from the National Clearinghouse for Drug Abuse Information.

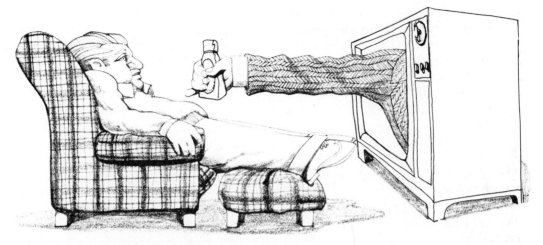

Fig. 22-3 ■ The BIG SELL of OTC medicines.

From FDA Consumer, December 1973-January 1974.

NONPRESCRIPTION DRUGS

Nonprescription, or over-the-counter (OTC), drugs—antacids, vitamin pills, headache remedies. laxatives, and the like—may not be a threat to life, but they certainly do threaten the pocketbook (Fig. 22-3). There are about 250,000 OTC drugs on the market. Each year the American public pays out over $5 billion for these products, many of which the Food and Drug Administration (FDA) has determined are largely ineffective. Put another way, it is essentially money down the drain. The FDA and other agencies are valuable in protecting against quackery, but it is the individual citizen who can do most to put quackery out of business. This means education, and we need a lot of it. For example, according to a recent FDA survey three fourths of the American public believe that extra vitamins provide more pep and energy. This is false. The body needs and can use only a certain amount of any vitamin and merely stores or excretes any excess. Furthermore, protracted megadosing of some vitamins—namely, A and D—can prove dangerous.

The admonitions against OTC drugs, however, must be tempered by common sense. That is, there are indeed OTC drugs—typically the least expensive—that have established value. Plain aspirin is an excellent analgesic; tincture of iodine is an excellent antiseptic; witch hazel is an excellent rubbing lotion; ipecac syrup is an excellent antidote; and so on. Such items are useful to have in the medicine cabinet.

DMSO

Dimethyl sulfoxide (DMSO) is a colorless by-product of wood pulp and paper manufacturing that has won a place in medicine cabinets across the land as a sort of all-purpose liniment for pulls, sprains, bruises, and the pain and swelling of gout and arthritis. Smeared on a sore ankle or stiff shoulder, DMSO finds its way into the bloodstream within minutes. To some doctors it is a wonder drug; others liken it to snake oil. All agree that under some circumstances it can be dangerous; it can carry poisons into the bloodstream or perhaps disrupt the body's immune system. Above all, the long-term effects of the chemical are simply not known. The Food and Drug Administration has refused to approve DMSO for any human use except to relieve the pain of a rare bladder disease called inter-stitial cystitis. Nonetheless, a number of states have passed special laws to allow doctors to prescribe DMSO for a variety of conditions and disorders. Perhaps the best advice is en-capsulated by the Latin phrase "caveat emp-tor," or "let the buyer beware."

SELF-TEST

1. __B__ opium
2. __H__ morphine
3. __O__ mescaline
4. __I__ barbiturate
5. __A__ tranquilizer
6. __M__ marijuana
7. __K__ phencyclidine
8. __J__ inhalant
9. __L__ amphetamine
10. __N__ local anesthetic
11. __D__ caffeine
12. __E__ increased dosage
13. __G__ psychologic dependence
14. __F__ physical dependence
15. __C__ narcotic treatment

a. Valium
b. codeine
c. methadone
d. Pepsi
e. tolerance
f. addiction
g. habituation
h. heroin
i. "downer"
j. model glue
k. "angel dust"
l. "upper"
m. THC
n. cocaine
o. peyote

STUDY QUESTIONS

1. What is the difference between "drug abuse" and "drug misuse"?
2. The effects of a drug depend on a number of variables. Name three such variables and dis-cuss each.
3. What is the difference between "drug habitu-ation" and "drug addiction"?
4. What is the significance of "drug tolerance"?
5. In your personal view why do people take drugs?
6. Do you see any difference between drinking alcoholic beverages and taking drugs?
7. What is the relationship among the following: opium, morphine, codeine, and heroin?
8. Sedatives and hypnotics are often one and the same drug. Explain.
9. What is the difference between a "minor tran-quilizer" and a "major tranquilizer"?
10. What is the relationship between hallucino-gens and psychedelic drugs?

11. What do all drugs classed as hallucinogens have in common?
12. Discuss the chemistry and effects of LSD and PCP.
13. What is the relationship among the following terms: *Cannabis sativa*, marijuana, hashish, delta-9-tetrahydrocannabinol, and THC?
14. In terms of acute poisoning inhalants probably are the most dangerous of abused chemicals. Why?
15. What do all stimulant drugs have in common?
16. Compare the effects of amphetamines and co-caine.
17. What are the major effects of caffeine?
18. A number of over-the-counter medications contain caffeine. Why?
19. Tea leaves contain more caffeine than ground coffee. How, then, do you explain the greater amount of caffeine in a cup of coffee than in a cup of tea?

20. On a typical day (referring to Table 22-1) about how much caffeine do you consume?

21. Several points were raised in the text concerning drug abuse prevention. What are your views on the points raised, and do you have further suggestions?

22. What are your views on the legalization of marijuana?

23. What are your views on the use of nonprescription, or over-the-counter, drugs?

24. What are your views on prescription drugs (those that the doctor prescribes)? For example, are they always prescribed wisely?

25. Do you have any comment on drug use—legal or illegal—not mentioned in the text or suggested in the questions?

CHAPTER 23

Medical care

The first requirement in the maintenance of the human mechanism, as in the case of a less complicated automotive or engineering mechanism, is proper operation and care. But similar also is its need for an occasional checkup and for repair in case of accident or the partial or complete breakdown of a part. In the rapidly changing world of medicine what is the patient-physician relationship? Who are the people involved in the medical care of the nation? What is the best procedure for securing and financing the medical care needed by the individual and the family? What advance planning is needed against the eventuality of illness? What dangers are involved when planning is unwise or neglected? What steps are being taken by government or society in the organization and provision of medical care? What about the use of drugs, prescription and nonprescription? What about good medical care for all of our older citizens? In the present chapter we are going to take a look at the answers to these and other questions related to our medical care.

Health care professionals

The medical checkup

Hospitals

Drugs and medical devices

Medical costs

Private health care

Tax-supported health care

National health insurance

The older generation

Nursing homes

Cults and quackery

Acupuncture

Holistic health care

Medical care is a vast business, and all of us have much to learn about the various services involved and about the people who deliver these services. This is especially true when we consider the fact that just about everything tends to change. That is to say, we must keep up with new developments. Furthermore, medical care involves topics beyond the services per se, for example, insurance, proper drug use, cults and quackery, and medical devices. These and other topics are discussed in the following pages.

HEALTH CARE PROFESSIONALS

Professional manpower in the field of health care includes chiropractors, dentists, dental hygienists, licensed practical nurses, pharmacists, physical therapists, physicians, podiatrists, registered nurses, and a host of others (Table 23-1). In the United States counts of these professionals include only those licensed in the state where they practice, with licensure usually requiring the completion of an appropriate degree or certificate program for that profession (Fig. 23-1). In international counts prepared by the World Health Organization only those professionals active in their profession are counted. Professionals may be classified according to specialty, place of practice, or other criteria.

Physicians are at the top of the manpower pyramid, and for most purposes they lead the health team in the delivery of medical care. There are over 400,000 active physicians in the United States, or two thirds more today than there were in 1960. The long-term trend toward increased physician specialization has meant a decline in general practice and an increase in specialty practice. In 1930 fully 75% of physicians were engaged in delivering primary care, including general practice, general internal medicine, and pediatrics. By 1969

the proportion of physicians delivering primary care dropped to a low of 38%, roughly where it remains today. This development has been an outgrowth of (1) the vast expansion of knowledge and the introduction of new technology in medical fields, (2) the active support of medical research on the part of medical schools, and (3) the clinical training physicians receive in the hospital setting, among other factors. About 92% of physicians are involved in direct patient care, and the remain-

TABLE 23-1

Estimated number of persons active in selected health occupations, 1983

Occupation	Number of persons active
Clinical laboratory services	300,000
Dentistry and allied services	375,000
Dentist (D.D.S)	125,000
Dental hygienist	40,000
Dental assistant	150,000
Dental laboratory technician	50,000
Dietetic and nutritional services	90,000
Health education	30,000
Medicine	430,000
Doctor of medicine (M.D.)	410,000
Doctor of osteopathy (D.O.)	20,000
Midwifery	5,000
Nursing and related services	3,000,000
Registered nurse (RN)	1,065,000
Pratical nurse (LPN)	525,000
Nursing aide, orderly, attendant	1,100,000
Home health aide	125,000
Occupational therapy	26,800
Optometry	37,000
Pharmacy	140,000
Physical therapy	33,000
Physician extender services	10,000
Podiatric medicine	10,000
Psychology	110,000
Respiratory therapy	30,000
Specialized rehabilitation services	15,000

Data from U.S. Department of Health and Human Services, National Center for Health Statistics: Health-resources and utilization statistics.

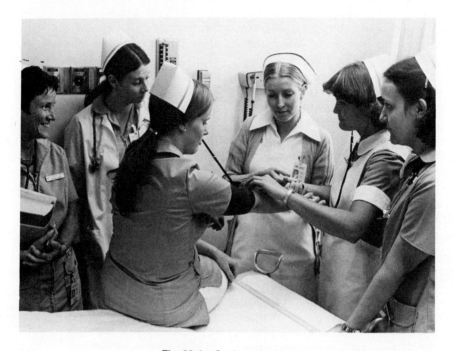

Fig. 23-1 ■ Student nurses.

der are engaged in administration, research, teaching, and other activities. An estimated 10% percent are women.

A physician is either a licensed doctor of medicine (M.D.) or a doctor of osteopathy (D.O.). A physician's specialty is any specific branch of medicine that a physician may concentrate in. The specialty classification used by the Bureau of Health Professions and the National Ambulatory Medical Care Survey (NAMCS) follows the American Medical Association categories. **Primary care** specialties include general practice (or family practice), internal medicine, and pediatrics. **Medical specialties** include, along with internal medicine and pediatrics, the areas of allergy, cardiovascular disease, dermatology, gastroenterology, pediatric allergy and cardiology, and pulmonary diseases. **Surgical specialties** include general surgery, neurologic surgery, obstetrics and gynecology, ophthalmology, orthopedic surgery, otolaryngology, plastic surgery, colon and rectal surgery, thoracic

surgery, and urology. Other specialties covered by NAMCS are geriatrics, neurology, preventive medicine, psychiatry, and public health. Other specialties covered by the Bureau of Health Professions include aerospace medicine, anesthesiology, child psychiatry, neurology, occupational medicine, pathology, physical medicine and rehabilitation, psychiatry, public health, and radiology.

■■■■ THE MEDICAL CHECKUP

The medical checkup is the key to preventive medicine; that is, it is the opportunity for the physician to advise during health and to check early signs of deviation from the normal. Larger numbers of persons are visiting their physicians than ever before (private and public health insurance is a contributing factor inasmuch as it helps to pay the bills), and as a result we are seeing a major decline in neonatal, postnatal, and infant mortality (Fig. 23-2) as well as a decline in death rates in in-

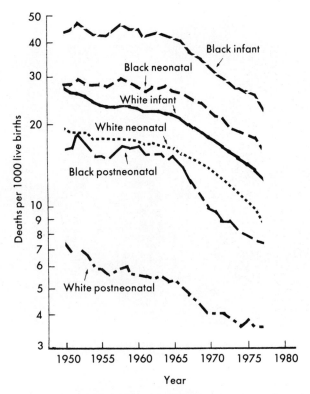

Fig. 23-2 ■ Infant, neonatal, and postneonatal mortality, according to race, in the United States, 1950-1977.

Computed by the National Center for Health Statistics, Division of Analysis, from data compiled by the Division of Vital Statistics.

fluenza, pneumonia, heart disease, diabetes, and a number of other diseases.

Typically, the initial visit to the **primary care physician** (an internist, a specialist in adolescent and adult medicine; a pediatrician, a child care specialist; or a family practitioner) involves establishing a "rapport" between doctor and patient. A good doctor-patient relationship is based on mutual respect and open communication. The patient owes the doctor cooperation and honesty in order to receive expert advice and/or treatment. If the doctor does not seem competent, thorough, and willing to listen, the patient should not hesitate to find someone else. Indeed, "shopping for a doctor" is not an uncommon practice.

At the first meeting the patient's **health history** is taken (past health problems, childhood diseases, parents' health status, etc.), and his or her eating, drinking, smoking, and sleeping habits, allergies, and any medications being taken are recorded and kept on file. This information is usually gone over by doctor and patient together. A complete **physical examination** follows (including measurement of height and weight [Fig. 23-3], blood pressure, and pulse, as well as blood screening, urinalysis, electrocardiogram, and sometimes chest x-ray). When the **laboratory reports** are completed, the doctor sends a summary to the patient and points out any abnormalities or problems that deserve further attention.

At the time of the first visit the patient should not be reluctant to inquire about office procedures: office hours, how to make an appointment, routine fees, method of payment

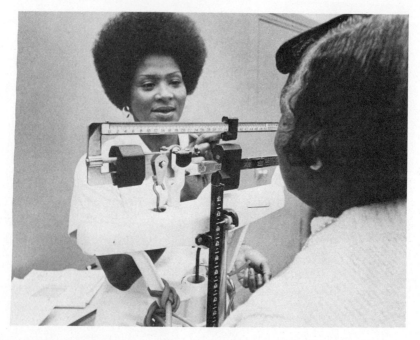

Fig. 23-3 ■ Measurement of weight is a basic feature of the physical examination.

Courtesy Johns Hopkins Medical Institutions.

of bills, whether or not the physician makes house calls, and what to do in an emergency. In addition, on this and subsequent visits the patient should bring along a list of any questions and specific information the doctor might need in order to make a proper diagnosis.

The primary care physician may practice alone or with a group. Oftentimes in large cities and suburbs doctors pool their services and share common offices, laboratory equipment, and other facilities. One doctor from the group continues a certain patient's medical care, and when that doctor is unavailable, one of the others of the group will be the "covering" physician. In this manner health care services become available twenty-four hours a day.

How often an individual should have a checkup usually turns out to be a matter of personal choice. Many physicians recommend the "yearly checkup" while others feel the frequency depends on a combination of factors, such as a person's age and general health. In any case it is a good idea for an adult to maintain a doctor-patient relationship with a regular 1-, 2-, or 3-year checkup (and put preventive medicine into practice). Medical supervision is a must for expectant mothers, infants, and very young children. And, certainly, chronic conditions should not be neglected.

Unfortunately, approximately 10% of Americans seeking medical help are unable to get it for one reason or another. Aside from the high cost, one of the most important reasons is the uneven geographic distribution of physicians. For example, the highest ratios of physicians to population are found in the District of Columbia, New York, Massachusetts, Maryland, and Connecticut, in that order; the lowest ratios are found in South Dakota, Mississippi, Wyoming, and Ohio. Hospital personnel and local medical societies (listed in the telephone directory) can direct the newcomer to the type of physician he is seeking.

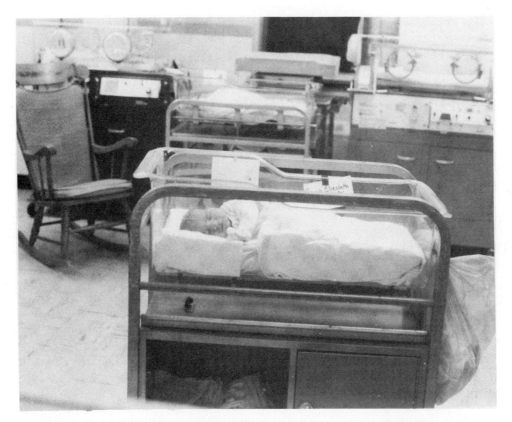

Fig. 23-4 ■ Special care for the newborn is provided in the typical general hospital. Rocking chair underscores confluence of the old and the new.

HOSPITALS

There are approximately 7000 general hospitals in the country that must meet standards set by the National Commission on Accreditation of Hospitals. Hospitals may be classified by type of service, ownership, and length of stay.

General hospitals provide both diagnostic and treatment services for patients with a variety of medical conditions, both surgical and nonsurgical. According to the World Health Organization, these are hospitals that provide medical and nursing care for more than one category, or medical discipline (for example, general medicine, specialized medicine, general surgery, specialized surgery, obstetrics,

and so on) (Fig. 23-4); excluded are hospitals, usually in rural areas, that provide a more limited range of care. **Specialty hospitals** provide a particular type of service to the majority of their patients (for example, there are hospitals for psychiatric illness, tuberculosis, chronic disease, rehabilitation, maternity care, and alcoholic or narcotic addiction).

Proprietary hospitals are operated by individuals, partnerships, or corporations for profit. **Voluntary nonprofit hospitals** are operated by a church or other nonprofit organization. **Federal hospitals** are operated by the federal government. **Nonfederal government hospitals** are operated by state or local governments.

Short-stay hospitals in the National Hospital Discharge Survey are those in which the average length of stay is less than 30 days. The American Hospital Association and National Master Facility Inventory define short-term hospitals as hospitals in which more than half the patients are admitted to units with an average stay of less than 30 days, and they define **long-term hospitals** as those in which more than half the patients are admitted to units with an average stay of 30 days or more. The National Health Interview Survey defines the short-stay hospital as any hospital or hospital department in which the type of service provided is general: maternity; eye, ear, nose, and throat; pediatric; or osteopathic.

◼◼ DRUGS AND MEDICAL DEVICES

According to the United States Food and Drug Administration, consumers spend billions and billions of dollars each year on all sorts of drugs and devices, including items such as food supplements, cures for "tired blood," cures for baldness, cures for impotency, cures for arthritis, cures for cancer, preparations for anemia, preparations to eradicate wrinkles, preparations to erase freckles, cold remedies, sleeping aids, weight-loss products, muscle builders, waist trimmers, and bust developers. The list is endless. Often these items produce questionable results, and some are hazardous to health as well as a waste of money.

◼ Drugs

Drug use constitutes a major problem in the United States. This does not mean that people should not use medications when necessary; rather, they should be more knowledgeable in the proper use. A person's health can be protected, and accidents or illness can be prevented by knowing the best ways to buy and use drugs.

There are two basic types of drugs (Chapter 22): over-the-counter (OTC) and prescription (℞). OTC drugs (also known as patent medicines) include common remedies such as aspirin, laxatives, and antacids. If used according to the directions on the label, they are relatively safe. OTC drugs can be purchased without a prescription in drug stores and in many supermarkets. Prescription drugs (which bear the symbol ℞) can be ordered or prescribed only by a physician and sold only by a registered pharmacist (druggist). Generally more powerful than OTC drugs, prescription items are also more likely to cause side effects.

Before purchasing an OTC medicine, a person should decide whether or not he or she needs it and should scrutinize the labels carefully, asking the pharmacist for advice if necessary. Pharmacists are well-trained professionals who can help their customers understand how to buy and use drugs. People should not be reluctant to ask for help—their health may be at stake.

The following information is required by federal law on all OTC drug labels: name of the product; name and address of the manufacturer, packer, or distributor; active ingredients; directions for safe use; and cautions or warnings. (These latter tell what side effects might occur and what persons should not take the drug at all.)

When the doctor gives a prescription, the patient should write down the name of the drug and when and how often it should be taken. Also, the patient should ask whether this is the least expensive form of the medicine, whether it can be taken along with other drugs, what effects can be expected, and what precautions can be taken. It should also be established if the prescription can be refilled and whether or not all of the medicine should be taken.

Some basic rules for drug safety include the following:

1. Take exactly the amount of drug prescribed by the doctor and follow the dosage schedule as closely as possible.
2. Never take drugs prescribed for a friend or relative, even though your symptoms may be the same. (Medicines do not produce the same effects in all persons.)
3. Always tell the doctor about past problems you had with drugs and be sure to mention other drugs, including OTC drugs, that you are taking.
4. Keep a daily record of the drug you are taking, especially if your treatment schedule is complicated or you are taking more than one drug at a time.
5. Keep easy-to-open containers out of the reach of children.
6. Be sure that you understand the directions printed on the drug container and that the name of the drug is clearly printed.
7. Throw out old medicines, particularly prescription drugs. If your doctor takes you off a medicine before it is used up, destroy what is left.
8. Ask the doctor about special rules for storage and about which foods or beverages, if any, to avoid.
9. Always call your doctor promptly if you notice unusual reactions.
10. When traveling, be sure you take enough prescription drugs to last on a long trip.

■ Medical devices

There are all kinds of testimonials used in magazine, newspaper, radio, and television advertising that promise new shapes, new looks, and new happiness to those who buy the preparation, the device, or the prescribed program of action. The promoters of such products make claims that often are nothing more than money-making schemes and hazards to a person's health as well as to the pocketbook.

When it comes to any treatment, device, program, or product being promoted to make the body beautiful, buyers should beware. They should learn all the facts—potential hazards as well as potential benefits. They should be especially cautious of products or treatments that promise amazing results in a very short time.

In 1976 the public began to receive some protection when the Medical Devices Amendments were enacted by the federal government. Up until that time the Federal Drug Administration (FDA) had no authority to require premarket approval of medical devices for safety and effectiveness. The 1976 amendments gave the FDA significant new authority to regulate these devices. All devices that are implanted in the body and all life-supporting devices now require premarket approval by the FDA, and the FDA can ban devices that are deceptive as well as a risk or impairment to health. The FDA can also ban a product if the manufacturer fails to substantiate claims about what the product will do. But with some 8000 different types of medical devices in use, it will be some time yet before every one can be brought under scrutiny. Of course, those that are most vital to human health have been given top priority.

In addition to the FDA watchdog agencies, there are the Federal Trade Commission (FTC) and the United States Postal Service. The public at large can help combat the problem by reporting to one of these agencies any product that has not lived up to its promise or has caused any injury to a person's health.

■■■ MEDICAL COSTS

Spending for personal health care in the nation amounted to about $287 billion in 1982 (or more than $1200 per person). This sum includes all outlays for health and medical services for the direct benefit of the individual, including both public and private spending. The largest portion of the personal health care dollar is financed by third-party sources. Private health insurance, philanthropy, industry, and the government paid 70% of all expenditures for personal health care in 1982. Personal health care figures include expenditures of all consumers, whether insured or not. Included are expenses for nonprescription drugs and medicines, household supplies such as tissues and rubbing alcohol, and other items not covered by insurance. In terms of the growth of personal health care components, hospital care has been one of the fastest growing categories of expenditures. In 1965 monies spent for hospital care represented 39% of personal health care expenses. By 1982 the proportion rose to 45%.

The demand is growing for expensive professional and technical services as the population becomes better educated and continues to spend more for personal health care. Utilization of care is increasing with the growth and aging of the population. Incomes are higher, and health insurance coverage is better. The nature of health care itself is changing as medical technology advances, bringing with it expensive equipment, costly techniques, and innumerable skills of the highest order. Modern scientific medical diagnosis and treatment come with a high price tag that everyone must face sooner or later.

▮▮▮▮ PRIVATE HEALTH CARE

Health insurance protects against accidents and illness. It may cover all or part of major hospitalization expenses and the cost of physicians' services. It may cover dental care, prescription drugs, and nursing care. Approximately 169 million Americans, under age 65, or nearly 9 out of 10, carry **private health insurance**. Many persons over 65 years supplement or extend their benefits from Medicare (p. 348) with private insurance. It is estimated that 18 to 26 million individuals do not have any private health insurance. There are a variety of reasons for this, and not all are economic. Some think it is too expensive (even though they could easily afford it). Others believe there is no need for it because they have always been in "good health." A substantial number do not have insurance because they are unemployed. According to the U.S. Congressional Budget Office (report on the uninsured population), young adults are almost twice as likely as any other group to be without coverage, and among employed persons those earning lesser incomes are most likely to be without coverage.

Various forms of private health insurance coverage are available from several types of insurers: insurance companies; hospital and medical service plans, such as Blue Cross and Blue Shield; group medical plans operating on a prepayment basis, such as Health Maintenance Organizations; and others.

Over 1200 private insurance companies in the United States write individual and/or group health insurance policies covering more than 104 million persons annually. Policies issued by insurance companies provide for payment directly to the insured or, if assigned by the insured, to the provider of services for reimbursement of expenses incurred. Health insurance coverage made available by insurance companies can be divided into two basic categories: medical expense insurance and disability income insurance. Medical expense insurance is a "reimbursement type" of coverage that provides broad benefits for virtually all expenses connected with hospital and medical care and related services. Disability income insurance provides periodic payments when the insured is unable to work as a result of sickness or injury.

The Blue Cross Association and the Blue Shield Association are coordinating bodies for the nation's Blue Cross and Blue Shield plans. These nonprofit member plans serve statewide and other geographical areas, offering both individual and group coverage. Blue Cross plans provide hospital care benefits on essentially a "service type" basis, under which the organization, through a separate contract with member hospitals, reimburses the hospitals for covered services rendered to the insured. Blue Shield plans provide benefits for surgical and medical services performed by a physician. The typical Blue Shield plan provides benefits similar to those provided under the benefit provisions of hospital-surgical policies issued by insurance companies. Today there are some 68 Blue Cross plans and 67 Blue Shield plans in the country. Of these, many are joint plans, making a total of well over 100 Blue Cross and Blue Shield plans.

Health care coverage is also provided through Health Maintenance Organizations (HMOs), which provide comprehensive health care services for their members (9.2 million) for a fixed periodic payment. In such plans a group of physicians, surgeons, dentists, or optometrists furnish needed care as specified in the contract to subscribers. The Ross-Loos Clinic, established in 1930 in Los Angeles, California, paved the way for the almost 200 certified HMOs in existence today (there are scores of others in the process of becoming established). In 1973 the federal government began to subsidize HMOs (through the Health Maintenance Organization Act) as a measure to stem the tide of rising health care costs by keeping people out of hospitals. Once an HMO is financially self-sufficient, the government withdraws its support.

Certain types of health insurance coverage are also made available by plans that are administered by employers or labor unions, fraternal societies, communities, or rural and consumer health cooperatives. Usually the protection provided by these groups is the amount desired and affordable by a specific group of people.

It is estimated that some 20% of group coverage is represented by Administrative Service Only (ASO) arrangements and Minimum Premium Plans (MPPs). Under these systems corporations and other organizations can establish self-funded health plans. Insurance carriers or private organizations are paid a fee by the self-funding group to process the claims and benefits paperwork and insure against a certain level of large, unpredictable claims. These types of arrangements represent approximately 18% of total insurance company group coverage.

◼◼◼ TAX-SUPPORTED HEALTH CARE

Medical and health care services are provided through a variety of public programs by all levels of government. In addition, the federal, state, and local government agencies often fund research projects and construct medical facilities with public funds. Of the more than 200 billion dollars spent each year on national health care, some 91 billion covers health and medical care programs at all levels of government. As the number of programs funded by public monies has multiplied and expanded, so, too, has the public share of national health expenditures (about 45%). The introduction of Medicare produced the largest single-year increase in 1967, during which governmental expenditures rose from 25% to over 33% of national health expenditures. Before 1967 state and local expenditures for health care exceeded those of the federal government. In 1979 federal expenditures were double those of state and local governments. Most of this federal health spending is for health services to persons over 65 years of age (Medicare), to low-income individuals and others eligible for Medicaid services, to federal civilian employees, to native Americans, to military personnel and their dependents, and to veterans.

Federal medical care for the indigent was first provided in 1935 under the federal **Social Security Act**, which established medical services for aged persons, blind persons, and dependent children; subsequently these benefits were extended to the permanently disabled. Under this act the aged included any person 65 years of age or older whose income was below a specified amount deemed adequate for self-support or support of the person's family. In 1960 the **Kerr-Mills Act** broadened federal medical assistance to include persons over 65 not on relief but who were unable to meet their medical expenses. Federal grants were made to states that enacted medical programs that met certain conditions set by the federal legislation.

■ Medicare

On July 30, 1965, monumental legislation was passed by Congress that appreciably expanded the Kerr-Mills program. Effective July 1, 1966, **Health Insurance for the Aged** (Title XVIII), popularly known as **Medicare**, provided certain benefits for those persons 65 years of age, regardless of income, and for certain persons under 65 years with severe disabilities and chronic kidney disease. Administered by the Social Security Administration (Fig. 23-5), the program is divided into two parts: (1) compulsory hospitalization insurance (Part A, or HI) and (2) voluntary supplementary medical insurance (Part B, or SMI). Part A is financed by contributions from employees, employers, and self-employed persons to Social Security. Part B is voluntary and financed by monthly premiums paid jointly by those who choose to enroll and by the federal government.

Part A helps pay the cost of hospital care for up to 90 days, the patient paying a certain amount for the first 60 days; for days 61 to 90 the insurance covers all services except for another small amount per day. The hospital insurance also provides for 100 days of care in a nursing home, visits to the patient's home by a part-time nurse, and certain diagnostic tests. These basic benefits do not cover private-duty nurses, services or supplies that are not necessary for diagnosis or treatment of an injury, physicians' fees (which may be covered under Part B), or convenience items (television, radio, and the like).

Part B extends the individual's Medicare benefits to include surgery and some other physician's services. A fixed monthly premium is paid for this but changes when there is an increase in Social Security cash benefits. Eighty percent of the physician's and surgeon's bills, certain specified nursing care, and some other benefits are covered. The insured individual pays the first $60 of expenses in each calendar year. Not covered are services or supplies that are not necessary for diagnosis

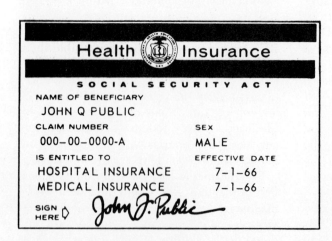

Fig. 23-5 ■ Medicare identification card.

or treatment of an illness or injury, routine physical checkups, prescription drugs, patent medicines, eyeglasses and eye examinations to fit glasses, hearing aids and examinations for hearing aids, dentures and routine dental care, and so on.

■ Medicaid

Medicaid is provided for under Title XIX of the Social Security Act. This program, which supplies medical assistance for certain low-income individuals and families, became law in 1965. Medicaid is basically administered by each state within certain broad federal requirements and guidelines. It is financed jointly by state and federal funds and is designed to provide medical assistance to those groups or categories of persons who are eligible to receive payment under one of the cash assistance programs (that is, Aid to Families with Dependent Children and Supplemental Security Income). Additionally, states may provide Medicaid to the "medically needy," that is, to persons who fit into one of the categories eligible for public assistance, who have enough income to pay for their basic living expenses but not enough to pay for their medical care. According to present figures, thirty-one states, plus Guam, Puerto Rico, and the Virgin Islands, have granted Medicaid eligibility to their "medically needy" populations.

Many members of the Medicaid population are aged or disabled and are also covered by Medicare. In cases where this dual coverage exists, most state Medicaid programs pay for the Medicare premiums, deductibles, and co-payments, and for services not covered by Medicare. State participation in the Medicaid program is optional. Currently, all states except Arizona have Medicaid programs. The District of Columbia, Guam, Puerto Rico, and the Virgin Islands also provide Medicaid coverage.

■ Other programs

The Federal Employee Health Benefits program and the Retired Federal Employees Health Benefits program provide health insurance coverage for active and retired civilian federal workers. The premiums are paid by both the employer and the employee. More than 734,000 American Indians and Alaskan natives are entitled to medical care in Public Health Service hospitals. Military personnel on active duty or after retiring from the service receive free medical care, as do members of the U.S. Merchant Marine. Medical care is provided by the Veterans Administration for honorably discharged veterans for any condition incurred or activated while in service and for nonservice-inflicted disabilities on proof that the veteran is not able to pay for the treatment. All active and retired military personnel and their dependents are eligible for medical treatment at any Department of Defense (DOD) installation medical facility. Additionally, the Civilian Health and Medical Program for the Uniformed Services (CHAMPUS) provides medical care (in civilian facilities) to the wives and children of military personnel on active duty, to retired military personnel and their dependents, and to dependents of deceased military personnel.

The federal government each year pays millions of dollars in hospital and medical benefits and administrative expenses under Workers' Compensation laws in the various states. Hospital and medical costs amount to about one-third of all Workers' Compensation expenditures.

Medical services are provided by the federal, state, and local governments in the case of certain diseases. Tax-supported hospitals provide psychiatric care and clinics for alcoholism, drug addiction, and venereal disease. In Carville, Louisiana, the federal government operates a hospital for leprosy. Public health programs of state health agencies are concerned with personal health, environmental health, health resources, and laboratory services. The largest expenditures of the state health agencies fall into the following categories: general and supporting personal health, maternal and child health, communicable disease, handicapped children, dental health, chronic disease, mental health and related programs, state institutions, and other personal health services (home health care and services to special population groups such as migrants). There were some 3100 local health departments in the United States in 1981. The territories and possessions (with the exception of Puerto Rico), three states, and the District of Columbia are without local health departments.

▰▰ NATIONAL HEALTH INSURANCE

The United States faces a crisis in providing quality health care to every individual at a reasonable price. Many persons face financial disaster in the wake of serious illness. National health insurance has become more visible as an issue each year.

In 1945 the Wagner-Murray Dingell Bill introduced for the first time in American history a proposal for health insurance for the entire American populace. After its defeat and the defeat of several other bills, President Truman created the President's Commission On the Health Needs of the Nation in 1951. This was another "first" in the nation's history, and in 1952 the commission presented the historic report, "Building America's Health." Various proposals (the Kennedy-Mills Bill, Corman-Kennedy Bill, Long-Ribicoff Bill) have been offered to policy makers in recent decades, differing essentially in the means of financing such a health program.

According to surveys conducted by the Health Insurance Institute, the number of persons who have heard a fair amount or anything at all about national health insurance increased from 25% in 1978 to 32% in 1980.

While awareness has risen, it is noteworthy that 68% of the public had heard little or nothing at all about the issue in 1980. This suggests that for the majority of the population national health insurance is not a salient issue. Predictably, awareness of national health insurance as an issue is strongly related to education and income. Fifty-nine percent of college graduates (in the same survey) had heard something about national health insurance, compared to 18% of those persons who had not completed high school and 30% of high school graduates.

The survey also showed that people with family incomes above average are more likely to have heard about national health insurance (43%) than those with lesser yearly incomes. Age is also a factor: young people between the ages of 18 to 24 showed significantly less awareness of national health insurance (15%) than did the rest of the population (35%). The Health Insurance Institute survey indicated that 41% of the people supported a national health insurance program that would be accompanied by an increase in taxes, 24% opposed such a program, and 36% had no strong opinion. Of this latter group, more than half leaned toward supporting a national health insurance program.

Perhaps even more significant than support for national health insurance is the issue of just what kind of program would be supported by the public. While there are many different elements to be considered (for example, who should be covered, how should such a program be administered, what type of services should be covered), one basic distinction to be made is between (1) a program that would cover people only for catastrophic medical expenses and (2) a comprehensive plan that would cover people for nearly all their health care costs. Surveys show that since 1979 there has been a significant decline in public support for a comprehensive health insurance program and an increase in support for a catastrophic program.

An American Medical Association survey showed recently that support for national health insurance is sensitive to cost considerations. When costs are not considered, 67% of the public in the 1979 survey said there was a need for national health insurance. When costs were considered, support dropped to 42%.

A Louis Harris survey found that 48% of the public favor a program that would be run by both the government and private health insurance companies. Twenty-one percent of the persons interviewed in the survey wanted the program to be run completely by the federal government, and 18% said it should be run solely by health insurance companies.

Although these surveys phrase their questions differently, the results taken together confirm a public mood that has reservations about a major health insurance program if it is costly, raises taxes, or is run entirely by the federal government.

■■■ THE OLDER GENERATION

Thanks to modern medicine and public health, most of us can expect old age to come to our parents and eventually to us. Today (and in the future) we need an abundance of understanding of and consideration for the burgeoning personal and social problems that accompany the growing elderly population. Just a quick look at the figures is proof enough of what we face today and what lies ahead. In 1900, 4% of the population in the United States was age 65 and over. In 1980 this figure jumped to 11%, and the United States Census Bureau projects that by the year 2030 the age group 65 and over will constitute 20% of the population. Medical care, medical costs, nutrition, nursing homes, housing, social relations, and community status are a few of the problems facing the elderly that need to be dealt with not only by government agencies but also by society itself.

Finding the best possible medical (and den-

tal) care, a difficult search at any time of life, becomes more difficult just when people begin to need it most: after they reach age 60 or 70. The older person needs a doctor who is aware of the special needs and problems of the elderly. But finding such a physician may not be easy because doctors in the United States do not routinely receive special training in the care of the elderly. **Geriatrics**, the study of the care of the aged, has only recently begun to be included in medical school curricula (Fig. 23-6). Geriatrics is not a separate medical specialty such as pediatrics or cardiology. As a start toward finding a doctor who has a special interest in treating older persons, the county medical society or state agency on aging can be helpful. Other possible sources of information include local referral services, medical schools, and university medical centers.

After establishing a doctor-patient relationship, the older person should consult the doctor about eating habits, especially if any chronic illnesses might require changes in the person's diet. Good nutrition is important to people of all ages, but older persons in particular may have questions about what they should eat to maintain their health. Many health problems of the elderly are the result of poor nutrition. Researchers supported by The National Institute on Aging (p. 352) are studying nutrient intake and requirements of older persons, changes in taste and smell with aging, behavior aspects of dietary habits, and the influence of nutrition on health in the "golden years." Through such research they hope to gain a better understanding of how diet and the aging process affect one another.

The financial barriers to medical services for the older citizen have been broken down substantially through Medicare (p. 348) and Medicaid (p. 349) along with coverage from private health insurance plans. Income no longer determines utilization of medical services. The result has been a substantial de-

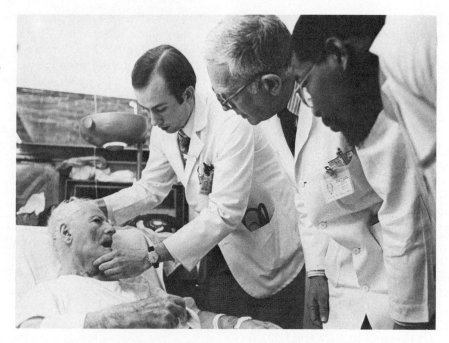

Fig. 23-6 ■ Geriatrics is a growing field of interest in medical education.

Courtesy Johns Hopkins Medical Institutions.

cline in heart disease, the leading cause of death among the elderly, and in cerebrovascular disease, the third leading cause of death in the United States. Consequently, mortality for older people has declined. Hospital and physicians' costs are borne for the most part by the federal government and other public agencies. Nursing home costs are paid for in part by public funds, in certain instances, but the patient's private resources, if available, must be utilized in the bulk of cases for items such as dental care, drugs, eyeglasses, and hearing aids. These latter constitute the largest out-of-pocket expense for the elderly citizen in the community.

It has gradually become apparent that in addition to physical infirmities resulting from advanced age certain economic, social, and psychologic factors combine to exclude millions of Americans from the fullness of life and from the places in our society to which their years of service and experience entitle them.

In 1974 the study of the aging process was given a tremendous boost when Congress created the National Institute on Aging (NIA). NIA was authorized to conduct and support biomedical, social, and behavioral research and training related to the aging process and to diseases and other special problems and needs of the aged. For example, one of the goals of the Geriatric Research Section of NIA is to prepare future physicians and dentists to deal with these special problems and needs of the growing population of the elderly in the United States. Other goals of NIA are to improve the diagnosis, treatment, and management of certain diseases (for example, neurologic conditions such as senile dementia, stroke, and Parkinson's disease) and common problems such as dizziness, tendency to falls, incontinence, urinary tract infection, and impotency. NIA is studying the pharmacologic effects of drugs (for example, the optimum drug dosage levels), since the elderly may respond very differently to a drug than do younger people. Most pharmacologic information in the past has been obtained in young subjects, and therefore adverse drug reactions and interactions are only beginning to be studied in the elderly.

Under NIA the Social and Behavioral Research (SBR) program is studying the social, cultural, economic, and psychologic factors that affect both the process of growing old and the place of older persons in society. Studies are probing links between the changing social environment and potentially preventable or reversible decrements of old age such as memory loss, chronic ill health, sensory impairments, low self-esteem, and withdrawal from active participation in social and economic roles.

In 1978 President Carter signed into law a bill forbidding forced retirement at age 65. (An arbitrary number, "65" marks the beginning of old age mostly for legislative reasons, such as Social Security.) As a result of that bill, millions of Americans were given the right to choose to continue working until age 70.

In addition to NIA, the U.S. House of Representatives has a federal funds watchdog committee (the House Aging Committee), and the U.S. Senate's Senate Special Committee on Aging is designed to keep an eye on the needs and interests of the elderly citizen. The Supplemental Security Income (SSI) is a program that provides funds to persons over 65 years of age who have very little or no cash income.

Organizations such as Operation Mainstream, the Retired Senior Volunteer Program (RSVP), the Gray Panthers, National Council of Senior Citizens (NSC), American Association of Retired Persons (AARP), Green Thumb, and Action provide a variety of useful community services for the older citizen. State welfare departments and local community agencies provide intellectual and cultural programs as well as assistance in housing and homemaking needs.

◼◼◼◼ NURSING HOMES

An estimated 1.4 million persons are in nursing homes (and it is believed that 10% to 20% of these individuals could live at home if they had adequate help). This accounts for approximately 5% of the persons in the United States who are 65 years of age and over. The number of elderly residents in state and county mental hospitals has decreased dramatically in the past 20 years or so. This decrease is a result, in part, of new methods of treatment, especially the use of psychotropic drugs. If nursing homes were not available, however, large numbers of elderly would remain in mental hospitals or would enter them for the first time.

The minimum standards and regulations for nursing homes vary among the states so that no uniform definition is possible. However, the National Master Facility Inventory includes in its count only facilities licensed by the states in which they are located. The homes are then classified according to the level of care they provide. There are four categories as follows:

Nursing care homes employ one or more full-time registered or licensed practical nurses and must provide nursing care to at least half the residents. **Personal care homes with nursing** have fewer than half the residents receiving nursing care. In addition, such homes must employ one or more registered or licensed practical nurses or must provide administration of medications and treatments in accordance with a physician's order, supervision of self-administered medications, or three or more personal services. **Personal care homes without nursing** have no residents receiving nursing care. These homes provide administration of medications and treatments in accordance with a physician's order, supervision of self-administered medications, or three or more personal services. **Domiciliary care homes** primarily provide domiciliary, or residential, care, but they also provide one or two personal services.

CULTS AND QUACKERY

A cult, according to Webster, is a "system for the cure of disease based on the dogma, tenets, or principles set forth by its promulgator to the exclusion of scientific experience or demonstration." There are many "healers" of different kinds and many "cures" advertised in many places. Cultists commonly advertise secret methods of diagnosis and treatment.

A quack, according to Webster, is "a pretender to medical skill." Quacks and their immediate cures for diseases that are incurable cost the American public untold millions of dollars each year. In advertising the quack preys on the fears and emotions of the victim. Hypnosis may be a useful and legitimate tool in medicine, but the consumer should be aware of the phony "hypnotherapist" or "hypnotist" who has no professional qualification. "Psychic surgery" may be advertised as "bloodless," but is another form of quackery and not a legitimate medical procedure. The list can go on and on.

Aside from defrauding the public, health quackery's most devastating effect is that it may delay or prevent an individual from seeking sound medical advice and treatment; thus it may even make the difference between life and death. Miracle drugs, secret remedies, special devices, faith healers, and the like can only lead, at best, to an empty pocketbook and at the very worst, to disaster. To be on the safe side, the consumer should contact his or her local medical society or better business bureau if there are any doubts concerning the legitimacy of any practitioner, procedure, or product.

ACUPUNCTURE

Controversy over the use of **acupuncture** and its efficacy has existed since its appearance in the United States in the 1960s. Originating in China, acupuncture is the practice of piercing specific peripheral nerves with needles to relieve the discomfort associated with painful disorders, to induce surgical anesthesia, and to provide therapy. Medical associations are somewhat noncommittal about the use of acupuncture in the United States. The legal status varies from state to state concerning who can practice it; therefore, the consumer takes a large risk unless there is valid proof that the person performing the treatment has had proper training at a legitimate institution. If a medical physician is not performing the treatment, it would be wise at least to have a physician in attendance.

HOLISTIC HEALTH CARE

In recent years the health care system has been criticized for focusing too much on the treatment of disease, rather than its prevention. According to a 1980 Harris Survey, 60% of the public agree that "the trouble with the health care system in the United States is that it is designed to treat disease rather than prevent disease." Advocates of **holistic health** go even further and suggest that more attention should be paid to enhancing health and **wellness** rather than preventing or curing illness. Indeed a basic tenet of the holistic approach is that health care is not exclusively the province or responsibility of orthodox medicine. Holistic medicine teaches that the patient and the health practitioner share the responsibility for the health process. True holistic advocates believe all of us should accept routine management of our own bodies. In a word, holistic medical care centers on self-reliance, and there is certainly nothing wrong with this. Other things being equal, healthy self-reliance can lead to a healthier body—and a healthier bank account.

SELF-TEST

1. _____ adult care		a. wellness
2. _____ child care		b. pediatrician
3. _____ holistic medicine		c. Blue Shield
4. _____ practical nurse		d. HMO
5. _____ registered nurse		e. pharmacist
6. _____ druggist		f. 65 and over
7. _____ osteopath		g. LPN
8. _____ dentist		h. internist
9. _____ acupuncture		i. aspirin
10. _____ group practice		j. "weight-loss belt"
11. _____ OTC		k. D.O.
12. _____ prescription		l. ℞
13. _____ medical device		m. needle manipulation
14. _____ surgical insurance		n. RN
15. _____ Medicare		o. D.D.S.

STUDY QUESTIONS

1. What are the qualifications for entrance into medical school?
2. What are the qualifications for the legal right to practice medicine in the United States?
3. What is a primary care physician?
4. Name five medical specialties.
5. What should a good medical checkup include?
6. Compare the training and function of a physician's assistant (PA), registered nurse (RN), and licensed practical nurse (LPN).
7. Compare the training and function of a Doctor of Osteopathy and Doctor of Chiropractic.
8. Does a dentist have the legal right to write a prescription?
9. Name the various professional duties and responsibilities of the pharmacist at the typical "corner drugstore."
10. Distinguish among the terms ophthalmologist, oculist, optometrist, and optician.
11. What is the legal status of acupuncture in your state?
12. The modern general hospital brings together a host of diverse areas of medical, paramedical, and nonmedical expertise. Name as many as you possibly can (and don't forget the accounting department).
13. Describe any and all professional contacts you have had with the medical health team within the past year. Be specific, for example: internists, optometrists, and druggists.

14. Describe any personal contacts you have had with medical cults and/or quacks.
15. What are your personal views on over-the-counter drugs?
16. A number of rules of drug safety are presented on p. 345. Can you think of any others?
17. Distinguish between generic drugs and brand name drugs.
18. Describe any experience you have had with private health insurance.
19. Blue Cross and Blue Shield are characterized as nonprofit organizations. In as much as the people who work for these plans are receiving a salary, are the organizations really "nonprofit"? Discuss.
20. Health Maintenance Organizations (HMOs) are becoming very popular throughout the United States. What is their special appeal?
21. Distinguish between Medicare and Medicaid in regard to eligibility and benefits.
22. What are your views on national health care?
23. What are your views on "socialized medicine," as in England, where the government owns the medical facilities and physicians are employees of the government?
24. Since 1930 women have outlived men at an increasing rate. Why?
25. What are your views on nursing homes?

CHAPTER 24

Accidents and safety

In the United States accidents are the fourth leading cause of death, close on the heels of heart disease, cancer, and stroke. In people from 1 to 38 years of age accidents pose a greater threat to life than all other causes combined. Accident prevention obviously deserves consideration in the student's health program. Also, knowing what to do when an accident occurs is crucial. For example, one single, simple measure—the Heimlich maneuver—can save a person from choking to death. This and other first aid measures are discussed in the present chapter.

Motor vehicle accidents

Home accidents

Public accidents

Sports and recreational accidents

Work accidents

Radiation

Accident prevention

First aid

The twentieth century is a power-packed era; therefore it is not too difficult to see how accidents have become an important concern to the federal and state governments as well as to individuals and industries. We step on the automobile starter and "200 horses" leap forward. Millions commute to and from work daily. In both the country and city occupational accidents are common. The home is equipped with a wide variety of accident-causing products. Recreational activities lend themselves to fatal and nonfatal accidents. The environment in which we live also plays the devil's disciple.

The personality of the individual and the existing social customs or pressures play an important role in accidents. To be effective, accident prevention must change one or more of these factors. We can prevent accidents by providing a safe environment, by becoming emotionally stable and safety conscious, and by making safety practices socially acceptable. To avoid automobile accidents, for example, we must have safe roads and automobiles, careful drivers, and social support for traffic control.

Accidents are commonly divided into four major groups: **motor vehicle, home, public,** and **work**. In the United States accidents yearly cause about 100,000 deaths and an estimated 10 million nonfatal injuries sufficiently severe to cause either temporary or permanent impairment. The cost to the American people—about $83 billion annually—is reflected in medical fees, hospital expenses, lost wages, insurance costs, property damage (in motor vehicle accidents), property loss (in fires), and certain indirect costs (in work accidents). As most of us probably know, home accidents are by far the most numerous; however, the number of deaths resulting from home accidents is not so great as those resulting from motor vehicle accidents. The encouraging element is that accidents are preventable. Accident rates have been and can be reduced. For example, the National Safety Council reported a drop in the death rate for all accidents from 85.5 deaths per 100,000 population in 1913 to 48.1 in 1977.

▇▇▇ MOTOR VEHICLE ACCIDENTS

In 1915, the first year the automobile caused more deaths in the United States than the horse, there were 3 million motor vehicles and 4 million drivers in this country. Ten years later the number of motor vehicles and drivers had increased more than six times, and traffic deaths had more than tripled. Clearly, a national problem of immense proportions had developed within a relatively short period of time. Today we can report the staggering fact that more deaths have occurred from automobile accidents in the United States than from all the wars the country has fought since its beginning. In 1966 the Department of Transportation was created under whose jurisdiction the National Highway Traffic Safety Administration (NHTSA) sets and enforces safety standards that set minimum performance levels for motor vehicles. In addition, this commission is on the alert for motor vehicle defects.

■ Fatalities

Every day in America an average of 140 persons die (about one death every 10 minutes) and an additional 5000 are maimed or seriously hurt in motor vehicle accidents. Motor vehicle accidents cause about 65% of all accidental deaths within the age group of 15 to 24 years (Fig. 24-1) and are the leading cause of childhood deaths (once the critical weeks immediately following birth have passed [Fig. 24-2]). Each year an estimated 1000 children are killed and 70,000 are injured in automobile accidents (Fig. 24-3). According to the National Safety Council, men are twice as likely as women to be involved in fatal acci-

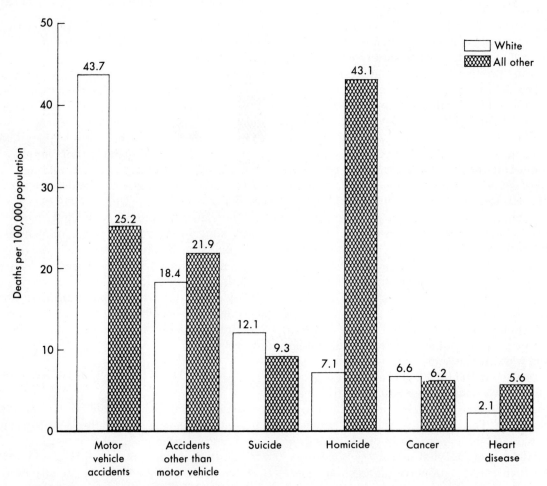

FIG. 24-1 ■ Major causes of death among persons 15 to 24 years of age in the United States, 1980.

From Office of the Assistant Secretary for Health and the Surgeon General.

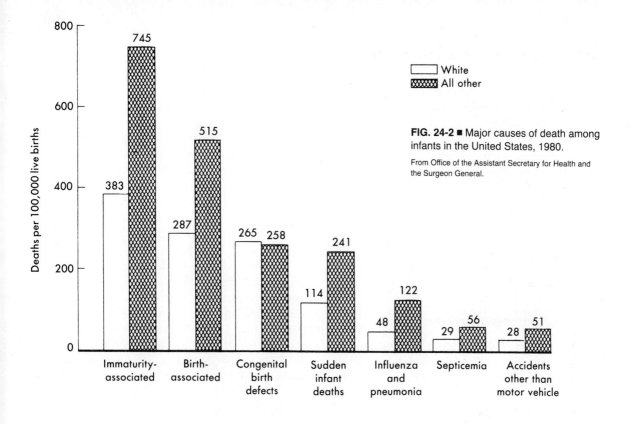

FIG. 24-2 ■ Major causes of death among infants in the United States, 1980.

From Office of the Assistant Secretary for Health and the Surgeon General.

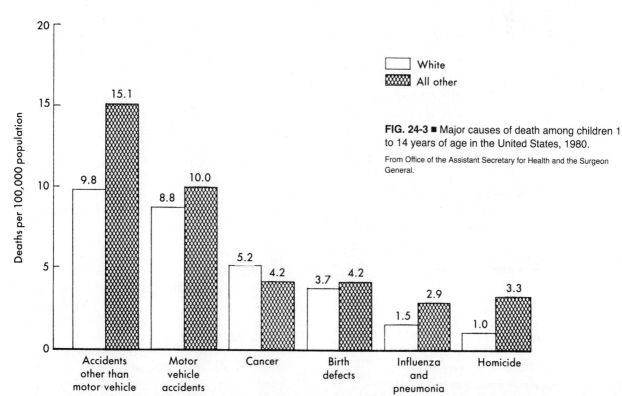

FIG. 24-3 ■ Major causes of death among children 1 to 14 years of age in the United States, 1980.

From Office of the Assistant Secretary for Health and the Surgeon General.

dents, mainly because they drive in riskier situations (for example, more men drive at night than women).

Although the total number of annual deaths from motor vehicle accidents has increased over the years, **deaths per million vehicle miles** have decreased. For example, the number has declined from 15.6 deaths per 100 million vehicle miles in 1933 to 3.53 in 1980. Some credit for this decrease is attributed to our modern superhighways that are considered to be about three times safer than conventional roads (for example, the two-lane highway).

■ The automobile driver

There were an estimated 145.1 million automobile drivers in America in 1981, and the number of new operators is increasing daily. Most of these persons, fortunately, realize the tremendous responsibility they assume the moment the ignition is turned on. They realize that not only their own lives and those of their passengers depend on their driving ability and caution but also the lives of pedestrians and other persons whom they will be confronting in other cars.

The good driver is a **defensive driver** (as compared with the offensive driver) and is the person who has developed fundamental driving skills, good driving habits, precise coordination, and sound judgment. These latter

TABLE 24-1
Kinds of improper driving in order of frequency

Speeding
Right of way
  Failing to yield
  Passing stop sign
  Disregarding signal
Driving left of center
Improper overtaking
Making improper turn
Following too closely

From National Highway Traffic Safety Administration.

go together with mental and physical fitness. Beyond that, an attitude of responsibility and carefulness is of the greatest importance. The cautious, defensive driver never assumes that the other person, either pedestrian or driver, will do the right thing or take proper safety precautions. A margin of safety should always be maintained and allowances made for possible foolish, selfish, or erratic driving on the part of others, as well as for adverse driving conditions such as slippery roads.

A number of drivers (fortunately these are in the minority) are not so careful and throw caution to the wind (Table 24-1). In particular, accident figures are not very complimentary to the young, white male driver 15 to 24 years of age. The accident rate is higher for this age group than for any other. (The safest drivers are persons 65 to 74 years of age.) In some states automobile liability insurance rates are higher for persons under 25 years. Yet this is an age group that should have a good accident record. The young person's health is good, coordination is excellent, and the mind is keen.

■ Speeding

According to the National Safety Council, excessive speed is the most common violation in driving (and the highest in the 15- to 24-year age group), and speeding violations are 87% higher in rural areas than in urban settings. Evidently, speed warnings are disregarded, especially after midnight. Many persons put on bursts of excessive speed after passing through a congested area so as to make up for lost time. Others speed dangerously in passing other vehicles. Many weave back and forth at accelerated rates between lanes on superhighways. The likelihood of being killed in an automobile accident increases dramatically with higher speeds. Interestingly, in 1974, when the mandatory 55 mile per hour speed limit went into effect across the country, the yearly death rate dropped below the "50,000 plus" figure, where it hovered for many years.

However, the rate has gone up again, above 50,000, and the rise is attributed by some experts to the popularity of the compact and subcompact cars. The rate is expected to continue to rise in future years inasmuch as, it is predicted, small cars will constitute the major portion of the nation's autos by 1986.

■ Alcohol and other hazards

Along with excessive speed, the major threat in driving today is the effect of alcohol. It is estimated that in nearly one out of two fatal accidents alcohol is involved. Put another way, alcohol is responsible for killing at least 25,000 persons a year (and seriously injuring a million others). It is further estimated that one out of every two Americans will be involved in an alcohol-related automobile crash during his or her lifetime. Drinking interferes with the driver's judgment, reaction time, and ability to make quick decisions. The person who has been drinking tends to disregard usual safety practices, often without being aware of it. Judgment of speed is poor, and vision is likely to be blurred. "If you drive, don't drink. If you drink, don't drive." It is also a wise decision not to drive with someone who has been drinking. An individual is putting his or her safety in the hands of another who is not fully responsible. The taking of drugs also incapacitates the person who is driving. The physiologic and psychologic effects of drugs in this instance are described in Chapter 22. Driving when fatigued or sleepy can be as hazardous as driving under the influence of liquor or drugs. The wise driver will pull over to the side of the road and nap until able to stay awake and alert.

Anyone under emotional strain should not drive. If a person's eyesight is poor, corrective lenses should be worn, or, if necessary, driving should be curtailed altogether. Driving should be left to someone else if a person has a temporary medical impairment such as hay fever, with bouts of sneezing. The elderly should discuss with a doctor the problem of driving, as should anyone with a severe or chronic illness. Other sources of danger include carrying on a conversation, especially with those in the back seat, showing off, hogging the road, tailgating, listening to the radio or tape deck too intently, and behaving indecisively. Driving is a full-time, serious, responsible job. There is no time for inattention.

Accidents occur frequently when a person, an animal, or a vehicle suddenly appears in front of an oncoming automobile, and the driver is unable to stop quickly enough. A varying distance is required in which to stop a car, according to the speed at which it is moving. Two factors determine stopping distance: (1) **reaction time** of the driver in stepping on the brake, and (2) **brake time**, the time it takes the car to stop after the brakes are applied (Table 24-2). For example, a car traveling 30 miles per hour will move 33 feet before the average driver can apply the brakes

▬▬▬▬▬▬▬▬▬▬ **TABLE 24-2**
Stopping distances for different speeds

Miles per hour	Reaction time distance (ft.)	Braking distance (ft.)	Total stopping distance (ft.)
5	5.5	4	9.5
10	11	9	20
15	16.5	15	31.5
20	22	23	45
25	27.5	33	60.5
30	33	45	78
35	38.5	61	99.5
40	44	81	125
45	49.5	105	154.5
50	55	133	188
55	60.5	167	227.5
60	66	206	272
65	71.5	252	323.5
70	77	304	381

Prepared by the American Automobile Association.

and 45 feet after the brakes are applied. This provides a stopping distance of 78 feet.

Poor maintenance of a motor vehicle is a hazard that could be the cause of an accident. The responsible person is conscientious in maintaining top-notch mechanical condition of the vehicle at all times. This involves periodic check-ups by a reliable service station. It goes without saying that brakes, tires, steering mechanism, exhaust system, and windshield wipers, to name a few, should be in good working order.

■ Seat belts

Improved car design, the collapsible steering wheel, shatterproof windows, and seat (safety) belts have been demonstrated to reduce serious injuries. However, in the instance of **seat belts**, only one in nine drivers uses them. The force generated by a collision is so great and so sudden that it is nearly impossible for a person to control the movement of his or her body. It is not unusual for an unbelted person to be thrown against and injure another person. In a minor accident a seat belt can prevent the driver from being thrown out of position and thus can help him maintain control of the car and avoid a more serious accident.

Accidents to infants and young children can be prevented to a large extent if restraints are used. Infants should be put in semireclining carriers, and very young children should use special car seats or harnesses. For these devices to be effective, the manufacturer's instructions on installation and use must be followed exactly. Older children should be encouraged to wear seat belts—both lap and shoulder belts, never just the shoulder belt alone—for not only will they be protected, but they will also learn a lifelong habit through consistent use.

In 1966 the National Traffic and Motor Vehicle Safety Act was passed by Congress in the interest of reducing highway fatalities and injuries. Among other standards, the act declared "auto makers would have to equip their cars with passenger restraints (either seat belts or air bags) without the need for action by passengers." The target date was 1972, a date that was not met, and eventually 1983 was set as the mandatory deadline for manufacturers to install **air bags** or seat belts that would automatically envelop the passenger in time of need. Once again, the government put off the enforcement of this requirement and in 1981 began to "re-evaluate the entire restraint system."

■ Pedestrians

Pedestrians, as well as drivers, should be concerned with safety. Pedestrians violate some rules that could help prevent the approximately 10,000 yearly deaths that occur as a result of carelessness or ignorance. In urban centers streets should be crossed at crosswalks, and jaywalking should be avoided (Fig. 24-4). It should not be taken for granted that a driver will see the pedestrian or anticipate his or her movements. Before crossing the street a person should look both ways and allow plenty of time for any oncoming car. Allowances should be made for cars picking up speed. On roads without sidewalks a person should walk on the left side so that oncoming traffic can be watched. If possible, at night the pedestrian should wear an article of light-colored clothing or carry a white handkerchief, a folded newspaper, or a flashlight.

■ Insurance

Most states require automobile owners to hold **insurance** policies that protect the driver from **liability** in cases of bodily injury and collision. Even if the insurance is not required, the owner should have adequate protection. The legal fees, indemnities, and compensa-

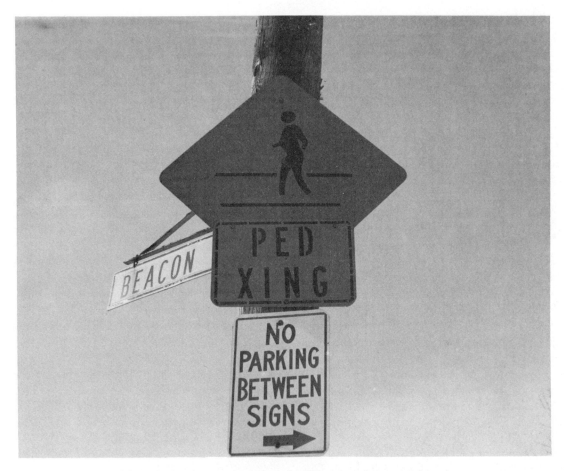

FIG. 24-4 ■ In urban centers streets should be crossed at crosswalks only.

tion for a single accident could put an end to a college career by exhausting the student's and even the family's finances.

■■■■■■ HOME ACCIDENTS

Home accidents commonly occur from carelessness or ignorance in the use of many consumer products. Thousands of persons meet their deaths each year, and thousands more receive hospital emergency room treatment each year as a result of falls, fires and burns, poisoning, suffocation, firearms,

drowning, and contact with electric current or with explosive materials, to name several types of accidents at the top of the list.

For the population at large, falls of all kinds account for nearly one third of accidental deaths in the home. An estimated 710,000 falls occur on stairs each year. Highly polished floors and other slippery surfaces, as well as ladders and stepladders, contribute to the number of falls.

Fires and burns are caused by the careless use of matches, by smoking in bed, etc. Faulty or poorly constructed space heaters and fireplaces also create hazards. Some precautionary measures are as follows:

1. Every home should be equipped with smoke detectors.
2. Every family should have periodic fire drills.
3. All stairs, hallways, corridors, etc. should be kept free and clear at all times.
4. Living accommodations should be checked periodically for faulty wiring, frayed cords, exposed wires, and defective electric appliances.
5. Efficient housekeeping and regular disposal of easily combustible material and substances that are of no further use can do a lot to make a home safe from fire.
6. The emergency number of the fire department should be kept near the telephone.

Poisoning occurs from ingestion of such solids and liquids as drugs, medicines, mushrooms, and shellfish, as well as the commonly recognized poisons; poisoning occurs from gases and vapors, principally **carbon monoxide** (CO), a product of incomplete combustion involving cooking stoves, heating equipment, and standing motor vehicles.

Poisoning of young children who find and swallow household or prescription medicines is very common. They also ingest detergents, bleaches, soaps, wax polishes, lighter fluids, cosmetics, insecticides, and other toxic products. To reduce injury and death, parents should take care in the handling and storage of many consumer products and should keep the telephone number of the nearest **poison control center** (PCC) by the telephone. There are over 500 poison control centers coordinated by the National Clearinghouse for Poison Control Centers of the Public Health Service. Manufacturers of drugs and household supplies inform the Clearinghouse of the toxic ingredients in their products and the antidotes for them. This information is available by telephone to parents or physicians when needed.

Accidental ingestion or inhalation of objects or food often results in the obstruction of respiratory passageways. Suffocation from bed clothes or thin plastic materials (such as the type used in dry cleaning bags) and suffocation by confinement in closed spaces (discarded refrigerators, freezers, etc.) are home accidents that occur all too frequently. Firearms accidents occur mainly while someone is cleaning or playing with the guns. Drownings occur oftentimes when a person swims alone or dives into a shallow pool. Small children should never be left unattended near a swimming pool. Swimming pools should be enclosed by a fence and should have safety equipment near at hand. Electric hazards can be avoided by avoiding the use of appliances in wet areas (for example, vacuum cleaning while washing the car or mowing wet grass with an electric mower). When raising an antenna or placing a ladder against a tree, it is wise to be aware of power lines. Children should be taught not to fly kites near power lines and not to climb trees around power lines. Accordingly, a multitude of home accidents may be prevented through safety education plus the removal of possible hazards.

■ PUBLIC ACCIDENTS

According to the National Safety Council, in 1980 21,000 persons died and 2,600,000 persons were injured (some permanently disabled) as a result of nontransport-related accidents in public places, privately or nonprivately owned (such as playgrounds, parks, beaches, restaurants, stadiums, and theaters) and as a result of accidents on public carriers (aircraft, buses, and trains). Falls in public places accounted for some 6000 deaths; fire-related injuries resulted in an estimated 1500 deaths; drownings accounted for 7000 deaths; and firearms (rifles, handguns) were involved in approximately 1000 deaths (in the "public accident" category).

Prevention of public accidents depends on

a combination of factors, not the least of which is common sense. Simply watching one's step and not hurrying can eliminate hazards associated with falling. Becoming familiar with the location of the nearest fire exit on entering a public establishment, such as a restaurant, theatre, or hotel room, can spell the difference between life and death. In the opinion of many persons gun control legislation can reduce the number of fatalities and injuries resulting from firearms. Gun control laws would require that all firearms be registered and that owners be tested for proficiency and qualification.

The amount of sensational publicity given to aircraft, bus, and train accidents might lead a person to believe that travel by public carrier is far more dangerous than travel by automobile. But statistics tell us that travel by public transportation is much safer than driving one's own car (or, for that matter, safer than being a passenger in a car). Interestingly, in 1978, according to the National Safety Council, in domestic air travel the passenger death rate per 100 million passenger miles was 0.01 as compared with 1.32 for automobiles. (For buses the rate was 0.72 and for passenger trains 0.13 per 100 million passenger miles.)

Even so, considering the relative safety of public carriers, it's a good idea to keep certain safety rules in mind. For example, the National Safety Transportation Board advises air travelers to pay close attention to the flight attendant's instructions regarding seat belts and emergency exits and to store only coats or soft belongings overhead. No matter whether on a plane, bus, or train, everyone should take note of the nearest emergency exit and should decide how to get to it and how to open it.

■ SPORTS AND RECREATIONAL ACCIDENTS

Sports and recreational activities account for an increasing number of mishaps (Table 24-3)

■ TABLE 24-3

Sports activities and sports equipment injuries (1980)

Bicycles	504,000
Football (organized and informal)	464,000
Baseball (organized and informal)	443,000
Basketball (organized and informal)	422,000
Skating (roller, ice)	241,000
Mopeds, minibikes	240,000
Swimming (scuba diving, swimming pools, diving and diving boards, swimming pool slides, swimming)	140,000
Soccer (organized and informal)	94,000
Skateboards	87,000
Tennis, badminton, squash, racquetball, paddle ball	77,000
Volleyball	74,000
Wrestling	68,000
Hockey (ice, street, field)	59,000
Gymnastics	58,000
Skiing (downhill, cross country)	54,000
Exercise equipment (including weight lifting)	46,000
Horseback riding	43,000
Snowmobiles	19,000
Trampolines	6,000

Data from U.S. Consumer Product Safety Commission (annual estimated number of injuries treated in hospital emergency rooms).

and fatalities every year. In 1980, for example, there were an estimated 35,000 mishaps, fatal and nonfatal, associated with pleasure boating; a large number of the fatalities were caused by drowning. Boating accident prevention demands proper instruction in handling the vessel (regardless of size), the use of life preservers, knowledge of passenger capacity (overloading is a common hazard), and familiarity with the location of the body of water.

Each year finds new threats to a person's safety in recreational and sports activities as certain activities become popular and readily available to the public. Mountain climbing, for instance, is fast becoming an activity that more persons pursue than ever before in the United States, with the result that there are numbers of injuries and fatalities associated with it.

Safety, once again, in all activities lies in common sense plus knowledge. Accidents can be prevented by proper instruction in the use of equipment, by wearing proper clothing and protective gear, and by having properly maintained equipment and experience in whatever the activity may be. These can make the difference between pleasure and pain—or possibly, death.

■ Bicycling

In 1981 an estimated 105 million Americans bicycled for pleasure or commuted to work or school on bicycles. This figure compares to about 75 million in 1970. Since so many Americans are taking to the road on their wheels (bicycling enjoys worldwide popularity), the number of injuries and deaths is also on the rise. The National Safety Council estimates at least one-half million persons are injured each year, and 1300 deaths are the result of bicycle-related accidents. Unfortunately, the majority of these accidents involve youngsters bicycling their way to and from school. Therefore bicycle safety should be included in the school curriculum. Many schools are providing courses today for elementary school children. Various organizations are more than happy to provide safety and maintenance information to persons of all ages. Accident prevention depends also to a large extent on compliance with the U.S. Cycling Federation's "Rules of the Road" (Fig. 24-5).

According to the U.S. Cycling Federation, the seven "Rules of the Road" are as follows:

1. Obey all traffic signs and signals.
2. Ride on the right side of the road, single file, and never ride against traffic.
3. Watch out for car doors opening into traffic.
4. Do not have more than one rider on a bicycle at a time, and never hitch a ride on another vehicle.
5. Watch out for road surface hazards.
6. Be careful at intersections, especially when making a left-hand turn; over half of all bicycle-car accidents occur at intersections. (Use hand signals.)
7. Ride your bike defensively. Watch out for the other person.

■ WORK ACCIDENTS

More than 90 million Americans spend their days on the job. They are our most valuable national resource, yet job-related accidents claim the lives of more than 14,000 workers and disable about 2½ million every year. In terms of lost production and wages, medical expenses, and disability compensation, the burden on the nation's commerce is staggering and the human cost beyond calculation.

On the positive side, through the combined efforts of leaders in industry and small business management and the Office of Occupational Safety and Health Administration, the number of work-related accidents has been declining in recent years. This decline is undoubtedly due in no little part to steps taken to safeguard machinery and eliminate certain work hazards. In addition, many plants now have a strong safety education program on the job. The use of items such as protective headgear and clothing plus mechanical safeguards has also played an important role in reducing workers' accidents.

■ Occupational Safety and Health Administration

In 1970 the United States Congress passed the Occupational Safety and Health Act, which provided for the Occupational Safety and Health Administration (OSHA). Its objectives, as stated, were "to assure so far as possible every working man and woman in the nation safe and healthful working conditions and to preserve our human resources." Taking effect in 1971, the act provided that any busi-

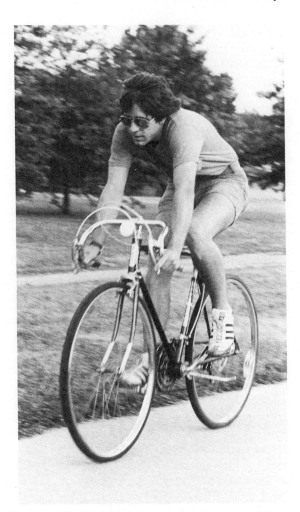

Fig. 24-5 ■ This cyclist knows what he is doing and obeys the "Rules of the Road."

ness with one or more employees that affects interstate commerce must provide a safe and healthful place in which to work. The workplace must be free from any recognized hazards likely to cause death or serious harm. The standards, rules, and regulations for safety are set up by the Department of Labor and enforced by OSHA. Inspection of a workplace is made by "Compliance Safety and Health Officers" who make visits that are usually unannounced.

In general OSHA coverage extends to all employers and their employees in the 50 states, the District of Columbia, Puerto Rico, and all territories under federal government jurisdiction. Federal agencies are also covered by OSHA. Individual states may develop and operate their own plans for OSHA approval and thereby receive federal funding for 50% of the program's operating costs.

Included under OSHA's coverage are employers and employees in such varied fields as construction, longshoring, agriculture, law and medicine, charity and disaster relief, orga-

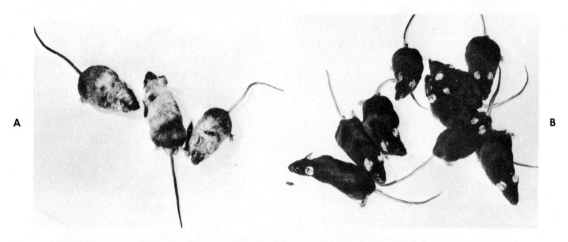

FIG. 24-6 ■ Originally there were nine 14-month old mice in each group. One group, **A**, received large but nonlethal dose of radiation as young adults; the other, **B**, did not. Untreated group is healthy; only three irradiated mice survive, and they are senile and gray.

Courtesy Howard J. Curtis, Brookhaven National Laboratory, Upton, N.Y.

nized labor, and private education. Religious groups are included to the extent that they employ workers for secular purposes. Not covered are self-employed persons, farms at which only immediate members of the farmer's family are employed, and workplaces already protected by federal agencies under other federal statutes. There are 10 OSHA regional offices: Boston, New York, Philadelphia, Atlanta, Chicago, Dallas, Kansas City, Denver, San Francisco, and Seattle.

■■■■■ RADIATION

Radiation is the emission and propagation of waves or subatomic particles. Except for light, the various forms of radiation are invisible. So-called **ionizing radiation** is the kind most damaging to living things. Forms of ionizing radiation of chief concern include **x-rays, gamma rays, alpha rays,** and **beta rays.** Either directly or indirectly such rays produce ionization in tissues; that is to say, they dislodge electrons from atoms and molecules and

thereby create electrically charged particles, or **ions.** Ions cause biochemical lesions that initiate a series of histologic changes, symptoms, and signs that vary with the dose of radiation and the time after exposure. In addition to the early somatic effects of large doses (observable within days), changes in the DNA of rapidly proliferating cells may become manifest as a disease or as a genetic effect in offspring many years later. The effect of a large dose of radiation on mice is dramatically evident in Fig. 24-6.

The units of measurement commonly used in expressing radiation intensity are the **rad** (**r**adiation **a**bsorbed **d**ose) and the **rem** (**r**oentgen **e**quivalent in **m**an). The dose rate is the radiation dose per unit of time. From the very low dose rates of unavoidable natural background radiation, where no effect can·be observed, the detectable effects increase as the dose rate climbs. Roughly, an observable effect is certain (in humans) with dose rates greater than 4 rads/min. As a rule of thumb, large doses are of concern because of their immediate effects, whereas small doses are of concern because of potential long-term genetic effects. A total whole-body dose of 600 rads received in a very short time almost always proves fatal. By contrast, many thousands of rads delivered over a long period of time (as in cancer treatment) can be tolerated by the body when small volumes of tissue are irradiated. This is certainly not to say, however, that such exposure is tolerated genetically.

The only certain way to avoid fatal or serious overexposure to radiation is the rigorous enforcement of protective measures and adherence to the **maximum permissible dose** (MPD). As determined by the International Commission on Radiological Protection, the MPD for the public at large is 500 millirems/year. Scientists estimate that the average American is exposed to 100 to 200 millirems of radiation per year from natural and manmade sources. Diagnostic x-rays currently constitute the largest single source of manmade radiation, a normal chest x-ray exposure delivering about 25 millirems. Although these x-rays can be valuable, life-saving tools in helping to diagnose and prevent disease, they obviously can also be dangerous. This is especially important to keep in mind in light of the fact that over half of the annual x-ray exposure received in this country is unnecessary.

■ Microwaves

Microwaves fall into the radio frequency band of electromagnetic radiation. They are **nonionizing** and much less dangerous than the forms of radiation just discussed. They are used to detect speeding cars, to send telephone and television communications, and to treat muscle soreness. Industry uses microwaves to dry and cure plywood, to cure rubber and resins, to raise bread and doughnuts, and to cook potato chips. But the most common consumer use of microwave energy is in **microwave ovens**.

Microwave cooking can be more energy efficient than conventional cooking because foods cook faster, and the energy heats only the food, not the oven compartment. Microwave cooking does not reduce the nutritional value of foods any more than conventional cooking. In fact, foods cooked in a microwave oven may keep more of their vitamins and minerals, because microwave ovens can cook more quickly and without water. On the basis of current knowledge about microwave radiation, the Food and Drug Administration believes that ovens that meet FDA standards and are used according to the manufacturer's instructions are safe for use. There have been allegations of radiation injury from microwave ovens, but the injuries known to the FDA could have happened with any oven or cooking surface. At one time there was concern that leakage from microwave ovens could interfere with certain electronic cardiac pacemakers. Because there are so many other products that also could cause the problem, the FDA does not require microwave ovens to carry warnings for people with pacemakers. The problem has been largely resolved, since pacemakers are now designed so they are shielded against such electronic interference. However, patients with pacemakers may wish to consult their physicians about this.

■ Laser light

Laser light is a nondivergent, monochromatic beam of light capable of mobilizing intense heat and power. Some lasers can produce a beam of light that, even miles away, can be thousands of times brighter than the sun's surface appears from earth. The fact that a laser beam can retain such high power, even over long distances, partly accounts for its use in light shows and its many other applications. But this same fact also accounts for its potential hazard. The high-powered lasers that are increasingly used in laser shows can produce enough light radiation to cause permanent eye damage as well as severe skin burns. It only takes a fraction of a second to cause serious injury. With some lasers, you can light a cigarette merely by putting the end of it in the laser beam. The Food and Drug Administration regulates the manufacture and assembly of lasers, requiring corrective action for those that do not comply with the safety regulations. In addition, the FDA is working to educate people about laser safety. Several state radiation agencies are also active in the control of laser products and their use. But such efforts cannot ensure absolute safety. It is up to the laser operator and other responsible parties to see that the laser is used in a safe manner. If there is reason to believe that a laser show is not being run safely, the FDA or appropriate state authority should be notified forthwith.

ACCIDENT PREVENTION

Much can be done to prevent accidents from happening. It is probably easier to avoid having an accident than to avoid catching a cold. Safety habits, however, are based on individual attitude. Of course a person does not place safety above all else in life. It has been suggested that "Choose Your Adventure" might be a better slogan than "Safety First." If we carried the "safety first" idea to the extreme, we would wrap ourselves up in cotton batting and sit still. We all do things that involve accident risk. Adventure is desirable. Safety education urges us to avoid stupid and needless risk to ourselves and others, to give attention to the safety of our environment and our equipment, and to use skill and science in accident prevention.

The National Safety Council has rendered a valuable service to the public by spearheading, organizing, and promoting accident prevention. Just about everyone is familiar with

its holiday weekend admonitions for safety appearing in the news media. The Council has a broad program. Through its headquarters, its regional offices, and its state and local affiliated units, it carries on a continuous and unified program of accident prevention. It employs scientists, safety engineers, statisticians, psychologists, and health educators. It works cooperatively with other groups, such as the American Automobile Association, in industrial safety, traffic safety, home safety, and safety education in the schools.

Safety education programs in elementary and secondary schools rank high in reducing accidents and saving lives. Elementary schools are especially concerned with classroom and street safety (Fig. 24-7). In the secondary school increased emphasis is being placed on safety in sports and in transportation. Driver education courses are required by many insurance companies as a prerequisite for obtaining lower premium rates.

In their health education programs state and local health departments are devoting attention to safety. Special emphasis is being directed to the prevention of home accidents. In many communities several groups often work together in accident prevention: schools, police, health departments, parent-teacher associations, labor, and industry.

Safety and accident prevention in recreational activities should be of particular interest to the student. Swimming and diving accidents often occur when a person swims alone or dives into unfamiliar or shallow waters. Everyone should know how to swim and should be able to swim at least well enough to keep afloat. Racquet sports, such as tennis, racquetball, badminton, and squash, are causing a growing number of injuries, especially to the eye and head. Skiing, roller skating, ice skating, and skateboarding injuries are also on the rise as these sports grow in popularity. Most safety experts agree on the importance of having proper clothing and protective gear, checking equipment, learning how

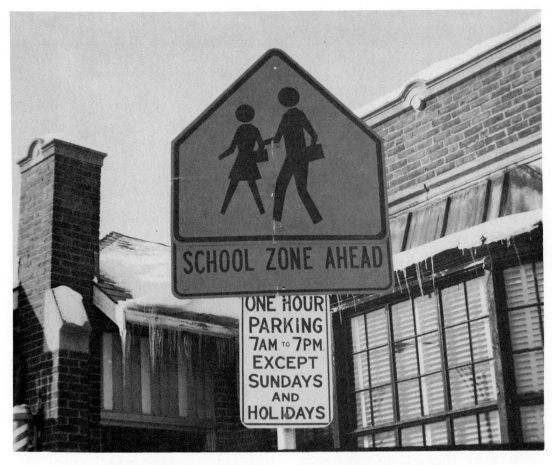

FIG. 24-7 ■ Elementary schools are especially concerned with street safety.

to fall, leaving an activity before becoming overfatigued, and staying within the limits of one's ability. These precautions coupled with adequate preparation (including expert instruction, if needed) and, in the instance of competitive sports, with good supervision and officiating will reduce accidental fatalities and injuries.

■ Physical attack

No matter how extensive a national, state, or local program of accident prevention may be, safety in the last analysis depends mainly on the individual citizen. And, unfortunately, in today's world safety preparedness should include being prepared for **physical attack**. Expert guidelines to keep in mind concerning physical attack are as follows:

1. Keep children with an adult when traveling. Never let them go anywhere alone when away from home. Be sure their whereabouts are known at all times.
2. Never hitchhike or pick up hitchhikers.
3. On public transportation sit near the driver or conductor.
4. Avoid dark alleys, deserted streets, and dark doorways.

5. If mugged (a) scream and run, if possible, and (b) don't resist a robbery by fighting the attacker.
6. Never accept rides from strangers.
7. When walking alone at night (a) walk near the curb, avoiding shrubs; (b) avoid dark doorways; (c) carry an object that can be used as a defensive weapon.
8. When driving stay on busy streets, if possible, and keep car doors locked and the windows rolled up.
9. At home don't open the door to strangers without a chain lock kept in place. Keep all doors and windows locked. If you come home and find a door or window broken, don't go in. Go to the nearest neighbor and call the police.
10. Always use common sense.

FIRST AID

First aid can work miracles, even save a life, but it must be proper. Above all, the person called on to render such aid—and by circumstances, that could be just about anybody—must remain calm and employ common sense. Furthermore, we should prepare for emergencies at home, on the job, and on the road. A crucial preparation is a list of emergency telephone numbers right next to the phone and in clear sight. Recommended numbers include doctor, hospital, ambulance, police department, fire department, druggist, poison control center, taxi, and neighbor. In some areas one number (for example, 911) takes care of any emergency: in all areas the "operator" (0) will respond. The National Safety Council stresses the following three points that should be covered clearly and quickly in an emergency call for help: (1) Tell where it happened. (2) Tell what has happened. (3) Tell who you are. This takes about 10 seconds. After you have finished, don't hang up immediately. Pause and give the person at the other end a chance to ask a question. Until help ar-

TABLE 24-4

First-aid items

Adhesive tape
Adhesive-type bandages (assorted sizes)
Alcohol
Aspirin
Calamine lotion
Cotton (sterile)
Cotton-tipped applicators
Elastic bandage
Gauze bandages (sterile)
Gauze pads (sterile)
Hydrogen peroxide (3%)*
Ice bag
Nose drops (aqueous, not oily)
Round-tipped scissors
Soap
Syrup of ipecac
Thermometer (both oral and rectal)
Tongue depressors (for small splints)
Tweezers

*Although weakly germicidal and very unstable, peroxide is gentle to the tissues and useful for cleansing wounds. (The mechanical action of the rapidly released oxygen aids in the removal of material from wound cavities.)

rives, calmly and expeditiously administer first aid. The following procedures and techniques were gleaned from standard sources, including the American Medical Association, American Red Cross, American Academy of Pediatrics, and National Safety Council. They should be studied carefully and, ideally, committed to memory. And by all means contact your local American Red Cross or comparable community service and sign up for a course in first aid. (Table 24-4 lists first-aid items to have on hand.)

Artificial respiration

Stoppage of breathing, whether from drowning, choking, electric shock, smoke inhalation, chemical fumes, asphyxiation, or from any other cause, calls for **artificial respiration** (Fig. 24-8). Act fast. Turn victim on back and,

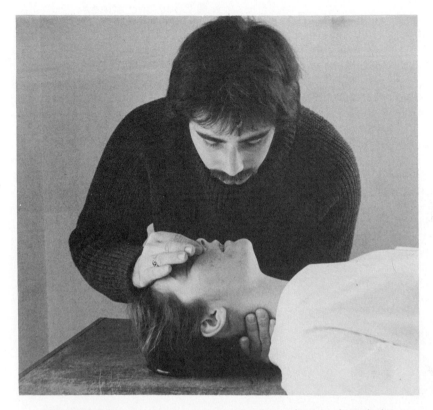

FIG. 24-8 ■ Preparing victim for opening airway in mouth-to-mouth respiration.

if necessary, quickly wipe out mouth. Place one hand under victim's neck and lift, tilting head back as far as possible with other hand. This provides an airway. Pinch victim's nostrils shut, take a deep breath, place your mouth tightly over his mouth, and blow until you see his chest rise. Remove your mouth, allowing victim to exhale. Continue rescue breathing at 12 times a minute. For a child or infant, cover nose and mouth tightly with your mouth. Blow gently 20 times a minute. If you are not getting an exchange, quickly recheck position of the head, turn victim on his side, and give several sharp blows between the shoulder blades to jar foreign matter free. Sweep fingers through victim's mouth to remove foreign matter. If one can observe the

chest to rise and fall, all within reason is being done.

■ Respiratory-cardiac arrest

Respiratory and cardiac arrest—the stoppage of both breathing and circulation—has a number of causes, including myocardial infarction ("heart attack"), pulmonary embolism, near-drowning, strangulation, suffocation, carbon monoxide inhalation, electrocution, and barbiturate intoxication. Successful **cardiopulmonary resuscitation** (CPR) calls for speed and efficiency. Delay may be fatal! Adequate amounts of oxygen must be distributed to the tissues constantly; tissue anoxia for more than 4 to 6 minutes results in irreversible brain damage or death. Resuscitation must be continued until victim recovers or is pronounced dead. Breathing and heartbeat have been restored in humans after as long as 3 hours of resuscitation. CPR is a combination of **artificial respiration** (p. 372) and **artificial circulation**; it should be started immediately as an emergency procedure when cardiac arrest occurs. It has been used widely and successfully by doctors, nurses, and other health professionals, and public health authorities strongly recommend that as many members of the general public as possible be trained in the technique. Your local Red Cross will be more than happy to train you.

■ Bites and stings

For animal bites wash with clean water and soap. Hold wound under running water for 2 or 3 minutes if it is not bleeding profusely. Apply sterile dressing. Call doctor immediately. If possible catch or restrain the animal and maintain alive for observation for signs of rabies. Notify police or health officer. For nonpoisonous snake bites treat as a cut. For poisonous snake bites enforce complete rest and apply a constricting band above the bite (not too tight). Get victim to doctor or hospital as soon as possible. For insect bites scrape out stinger if present with a scraping motion of the finger nail. Do not pull out. Apply cold compresses. Consult doctor promptly if there

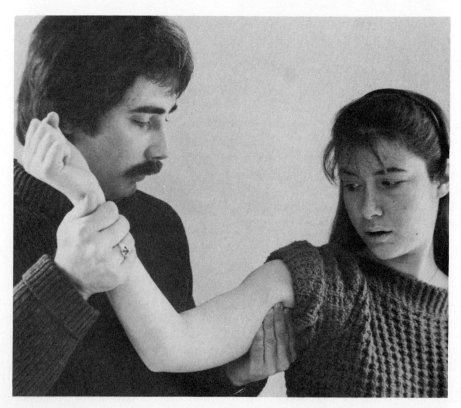

FIG. 24-9 ■ Brachial artery pressure point. To arrest severe bleeding of arm, pressure is applied to the upper arm as demonstrated.

is any reaction, such as hives, generalized rash, pallor, weakness, nausea, vomiting, tightness in chest, nose, or throat, or collapse.

■ Severe bleeding

Severe bleeding, unless checked immediately, results in circulatory failure and, ultimately, in death. Lay victim down; press sterile gauze dressing firmly over wound with your whole hand. If bleeding from an arm or leg cannot be stopped by direct pressure, shut off circulation in artery by pressing firmly against one of four **pressure points** (Figs. 24-9 and 24-10). Do not use arterial pressure for wounds of head, neck, or torso. Do not use tourni-quets unless you have been trained in their use. When bleeding stops, firmly bandage dressing in place without cutting off pulse. Watch for signs of shock. Call for help.

■ Burns and scalds

Burns and scalds are either of minor or major consequence. If caused by heat, minor burns of the extremities may be immersed in cold water, and an ice bag or cold, wet packs may be applied to areas on the trunk or face. Cooling must be constant until pain disappears. An adhesive dressing such as Telfapad should be used if available. Plastic film (Saran Wrap, etc.) makes an excellent nonadhesive

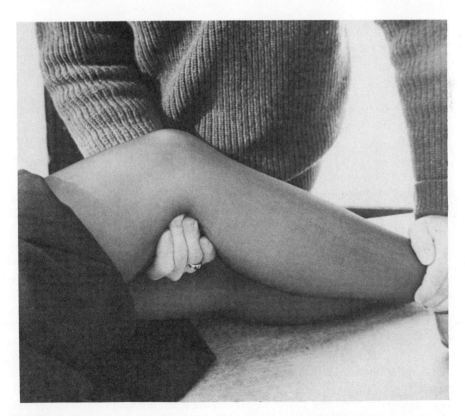

FIG. 24-10 ■ Popliteal artery pressure point. To arrest severe bleeding of the lower leg, pressure is applied behind the knee as demonstrated.

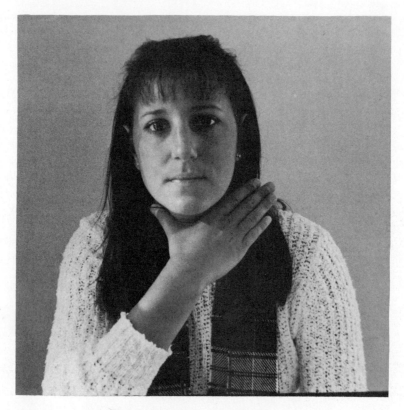

FIG. 24-11 ■ International sign to indicate choking.

emergency covering. Do not break the blisters. Consult your doctor. If the burn was caused by chemicals, wash burned area thoroughly with water. If an eye is burned by a chemical, flush the eye gently but thoroughly with water (preferably sterile) and cover with bandage or clean cloth. Get victim to hospital immediately. For major burns keep victim in flat position. Remove clothing from burned area (if it is adherent, leave clothing alone). Cover with clean cloth and keep victim warm. Get victim to hospital immediately. NOTE: Do not use ointments, greases, or powders. Electric burns accompanied by electric shock may require artificial respiration. Pull victim away from wires with nonconductive material. Do not use bare hands.

■ Choking

When a person is choking (Fig. 24-11), apply the **Heimlich maneuver** (Fig. 24-12) immediately. Stand behind the victim and put both arms around the person. Let the head, arms, and upper torso hang forward. Grab your fist with the other hand and place it against the abdomen (thumb side against abdomen) slightly above the navel and below the rib cage. Push into the abdomen with strong, quick, upward thrust to force diaphragm up and compress the lungs. Repeat as often as necessary. If the victim collapses or is too heavy to hold, lay the victim on the back and straddle the hips. With the heel of one hand pressing against the back of the other hand, push forward into the abdomen just above the navel.

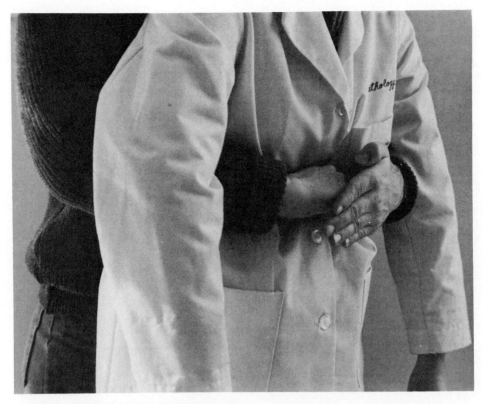

FIG. 24-12 ■ Administering Heimlich maneuver. *Note*: the rescuer's left hand is partially open in photograph to show thumb side of right hand against victim's abdomen.

A second person should be ready to remove the ejected food from the victim's mouth (especially when victim is on the back) with a spoon or finger. Give artificial respiration if necessary after food is removed. Transport victim to hospital. If you choke on something while you are alone, use the maneuver on yourself by pressing your fist rapidly up against your abdomen.

■ Convulsions

Convulsions are characterized by uncontrollable spasms. Also, the lips turn blue, the eyes roll upward, and the head is thrown back. Do not try to restrain convulsive movement. Place victim on floor, and turn the head to one side to allow saliva to drain. Move furniture to prevent injury. Put rolled handkerchief between the teeth to prevent victim from biting the tongue. Apply cold cloths to head and sponge with cold water. Give nothing by mouth. Call for medical help.

■ Cuts

Wash small cuts with clean water and soap. Hold under water. Apply sterile gauze dressing. For large cuts apply dressing, press firmly, and elevate injured area to stop bleeding. Use tourniquet only if necessary. Bandage. Secure medical care. Do not use iodine or other antiseptics.

Foreign bodies in eye

Do not rub eyes in response to a foreign body. Close both eyes for a few minutes to let tears wash out particle. If this fails, grasp lashes of upper lid and pull this lid down over bottom lid to dislodge particle. If this does not work, wash hands carefully and examine eye by pulling down lower lid and turning back upper lid. Remove speck with a moist cotton swab. Do not overdo it. Pain in eye from foreign bodies, scrapes, scratches, cuts, and so on can be alleviated by bandaging the lids shut until doctor's aid can be obtained. Immediate and abundant flushing out with plain water is the procedure for chemicals splashed in eyes. Do not use eye drops or ointment.

Fainting

Fainting may be caused by fatigue, hunger, emotional shock, stuffy rooms, and so on. Breathing is usually weak, face pale, forehead perspiring. Place victim on his or her back, head low. Loosen tight clothing and apply cold cloth to face and forehead. Do not splash water on the face. If it is available, let victim inhale aromatic spirits of ammonia. If fainting lasts more than a minute or two, cover victim warmly and call for help. If the person merely feels faint, he or she should bend forward in chair, head between legs and lower than knees. While in this position the person should breathe deeply.

Frostbite

Frostbite is caused by exposure of inadequately protected flesh to subfreezing temperatures. Tissue damage is caused by the reduced blood flow to the extremities, as opposed to hypothermia, which causes lowering of the body's rate of metabolism. The symptoms are loss of feeling and a dead white appearance. Restore body temperature as rapidly as possible, preferably by immersion in a bath of water at a temperature of less than 110° F or by other means. If it is necessary for the victim to be moved, the affected part should be kept covered and the victim moved to a location where effective treatment and vehicle evacuation can be obtained.

Head injuries

Any head injury may prove serious and consequently calls for complete rest as a first aid measure. Seek medical assistance if there is loss of consciousness, if you are unable to arouse victim from sleep, if there is persistent vomiting, if there is inability to move a limb, if there is oozing of blood or watery fluid from ears or nose, if there is persistent headache, if there is persistent dizziness for 1 hour after the injury, if the pupils are unequal in size, and if there is a pallid color that does not return to normal in a short time. The important thing is to keep on the alert for the development of these signs.

Heatstroke and heat exhaustion

Heatstroke and heat exhaustion may or may not be caused by direct sun rays. The symptoms of **heat exhaustion** include headache, dizziness, mental confusion, extreme weakness, pallor, and profuse sweating. The skin feels cool, and the pulse is weak and very rapid. Move the victim to a shady, cool place and apply cold towels to the head. Elevate the feet and gently massage the arms and legs to increase circulation. Give the victim as much water as he or she can comfortably take. **Heatstroke** is much more serious and a real medical emergency. The early symptoms are like those of heat exhaustion, but soon the victim stops sweating; the skin becomes hot, dry, and red, and the victim will probably lose consciousness or even go into convulsions. Act fast. Lay the victim in a shaded place and pour buckets of cool water over entire body, or wrap head and body in cold, wet towels or sheets. Do not give stimulants. Call for help.

■ Nosebleed

Nosebleed (epistaxis) occurs secondary to infection, drying of the nasal mucosa, trauma, hypertension, and bleeding tendencies associated with certain blood coagulation disorders. The American Academy of Pediatrics recommends the following first aid procedure: In sitting position blow out from the nose all clots and blood. Into the bleeding nostril insert a wedge of cotton moistened with any of the common nose drops. (If no nose drops are available, cold water or hydrogen peroxide may be used to moisten the pack.) With finger against the outside of that nostril, apply firm pressure for 5 minutes. If bleeding stops, leave packing in place and check with doctor. If bleeding persists, secure medical care.

■ Poisoning

Household poisons lurk in medicine chests, under kitchen sinks, and in laundry room cabinets. They kill hundreds of children (p. 364) each year—innocent victims of their own curiosity and adult carelessness. If poisoning occurs, the American Academy of Pediatrics recommends the following first aid until medical help is obtained. If the victim is unconscious or in convulsions, DO NOT force liquids and DO NOT induce vomiting. Provide artificial respiration if necessary, keep the victim warm and transport to hospital immediately. Take along poison container, remaining contents, or any vomited material to help identify poison. If the victim swallowed a corrosive or petroleum product, DO NOT induce vomiting. Dilute the poison with water or milk. (Dose: 1 to 2 cups for those under 5 years of age; up to 1 quart for those over 5 years old.) Transport victim to hospital at once.

If victim swallowed an overdose of a drug or a poison that is not a corrosive or petroleum product, dilute with water or milk. (Dose: 1 to 2 cups for those under 5 years; up to 1 quart for those 5 years old or older.) Induce vomiting. Every home with small children should have **syrup of ipecac** at hand (obtainable without prescription at pharmacies), for it is the most effective emetic. (Dose to induce vomiting: 1 tablespoon [½ ounce]). If no vomiting occurs in 20 minutes, dose may be repeated once only. If syrup of ipecac is not available, induce vomiting by placing the smooth handle of a spoon or your finger at the back of victim's throat. Do not use salt water.

■ Puncture wounds

All puncture wounds should be seen by the doctor because of the likelihood of **tetanus** (lockjaw). Proper first aid can be crucial. Gently squeeze wound to encourage bleeding. Wash hands and then clean wound with soap and water. Cover wound loosely with sterile dressing and apply ice bag to reduce swelling.

■ Shock

Shock is a state of circulatory collapse resulting from hemorrhage, heart failure, vasodilatation, or a combination thereof. The symptoms of shock include clammy skin and shallow or rapid breathing. Lay victim down, head lower than feet except in the case of head or chest injuries. For these latter injuries raise head and shoulders 10 inches higher than feet. (If breathing is difficult, lower head.) Loosen clothing and keep victim tightly covered. Victim should be warm without sweating. Do not apply heat. If victim is conscious and thirsty, give plain water (neither hot nor cold), a few sips at a time. Do not give water if victim is nauseated or has a deep abdominal wound. Do not give stimulants. Call for help.

■ Sprains and fractures

A sprain is an injury of a ligament; a fracture is a broken bone. For sprains, elevate injured part and apply cold compresses for half an hour. If swelling is unusual, do not use injured part until seen by the doctor. Severe sprains should be x-rayed for possible bone fractures. All sprains or strains of the back should be examined by a doctor. Any deformity of an injured part usually means a fracture. Do not move person if fracture of leg, neck, or back is suspected. Summon help at once. If victim must be moved, immobilize injured part with adequate splints.

■ SELF-TEST

1. _____ auto accidents
2. _____ defensive driving
3. _____ "reaction time"
4. _____ proper maintenance
5. _____ workplace hazards
6. _____ major home accident
7. _____ discarded freezers
8. _____ auto insurance
9. _____ good safety record
10. _____ auto exhaust
11. _____ cardiac arrest
12. _____ Heimlich maneuver
13. _____ pressure points
14. _____ cold water
15. _____ syrup of ipecac

a. airlines
b. falls
c. liability
d. choking
e. alcohol
f. burns
g. CPR
h. poisoning
i. CO
j. suffocation
k. bleeding
l. OSHA
m. braking
n. tires
o. judgment

■ STUDY QUESTIONS

1. The text states that "the personality of the individual plays an important role in accidents." Discuss at length and provide some examples, preferably from your own experience or from firsthand knowledge.
2. More deaths have occurred from automobile accidents in the United States than from all the wars the country has fought since its beginning. This is obviously a staggering statistic, yet society appears somewhat nonchalant. In your opinion, why is this so?
3. Based on deaths per million vehicle miles, statistics indicate that driving is safer today than in the 1930s. Given the great increase in both population and automobiles, how do you account for this?
4. The experts state that the defensive driver is the best driver. Do you have any evidence to the contrary?
5. Without question, alcohol is the major factor in motor vehicle accidents. Do you have any ideas or thoughts beyond those proposed in the text to remedy this highly dangerous situation?
6. Statistics show that the most dangerous drivers are white males between ages 15 and 24, and the safest are those between ages 65 and 74. What are your explanations?
7. What in your view can be done to reduce death on the highway? Be as specific as possible.
8. Two factors determine stopping distance: "reaction time" and "brake time." Identify and discuss each.
9. The garage mechanic has a grave responsibility in auto safety, much more so than many people might imagine. Please discuss the obvious.

10. What are your specific views on "seat belts" and "air bags" in auto safety?

11. Studies show that many pedestrians involved in auto accidents are nondrivers. Does this surprise you? Discuss.

12. Do you have any suggestions for home safety other than those cited in the text?

13. Even though air travel is one of the safest modes of transportation, not a few people fear it. What is your explanation?

14. A number of points were raised in the text concerning public fire safety. Have you had any experience along this line? Do you have further suggestions?

15. The United States Cycling Federation sets forth seven safety points in their "Rules of the Road" (p. 366). Do you have any further suggestions?

16. OSHA has had considerable impact on workplace safety and is often in the news. Do you happen to know of any recent developments?

17. The National Safety Council renders a valuable service to the public in promoting accident prevention. But there are also other such organizations. Cite three or four and state their purposes or functions.

18. In rendering first aid we must, above all, remain calm and employ common sense. Elaborate in detail and, if possible, cite first hand experience to underscore the importance of this dictum.

19. Artificial respiration ("rescue breathing") specifies a rate of about 12 times a minute for adults and 20 times a minute for infants and children. Why the difference?

20. In relation to severe bleeding, what are "pressure points"?

21. For burns and scalds we are admonished not to use ointments, greases, powders, and so on. Why?

22. What is the principle of the Heimlich maneuver? That is, how does it work?

23. In the first aid care of cuts we are told not to use iodine or other antiseptics. Why?

24. How does one distinguish between heat exhaustion and heatstroke?

25. We are told not to induce vomiting in the event the victim has swallowed a corrosive chemical or petroleum product. Why?

CHAPTER 25

Evolution of public health

With the development of organized society it became increasingly evident that factors beyond individual control were important in the maintenance of health and that the community as well as the individual must take steps for health protection. Most important in developing this realization were the terrifying epidemics. It is difficult for us today to realize the death toll taken by communicable diseases in times past. For example, an epidemic of plague swept over Europe in the middle of the fourteenth century, killing 25 million people, or about one fourth of the population. And history tells us that in our not-too-distant past there were many other waterborne, milkborne, and foodborne epidemics. The need for social effort to strengthen medical and allied professions, to learn more about diseases, and to provide facilities for their treatment eventually became very evident. In the present chapter we shall witness the development of health knowledge, the establishment of the basic sciences involved, and the emergence of public health as an entity in itself.

Infection and communicable disease

Immunology

Epidemiology

Communicable disease control

Achievements in disease prevention and control

The broadening and changing public health program

Legal basis for public health work

Legal procedures

Medicine is constantly finding new means of restoring health, and the health and medical sciences have been developed on a broad front. There is now extensive and organized knowledge about the functions of the body (**physiology**), the nature of disease (**pathology**), organisms that cause disease (**microbiology**), and the way in which these organisms reach whole population groups (**epidemiology**). There is organized information concerning poisons and their sources (**toxicology**), the chemical substances needed by the body to maintain health (**nutrition**), the function of hormones in maintaining health (**endocrinology**), the ways in which heredity affects health (**genetics**), and various external and environmental factors affecting human well-being (**sanitation**). Society makes possible the continuing research that expands these areas of knowledge.

INFECTION AND COMMUNICABLE DISEASE

In 1839 Johann Schönlein showed that a moldlike plant was the cause of **favus**, a fungal infection of the scalp. This was the first demonstration that a parasite caused human disease. As our knowledge has grown, we have found hundreds of other plant and animal pathogens, and we have discovered that most communicable diseases are caused by bacteria and viruses.

Louis Pasteur (Fig. 25-1) laid the foundation for the modern program of disease prevention. From 1857 to 1863 he studied **fermentation** and showed that "diseases" of beer and wine (abnormal sour and bitter tastes) were produced by bacteria that had invaded the liquid and disturbed the usual alcoholic (yeast) fermentation by producing undesirable fermentations of their own. From 1865 to 1868 he studied the silkworm disease, pébrine. He showed that this disease was caused by a particular organism that could be grown by

itself in suitable liquids. The foundations for bacteriology and a scientific attack on germ diseases caused by organisms were securely laid.

Basic methods of studying the bacteria were developed by Robert Koch. He isolated bacteria in pure cultures by growing them in a medium that could be solidified (gelatin or agar-agar). Koch further discovered how to kill and fix bacteria and stain them on a glass slide for more effective study. In his study of anthrax he found the bacillus in diseased animals, grew it for several microbic generations in sterile aqueous humor from the eye of an ox, and reproduced the disease by introducing these remote descendants into healthy animals. In other words, the chain of proof had been made complete. A specific organism had been found in animals having a particular dis-

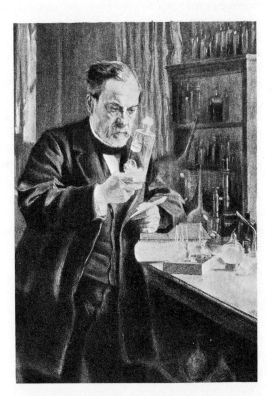

FIG. 25-1 ■ Louis Pasteur (1822-1895).

ease; it had been isolated and grown by itself in pure cultures; it had been introduced into healthy animals in which it produced the disease resulting in the death of the animal; and after the death of the animal it had been recovered from the tissues. These four steps in establishing the cause of an infectious disease constitute what are aptly referred to as **Koch's postulates**.

From such beginnings the science of microbiology has developed with its many applications in industry, dairying, farming, and food preservation, as well as in public health and medicine.

■■■■■ IMMUNOLOGY

Some knowledge of immunology, as well as some knowledge of epidemics, preceded the discovery that microorganisms can cause disease. As early as 1717 Lady Mary Wortley Montagu, the wife of the British ambassador at Constantinople, wrote to friends at home about the Turkish custom of "inoculating" against **smallpox**. In this inoculation some "matter" obtained from the pustule of a patient with smallpox was introduced under the skin of a healthy person. Such an individual, by choosing to contract smallpox by inoculation when in good physical health and by taking good care of himself or herself from the onset of the disease, usually had a mild attack and was immune thereafter. The general adoption throughout Europe of this strenuous method of securing immunity speaks for the horror with which the disease was regarded. Previous to that time smallpox was the great scourge and destroyer of humanity. Scarcely one person in a thousand escaped it. So common was it during childhood that smallpox was regarded as a children's disease.

Then came the discovery of **vaccination** by Edward Jenner in 1796 (Fig. 25-2). As a medical student Jenner had been impressed by the remark of a patient who said, "I cannot take smallpox because I have had cowpox." Testing this belief in his classic experiment, Jenner transferred some of the fluid from a typical cowpox sore on the hand of Sarah Nelms, a dairymaid who had contracted cowpox from her master's cow by infection through a scratch on the hand, to the arm of James Phipps, a boy about 8 years old. This successful vaccination was followed by exposures that showed the boy to be immune to smallpox.

At that time it was only known that "having cowpox" either by accidental or intentional vaccination (Lat. vacca, cow) would prevent smallpox. Now we know that the virus of smallpox is changed in some way by its life in the body of the cow. When reintroduced into the human body, the virus stimulates the body to develop immune substances against the disease but it produces only a local reaction instead of characteristic smallpox. As a result of vaccination smallpox has been virtually eliminated throughout the world. So rare has smallpox become in the United States that routine vaccination is no longer considered necessary.

Contributions of Pasteur to immunology were based on an application of the principle of germ disease to the experience with vaccination. He reasoned that if infectious disease is a struggle between an individual and a microbe and if the smallpox germ was weakened in the body of the cow, it should be possible to weaken, or "attenuate," other germs by heat, cold, starvation, or other means. Pasteur's demonstration of the protection of animals against anthrax by inoculation with attenuated anthrax germs is a thrilling episode in the annals of immunity.

Equally exciting was Pasteur's development of a vaccine for rabies. In this case the causative organism was attenuated by being dried in spinal cords taken from rabbits that had been infected with the disease. Emul-

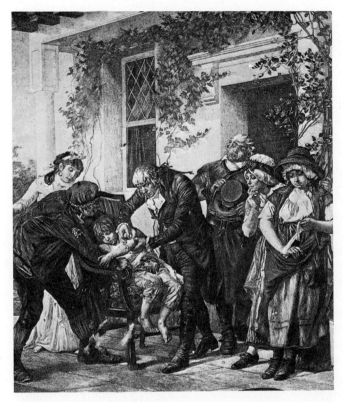

FIG. 25-2 ■ Edward Jenner (1749-1823). An old print showing Jenner performing the first vaccination on James Phipps.

sions of these dried spinal cords were injected into the person who had been bitten by a rabid animal. In this situation, also, attenuated germs enabled the body to develop protection against the more virulent organisms.

From these beginnings the science of immunology has developed. Essentially, this specialty involves the development of vaccines and their use to provide active immunity in susceptible individuals.

■ EPIDEMIOLOGY

Primitive beings sought the explanation of epidemics in supernatural causes. Civilized people began looking for natural causes. It is not surprising that an epidemic had been studied before microorganisms were known to cause disease. The study of the cholera epidemic of the Broad Street Well by Dr. John Snow of London in 1854 may be regarded as the beginning of the science of epidemiology. His report said, in part:

With regard to the 73 deaths occurring in the locality belonging, as it were, to the pump, there were 61 instances in which I was informed that the deceased persons used to drink water from the pump in Broad Street, either constantly or occasionally. In six (6) instances I could get no information, owing to the death or the departure of every one connected with the deceased individuals; and in six (6) cases I was informed that the deceased persons did not drink the pump water before their illness.

The result of the inquiry consequently was that there had been no particular outbreak or increase of cholera in this part of London, except among the persons who were in the habit of drinking the water of the above-mentioned pump well.

I had an interview with the Board of Guardians of St. James Parish on the evening of Thursday, 7th of September, and represented the above circumstances to them. In consequence of what I said the handle of the pump was removed on the following day.

Further investigation showed that the well had been polluted from a leaking cesspool that had received the excrements of cholera patients.

Epidemiology, formally defined, is the study of the relationships of the various factors determining the frequency and distribution of diseases in a human community. Frequency is expressed in terms of **rates**—that is, the number of persons with a disease per unit of population per unit of time. These rates express either **morbidity** (frequency of disease) or **mortality** (frequency of death). **Prevalence rates** measure the number of people in a population who have a disease at any one time; **incidence rates** measure the number of people who develop a disease during a specified period of time. Incidence of infection is characterized by the expressions sporadic, endemic, epidemic, and pandemic. **Sporadic diseases** occur infrequently and only in isolated or single cases; **endemic diseases** are those that are continually present in the population; **epidemic diseases** are those that spread rapidly and attack a large number of people in one location at any one time; **pandemic diseases** are worldwide or affect many countries.

To maintain itself in nature a parasite must be transmitted from host to host. This can occur either directly or indirectly. **Direct transmission** includes sexual contact (venereal disease), contact with respiratory secretions from sneezing (Fig. 25-3) and coughing, and congenital transfer (mother to child). **Indirect transmission** encompasses contaminated articles, or fomites; contaminated food, water, and milk; contaminated airborne particles; and insect vectors. Vectors are said to be mechanical or biologic. A **mechanical vector** transmits an infectious agent from one host to another but is not essential to the life cycle or survival of the parasite; a **biological vector** is one in whose body the infectious agent develops or multiplies before becoming infective to the recipient individual. The chief vectors of concern in community health include flies, mites, lice, fleas, ticks, and mosquitoes (Fig. 25-4).

COMMUNICABLE DISEASE CONTROL

Our constantly growing knowledge of disease-producing organisms and the way in which they are spread enables us to develop various measures to prevent and control communicable diseases. In personal hygiene the use of common drinking cups (Fig. 25-5), the eating of food prepared and served by persons with unclean habits whose freedom from infectious disease cannot be vouched for, and many other unhygienic procedures are automatically condemned. Immunization, sanitation, and public health administrative procedures are used in the protection of community health.

In addition to these public health measures we have the invaluable assistance of curative medicine in general and **chemotherapy** in particular. Penicillin, still the most widely used antibiotic, was discovered by Alexander Fleming in 1929. Fleming observed that on a culture plate a blue-green mold (*Penicillium notatum*) checked the growth of a culture of staphylococci. The therapeutic possibilities of penicillin, the substance produced by the mold (Fig. 25-6), were not appreciated until the work of Oxford researchers in 1940.

There are in use today many antibiotics, in addition to the various forms of penicillin, that are produced from different molds and nonpathogenic bacteria as well as by synthetic

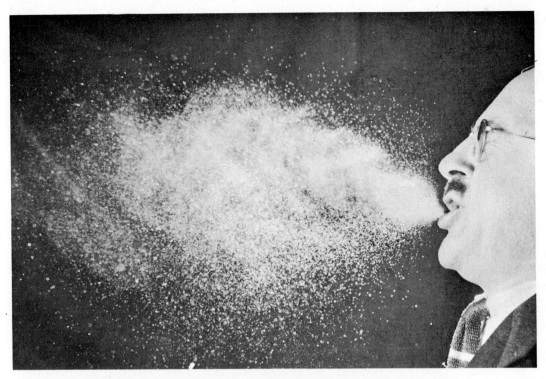

FIG. 25-3 ■ Photograph of a sneeze taken with an exposure of 1/30,000 of a second.

Courtesy M.W. Jennison.

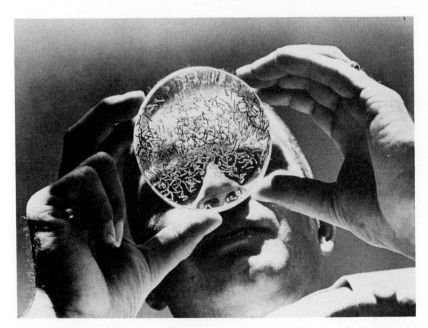

FIG. 25-4 ■ The larval forms of the mosquito that transmits yellow fever.

Courtesy Eli Lilly & Co., Indianapolis, Indiana.

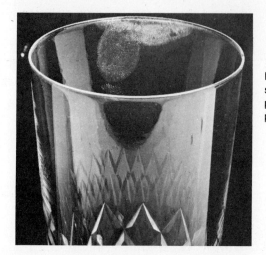

FIG. 25-5 ■ Photograph of a thumb print and lipstick smears on an otherwise clean glass shows the need for properly cleansed (sanitized) glassware or the use of paper cups at public eating places.

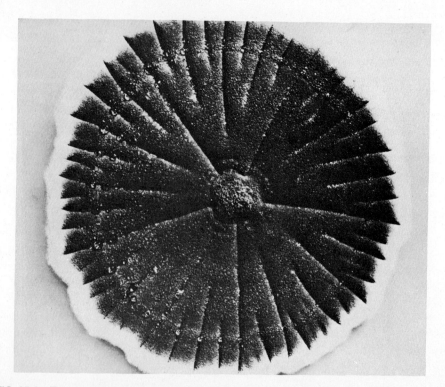

FIG. 25-6 ■ The mold shown here is *Penicillium chrysogenum*, a mutant form from which almost all the world's supply of penicillin is obtained.

Courtesy Pfizer, Inc., New York, N.Y.

means. These include tetracyclines, erythro-mycins, cephalosporins, chloramphenicol, and antifungal drugs. Different antibiotics are effective against different disease-producing microbes, but they are not effective against the common viral diseases. Nor are the **sulfonamides** (sulfa drugs) effective. Often, however, antibiotics are used in viral infections that are complicated by bacterial infections.

A close look at some of the classes of chemotherapeutic drugs in existence today will provide the reader with some insight into the astonishing strides medical science has made in the twentieth century, let alone since the time of Jenner, Schönlein, Pasteur, Koch, and even Fleming. There are **antiinfectives** (including antibiotics and sulfonamides, antiseptics, disinfectants, germicides, fungicides, pediculicides, and scabicides), **biologicals** (allergens, antitoxins, antivenins, immune serums, toxoids, and vaccines), **antivirals** (drugs that destroy or prevent the replication of viruses), **antiprotozoals** (drugs used in infections caused by protozoa—malaria, amebiasis, trichomoniasis, giardiasis, and trypanosomiasis), **antituberculotics** (used in the treatment of tuberculosis), and **diagnostics** (used to signal a specific infection).

■■■ ACHIEVEMENTS IN DISEASE PREVENTION AND CONTROL

Throughout the history of the United States, improvements in the standard of living, advances in medical science, and programs of public health have combined to produce almost unbelievable results in the prolongation of human life. The average length of life of persons living in the United States has more than doubled since 1850, when it was about 35 years (which is still the average length of life in some parts of the world). In 1900 the death rate (mortality) in the United States was 17.2 per 1000 people. Today it is less than 10

TABLE 25-1

Maternal mortality, 1915-1977

Period of time	Deaths per 100,000 live births
1915-1919	727.9
1935-1939	493.9
1956	40.9
1976	12.3
1977	9.4

From U.S. National Center for Health Statistics, U.S. Public Health Service.

per 1000. The death rate has dropped more rapidly for women than for men and more rapidly at the younger ages than at the older ages. Infant mortality has dropped drastically in the most recent decades (Chapter 14). Perhaps the most phenomenal change in mortality statistics in this century has occurred in the number of maternal deaths attributed to pregnancy and childbirth (Table 25-1). The mortality differential between the white and nonwhite populations has narrowed. Most of the gains in life expectancy are the result of health improvements in the early years of the life cycle, particularly for children and infants. For example, a person born in 1976 (with a life expectancy of 72.8 years) will live an average 25 years longer than a person born in 1900; someone who was 60 years old in 1976 can expect to live only 5 years longer than a person born in 1900.

The chief reason for the rapid decline in mortality during the first half of this century has been the control of communicable diseases, which were the major cause of death in 1900 (Table 25-2). World health data clearly show that active immunization and "wonder drugs" have saved millions of lives. Deaths for some diseases have been reduced almost to the vanishing point. The death rates for tuberculosis, pneumonia, and influenza, for

TABLE 25-2

The ten leading causes of death in the United States, 1900 and 1980

1900	1980
Influenza and pneumonia	Heart disease
Tuberculosis	Cancer
Diarrhea and enteritis	Cerebrovascular disease
Heart disease	Accidents
Cerebral hemorrhage	Influenza and pneumonia
Nephritis	Diabetes mellitus
Accidents	Cirrhosis of liver
Cancer	Arteriosclerosis
Diseases of early infancy	Suicide
Diphtheria	Asthma, bronchitis, emphysema

From U.S. National Center for Health Statistics, U.S. Public Health Service.

TABLE 25-3

Population of the United States (millions) in 1980 compared to 1970

Years of age	1970	1980
Under 5	17.2	16.3
5-14	40.7	34.9
15-24	35.4	42.5
25-34	24.9	37.1
35-44	23.1	25.6
45-54	23.2	22.8
55-64	18.6	21.7
65 and older	20.0	25.5
Total	203.1	226.4

From the Bureau of the Census, 1980.

example, have dropped dramatically; the death rate for diphtheria is virtually zero. The reduction in deaths from communicable diseases of children has been especially significant in extending expectation of life and average age of the population (Table 25-3).

THE BROADENING AND CHANGING PUBLIC HEALTH PROGRAM

Government and voluntary activities in public health in the United States began with an attack on communicable diseases. Quarantine, sanitation, and immunization were and still are major activities. As a result, today the control and prevention of communicable diseases is fairly well in hand. But now we face serious problems of pollution control, accident prevention, noncommunicable diseases, nutrition, mental health, drug abuse, alcohol abuse, caffeine abuse, alcoholism, and so on. To combat these growing threats to our personal health, schools of public health have come into existence and have grown along with

expanding public health organizations on all levels—government, private, and voluntary. Public health professionals, as well as private physicians and others in the health care field, are interested in the promotion and availability of vigorous positive health care for infants, mothers, schoolchildren, workers, the physically and mentally handicapped, and the general population.

Preventive medicine and personal health are both based on the application of health knowledge by the individual, and therefore organized health education in the school and in the community has become an important factor in public health programs. The first graduate program for the preparation of specialists in health education to be established in a **school of public health** was offered in 1921 in the school conducted jointly by Harvard University and the Massachusetts Institute of Technology. Accredited programs for the professional education of health educators are now in existence. Techniques and skills have been highly developed, and health departments, school systems, and private health agencies have added health educators to their staffs. With the understanding and support of social-minded and knowledgeable citizens, leaders in health administration and in the health and medical sciences are planning education programs for the future based on our best present practices, but attuned to changing needs.

▆▆▆ LEGAL BASIS FOR PUBLIC HEALTH WORK

The division of the responsibilities for administering public health among national, state, and municipal governments is dependent on the relationship that these bodies bear to each other under the Constitution of the United States and under the various state constitutions. Ours is a federal government, and each state has supreme power in those questions that affect that state alone. In such matters the state may, if it chooses, direct the individual community, and it may not be interfered with by the federal government. Each state bears the responsibility for its health conditions, and this responsibility rests primarily on the state legislature as the supreme power of the state. The legislators, limited only by the state constitution and responsible only to the electorate, have supreme power to determine how health regulations shall be made and what official organizations shall be provided by municipalities and by the state at large to administer public health.

Legislatures sometimes delegate a limited amount of "law-making power" to state departments of health. This delegation of power is wise, since only a body of experts is qualified to work out the details of public health regulations. Under this power a **sanitary code**, consisting of rules and regulations affecting the security of life or health, is enacted. The provisions of this code have the force and effect of law in all parts of the state. In enforcement they supersede any local ordinances that may be inconsistent with them.

The desirable relationship between state and local **health departments** leaves the basic responsibility for community health with the local or municipal officials, but it gives power to the state health officer to protect the health of the whole state whenever it may be endangered by local inefficiency. The division of authority between the state and local health departments in each state is determined by the state laws that established these departments. The national government has only such powers as are granted to it by the Constitution. In these matters state law must give way, but when power is not specifically given to the national government, it is assumed that the power lies within the state.

There is no specific mention of any power over the public health in our federal Constitution, but power to regulate commerce, to provide for the common defense, and to carry out treaty agreements are specifically granted to the national government. The federal government is also given direct jurisdiction over territories, national parks, and other federal domains and power to "promote the general welfare." Certain public health activities are very properly carried on under these broad powers.

Under the "power to regulate commerce" the federal government has the authority to prohibit, under criminal penalty, the interstate transportation of persons or articles. This includes the power of **quarantine** against persons or things to prevent their entrance from one state to another when such an entrance may be judged to endanger the public health or safety. An important use of this power was the enactment of the Food and Drug Act (p. 403), which forbids the transportation from one state to another of adulterated food products and certain drugs.

Under the "power to provide for the common defense," the federal government raises and supports armed forces and does whatever is necessary to protect the health of the United States Army, Navy, and Air Force, even within state lines. In the District of Columbia and on reservations the federal government has complete health powers at all times through its direct jurisdiction.

Under the "power to promote the general welfare," the United States government established a Public Health Service and other agencies authorized to assist state health authorities and to cooperate with them. Although the United States government may not interfere with the sanitary work within the states, it may have a far-reaching influence on state health administration through its power of appropriating money for health work in the form of grants-in-aid to states for specified public health activities.

LEGAL PROCEDURES

On the legal side of public health administration common and constitutional as well as statutory laws are involved. The **common law** consists of the court decisions made in the course of administering justice. The decision of a lower court or the opinion of an attorney has little value as a precedent, but the decision of the Supreme Court is binding on subordinate courts until overruled. **Constitutional law** has to do with the interpretation of federal and state constitutions. **Statutory laws** are enacted by legislatures.

All authority for the protective operations of government, including the preservation of public health, is derived from **police power**, an inherent function of government. It is the right of government to protect the health, morals, and safety of the public. In its exercise is sanction for otherwise illegal acts, for example, the violation of personal or property rights to protect the safety of the people in great epidemics. It is a fundamental social principle that personal liberty ends when individual action menaces public safety. On this

principle are based many public health procedures, such as the prevention of nuisances and the control of communicable diseases.

The issuing of licenses is done under police power. A license may be issued on payment of a slight fee, as in licensing milk dealers, where it is the need for a license rather than the fee that restricts or regulates the business. On the other hand, the issuance of licenses at a very high cost has been a reasonable use of police power in restraining and controlling the marketing of liquor.

In enforcing the public health law the health officer is given considerable power of discretion as to what shall be done. The health officer is entitled to perform any act within that discretion, and all such actions will be held to have been done with the express authorization of law. The health officer who abuses this power of discretion is amenable to prosecution, but the act, to be criminal, must be willful and corrupt, and proof of this rests on the complainant. If discretion is left entirely to the administrative officer, there is no way in which that person can be forced to act. An officer cannot be sued personally for neglect of an exclusively public duty, even if someone is specially injured thereby. If a law prescribes specific duties for a health officer (if it is mandatory), those duties must be performed.

Injunction (a restraining order issued by the court) can be used to prevent executive action, the taking or impairment of property, or the creation of nuisances. It is not used to direct or to restrain the exercise of discretionary authority. A public health **nuisance** is a state of affairs that is dangerous to public health. Obviously something may be a nuisance under either common or statutory law. In exigencies the health authorities may summarily abate the nuisance, but the property owner who cannot get a formal trial before the abatement is entitled to a hearing afterward. The burden then falls on the authorities to justify their action.

■■■■■■   **SELF-TEST**

1. _____ study of disease   a. genetics
2. _____ study of microbes   b. immunology
3. _____ study of population group   c. sanitation
4. _____ study of food   d. infection
5. _____ study of heredity   e. chemotherapy
6. _____ pollution control   f. sporadic
7. _____ Koch's postulates   g. vectors
8. _____ vaccination   h. nutrition
9. _____ frequency of death   i. epidemic
10. _____ frequency of disease   j. endemic
11. _____ continually present   k. epidemiology
12. _____ isolated cases   l. mortality
13. _____ large outbreak   m. microbiology
14. _____ insect transmission   n. morbidity
15. _____ antibiotics and sulfonamides   o. pathology

■■■■■■**STUDY QUESTIONS**

1. Strictly speaking, the terms communicable, contagious, and infectious are not synonymous. Discuss and give examples.
2. What value is the subject of epidemiology in public health programs? Give examples.
3. What does sanitation mean in the context of public health?
4. Discuss the subject of immunology in relation to public health.
5. Distinguish between vaccine and vaccination.
6. Distinguish between prevalence and incidence in relation to public health.
7. Discuss the topic of disease transmission and cite appropriate examples.
8. What is the meaning of chemotherapy?
9. Since 1900 the death rate for females has dropped more rapidly than for males and more rapidly at the younger ages than at the older ages. In your view, what are the reasons for this?
10. Infant mortality has dropped drastically since 1900. How do you account for this?
11. What is the meaning of quarantine?
12. The purview of public health now goes well beyond communicable disease. Cite a number of other areas of concern and discuss each.
13. What role do you think schools (at all levels) should play in public health?
14. In your own words discuss the interplay of the federal, state, and municipal governments in the administration of public health.
15. What does the expression "community health" mean to you?

CHAPTER 26

Health programs

Knowledge is one thing, but putting it to proper use is something else again. Indeed, unless we put to use what we know, we may, with excellent reason, question the logic of acquiring knowledge. Pasteur and Koch demonstrated that microbes cause disease, and Jenner unlocked the door to prevention, but just suppose that these great revelations had not been acted on. Stated otherwise, medical and scientific knowledge must be put to use to benefit the community in general and the individual in particular. And this means establishing a system of public health, which in turn calls for well-conceived laws, ordinances, and programs at all levels of government—federal, state, county, and municipal. What is more it calls for voluntary organizations and agencies to complement and supplement "the law," and, ultimately, it calls for individual initiative. In the present chapter we shall take a good look at the various government programs, voluntary agencies, and professional organizations dealing with public health. Furthermore, we shall consider international programs and, most especially, the World Health Organization.

State public health programs

City health departments

County health units

Federal health programs

International health programs

Occupational health programs

Voluntary health agencies

Professional organizations

Public and community health programs encompass the full spectrum of government, voluntary, and professional organizations dealing with every aspect of health and disease. The areas of jurisdiction and concern include state health programs, city health departments, county health units, federal programs, occupational health programs, voluntary health agencies, and professional groups. The very special role of school health programs is treated in Chapter 27.

■■■■ STATE PUBLIC HEALTH PROGRAMS

The central agency for public health in the state is the **department of health**, although there are other health activities carried on by many different types of agencies, such as the state departments of education, welfare, agriculture, safety, conservation, and civil service. In addition, there may be specific commissions dealing with drug abuse, pollution, and dairy and food products.

State health departments characteristically consist of a state commissioner of health or state health officer, who is a physician with special public health training, together with the staff and an advisory public health council. The state health department has some statewide regulatory functions and usually some extremely limited personal service in the form of traveling diagnostic and immunization clinics. Important functions are statewide planning and guidance and assistance to local health departments.

The general plans of organization in the 50 states are similar, but no two state health departments are exactly alike. Moreover, these plans change from time to time as changing public health needs require placing emphases in different areas. For example, problems of drug abuse, venereal disease, air and water pollution, and health problems related to welfare activities are now demanding much at-

tention, whereas activities for the control of tuberculosis and other communicable diseases demand less attention than they did a few generations ago. Nevertheless, several divisions may be found in the majority of health departments: (1) administration, including finance, personnel, hospital administration, health education, and vital statistics; (2) preventive medicine, including chronic diseases and adult health; (3) local health services, usually including public health nursing; (4) dental health; (5) maternal and child health; (6) environmental health; and (7) laboratories.

The office, or division, of administration is presided over directly by the health officer and includes activities for drafting legislation, for licensing certain operations, for budgeting and accounts, and for the employment and management of personnel.

The maintenance of **vital statistics**, which is sometimes handled in the office of administration and sometimes in a separate division, includes recording and analyzing data concerning deaths, births, marriages, population, and diseases. If disease is to be prevented and lives are to be saved, careful records must be kept to show where, when, and how diseases and deaths occur. The recording and interpretation of vital statistics require skill, and highly trained vital statisticians are employed for this work. The most commonly computed rates are discussed as follows.

The **crude birth rate** is the ratio of 1 year's births to the total population. It is usually expressed as the number of births per 1000 population. The **true birth rate** is the ratio of births to the female population of child-bearing age. The **death rate** (**mortality rate**) is the number of deaths annually per 1000 population. **Specific death rates** state the number of deaths per 100,000 population for specific diseases. The **morbidity** is the number of cases of a specific disease per 1000 population (sometimes expressed as the number per 100,000 population). The **fatality rate** is the number of deaths annually from a specific disease per 100 cases (the percent fatality). When we realize that such rates show whether we live in a safe and healthy community or in a dangerous and unhealthy one, the statistics of our state and local health departments become most interesting reading. The registration of births, marriages, and deaths is also important for legal, social, and property rights.

The division of environmental affairs is headed by a state sanitary engineer and staffed by persons skilled in water purification, sewage disposal, food sanitation, and the control of air pollution. These persons also work in the fields of housing, rodent and insect control, industrial hygiene, and hazardous waste disposal.

In **communicable disease control** the state health department works to limit the spread of communicable disease. It promotes immunization and investigates incipient epidemics. The division may provide trained epidemiologic teams who offer assistance in diagnosis as well as in control measures. Laboratories provide diagnosis of communicable diseases and in the larger states may prepare vaccines and antitoxins. The laboratories also carry out chemical and bacteriologic examinations of water, milk, food, air, drugs, and other substances.

In maternal and child health trained workers make surveys, develop special state and local campaigns to improve the hygienic conditions of maternity, infancy, and childhood, and cooperate with private child health agencies and physicians throughout the state. In many states a special program for handicapped children has been added. Its purpose is to learn the prevalence of crippling conditions and to provide supplementary aid in rehabilitation of the children affected.

In public health nursing the state health department determines the qualifications of the public health nurse, employs a corps of nurses

to assist district health officers, and strengthens the work of those nurses who are employed in various communities in the state by affording them advice, assistance, and cooperation.

Unless there is a separate division of mental health, the state department of health directs the operation of mental hospitals, establishes mental health clinics, helps to ascertain the extent of mental health services needed in a community, and carries on educational programs for other professional and community workers, including social workers, teachers, and public health nurses.

The office of public health education provides educational material, including pamphlets, news releases, radio and television programs, and movies. It assists local health workers in the development of educational activities and in community organization for health education.

Highly industrialized states may have a division of industrial hygiene in the state health department. In other such states these activities are carried on in a state board of labor and industries. The industrial hygiene agency maintains a staff consisting of physicians, engineers, chemists, and inspectors. Central laboratories equipped to make chemical and physical tests are usually established. Intensive surveys of special industries and routine inspections are made. Factory inspection involves the enforcement of laws regulating items such as ventilation, dusts, gases, odors, temperature, moisture, light, cleanliness, overcrowding, water supply, washing facilities, water closets, lockers, fire prevention, safeguarding machinery, first-aid facilities, hours of labor, employment of women and children, and ages of employment.

■■■ CITY HEALTH DEPARTMENTS

The local health organization usually consists of a board of health and a health officer

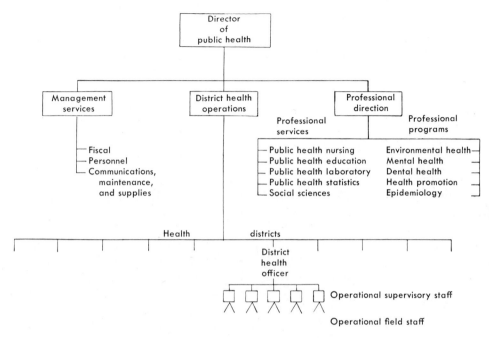

FIG. 26-1 ■ Organization of a decentralized city health department.

From Hanlon, J.: Public health: administration and practice, ed. 7, St. Louis, 1979, The C.V. Mosby Co.

(Fig. 26-1). The board determines policies and procedures. The health officer employs a staff with the approval of the board and is responsible for administration of the organization. The board of health is either elected or appointed by the mayor. The health officer is usually appointed by the board. In some instances legislation provides for a type of local organization with a health commissioner and an advisory committee. The scope of local health work in a large city is comparable to that of a state health department and usually embraces such activities as those listed in Table 26-1. It is the city health department, rather than the state, that renders direct service to the individual, the family, or the business group. The state health department aids in planning and in the development of quality service.

Health centers (Fig. 26-2) for public health work may house facilities for the physical examination of well people, health consulta-

tions, well-baby clinics, venereal disease clinics, special classes, and health education. In many cases activities of voluntary agencies such as the Red Cross and the Visiting Nurse Association are carried on in these centers.

■■■ **COUNTY HEALTH UNITS**

County health programs began with the establishment of the first county health department in the United States in Yakima County, Washington, in 1911. A unit of rural population of some 25,000 to 100,000 people may be conveniently served by a county health department. In some cases a department covers more than one county in order to have a suitable population group. Small cities up to 20,000 people are usually included in county health department projects, but large cities usually have their own health department

▰▰▰▰▰▰▰ **TABLE 26-1**
Typical activities of a large city health department

VITAL STATISTICS
Births
Deaths
Morbidity
Maps
Charts
Records

COMMUNICABLE DISEASE CONTROL
Isolation
Quarantine
Release
Home instruction
Diagnostic aid
Epidemiology
Hospitalization
Immunization
Biological products

ENVIRONMENTAL QUALITY
Air pollution
Water pollution
Hazardous wastes

MATERNAL AND CHILD HEALTH
Clinics
Nursing
Midwives
Education
  Infant hygiene
    Well-baby clinics
    Nursing
    Institutional care
  Preschool hygiene
    Clinics
    Immunization
    Dental hygiene
    Mental hygiene
    Nutrition
    Correction of defects
    Nursing
    Municipal hospitals

SCHOOL HYGIENE
Sanitation
Communicable disease control
Examinations
Follow-up
Clinics
Special classes
Health education
Dental health

SANITATION
Housing
Vermin and insects
Milk
  Standards
  Dairy inspection
  Pasteurization
  Laboratory testing
Food and drugs
  Food handlers
  Food establishments
  Drug control
Water and sewage
  Inspection
  Laboratory control

LABORATORIES
Diagnostic
Food
Water
Air

PUBLIC HEALTH EDUCATION
  (Serving many parts of the program)

INDUSTRIAL HYGIENE
Education
Engineering
Toxicology

PUBLIC HEALTH NURSING
  (Serving many parts of the program)

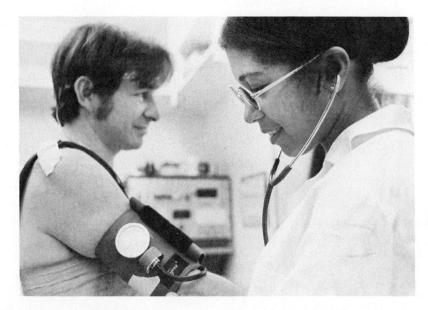

FIG. 26-2 ■ Hypertension screening programs may be conducted by public health workers at community health centers.

Courtesy Johns Hopkins Medical Institutions.

separate from that of the surrounding rural areas.

The modern county health department has trained full-time personnel consisting of a health officer, public health nurses, a sanitary engineer, sanitary inspectors, a clerk, and a health educator (Fig. 26-3). Frequently a nutritionist and a social worker are included. In addition, part-time physicians and dentists are commonly employed to staff such clinics as may be operated. Immunization clinics, venereal disease clinics, and dental clinics for children are commonly organized in cooperation with the county medical and dental societies. Prenatal clinics and well-baby clinics are sometimes provided.

The county board of health may consist of three to five citizens, some but not all of whom may be physicians. A position on the board is honorary and carries no remuneration. The board makes general policies, approves the budget, and selects the specially trained health officer. It does not have administrative responsibility. The work of a county health unit is similar to that of other local health departments.

■ FEDERAL HEALTH PROGRAMS

The first activity of the federal government in the field of health began with an act creating a Marine Hospital Service (Fig. 26-4). This act was signed into law on July 16, 1798, by President John Adams. It provided medical care and hospitalization for merchant seamen. The service was located in the Treasury Department because a small tax was collected from each sailor by the Collector of Customs. This agency gradually took on public health activities and in 1912 became the United States Public Health Service. In 1953 the agency was placed under the jurisdiction of the newly created Department of Health, Education, and

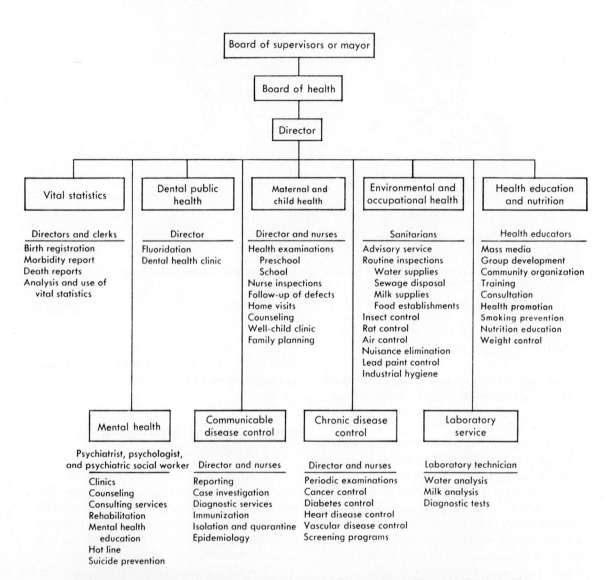

FIG. 26-3 ■ Organization and services of a city or county health department. Many variations in health department organization exist, and services vary from one health department to another, but the services listed in this chart represent the core of local health department activities.

From Green, L.W., and Anderson, C.L.: Community health, ed. 4, St. Louis, 1982, The C.V. Mosby Co.

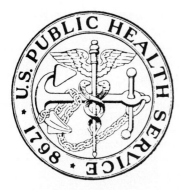

FIG. 26-4 ■ The seal of the United States Public Health Service reflects its medical and health activities and its origin as the Marine Hospital Service.

Welfare (HEW). HEW was completely reorganized in 1979 under the Department of Education Organization Act, which set up a separate Department of Education and a Department of Health and Human Services (HHS) (see below). Each of these departments is headed by a secretary who is a member of the President's cabinet.

In addition to the Department of Health and Human Services, cabinet-level agencies with health responsibilities include the Department of Agriculture (p. 405); Department of Commerce (Bureau of the Census); Department of Transportation (National Highway Traffic Safety Administration, Federal Aviation Agency, and the U.S. Coast Guard [Office of Boating Safety and Office of Merchant Marine Safety]); Department of Labor (Occupational Safety and Health Administration, p. 366); Department of the Interior (Bureau of Mines); Department of Energy (p. 441); and Department of Justice.

Other federal agencies associated with health include the Veterans' Administration (VA), Federal Trade Commission (FTC), Interstate Commerce Commission (ICC), U.S. Postal Service, Federal Communications Commission (FCC), U.S. Consumer Product Safety Commission (CPSC), Department of Housing

■ TABLE 26-2
The Department of Health and Human Services (HHS)

Administrators
Secretary of Health and Human Services
Assistant Secretaries (7)

Operating programs
Public Health Service
Health Care Financing Administration
Office of Human Development Services
Social Security Administration
Office of the Inspector General
Office of Civil Rights
Office of Refugee Settlement

Regional offices

Boston	Kansas City
New York	Dallas
Philadelphia	Denver
Atlanta	San Francisco
Chicago	Seattle

and Urban Development (HUD), and Environmental Protection Agency (EPA) (Chapter 28).

■ Department of Health and Human Services (HHS)

The Department of Health and Human Services is organized into 7 agencies (Table 26-2) that carry out its work in 10 regional offices across the United States in conjunction with state and local agencies. These are discussed as follows.

United States Public Health Service (USPHS). The United States Public Health Service (Table 26-3), headed by the Surgeon General, is responsible for the maintenance, protection, and advancement of the health of the American people via its six programs.

The **National Institutes of Health (NIH)** (Table 26-4), the largest research operation in

TABLE 26-3
The United States Public Health Service (USPHS)

National Institutes of Health (NIH)
Food and Drug Administration (FDA)
Centers for Disease Control (CDC)
Health Resources Administration (HRA)
Health Services Administration (HSA)
Alcohol, Drug Abuse, and Mental Health Administration
   (ADAMHA)

TABLE 26-4
The National Institutes of Health (NIH)

National Cancer Institute
National Institute on Aging
National Institute of Child Health and Development
National Institute of General Medical Sciences
National Heart, Lung, and Blood Institute
National Institute of Allergy and Infectious Diseases
National Institute of Dental Research
National Institute of Neurological and Communicative
   Disorders and Stroke
National Library of Medicine
National Institute of Arthritis, Metabolism, and Digestive
   Diseases
National Institute of Environmental Health Sciences
National Eye Institute

TABLE 26-5
Food and Drug Administration (FDA)

Bureau of Foods
Bureau of Biologics
Bureau of Drugs
Bureau of Medical Devices and Diagnostic Products
Bureau of Veterinary Medicine
National Center for Toxicological Research
Bureau of Radiological Health
Executive Director of Regional Operations

the world, spends some 90% of its budget on subsidizing research carried out in hospitals, medical schools, and nonprofit research centers.

The **Food and Drug Administration (FDA)** (Table 26-5), staffed by chemists, nutritionists, microbiologists, pharmacologists, and physicians, is responsible for enforcing the responsibilities delineated in the **Federal Food, Drug, and Cosmetic Act (as amended January, 1980)**; the **Public Health Service Act, Biological Products**; the **Radiation Control for Health and Safety Act**; and the **Fair Packaging and Labeling Act**. In coordination with federal, state, and local agencies, the FDA performs the following services:

1. Makes periodic inspections of food, drug, device, and cosmetic establishments and examines samples from interstate shipments of these products.
2. Assists industry to voluntarily comply with the law by setting up controls to prevent violations.
3. Requires manufacturers to prove the safety and effectiveness of new drugs before they are put on sale to the public.
4. Tests every batch (except for exemptions) of drugs and biologicals for human consumption and use for safety and effectiveness before they are put on the market.
5. Enforces the law against illegal sales of prescription drugs.
6. Investigates medical devices for safety and truthfulness of labeling claims.
7. Sets up standards of safety and wholesomeness of foods and standards of identity, quality, and fill of containers for food products as well as the honest, informative, and accurate labeling of foods and products.
8. Passes on the safety of food additives, and checks to see that safety rules are followed.
9. Sets safe limits on the amount of pesti-

cide residues that may remain on food crops, and checks shipments to see that these limits are observed.

10. Passes on the safety of colors for use in foods, drugs, and cosmetics, and tests and certifies each batch manufactured when necessary.

11. Protects the consumer from hazardous exposure to radiation (from products such as color television sets, x-ray machines, and microwave ovens).

12. Checks imports of foods, drugs, devices, and cosmetics to make sure they comply with United States law.

13. Cooperates with state and local officials in the inspection of foods and drugs contaminated by floods, hurricanes, explosions, and fires and assists in the removal of damaged items from the market.

14. Sets up standards for milk and shellfish sanitation, as well as restaurant operations.

The need to protect the quality of the food supply in behalf of the consumer has long been recognized by governments. In England, for example, the first food law was proclaimed by King John in 1202. It was called the Assize of Bread and prohibited the adulteration of bread with ground peas or beans. The first general food law in the United States was enacted in Massachusetts in 1784. In the ensuing years several state laws and local regulations were enacted, and various acts touching different phases of the problem were enacted by Congress. It was not until 1906, however, that the first broad national legislation was enacted for food and drug control.

Before the Pure Food and Drug Act of 1906 came into existence, a high percentage of processed food sold in the United States was adulterated. Food adulteration had become a specialized art. There was little control over the contents and labeling not only of foods but also of drugs. The act of 1906 was the first step

TABLE 26-6

Centers for Disease Control (CDC)

Center for Environmental Health
Center for Health Promotion and Education
Center for Prevention Services
National Institute for Occupational Safety and Health
Center for Professional Development and Training
Center for Infectious Diseases

in correcting this situation, and, as a result, food adulteration and drug addiction were reduced. In 1938 the act was completely rewritten, modernized, strengthened, and renamed the Federal Food, Drug, and Cosmetic Act. With the years the FDA expanded to include legislation mentioned on p. 402 to control problems associated with medical devices, diagnostic products, pesticides and other chemicals, veterinary medicine, and radiation. However, its activities, especially in the area of screening new drugs and food additives seen as possible carcinogens, have been criticized from time to time by the food and drug industries. For example, the drug industry has argued that the 7 to 10 years it takes to get a new drug approved and on the market deprives consumers of beneficial medicines. But in 1962 the FDA received national acclaim when it became known that sleeping tablets containing **thalidomide**, which had been associated with the birth of thousands of malformed babies in Western Europe, had been kept off the American market because the FDA had not approved it for sale.

The **Centers for Disease Control (CDC)** (Table 26-6) was established in 1946 under the name Communicable Disease Center and in 1970 was retitled Center for Disease Control. In 1973 CDC became a major agency under the Public Health Service. In 1980, with increased work measures, CDC was greatly enlarged and renamed (this time with an "s" added to its name—"Centers"), and it was re-

TABLE 26-7
Health Resources Administration (HRA)

National Center for Health Statistics
National Center for Health Services Research
Bureau of Health Manpower
Bureau of Health Planning and Resources Development

TABLE 26-8
Health Services Administration (HSA)

Bureau of Community Health Services
Bureau of Medical Services
Bureau of Quality Assurance
Indian Health Service
National Health Service Corps

TABLE 26-9
Alcohol, Drug Abuse, and Mental Health Administration (ADAMHA)

National Institute of Alcohol Abuse and Alcoholism
National Institute on Drug Abuse
National Institute of Mental Health

organized into six operation units. CDC places particular emphasis on working closely with state and local health departments in the prevention and control of chronic and infectious diseases; the prevention of disease, disability, and death associated with environmental hazards; the prevention of occupational diseases and accidents; and the dissemination of health information and assistance in family planning.

The **Health Resources Administration (HRA)** (Table 26-7) concerns itself with availability and use of health manpower. It provides financial assistance to health professionals and institutions that have health care courses. It supports and works with state and local health agencies to improve the availability and quality of health care. In addition, it gathers information that will be helpful in determining how to better the health of the nation—data on illness and disability, vital statistics, and health survey programs, etc.

The **Health Services Administration (HSA)** (Table 26-8) funds community health programs such as health centers in areas where health services were once scarce or nonexistent; it gives assistance to migrant workers and their families and operates the National Health Service Corps, an agency whose goal is to see that health care is available to all citizens, especially those in underserved communities.

The **Alcohol, Drug Abuse, and Mental Health Administration (ADAMHA)** (Table 26-9) works through funded programs of research, prevention, and training projects on the community level. The agency also conducts research in its own biochemical and clinical laboratories. The goal of ADAMHA is to reduce and eliminate major health problems of alcoholism and alcohol abuse, drug abuse, and mental and emotional illness.

Health Care Financing Administration. The Health Care Financing Administration (Table 26-10) manages the Medicare and Medicaid programs (described in Chapter 23). This administration is also responsible for enforcing and developing standards of high-quality health care in federally funded programs.

Office of Human Development Services. The Office of Human Development Services (Table 26-11) is set up to meet the needs of the following groups of persons: abused children, battered women and their families, and working parents. In addition, it is concerned with the special economic and social needs of American Indians, Alaskan natives, and native Hawaiians, as well as com-

TABLE 26-10
The Health Care Financing Administration

Medicare
Medicaid

TABLE 26-11
Office of Human Development Services

The Administration for Children, Youth and Families
The Administration for Native Americans
The Administration on Aging
The Administration on Developmental Disabilities
The President's Committee on Mental Retardation
Work Incentive Program (WIN)

TABLE 26-12
Programs administered by the Social Security
Administration

Supplemental Security Income (SSI)
Aid to Families with Dependent Children

munity services for our older citizens. Working with state agencies, this agency aims to improve services to severely handicapped persons. Funding is provided the individual states for services such as counseling, homemaking, foster care, and family planning. The Work Incentive Program (WIN), operated jointly by HHS and the Department of Labor, has as its goal to assist persons on welfare to become self-sufficient.

Other agencies of HHS. The **Social Security Administration** (Table 26-12) distributes financial benefits to certain eligible persons in addition to the responsibility of the programs cited in the Table. The **Office of the Inspector General** has the duty to keep a watchful eye on HHS to be sure that all its programs are operated honestly and efficiently. The **Office of Civil Rights** is charged with the task of seeing to it that no person or institution is discriminated against on a basis of race, color, creed, or physical or mental handicap, insofar as receiving federally funded

medical assistance is concerned. The **Office of Refugee Settlement** was organized as a result of passage by Congress of the Refugee Assistance Act of 1980; it provides many kinds of assistance, including medical care, to refugees. The **Office of Child Support Enforcement**, self-explanatory by its title, is also under the wing of HHS.

■ The Department of Agriculture

The Department of Agriculture today deals with agricultural chemistry, inspection and grading of animal and dairy products, human nutrition, food stamps for the needy, labeling of certain foods, educational programs for the consumer, and entomology. The department in 1906 began inspecting meat intended for interstate trade, a responsibility carried on today. Meat that is to be consumed locally is inspected by the state or local health department. Maintenance of disease-free animals, controlled meat and poultry handling and storage, and inspection of meat at the various processing and distribution points where contamination and deterioration may take place are essential phases of a program to provide a safe meat and poultry supply.

■ Drug Enforcement Administration

The Drug Enforcement Administration, a division of the Department of Justice, is responsible for the execution of the provisions of the Drug Abuse Prevention and Control Act of 1970. This law deals with registration requirements, procurement, storage and security, distribution, administration, records and record keeping, and penalties for noncompliance. The law encompasses all narcotic and nonnarcotic drugs that have a potential for abuse and places these drugs in five categories, or **schedules**, according to the extent of their potential. Some states have enacted their own laws and created additional schedules; when such regulations are more stringent than the federal laws, the local regulations take precedence. The federal schedule runs as follows: Schedule I includes drugs of highest abuse potential with no legal medical use (for example, heroin and LSD); Schedule II includes drugs of high abuse potential that may lead to severe psychologic or physical dependence, but with less abuse than those of Schedule I (for example, narcotics and amphetamines); Schedule III includes drugs with

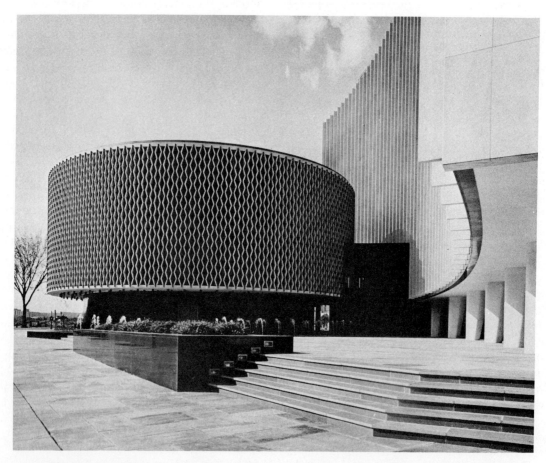

FIG. 26-5 ■ This building in Washington houses the Pan American Health Organization (PAHO) and is the headquarters of WHO in the Americas.

an abuse potential less than those of Schedules I and II (for example, codeine combinations and butabarbital sodium); Schedule IV includes drugs with a lower potential abuse than those of Schedule III (for example, phenobarbital and diazepam); Schedule V includes drugs with an abuse potential less than those of Schedule IV (for example, cough syrups containing codeine). Prescriptions for controlled drugs (Schedules II to V) must contain the full name and address of the patient, the Drug Enforcement Agency number of the prescribing physician, the signature of the prescribing physician, and the date. Prescriptions for Schedule II drugs are not refillable; Schedule III and IV drugs may be refilled up to five times within 6 months of issuance; Schedule V drugs may be refilled as authorized by the prescribing physician.

■■■■■ INTERNATIONAL HEALTH PROGRAMS

The oldest existing international public health organization is the Pan-American Health Organization (PAHO). Organized in 1902 as the Pan-American Sanitary Bureau (PASB) it was supported by annual financial quotas contributed by each of the American republics. It has had a notable experience of technical assistance in public health to the member countries, in the financing of fellowships and in the promotion of research. Since the establishment of the World Health Organization it has become the regional office for the Americas (Fig. 26-5), although maintaining its own identity.

■ World Health Organization

The United Nations has several agencies concerned with health, but the agency that carries on public health activities directly is the World Health Organization (WHO), established in 1948. There are 125 member states and its headquarters are in Geneva, Switzerland. WHO has a large measure of independence and reports annually to the United Nations Economic and Social Council. Its budget is funded by assessments of member states and by contributions from various other sources, including individuals.

The controlling body of WHO is the World Health Assembly, composed of delegations from the member states (Fig. 26-6). It meets annually to determine broad policies, decide on programs, and adopt international health regulations. The assembly has an Executive Board, made up of 24 health specialists from as many countries, who serve on the board in an individual capacity for terms of 3 years. The Secretariat in Geneva comprises a Director-General and a staff including physicians, nurses, engineers, administrators, scientists, statisticians, health educators, interpreters, translators, and secretaries. Technical divisions relate to vector biology, health protection and promotion, epidemiology, public health services, education and training, communicable diseases, environmental health, malaria eradication, health statistics, biomedical sciences, pharmacology and toxicology, coordination and evaluation, and editorial and reference services.

Each division is made up of several units. For example, the units in the division of public health services are health education, health laboratory services, maternal and child health, nursing, organization of medical care, and public health administration. Field operations are carried out through six regional offices: Brazzaville, Africa; Washington, D.C., the Americas; Copenhagen, Europe; Alexandria, Egypt, Eastern Mediterranean; New Delhi, Southeast Asia; and Manila, Philippines, Western Pacific.

At the organization of WHO the following

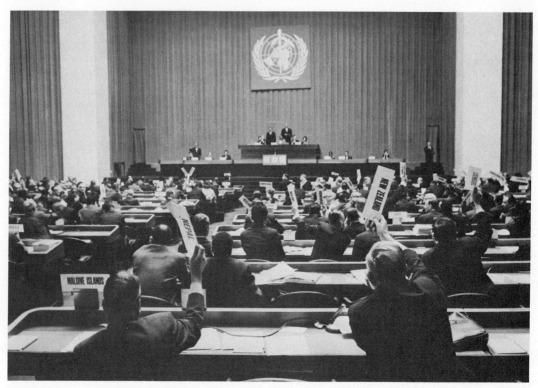

FIG. 26-6 ■ An assembly meeting of the World Health Organization.
Courtesy World Health Organization.

initial priorities were set for the work of the organization:

1. Malaria, tuberculosis, and venereal disease control; maternal and child health; nutrition; and environmental sanitation
2. Public health administration and other technical education
3. Parasitic diseases control
4. Viral diseases control
5. Mental health, including alcoholism and drug addiction
6. Cancer, rheumatoid diseases, leprosy, and cardiovascular diseases

These areas continue to receive major attention.

In terms of operating procedures WHO maintains epidemiologic intelligence on a world basis, carries on research in specific diseases, sends expert consultants and demonstration teams to various countries, promotes special campaigns in such fields as child health, nutrition, disease control, and mental hygiene, promotes programs of health education, and operates a fellowship program for training public health workers. This program provides fellowships each year, distributed among the fields of public health administration, sanitation, nursing, maternal and child health, communicable diseases, clinical medicine, mental health, dental health, health education, health statistics, and nutrition.

WHO collaborates with other United Nations agencies that include health activities in their respective special fields. These include

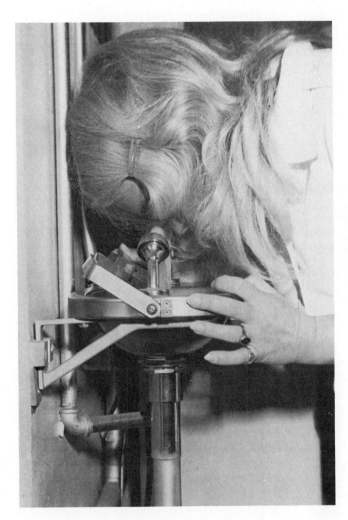

FIG. 26-7 ■ Technician demonstrates the safety eyewasher used when acid is splashed into eyes.

From Lee, L.: The lab aide, St. Louis, 1976, The C.V. Mosby Co.

the United Nations International Children's Emergency Fund (UNICEF), the Food and Agriculture Organization (FAO), the United Nations Educational, Scientific, and Cultural Organization (UNESCO), and the International Labor Organization (ILO).

■ OCCUPATIONAL HEALTH PROGRAMS

Workers in construction, manufacturing, mining, agriculture, public utilities, services (fire, police, and others), and so on are confronted with a variety of dangers to their health and safety. Government, unions, industry, and the workers themselves share the responsibilities of occupational health (Fig. 26-7). Early industrial history shows many exceedingly poor working conditions that have been greatly improved or altogether eliminated. However, there will always remain a need for minimal standards for safety and health, and probably the greatest impact felt by industry in this direction was with passage of the Occupational

Safety and Health Act (OSHA) in 1970 (Chapter 24). The maintenance of an industrial health and welfare program that protects the worker, ensures suitable job placement, and promotes physical and mental well-being is of benefit to the worker, to industry, and to the community. A typical health program in a large industry might be as follows:

Health and sanitation division

(a) **Medical section:** physical examination on entrance; follow-up on remedial work; first aid work; occupational disease research and treatment; epidemic prevention; health education; statistics and records; home nursing when applied for; visiting nurse used in absentee investigation. Many industrial medical departments treat employees for such minor ills as headache, toothache, stomach cramps, and the like. Periodic reexamination after employment is important, particularly for individuals working in dangerous occupations. (b) **Dental section:** examination on entrance; periodic follow-up; emergency treatments and referrals to outside practitioners. (c) **Sanitary section:** building cleanup; grounds cleanup; care of drinking water supply; supervision of washrooms, ventilation, heat, and light; general supervision of all plant facilities and working conditions as they apply to sanitation.

Safety service division

(a) **Accident prevention:** setting safety standards for all operations; mechanical safeguard requirements in construction or operation; safety education; inspection and report of plant hazards; investigation of all lost time accidents; cooperation with health division in reduction of disability hours; statistical report on all phases of accident prevention; reports and follow-up of state industrial cases; follow-up of compensation cases of any kind. (b) **Fire protection:** organization of volunteer associations; regular drills; regular inspection of fire fighting equipment and plant hazards; reports on conditions; complying with insurance requirements; advisory survey of all new installation to prevent fire hazards. (c) **Plant protection:** layout of watchmen's routes and supervision; gate inspection of parcels; control of admission of employees and visitors.

Employees' service division

Investigation of complaints; supervision of relief committee; legal and personal aid; transportation facilities; employees' clubs and associations (mutual benefit, thrift, musical, dramatic and athletic); community gardens and similar activities; employees' magazine; bulletin board service exclusive of safety information; miscellaneous publicity and exhibits.

Training and education division

Classes on elementary subjects; specialty classes (mechanical drawing, electrical engineering, chemistry, salesmanship, and the like); production classes for foremen and minor executives; supervision of shop training; lectures; library; cooperation with dental, medical, safety, and other departments in giving this work publicity; health education.

■ VOLUNTARY HEALTH AGENCIES

Public health is profiting increasingly from the services of volunteers. Innumerable individuals with the ability, time, and capacity for leadership enjoy serving voluntarily in agencies for community well-being. Voluntary health organizations are associations made up of lay and professional persons, dependent for funds on voluntary donations and dedicated to the prevention or solution of health problems. They carry on educational, research, and service programs in many different health fields. Their interests cover such health problems as tuberculosis, cancer, poliomyelitis, heart disease, birth defects, and family planning. Their support comes mainly from individuals, many of whom are interested in the agency's work because of personal or family experiences. They are a part of the American way of life. From small beginnings in the early 1900s they have increased until there are over 25,000 local units. The American public contributes several billion dollars annually to voluntary health organizations.

Voluntary health organizations have often led the attack on public health problems. They have set up research projects to ascertain needs and solutions and have sponsored demonstration control programs. Voluntary agencies also bolster existing official health programs by supplying funds and personnel. Their national organizations, through state and local chapters, carry on education programs for the improvement of personal and community health. Broad community participation makes these agencies valuable for increasing understanding of health needs and programs.

Information concerning specific purposes and programs of voluntary health organizations may be obtained by writing to their local, state, or national headquarters. Most national offices prefer that their local or state office be contacted in the interest of prompt and personalized service. Some of these organizations include:

Alan Guttmacher Institute
Alcoholics Anonymous
American Cancer Society
American Council on Science and Health
American Association for Voluntary Sterilization
American Heart Association, Inc.
American Lung Association
American National Red Cross
American Social Health Association
Arthritis Foundation
Association for the Study of Abortion
Muscular Dystrophy Association
National Association for Mental Health, Inc.
National Association for Retarded Children
National Cystic Fibrosis Research Foundation
National Foundation
National Health Council
National Multiple Sclerosis Society
National Safety Council
National Society for the Prevention of Blindness
Planned Parenthood Federation of America
Rutgers Center on Alcohol Studies
SIECUS (Sex Information and Education Council of the United States)
United Cerebral Palsy Association

Through national, state, and local health councils, voluntary health agencies work cooperatively with each other and with official health departments for the promotion of the total health program. The National Health Council was organized in 1920 with an initial membership of 10 agencies. It now has a membership of 65 national voluntary organizations. Its three principal functions are (1) to help member agencies work together more effectively in the public interest, (2) to identify and promote the solution of national health problems of concern to the public, and (3) to further improve governmental and voluntary health services for the public at the state and local levels. Its activities are guided by a 43-member board of directors elected by delegates from the member organizations. Major activities have included the conduct of an annual health forum, the promotion of information to combat health quackery, the promotion of recruitment of needed young people in the health field, and the coordination of a program of continuing education for the administrative staffs of state and local health agencies. The council does not participate in policy decisions of its member agencies, nor can it commit them to specific projects; but it has been instrumental in unifying voluntary efforts.

▇▇▇ PROFESSIONAL ORGANIZATIONS

Many **professional associations** in the broad areas of health, medicine, education, and social work have independent and cooperative programs for health promotion. Every profession has for its prime purpose the rendering of a public service. The health-medical professions serve the public in the field of health through the elevation of their own professional skills, special public health projects, and cooperation in governmental and nongovernmental health activities.

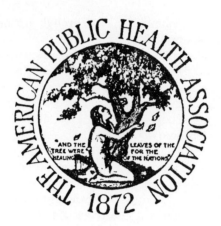

FIG. 26-8 ■ The seal of the American Public Health Association.

The United States has one association whose interests cover the whole broad field of public health. Established in 1872, the American Public Health Association (Fig. 26-8), has a membership of more than 25,000 public health workers, including statisticians, physicians, nurses, educators, engineers, bacteriologists, sanitarians, dentists, veterinarians, laboratory technicians, and nutritionists. The association has affiliated societies and branches in different states, which give attention to the following concerns: health officers, laboratory, statistics, engineering and sanitation, occupational health, food and nutrition, maternal and child health, public health education, public health nursing, epidemiology, school health, dental health, medical care, mental health, and radiologic health.

Membership of most professional health associations is composed of workers in a single field. These associations included, among a host of others:

American Academy of Pediatrics
American Alliance for Health, Physical Education
   and Recreation
American Dental Association
American Dietetic Association
American Home Economics Association
American Hopsital Association

American Medical Association
American Nurses Association
American Physical Therapy Association
American Public Health Association
American School Health Association
National Association of Sanitarians
National Education Association
Society of Public Health Educators

There are several hundred foundations in the United States. Many of them contribute funds for research, training, and demonstrations for the improvement of health. Some confine their contributions to programs in specific areas, such as nutrition or rural health. Others lend assistance to the broad program of public health. Especially well-known are the Rockefeller Foundation, W.K. Kellogg Foundation, Milbank Memorial Fund, and Commonwealth Fund.

International societies or **unions** have been organized by many of the health-medical professions, including medicine, public health, dentistry, nursing, biometrics, sanitary engineering, social work, health education, and pharmacology. They are federations of national professional societies banded together for international collaboration. Many of them also have official relationships with the appropriate United Nations organizations.

SELF-TEST

1. _____ city department
2. _____ morbidity/death rate
3. _____ hazardous wastes
4. _____ health education
5. _____ county health department
6. _____ Department of Agriculture
7. _____ Cabinet Secretary
8. _____ Surgeon General
9. _____ hospitals and medical schools
10. _____ food and drugs
11. _____ infectious diseases
12. _____ mental illness
13. _____ professional organization
14. _____ United Nations
15. _____ industrial health

a. meat inspection
b. radio and TV
c. OSHA
d. vital statistics
e. WHO
f. CDC
g. NIH
h. AMA
i. FDA
j. ADAMHA
k. board of health
l. HHS
m. environmental quality
n. USPHS
o. rural areas

STUDY QUESTIONS

1. Discuss the management of public health at the national, state, city, and county levels.
2. Discuss the relationships among the above levels.
3. Discuss the importance of vital statistics in public health.
4. Is it fair to say that most cabinet-level federal agencies are in one way or another associated with public health? Explain your answer.
5. Discuss the organization of the Department of Health and Human Services.
6. The passage of the Pure Food and Drug Act of 1906 was a monumental development in public health. Why?
7. In broad terms what is the function of the United States Public Health Service?
8. What basic roles do Medicare and Medicaid play in public health?
9. What functions of the Department of Agriculture directly relate to public health?
10. Discuss the structure and function of the World Health Organization.
11. Modern industry plays an important role in public health. Discuss and give examples.
12. Cite a major role for each of the voluntary organizations listed on p. 411.
13. Cite a major public health role for each of the professional organizations listed on p. 412.
14. Discuss the role education plays or should play in public health.
15. Your local community protects your health directly and indirectly in a number of ways. Name as many as you can.

CHAPTER 27

School health

The school is the most important agency outside the home in shaping the health and personality of the child. The promotion of mental and physical health is a joint enterprise of home and school. The parent wants to know what the school can do for the child, and the school must rely on the parents for cooperation and support for seeing that specific medical and health needs of the child are met.

Healthful school living

School health services

Health education

Physical education

School and community relations

The parents (or caretakers) are the persons primarily responsible for a child's well-being and health. It is their duty to secure all the necessary medical care, including immunizations. Additionally, they are the child's first health educators. Children's health habits—in eating, sleeping, playing, resting, cleanliness, and other phases of living—are established in the early years of life, from infancy through the preschool years. The secondary responsibility for a child's well-being lies with the school. There are many opportunities for cooperation between parents and school. Disaffection between home and school can be disastrous for the child. The parent is almost certain to have contact with one or more schools on a personal basis—at the student's school health examination, by informal visits to the classroom, and through participation in parent-teacher activities and other school functions.

The school health program may be divided into five areas: (1) healthful school living, (2) school health services, (3) health education, (4) physical education, and (5) school and community relations.

HEALTHFUL SCHOOL LIVING

Healthful conditions in the school building not only help to keep children well and happy, but the physical environment can also provide firsthand material with which to teach elements of hygiene in the home and elsewhere. Personnel at various levels can cooperate to make the school environment as desirable as possible. Children can be taught to take pride in their school building and to cooperate in keeping it and its environment clean (Fig. 27-1).

The school schedule contributes to a daily regimen that is sensible for the student: activity, study, regular food intake, and other phases of healthful living. The student's relationships and experiences at school should be as whole-some and constructive as possible. The length of the school day and recitation periods vary widely with different schools and with different age and grade levels. The time allotment for physical education varies also.

The school lunch program has been greatly expanded in the United States. Studies indicate that many children who have participated in these programs show better health, growth, and nourishment. The school lunch may be used also to develop the student's interest in nutrition and to improve eating habits.

SCHOOL HEALTH SERVICES

The goals of school health services include health protection, correction of abnormalities, health conservation, and health promotion. The school health program in large school systems is usually administered by the city's health department. Services that may be included are preventive care (to diagnose potential health problems), referral and follow-up, and the teaching of healthy living habits. These services are meant to supplement the care provided by the family doctor or pediatrician. They are not intended to replace such care or meant to treat an illness. Working as a team, the health care professionals involved are the school doctor (who may be a pediatrician or family medicine specialist), school nurses (public health nurses, perhaps headed by a pediatric nurse practitioner), technicians in hearing and vision, and dental personnel.

In addition to all required age-appropriate immunizations (against measles, mumps, rubella, polio, diphtheria, and tetanus), a comprehensive physical examination is commonly recommended for all children on entrance to school and at a later time, often during a certain elementary grade. Some children may be referred for examinations between these periods on the basis of teacher observation or health inspection by the school nurse. The first

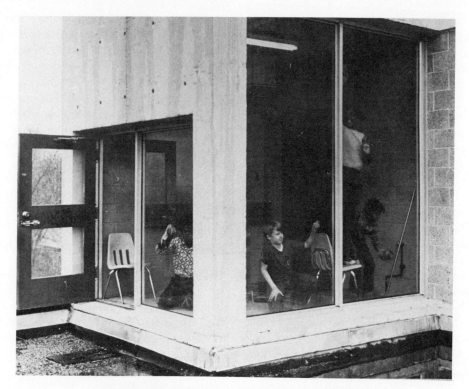

FIG. 27-1 ■ Student involvement in school housekeeping.

Courtesy School District of Philadelphia.

required examination is often given in the summer before the child enters kindergarten or the first grade in order to identify health problems that may influence school performance later on. Some health departments participate in a preschool screening program for 3- to 4-year-olds in conjunction with the school. Hearing and vision testing are carried out by technicians and public health nurses, and a health background is obtained on each child to identify medical or developmental problems that could influence future school performance.

Many school systems encourage children to secure a periodic physical checkup by their own physician. The results of the examination are reported to the school on a standard form.

In this plan the doctor is ready to proceed directly with any necessary corrections. In this way, also, children are taught the value of private medical service, although schools usually offer a comprehensive physical for those not seen for one reason or another by the family physician. The school physician who finds an apparent abnormality must refer the child to a private physician or clinic for reexamination.

The health appraisal may include yearly measurements of height and weight to monitor growth patterns and rule out abnormalities (Fig. 27-2). Growth and learning depend to a large extent on a child's ability to hear and see. Tests are conducted, especially in the elementary grades, to screen for hearing acu-

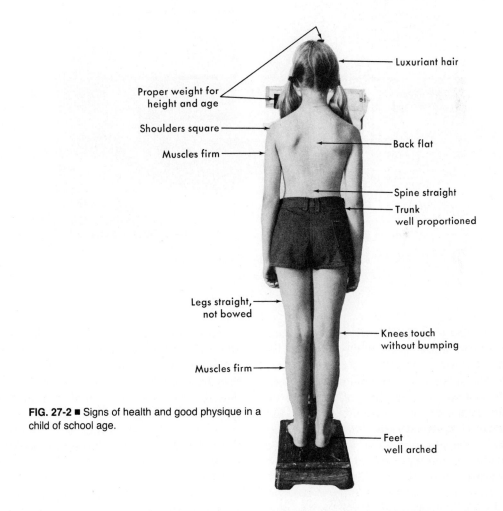

Luxuriant hair

Proper weight for
height and age

Shoulders square

Muscles firm

Back flat

Spine straight

Trunk
well proportioned

Legs straight,
not bowed

Knees touch
without bumping

Muscles firm

FIG. 27-2 ■ Signs of health and good physique in a child of school age.

Feet
well arched

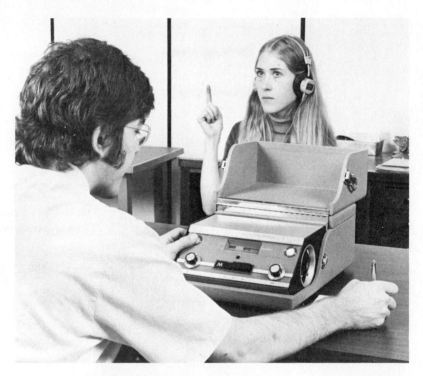

FIG. 27-3 ■ Testing for the sense of hearing—in this case pure-tone audiometry.
Courtesy Maico Hearing Instruments, Inc., Minneapolis.

ity and middle ear problems (Fig. 27-3) and for near and distant vision and eye muscle coordination. Many school systems perform annual scoliosis screening in grades five through nine. Scoliosis, or curvature of the spine, is common among adolescents but can be treated effectively if detected early. Progressive school systems provide screening for high blood pressure and cholesterol levels.

In the event an abnormality is discovered, the parents are notified and, if necessary, visited by the school nurse. Free clinics sponsored by local health departments, hospitals, and other community agencies provide services for those unable to pay for medical care. Problems of mental and emotional health may also be detected and dealt with in the same fashion.

Most authorities agree that the dentist should be visited at least once or twice a year. School personnel should encourage this practice; indeed, many school systems provide both dental screening and dental education programs in the elementary grades. If follow-up care is necessary, the children are referred to their own dentists, or, as the case may be, to a clinic.

A complete physical examination is usually required, as well as a medical history, for those students who desire to participate in interscholastic sports. The object is to detect any health problems or previous injuries that might be affected by sports activity.

Accidents, as we have already seen in Chapter 24, represent the major cause of death

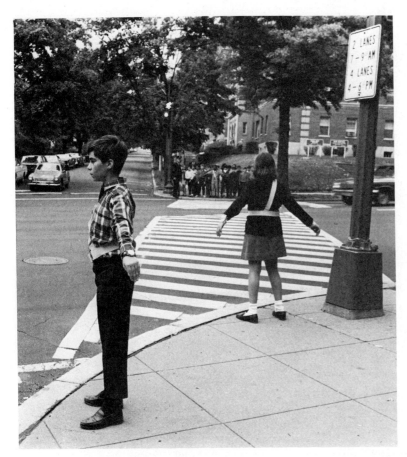

FIG. 27-4 ■ Safety patrol students.

Courtesy American Automobile Association.

in children. This means that a sound program of accident prevention and safety education is an extremely important part of the school health program. Safety precautions should be taken into consideration in the construction and equipment of the school plant. Precaution should be established in the operation of student transportation, as well as in physical education and other procedures. Plans should be on hand for the care of accidents when they occur. Safety education should be offered at all levels through student organizations and through direct instruction, including such courses as driver's education (Fig. 27-4).

Prevention of communicable disease is the responsibility of the local health department, and success in preventing epidemics rests on an effective and continuing disease control program. School doctors and nurses accept the control of communicable disease as one of their more important duties. In addition to the common cold and serious communicable diseases, the school must also combat various troublesome diseases such as pediculosis, impetigo, scabies, and ringworm. The health education program should develop sound knowledge and effective attitudes about immunization and should help students to become intelligent, reasonable, and cooperative in the control of disease.

◼◼◼ HEALTH EDUCATION

Health education in schools should provide a systematic program for the development of life-coping skills necessary to meet the students' needs in the present and future. Through direct health instruction, the correlation of health with other subjects, and motivational activities, the student can become well informed in personal health, growth and development, anatomy and physiology, disease, accidents and safety, environmental effects, consumer health, nutrition, drug abuse, alcohol abuse, tobacco abuse, mental and emotional health, and family health. Instruction should be based on student needs and adapted to the level of maturity of the class. On the secondary school level, health instruction may become more specific as well as more advanced. It may be presented in a separate course (as many educators believe) or in connection with another area of learning such as general science, biology, or physical education.

The teacher is or should be the most important member of the school health team, participating in all phases of the school health program. Through its health education activities the school, to a large extent, determines the health habits and attitudes of the nation. By the example of caring for his or her own physical, social, mental, and emotional health, as well as by the highest qualifications to teach health education, the teacher obviously plays an influential role in the student's health and attitudes toward health.

Health education may be further clarified by listing some of the underlying principles that pertain to educational psychology and philosophy. These are:

1. The same understanding of the child and of educational psychology is needed in teaching health as in other phases of education.
2. The child should think of health as a matter of conduct, not as a subject of instruction.
3. Motivation bridges the gap between knowledge and action.
4. That habits are acquired is recognized in health education.
5. Emphasis is placed on what to do, not on what not to do. The teaching is positive, not negative.
6. Children are commended for success.
7. Particular care is taken not to hold the child responsible for the improvement of conditions over which he or she has no control.
8. The teacher helps the child to see that the ultimate reward of health practices will be found in growth, in improved physical accomplishment, and in other concrete evidences of health.
9. The tendency of children to imitate those they admire is a force that may be used in developing improved health behavior.
10. Unhappy mental states are to be avoided.
11. The gaining of knowledge and the developing of a scientific attitude are important objectives in the higher grades.

Undoubtedly today the areas of drug, alcohol, and tobacco abuse and human sexuality are among the most important in the health education program in the public school system. And yet in a large number of instances these remain the most difficult of all to teach—if, indeed, they are in the curriculum at all. The teacher must be exceptionally skilled in helping the students identify for themselves the gross hazards that accompany drug, alcohol, and tobacco abuse and in bringing them to realize that human sexuality means more than sexual intercourse and sexual pleasures or perversion. The student should, in addition to learning the basic facts of the process of reproduction, come to grips with the fact that he or she is a unique being with the responsibility of caring for his or her own body. Also, attitudes should be developed that are personally satisfying and satisfactory to the family and society. Therefore, to attain a certain modicum of success the person who is shouldered with the task of teaching such a course must by all means be fully equipped to present the concepts of human sexuality so that the student will come away with both an understanding of the subject and positive, searching attitudes.

■ Sex education

The history of sex education portrays a long and arduous road that has not yet been fully paved. Despite the growing openness about sex in our everyday lives, the controversy still rages on: what should be taught; who should teach it; and where and in what grades should it be taught? Indeed, some groups want to have the subject thrown out of schools altogether. According to the National Education Association (NEA) there are several hundred extremely vocal organizations in America fighting sex education in the public schools. Opponents (found on school boards, in parent groups, and in conservative political and religious groups, to name a few) contend that sex should be taught at home or in the church, not in the schools. Many objections arise from the fact that major religious faiths are not in agreement on sexual ethics. It cannot be taught that premarital sex is right or wrong. Some parents fear that once sex has been introduced, their children will be pushed into sex for the sake of experimentation. Others feel the teaching of sex threatens their religious beliefs, and some find it an intrusion on the family itself.

In 1979 the only state teaching sex education on a mandatory basis was Maryland. Washington, D.C., also made the course mandatory in its public schools. New Jersey and Kentucky have only recently passed laws requiring sex education be taught, and New Jersey's law, which takes effect in 1983, faces the possibility of being overridden by certain opposing groups. Interestingly, a Gallup poll in 1980 showed that 77% of adults favored sex education classes, and in the same poll 82% of teenagers interviewed who had had sex education instruction indicated that they found these classes helpful. Another recent poll showed that 80% of all Americans favored the teaching of sex education.

In 1979 the Department of Health and Human Services completed a study indicating that in programs where sex education was being taught only about 10% of students received a truly comprehensive course. The average number of hours of instruction in sex education in the majority of courses was 10 hours. The study further indicated that a good sex education program helps improve communications between parents and their teenage children, and this in turn helps delay the beginning of the children's sexual activity. In the programs where sex education has been taught on an advanced level, the pregnancy and STD rates have significantly declined.

In 1973 in Anaheim, California, a program was instituted called "Family Life and Sex Education." Taught at the junior high and secondary high school levels, the program proved an immediate success and became the model for other programs across the country. In addition to presenting the students with the basic facts of the anatomy and physiology of the reproductive system, the program dealt with the relationship between the two sexes, the relationship between parents and their children, and moral behavior. The coordinator of the program was the school nurse. In 1979, after much controversy had been created by several groups opposing it, the program was dropped.

Today, in the majority of instances, little is taught regarding sex beyond basic anatomy. Menstruation and puberty may be taught in the sixth grade and reproduction and STDs in high school. Many schools disallow discussion of morality or emotion, abortion, contraception, masturbation, homosexuality, or human sexuality itself. Progressive courses deal with the family as a unit, the individual's responsibility to the family, and his or her place in the family unit; the uniqueness of the human body; behavior problems in sexuality (for example, masturbation, intercourse); the responsibilities of both partners in a relationship; the responsibilities and rewards of parenthood; methods of birth control; factors that influence marriage (such as age, religion, and finances); and child abuse.

There are several organizations striving to strengthen sex education programs at all levels. One of these is the Sex Information and Education Council of the United States (SIECUS). According to certain principles set forth by SIECUS, the "concept of sexuality refers to the totality of being a whole person"; that is, "sexuality refers to our human character, not solely our genital nature."

■■■■ PHYSICAL EDUCATION

Physical education in the school curriculum has both health and educational objectives. Leaders in physical education believe the aim of the physical education program is to help children and youth develop the habits and attitudes for maintaining a condition of physical fitness. And physical fitness as defined by The President's Council on Physical Fitness and Sports is "the ability to carry out daily tasks with vigor and alertness, without undue fatigue, and with ample energy to enjoy leisure-time pursuits and to meet unusual situations and unforseen emergencies." Furthermore, the council goes on to say, "the evidence is

mounting that physically fit persons live longer, perform better, and participate more fully in life than those who are not fit. Regular, vigorous exercise is essential to vibrant good health, and it enhances the capacity for enjoying it."

It is obvious that physical activities contribute to health directly and that the desire to succeed in physical accomplishment is a stimulus toward the development of health habits. However, the broad educational values of physical education are important enough that the program would be worth its while even if it did not make its contribution to health. Physical education and health education complement each other, but they are not identical, and neither can take the place of the other.

In building the physical education curriculum for elementary and secondary schools, a combination of activities is adapted to the needs and interests of the child and youth at each age and grade level. In the elementary school program desirable natural activities in the first three grades include running, chasing, throwing, catching, and jumping. Muscles are being developed, and vigorous activity is needed, although overexertion should be avoided. Games, rhythmic exercises, and stunts may be part of the program. Rhythmic activities include fundamental rhythms, creative rhythms, singing games, and simple folk dances (Fig. 27-5). Adequate attention to body mechanics is important.

In the intermediate grades the physical education periods are somewhat longer than in the earlier grades. Some activities may include folk, square, and social dancing and volleyball. Climbing, jumping, wrestling, racing, swimming, tumbling, stunts, rhythms, and team games test for strength, speed, and endurance. School camping is an excellent educational informal activity.

In junior high school desirable activities test physical strength, courage, and endurance and,

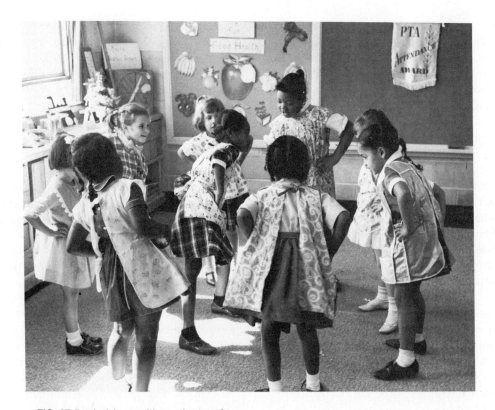

FIG. 27-5 ■ Activity provides a change of pace.

From Jenne, F.H., and Greene, W.H.: Turner's school health and health education, ed. 7, St. Louis, 1976, The C.V. Mosby Co.

at the same time, develop skills. The students may engage in stunts, tumbling, and major sports. Endurance is limited, and undue stress, both physical and emotional, should be avoided. Creative dancing can be a relaxing activity as well as an educational one.

The secondary school students take over more self-direction. The continuance of some form of physical activity depends largely on the degree of interest and the skills of the student. The program may include competitive games, gymnastics, conditioning activities, track and field sports, baseball, football, basketball, field hockey, ice hockey, tennis, softball, calisthenics, track sports, and creative dancing. Social dancing, square dancing, bad-

minton, and other recreational games may also be included in the program.

Competitive athletics require suitable regulations and policies. These sports have many values but alone do not constitute an adequate physical education program. Intramural sports have many of the same values and should be included along with the other activities.

SCHOOL AND COMMUNITY RELATIONS

Broad cooperative participation in planning both school health programs and community health programs is a common practice. Students, as well as teachers and parents, work on school health councils that plan and carry out school health measures. Likewise, school representatives are active in community health councils in which health programs coordinating school activities with those for the community as a whole are developed. Studies of health problems are made to determine immediate and long-range goals, and surveys are made of available local resources within the community.

In addition, school sanitation and school health services, which in some communities are administered by the health department, are educational as well as protective. Experiences with sanitary standards and with medical, dental, and nursing services are just as truly a part of the child's education in health as is direct health instruction.

As the child becomes older, experiences in the community, as well as at home and at school, shape health concepts and health behavior. Both governmental and voluntary agencies contribute to the child's health and to health education. The health department provides nursing and medical services, communicable disease control, and sanitary supervision in some schools. It may provide some clinical facilities for the correction of physical abnormalities and may send professionals into the schools for tuberculin testing, immuniza-

tion (vaccination), or other specific procedures. Such activities provide vital health learning experiences.

From the standpoint of the health department, school health education is important in raising the general standard of healthful living, in developing an appreciation of public health services, and in developing community support for special immunization programs and other health measures. Both the school system and the health department serve the child and the community better through mutual understanding and cooperation.

Voluntary health associations in the community furnish source material and conduct community-wide educational programs. The official and voluntary health agencies are actually solving the health problems of the community. No phase of health education can be more interesting to the child than some participation in this process. When schoolchildren and parents are both interested in solving the same health problem, health education is almost sure to be satisfying and effective.

For these reasons, schools have joined in community-wide efforts to improve various aspects of the public health. The school health program has become an integral part of the community health program. Closer coordination between school health education and public health education is under way.

SELF-TEST

1. _____ parents
2. _____ school lunch program
3. _____ safety education
4. _____ sex education
5. _____ physical education
6. _____ growth patterns
7. _____ spinal curvature
8. _____ vaccination
9. _____ drug abuse
10. _____ venereal disease

a. height/weight
b. alcohol
c. immunization
d. STD
e. accidents
f. scoliosis
g. SIECUS
h. caretakers
i. sports
j. nutrition

■■■■■■ **STUDY QUESTIONS**

1. What are the major elements of a school health program?
2. In what activities of the school health program are the understanding and cooperation of parents helpful?
3. What is important in the sanitary environment of the school?
4. What is the purpose of the health examination of school children? What follow-up takes place after the examination?
5. What is the role of the nurse in the school health program?
6. What steps in communicable disease control take place at the beginning of school?
7. Why and how should we provide special education for exceptional children?
8. What contributions to health are made by physical education?
9. What are some of the characteristics of a good program of health education?
10. What are your personal views on the teaching of sex education?

CHAPTER 28

Environmental protection

For well over a century hundreds of acres in Woburn, Massachusetts, a suburb 12 miles north of Boston, were used as chemical waste dumps for tanning, pesticide, and chemical companies as well as for general industries. Huge pits of toxic chromium, arsenic, and lead were identified in 1981, and chemicals such as benzene (a possible cause of leukemia) were found in the drinking water. This sort of situation, in one form or another and in varying degrees, prevails throughout America. We must act now because time, as noted, is already against us. No less pressing is the quality of the air we breathe and the water we drink. Furthermore, there are the perennial problems of refuse, garbage, and sewage disposal, not to mention radioactive waste, acid rain, and noise pollution. In short, the environment is in trouble, and our health is at stake.

Drinking water

Waste disposal

Hazardous waste

Radioactive waste

Air quality

Indoor air pollution

Acid rain

Noise pollution

The environment is the sum total of the external or extrinsic physical conditions that affect the growth and development of living things. Put succinctly, it is "our home." Accordingly, it must be protected. Indeed, it must be protected as never before because we are daily witnessing the ever-increasing side effects of modern technology. Protecting the environment essentially means implementing measures that promote community health and working hand in hand with public health programs (Chapter 26) and with what we learn in school (Chapter 27). The nuts and bolts of environmental protection deal with water, air, waste, and noise, each of which is discussed in some detail in this chapter.

DRINKING WATER

A century ago the United States had mainly a rural economy with an abundance of fresh water. Since then the population has increased fivefold, but the amount of rainfall has not increased. At the turn of the century some water supplies were becoming polluted, mainly from domestic sewage, and both sewage disposal and water purification were being undertaken. Today the difficulty of protecting our water supplies has become acute. The **pollution** of lakes and rivers from domestic sewage and industrial wastes (purified in varying degrees) has become so extensive that water must be increasingly recycled. Wastes are "purified" and released into a river or lake whose water is later purified for a city supply.

The amount of water used domestically and industrially in the modern city is great and increasing. The amount of available water in some parts of the United States is becoming more and more limited. Runoffs will have to be stored to conserve water; and perhaps water will have to be transferred from one river basin to another. Some lakes are becoming so highly polluted that their beauty is lost and they are no longer suitable for recreation.

Conservationists are joining in the demand for vigorous action against water pollution. Some regions of the ocean are being heavily polluted with fuel oil, pesticides, sewage, and industrial wastes.

The sanitation of public water supplies in the United States has been so efficient that the average person drinks water from the household faucet in any city with unquestioning assurance. This protection may make the individual less careful about the safety of drinking water from a lake or river, from a private roadside supply, or from a public supply in other countries. There is still an occasional waterborne epidemic of dysentery, diarrhea, hepatitis, typhoid, or paratyphoid fever. The majority of the epidemics are in communities of less than 5000 people. There are also occasional individual waterborne infections in rural areas, associated with the use of water from wells or springs.

Sources of water

The source of water is rainfall, or **precipitation**, (Fig. 28-1). A 1-inch rainfall over an acre of land is equal to 27,154 gallons of water. Some of this rain goes directly into ponds, streams, rivers, and lakes or washes over the surface of the earth into such bodies of water. Most of it percolates into the ground and becomes **groundwater**.

Surface water supplies. Surface water is one source of both domestic and public water supplies. Some cities have taken water directly from rivers and lakes. Others have constructed huge storage reservoirs. Today, safe surface water supplies are very rare. It is not safe for an individual to drink raw or unpurified water from the average lake, brook, or river.

Water taken from such a source must be purified, because surface water picks up dirt as it washes over the ground, and it may also pick up disease organisms. A concentrated

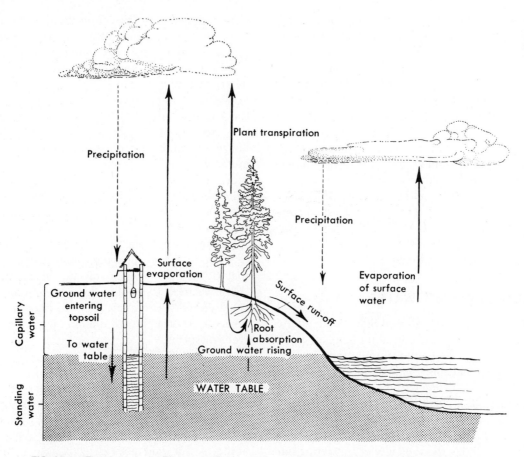

FIG. 28-1 ■ The water cycle. Plants contribute water vapor from transpiration and effectively increase atmospheric humidity in local areas.

From Arnett, R. H., and Bazinet, G. F.: Plant biology: a concise introduction, ed. 4, St. Louis, 1977, The C. V. Mosby Co.

sample of such water contains bits of wood, fibers of many kinds, minute plants and animals, particles of dirt, and bacteria, which can be seen with a microscope. Chemical analysis reveals many things besides H_2O. The water contains dissolved oxygen, which incidentally makes possible the respiration of fish and other animals. It also contains carbon dioxide, ammonia, salts, and traces of both natural and synthetic organic chemicals.

Groundwater supplies. Groundwater supplies are secured from subsurface or un-

derground water retained by the saturated soil. The upper limit of this zone of saturation is called the **water table.** It is found at various depths below the surface of the earth.

Groundwater dissolves salts and minerals as it passes through the soil. It is always in motion, moving from 0.2 to 20 feet per day toward either visible or underground rivers or in the direction of their flow. If the groundwater has passed through sand or gravel for a considerable distance, it will be clear, because microorganisms and particles of dirt will have been strained out; however, the dissolved mineral content may be high.

No definite figure can be set for the distance water must flow through soil in order to be purified. In general it may be said that passing through 100 feet of sandy soil will accomplish this. Sanitary precautions indicate that a well should be located at least 100 feet from a toilet or other source of pollution. The drainage from the source of pollution should be away from the well, not toward it. Even sandy soil may eventually become polluted. When instead of sand there is a broken formation, as in the case with limestone or some types of ledge, there is likely to be a brook by which pollution may reach the water supply directly.

Thus, although groundwater from a spring or well may be clear and cold, it is not necessarily safe, even though a family may have used this source of supply for a long time. Any student of bacteriology knows that a glass of water may contain thousands of bacteria without showing the slightest trace of sediment, and any student of chemistry knows that a glass of water may contain poisonous chemicals without showing a trace of sediment. Thus the safety of drinking water cannot be judged by the way it looks to the unaided eye.

An individual, or domestic, water supply for the family is most commonly a well or a spring. However, many towns and cities, especially those with a population under 25,000, use groundwater as a source of supply. About 50% of the United States population depends on groundwater. It is clear, cold, and easily protected, and it leaves surface water for other uses.

A spring is formed when groundwater reaches the surface through a rock fissure or through a layer of porous soil lying above an impervious layer of earth. The small springs like those found on the average farm have an output of only 200 to 300 gallons per day. On the other hand, 65 springs in the United States have an average yield of about 60 million gallons per day. Silver Springs, Florida, has a maximum discharge of 531 million gallons per day.

There are different types of wells to tap the groundwater supply. **Dug wells** are usually 3 to 6 feet in diameter and from a few feet to 30 or 40 feet deep. They are lined with stone, cement bricks, or other solid material to prevent cave-in. The top is of impervious material, preferably concrete, and large enough to extend several inches beyond the well itself. The ground around the top is graded so that drainage will be away from the well. A suitable and properly installed pump is important. The use of a bucket for drawing water is likely to permit pollution. **Driven wells** are deeper, but only a few inches in diameter. A "well-point" or pointed heavy metal end is attached to the end of the pipe that enters the ground. Above it is a section of perforated noncorrosible tubing known as the "strainer." The water passes through the strainer into the drop pipe, from which it is pumped to the surface. **Drilled wells** pass through an impervious layer of soil. The casing that forms the outer lining is usually driven down until it reaches an impervious stratum, and from there on the well is drilled to the necessary depth and water-bearing capacity. The casing is usually sealed into the rock or clay stratum.

All wells and springs should be protected from surface pollution, as suggested for dug wells. When the well is finished and before it is put into use, it is good practice to treat the water in the well and in the pump with chlorine to safeguard against any contamination that may have taken place while the well was being constructed.

There is always the danger of groundwater becoming polluted. Sanitarians recommend the chlorination of public groundwater supplies, but many cities do not carry out this extra precaution. The water from deep wells is usually more reliable than that from shallow wells because it has been in the ground longer and has worked its way through the soil for a longer distance. Moreover, it is less subject to pollution from surface water. If water in a well or spring becomes turbid or colored shortly after a rainstorm, the rain has apparently gained access quickly, and therefore the water may very possibly be polluted. Water from some domestic or family wells is chlorinated.

Converted seawater. A breakthrough in water supply was **desalination**, that is, the removal of salt from saltwater. Desalination is relatively expensive, but new technology will probably do much to whittle down the cost. Moreover, there are so many benefits that it may, in the long run, pay for itself. The largest desalination installation at present is in the capital city of Kuwait on the Persian Gulf. The first municipal plant in the United States was officially opened at Freeport, Texas, on June 22, 1961. The Freeport water supply is of excellent quality, and no complaints have been registered about hardness, chemical content, or any other factor. It is essentially distilled water and is very soft. This new source of potable water should prove of great importance to seacoast cities in arid regions. The Freeport plant uses a distillation process, but other methods are also being studied, including freezing in which the salt water is frozen and crystals of pure water are harvested.

■ Protecting and checking a water supply

Sanitary engineers, bacteriologists, chemists, and other scientists have developed methods for supervising and constantly checking the quality of a drinking water supply. For surface water supplies inspection and the prevention of pollution in "catchment areas" or "watersheds" are protective measures. Rivers, lakes, and reservoirs contain water that has run off ground surfaces covering many acres. The area draining immedi-

ately into a city water supply can be kept free of pollution through a regular inspection service. As a further precaution, cities usually obtain control of the watershed so that entrance into the area by unauthorized persons who might contribute to bacterial pollution can be restricted. Frequently these catchment areas are forested to reduce erosion and to retain rainfall.

Chemical examination of any water supply, whether surface water or groundwater, from either a public or a private source, will give information concerning its history and sanitary quality. The most important chemical tests from the point of view of sanitation are the tests for **nitrogen** in its various forms and the test for **chlorides(s)**. The nitrogen tests give us an index of the quantity, the nature, and the freshness of pollution by nitrogenous waste material. The test for chloride, under certain conditions, is an indicator of salt pollution.

When water is tested routinely for microbial pollution, bacteriologic tests for **coliform organisms** are used. These tests have largely replaced chemical tests in which only an index of pollution is desired. It is not easy to detect typhoid bacilli or other pathogens, but the coliform bacillus (*Escherichia coli*), which is a normal inhabitant of the intestinal tract, is easy to detect. The standards of the U.S. Public Health Service for certification of water to be used on ships, trains, planes, and other public carriers stipulate a requirement of not more than 1 coliform organism per 100 ml of water tested.

The standards of the U.S. Public Health Service are revised from time to time. Many of the individual states have adopted them as the standard for city water supplies. Limits are set not only on the bacterial content but also on turbidity, color, total solids, zinc, fluoride, lead, selenium, arsenic, mercury, cadmium, iron, sulfates, chlorides, and other chemicals and on radioactivity. The standards require that water should have no objectionable taste or odor and that lead must not be present in excess of 0.05 part per million.

In addition to the purity of the supply, certain other considerations are involved. Chemical treatment may be necessary to remove objectionable qualities and correct deficiencies. Some waters are so hard as to require a water-softening procedure. **Hard water** may be defined as water requiring an excessive amount of soap to form lather. The condition is caused by the presence of calcium and magnesium salts, which chemically react with soap to form a worthless, troublesome scum. Other water supplies have a corrosive action that must be neutralized, or they contain so much iron as to interfere with laundering. These industrial challenges are met by the sanitary engineer and are related to health only indirectly.

■ Purification

Nature's method of purifying water by filtration through soil has already been mentioned. Storage is another natural means of purification. Bacteria and other particles settle to the bottom of standing water, and the bacteria themselves die of starvation or are devoured by other organisms. Still water purifies itself more rapidly than running water

because in the latter case **sedimentation** is less effective, and the plants and animals that assist in the purification process are swept away.

Storage in large reservoirs, followed by **chlorination**, may be adequate if the initial quality of the water is good and the chance of pollution is slight. Most surface water supplies require more complete purification, especially if they are used for recreational purposes (Fig. 28-2). The process of **chlorination** (Fig. 28-3) kills pathogenic microbes. It is carefully controlled and involves the addition of chlorine in the amount of about 1 part chlorine per million parts water. The exact amount needed varies somewhat with different water supplies, and its addition is carefully regulated because an excess produces a chlorine taste and odor, whereas too little will not make the water safe. To be effective, the amounts must be adjusted to the water temperature and to the amount of organic matter present.

The acme of supply and purification is perhaps New Jersey's Wanaque Reservoir and **computerized filtration plant**. The reservoir is a 6-mile long, artificial lake (30 billion gallons), and the filtration facility can handle 100 million gallons per day—"more than enough" potable water for Newark, Paterson, Kearny,

FIG. 28-2 ■ Flowchart for water purification.

From Hunter, P.: General microbiology, the students' textbook, St. Louis, 1977, the C. V. Mosby Co.

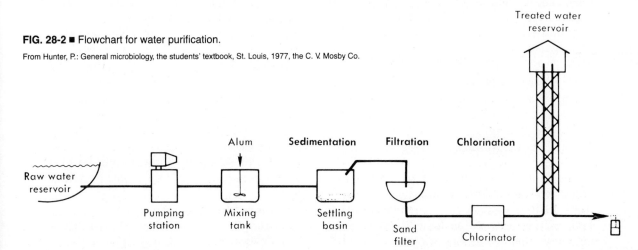

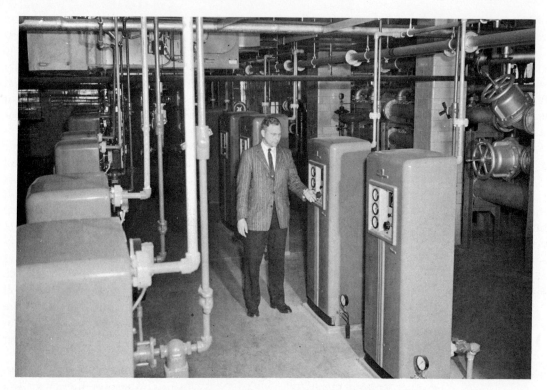

FIG. 28-3 ■ Master automatic chlorinators.
Courtesy Wallace & Tieman Co., Inc.

Passaic, Clifton, Montclair, Bloomfield, and Glen Ridge. These eight cities (partners in the North New Jersey District Water Supply Commission) divide the costs of operating the Wanaque water plant on the basis of their water consumption. Moreover, because the computer saves energy and manpower, the cost of water is the lowest per million gallons in the state.

■ Chemical pollution

The utilities have performed well in dealing with communicable diseases, but since the early 1970s scientists have become increasingly alarmed about the long list of organic chemicals that are finding their way into the water supply of the nation's communities. One chemical of major concern is **chloroform**, which produces cancer in animals. Almost all water supplies that use chlorination contain chloroform because it is created by the reaction between chlorine and the natural organic matter present in water. The Environmental Protection Agency (EPA) has set a standard for **trihalomethanes** (chloroform and related compounds) of no more than 100 parts per billion parts of water. Officials may reach the standard by any method—for example, lowering the chlorine content or using some decontaminant.

The second worrisome group of chemicals, aside from the trihalomethanes, is constituted by industrial wastes (p. 439). Known waterborne carcinogens of this kind include benzene, carbon tetrachloride, and vinyl chloride. Water systems subject to contamination by these chemicals filter the water through granulated activated charcoal, which removes most of the chemicals, along with unpleasant tastes and odors. The EPA has warned citizens against relying on home charcoal-filtering systems. Activated charcoal requires careful and constant maintenance and replacement, not only to ensure its effectiveness, but also to prevent the filter from becoming a breeding ground for bacteria.

■ Individual safety measures

Home methods of providing safe water may be necessary in emergencies. The simplest and safest method of disinfection is to boil the water for 15 minutes. Many people dislike the taste of boiled water, especially if it cannot be chilled after boiling. The flat taste is mainly due to the expulsion of the dissolved gases. Shaking the water to get some air into it will improve the taste.

The traveler, camper, or soldier may be faced with unsafe drinking water and may have no facilities for boiling it. For them chlorine tablets or iodine tablets, which can be carried in a pack or first-aid kit, provide a convenient means of disinfecting small quantities of water at a time. Or 2 drops of tincture of iodine may be added to a quart of water, mixed well, and allowed to stand for 30 minutes before using. However, there is no method for disinfecting small quantities of water that is as simple, safe, and sure as boiling.

■■■WASTE DISPOSAL

Many students of social problems suggest that population explosion leading to food shortages, famine, and armed struggle for land space is the world's most serious problem. Closely related to it in reducing the habitabil-

ity of the earth and caused by population explosion, urbanization, and industrialization are the rapidly growing problems of air and water pollution and the disposal of domestic and industrial wastes, including the startling accumulation of solid wastes. Our health is being threatened by air and water pollution, and we are in danger of being engulfed in trash.

These conditions are new in human history, and the general public has been slow in accepting their reality and still slower in taking the necessary corrective steps. It is at last being impressed on people that water, land, and air resources are fixed, whereas population size is not. The continuing processes of urbanization and industrialization are increasing the amount of waste products produced, resulting in an increasingly polluted environment that demands governmental action and citizen cooperation. Clearly, both research and activities for controlling pollution will have to be increased.

The Environmental Protection Agency (EPA) estimates that the total annual cost of pollution control in the United States is about $40 billion. Federal, state, and local government expenditures cover only about 35% of this figure, with the rest coming from private funds in the form of higher retail prices or lower stock dividends. However, the President's Environmental Quality Council believes that preventing further damage to the environment, to health, and to residential property is worth the price of pollution control.

■ Refuse disposal

Refuse includes all the solid waste materials from human habitations except sewage—primarily, rubbish, garbage, and ashes. Refuse also accumulates from industrial establishments. Ashes are now of minor importance in household wastes because of the use of oil, gas, and electricity for the heating of dwell-

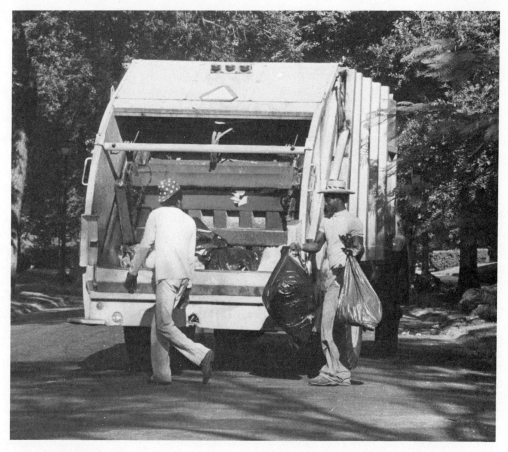

FIG. 28-4 ■ Refuse collection is a key sanitation measure in the health of the community.

ings. Garbage is the refuse (vegetable, animal, and food waste) resulting from the preparation, cooking, and serving of food. Rubbish includes all household and business refuse not classified as garbage or ashes (rags, paper, excelsior and other packing materials, wood, glass, crockery, metals, plastics, and other solid waste). In the United States rubbish amounts to the staggering figure of about 5 billion tons annually.

Most cities collect refuse at regular intervals (Fig. 28-4). In some cities all types of refuse are mixed and collected together. In other cities garbage and rubbish are kept in sepa-rate containers and collected separately. In some cases there is separation of the noncombustible from the combustible rubbish. The type of collection depends primarily on the final disposal of the refuse.

Various methods are used for the disposal of refuse. The most acceptable methods are incineration, sanitary fill, grinding, and composting. **Incineration** (burning) is an excellent method of refuse disposal from the sanitary standpoint. Rubbish and garbage are burned together. By heating the flue gases above 1250° F odor is avoided. The solids remaining after incineration are used to fill land.

Sanitary fill can be used in the disposal of mixed refuse. Each day as collections are made they are spread over strips of land or in trenches and packed down by bulldozers or other heavy equipment. The layer of refuse is covered with soil and rolled again. The packed surface keeps the garbage from being dug up by animals and also provides a solid fill, eventually making new land available for parks and the construction of buildings. Incineration and sanitary land fill may be combined with excellent results.

Garbage is sometimes disposed of separately by **grinding** and discharging it into sewers. Some communities have encouraged the use of home mechanical garbage grinders to cut down disposal costs. Before general disposal of garbage can be made through the sewerage system, tests need to be run to ascertain whether the extra load of sewage can be safely handled by treatment plants and disposal areas.

Some communities employ the principle of **composting** in the disposal of refuse. Noncompostable components such as glass, metals, and plastics are removed. The remaining materials are ground or shredded and placed in stacks, piles, or bins, where decomposition takes place. Some operators have added digested sewage sludge to enhance decomposition. Various enclosed units have been developed with agitation devices, vents to allow aerobic action, and devices for regulating moisture and temperature. When decomposition is complete, regrinding, screening, drying, and bagging make the product ready for sale for fertilizer. Because of the availability of cheap inorganic fertilizers in the United States, a widespread demand for compost has not yet materialized. At present it is sold principally to small users who have found it to be an excellent organic additive for agricultural soils.

Recycling. The future calls for and will demand the reuse (**recycling**) of refuse in the context of both health and economics (Fig. 28-5). The simplest method of recovery is to separate waste material prior to collection, and many communities now have deposition centers for cans, glass, and paper. Furthermore, some states have a mandatory deposit on containers made of glass or metal. As much as 20% of the fiber in new paper products is obtained from recycled material—1 ton of recycled paper saving an estimated 17 trees! More sophisticated recycling techniques are also under study, including **fermentation** and **pyrolysis**. Preliminary results indicate that yeast fermentation of organic waste produces yeast cells with sufficient nutritive value to serve as animal feed. Pyrolysis, or the heating of a substance to a high temperature in the absence of air, causes the organic wastes to break down into different, useful compounds. In pilot studies conducted by the United States Bureau of Mines, gas, liquid hydrocarbons, light oil, tar, pitch, and an assortment of other useful products have been produced.

■ **Sewage disposal**

Many areas of the world are without sanitary methods for the disposal of human and animal excreta. They have neither rural septic systems nor city sewerage systems. In these areas there exists a related prevalence of hookworm disease, typhoid fever, and dysentery. Experience has shown that the control of these diseases requires the sanitary disposal of human excreta. Scientific methods of disposal have been developed in all technologically advanced countries. Although **sewage** is about 99% water, it represents a galaxy of microbial forms and chemical compounds. Its sources include fecal wastes, industrial wastes, ground garbage, and washing compounds.

In actual practice two or more processes may be used in the treatment and disposal of sewage. For example, the sewage of a city might pass successively through screens, settling

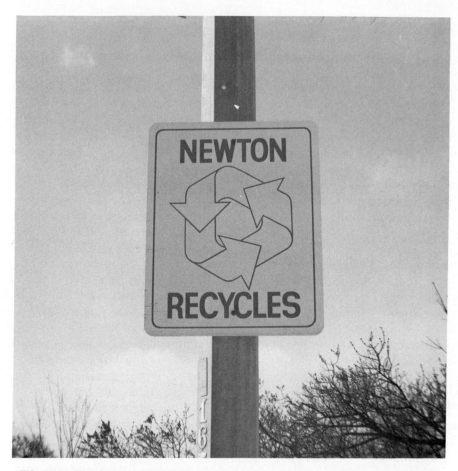

FIG. 28-5 ■ The city of Newton, Massachusetts, successfully recycles glass, cans, and paper.

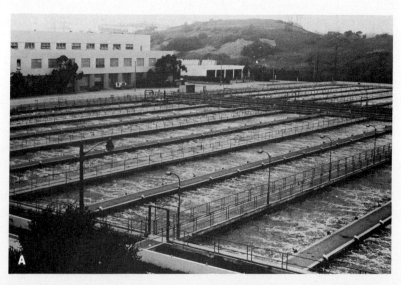

FIG. 28-6 ■ Major operational units, Hyperion Sewage Disposal Plant. **A,** Aeration tanks.

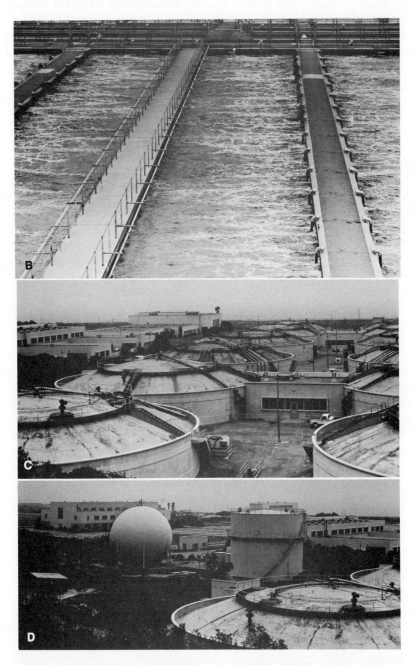

Fig. 28-6, cont'd ■ B, Close-up of aeration tanks. **C,** Sludge digestion tanks. **D,** Collection (cylindrical) and storage (spherical) tanks for gas from sludge digestion tanks.

tanks, and a trickling filter, after which the **effluent** (liquid sewage) might be disinfected with chlorine before being allowed to flow into a lake or river. In each case the sanitary engineer must propose a treatment that is adapted to the sewage itself and to the size and location of the city. It is possible to purify sewage and discharge the effluent into a stream that is to be used again some miles downstream as a city water supply, provided that the second city adopts proper methods of purification for its drinking water.

The Los Angeles Hyperion Sewage Disposal Plant at El Segundo on the Pacific Coast is a classic example of modern sanitation at its best (Fig. 28-6). Serving a population of some 3 million—and handling 300 million or more gallons of sewage per day—this plant combines **primary mechanical treatment** with highly sophisticated secondary treatment involving both **aerobic** and **anaerobic** ("air-free") processes. In the primary treatment raw sewage is passed through screens to remove large objects and then directed into a huge settling basin where grit and gravel fall to the bottom. The sewage then flows into a series of tanks to permit suspended organic matter to settle out. In the secondary treatment this **sludge** (solid sewage) is piped to digestion tanks, and the effluent flows into aeration holding tanks where air is forced through the effluent to stimulate bacterial decomposition. After about 6 hours this aerated sewage is piped into final settling tanks where the suspended organic matter settles to the bottom. The sludge is piped to the digestion tanks and the effluent, which flows from the top, is chlorinated and piped to the ocean. The anaerobic bacterial action in the digestion tanks continues for about a month until all decomposable compounds have been converted into simple compounds, including methane gas, which serves as the basic fuel for the operation of the entire plant. "Undigested matter" is discharged into the ocean via a 7-mile long pipe.

Biological oxygen demand. Since the basic idea of sewage disposal is to reduce organic matter, the concentration of the latter in the entering effluent and the concentration in the water after treatment together serve to assess the efficiency of a specific system. The test used to measure this concentration is called **biological oxygen demand**, or BOD. A sample of sewage or water is incubated with a known amount of oxygen for 5 days and the mixture then tested to determine how much oxygen was consumed by microorganisms present. The greater the level of organic matter, the greater the microbial activity and the more oxygen consumed (which is expressed as parts per million). The activated sludge treatment used at the Hyperion Sewage Disposal Plant can reduce the BOD as much as 96%.

Eutrophication. Even if sewage purification has been extensive, the effluent discharged into a river, lake, or ocean carries great quantities of nitrates, phosphates, and other plant nutrients that stimulate the unlimited growth of algae and other aquatic plants. This is called **eutrophication**. In sunlight these plants produce oxygen, but the sunlight cannot penetrate very far, and plants that settle a few feet below the surface are in relative darkness. They use up the oxygen dissolved in the water. Fish and the plants themselves die from lack of oxygen, and a nuisance is produced by the putrefaction that develops. This putrefactive condition may develop throughout a small pond, along the shallow margins of a big lake, or even in shallow tidal waters adjacent to sewer outfalls. The prevention of eutrophication centers on chemical processes directed at phosphorus and nitrogen. Removal of phosphorus, as phosphates, is relatively easily effected by the addition of aluminum sulfate or ferrous sulfate to the effluent contained in settling tanks. These chemicals produce precipitates, or flocculants, of insoluble phosphates that settle to the bottom along with the sludge. Nitrogen compounds are more

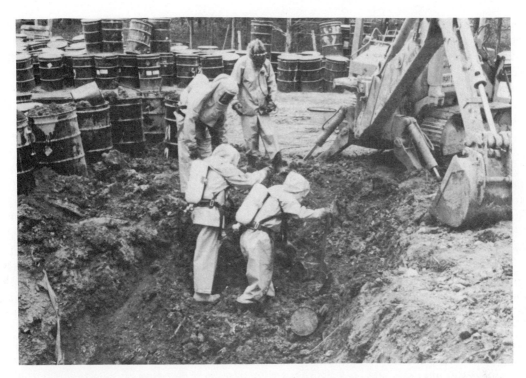

FIG. 28-7 ■ The exhumation of an abandoned hazardous waste site. Buried drums were rusting and leaking deadly chemicals.

Courtesy U.S. Environmental Protection Agency.

difficult to remove, especially nitrates and nitrites, and special, somewhat sophisticated procedures are necessary.

■■■■ HAZARDOUS WASTE

The U.S. Environmental Protection Agency (EPA) estimates that 60 million tons of the nation's total waste load can be classified as **hazardous**. About half of this is from the chemical industry, a broad industrial category that produces such common materials as plastics, synthetic fibers, synthetic rubber, fertilizers, medicines, detergents, soaps, cosmetics, paints, pigments, adhesives, pesticides, and explosives, as well as numerous other organic and inorganic chemicals used by various industries, commercial establishments, and laboratories. Especially hazardous are the **polychlorinated biphenyls** (known as PCBs) and **dioxin**, one of the deadliest compounds made by man. These are the substances society has "thrown away" over recent decades, only to find them returning—and making household words of "Love Canal" and "Valley of the Drums." These two incidents are historic but not unique. The EPA has on file hundreds of documented cases of damage to life and the environment resulting from the indiscriminate or improper management of hazardous wastes (Fig. 28-7). The vast majority of cases involve **groundwater**, the source of drinking water for about half of the United States population (p. 428). Other kinds of environmental damage include surface water pollution, air pollution, fires and explosions, and poisoning (either directly or indirectly through the food chain).

The proper handling of hazardous waste means more than just careful disposal. It means consideration of a range of options that depend on such factors as characteristics, volume, and location of the waste. According to the EPA, the desired options for managing hazardous waste are (in order of priority): (1) minimize the amounts generated by modifying the industrial process involved; (2) transfer the waste to another industry that can use it; (3) reprocess to recover energy or materials; (4) separate hazardous from nonhazardous waste at the source and concentrate it, thereby reducing handling, transportation, and disposal costs; (5) incinerate the waste or subject it to chemical treatment that renders it nonhazardous; (6) dispose of the waste in a secure landfill (one that is located, designed, operated, and monitored—even after it is closed—in a manner that protects life and the environment).

A relatively novel form of incineration is to use hazardous wastes as fuel in the manufacture of cement. Not only does this get rid of wastes but also substantially cuts energy costs by replacing coal, now the primary fuel. At the Alpha Portland cement plant (Cementon, New York) crushed limestone is fed into one end of a rotating kiln and, at the other end, a huge furnace, fed by a mixture of pulverized coal and waste solvents (from painting and printing industries) sends flames and gases heated to temperatures between 2700° and 3700° F into the kiln. The heat transforms the kiln's contents into "clinkers," small balls of cement that later are ground to a powder. Above all, the emissions from the kiln are no different from those resulting from the previous fuel.

Another example of economic common sense in the handling of hazardous wastes relates to lubricating oils. Waste lubricating oils need not be discarded. They can be recycled for reuse as a lubricating oil, for use as fuel oil, for dust control by spreading on roads, and for mixing with asphalt in road construction and repair. All of this can be effectively done at the local level at no cost. Indeed, it could very well yield a profit. But the central point with this type of operation (a form of recycling) is that it involves the community in general and the individual in particular. In the view of all experts on the subject we must begin as a nation to accept responsibility for working toward a solution of the hazardous waste problem. Money alone—and it will cost billions—is not enough. Every one of us must (1) dispose of wastes in the proper manner and (2) alert the appropriate authorities when we detect pollution.

■ Disposal sites

Although the state of New Jersey is the nation's second largest producer of petrochemicals—only Texas manufactures more—it did not, as of 1981, have a major toxic waste disposal facility, mainly because of staunch community resistance. Few New Jerseyans object to doing something to dispose of the more than 720,000 tons of dangerous wastes produced in the state each year, but apparently even fewer care to have it done in their communities. Clearly, hazardous waste facilities share a common characteristic with many other "undesirable" neighbors: prisons, highways, airports, and sewage treatment plants. However, we must act as a nation and learn to accept disposal sites as essential to community health. Obviously, such sites must be proper and scientifically sound. In the instance of New Jersey, a Hazardous Wastes Facilities Siting Commission (empowered in 1981 to select disposal sites) consists of three industry officials, three representatives of environmental groups, and three local representatives. Once the commission has made a selection, the city or town involved is free to voice objections and, if necessary, make an appeal to an administrative law judge. More or less this is the way the situation is being handled throughout the United States.

The major problem at present is correcting the mistakes of the past, especially the cleaning up of open storage "facilities" (the "Valley of the Drums" and a site in Lowell, Massachusetts, are flagrant examples). The Lowell site dated back to 1970, when a private corporation was set up to salvage and reprocess waste from area industries. In 1977 the company declared bankruptcy, leaving a staggering 20,000 barrels, many rusting and leaking, containing 1 million gallons of hazardous waste. Some of the barrels were only a few feet from a stream that flows into the Concord River, a tributary to the Merrimack. Several communities get their drinking water from the Merrimack River. Another 300,000 gallons were left in leaking storage tanks. With the company bankrupt, the state of Massachusetts had to appropriate 1.5 million dollars to clean up the site. This sort of thing is happening all across the country, and the total cost of cleanup is proving astronomic. This in itself should be enough to convince all of us that unless we dispose of hazardous wastes in the proper way at the outset, the country in the years ahead will, with inflation, face major financial as well as health hazards.

◼◼◼ RADIOACTIVE WASTE

Radioactive waste is also increasing. The nuclear industry has grown vigorously since 1942 when the first self-sustaining chain reaction was achieved. As of the end of 1980, there were 163 nuclear power plants in use or under review for construction in the United States, and there is increased use of radioisotopes in industry, agriculture, medicine, and scientific research. The great bulk of radioac-

tive wastes derives from the mining and use of nuclear fuels. Careful and scientific control in the disposal of radioactive waste (Table 28-1) is critical because of the somatic and genetic effects of radiation (p. 368). The number of radioactive isotopes (**radioisotopes**) is considerable, and their periods of activity, expressed as **half-life**, range from a few seconds to thousands of years. They differ, too, in the kinds of rays they emit: **alpha** (α) rays (a stream of helium nuclei, which can be stopped by a sheet of paper); **beta** (β) rays (streams of electrons strong enough to pass through aluminum foil); or **gamma** (γ) rays (electromagnetic energy traveling at the speed of light and capable of much greater penetration than x-rays) (Fig. 28-8).

A Department of Energy 1981 report estimated that 99,000 tons of highly radioactive spent fuel and millions of tons of other atomic wastes will have accumulated by the year 2000. To cope with this potentially dangerous situation the Nuclear Regulatory Commission (NRC) has proposed safety rules for long-term storage in a proposed underground repository. Specific standards are listed for the facility containment, controlled releases of radiation over the centuries, and groundwater containment risks. The packaging rule would prevent leakage for 1000 years. Actual radiation limits will depend on standards currently being developed for permanent waste repositories by the EPA. The Department of Energy has the job of selecting the repository site and developing the facility for eventual licensing by the NRC. The repository site is to be identified by 1985, and licensure for operation is scheduled for 1994.

◼◼◼ AIR QUALITY

The air we breathe is made up of 78% nitrogen, 21% oxygen, and 1% miscellaneous gases and particles of solids so small that they float around suspended in air. (These percentages

TABLE 28-1
Disposal methods for radioactive waste

Type of waste radioactivity	Source of waste	Form of waste	Typical isotopes	Type of radiation	Disposal methods
Natural activity	Mining of uranium ores	Solids	Uranium-238	α, γ	Pile in open
		Liquids	Thorium-230	α, γ	Seep into ground
		Gases and dusts	Radon-222	α	Ventilate mine
	Fuel fabrication plants	Solids	Uranium-238 Uranium-235	α, γ	Decontaminate
		Liquids (acid)	Uranium-238 Uranium-235	α, γ	Neutralize, concentrate, and bury residue
		Dusts	Uranium-238 Uranium-235	α, γ	Ventilate, filter, and disperse to air
Fission-product activity	Fuel irradiation and processing	Solids (from purposeful solidification)	Strontium-90 Cesium-137	β β, γ	Encase in container and store permanently (~600 years)
		Liquids (with strontium and cesium removed)	Technetium-99 Ruthenium-103 Cesium-144	β β, γ β, γ	Store in tanks for several years; then solidify in place
		Gases	Iodine-131	β, γ	React with chemicals to bind in solid, for example, silver iodine
			Krypton-85	β, γ	Disperse to air
Activation-product activity	Reactor materials unavoidably irradiated during operation	Solids	Aluminum-28 Manganese-56	β, γ β, γ	Package and ship for land burial
		Liquids (dissolved material)	Cobalt-58	β, γ	Evaporation or ion exchange; bury residue
		Gases	Nitrogen-16	β, γ	Hold for decay (very short life); then disperse to air
	Purposeful irradiation to produce useful isotopes	Solids	Cobalt-60	β, γ	Ship for burial when no longer useful (long life)
			Phosphorus-32	β	Store for decay to safe levels (short life)

Courtesy Nuclear Regulatory Commission.

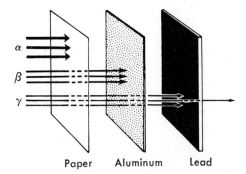

FIG. 28-8 ■ Diagram showing relative penetrating power of alpha, beta, and gamma rays—the three types of radiation associated with radioactive substances.

Reprinted with permission from Research Reporter, Chemistry 38:20, 1965. Copyright by the American Chemical Society.

are for dry air, ignoring water vapor.) When air pollution is considered as a fraction of all air, it seems very tiny—less than one tenth of 1%—but the total amount of pollution in the air over the United States at any given time is staggering. The five most pervasive pollutants—**sulfur dioxide**, **nitrogen dioxide**, **carbon monoxide**, **hydrocarbons**, and **particulates** (soot and dust)—spewed into the air each year in the United States are estimated to total about 200 million tons, nearly a ton for every man, woman, and child in the country. The major sources of this tonnage are vehicular exhausts (especially the automobile), power plants, refuse disposal plants, and, of course, industry (Fig. 28-9).

Our most serious difficulties usually arise from a mixture of gases, mists, and dusts in the form of **smog**. The term "smog" was originally used to mean a mixture of smoke and fog. As used today the term refers to photochemical smog produced by the radiant energy of the sun acting on the emissions of the automobile and other materials (Fig. 28-10). Nitrogen dioxide (NO_2) in the presence of hydrocarbons absorbs energy from the sun, producing nitric oxide (NO) and nascent oxygen (O). The latter reacts with oxygen molecules

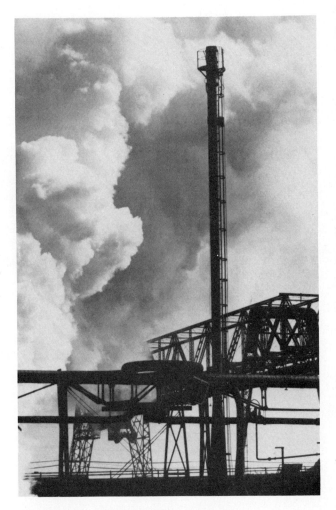

FIG. 28-9 ■ Atmospheric pollution at the source.

(O_2) and other constituents of automobile exhaust to produce **ozone** (O_3) and, in turn, formaldehyde, peroxyacetyl nitrate (PAN), and other chemicals. Ozone can cause choking, coughing, headache, and fatigue. It can fade colors, crack rubber, damage the leaves of plants, and deteriorate fabrics. PAN and formaldehyde are irritants to the skin, eyes, and respiratory tract.

Some of the earliest and best-known "attacks" of severe air pollution occurred in Lon-

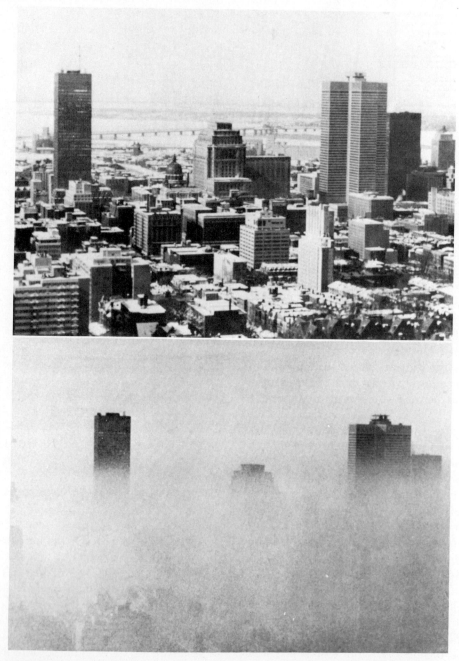

FIG. 28-10 ■ The top photo shows Montreal on a clear day. The bottom photo shows the city blanketed by smog following a period of atmospheric stagnation.

From LeBlanc, F., and De Sloover, J.: Relation between industrialization and the distribution and growth of epiphytic lichens and mosses in Montreal. Reproduced by permission of the National Research Council of Canada from the Canadian Journal of Botany **48**: 1485-1496, 1970.

don and Donora, Pennsylvania. In London during the month of December, 1952, 4000 persons died, and many thousands became ill as the result of smog. In 1948, during three days of fog and excessive air pollution in Donora, 5910 cases of illness and 20 deaths were ascribed to the poisoned air. Severe illness and death were more common in older persons and individuals with preexisting heart or lung difficulties, but younger persons in good health showed the typical symptoms of severe cough and irritation of the respiratory tract. Autopsies performed on three of the victims in the Donora episode revealed the presence of edema, hemorrhage, and purulent bronchitis.

Of all urban dwellers, one in five—more than 35 million people—because of age or health are at special risk from such illnesses as emphysema and bronchitis that result from exposure to air pollution. In general, industrialized, densely populated metropolitan areas have a higher cancer mortality than rural areas, especially for lung cancer. The presence of airborne pollutants, especially toxic chemicals, helps contribute to the deaths of many of the more than 400,000 Americans who die of cancer. The Ohio River Basin Energy Study of 1981 concluded that air pollutants from coal-fired power plants alone might be factors in the death of 8000 people a year in the Ohio Valley. It further indicated that 163,000 people there could die of heart and lung disease caused by pollution in the next 25 years if current trends continue. Stricter controls could reduce the figure by a third; weak enforcement could increase the toll to 200,000.

■ Pollution control

The control of air pollution depends, ultimately, on the people. Ordinary people must be aware of the problem and accept the methods developed to solve it. Public interest in clean air led Congress to pass the Clean Air Act and its amendments, and Congress built into the law provisions for citizens to take part in making the decisions and setting the rules to carry out the law. The President's Council on Environmental Quality estimates that the national benefits that have been realized from reductions in air pollution since 1970 lie in the range from roughly 5 billion dollars to 50 billion dollars per year. Such savings include reduced damage to human health, crops, forests, vegetation, buildings, and other property. The council further estimates that some 14,000 lives are saved per year as a result of air pollution control. But the Environmental Protection Agency (EPA) is the first to admit that there is still much to be done. Indeed, a great majority of the nation's air quality control regions have not achieved EPA standards. Clearly, the battle against pollution must intensify.

Research in methods of controlling air pollution is crucial. Special air-monitoring equipment built by the U.S. Public Health Service automatically measures and analyzes the levels of sulfur dioxide, nitrogen dioxide, carbon monoxide, ozone, and hydrocarbons. Information is gathered on particulate pollutant concentration, pollutants washed out of the atmosphere by rainfall and local wind turbulence. Chemical studies of the development of smog continue. Control measures have included the development of devices to reduce automobile exhaust pollution. The burning of rubbish within city limits has been forbidden. The use of high-sulfur–containing coal as fuel has been restricted. Devices to reduce the smoke and noxious gases coming from smokestacks have been developed (Fig. 28-11). Science is providing the tools to control pollution, but, as noted earlier, the people must supply the will to use them wisely.

■ Pollutant standards index

To avoid confusion and to provide clear, consistent advice to the public on air pollution the EPA, in cooperation with the Council

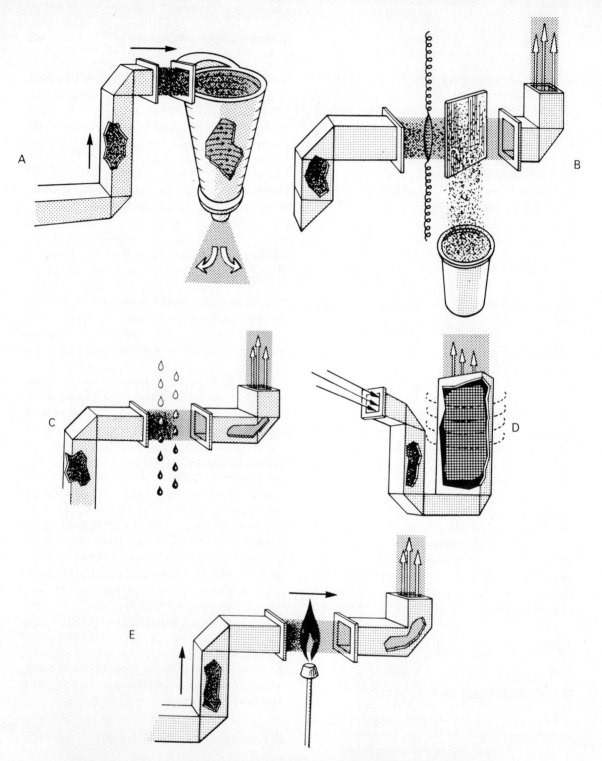

FIG. 28-11 ■ Principles of removal of particulate and gaseous pollutants. **A,** Mechanical dust collectors. **B,** Electrostatic precipitators. **C,** Wet scrubbers. **D,** Fabric filters. **E,** Combustion removal of gases through flame.

From Waldbott, G.L.: Health effects of environmental pollutants, ed. 2, St. Louis, 1978, The C.V. Mosby Co.

![table header bar] **TABLE 28-2**
Pollutant Standards Index (PSI)

Index value	Air quality	Cautions
0-50	Good	—
50-100	Moderate	—
100-200	Unhealthful	Persons with heart or respiratory ailments should reduce activity
200-300	Very unhealthful	Elderly persons and persons with heart or lung disease should stay indoors
300-400	Hazardous	Same as above plus general population should avoid outdoor activity
400-500	Very hazardous	All persons should remain indoors, keeping windows and doors closed

Data from U.S. Environmental Protection Agency.

on Environmental Quality (CEQ) and other agencies, developed the **pollutant standards index** (PSI). The PSI is a reporting tool that converts the pollutant concentrations measured in a community's air to a simple number on a scale of 0 to 500. As noted in Table 28-2, intervals on the PSI scale are related to the potential health effects of the daily concentration of major pollutants. The index value of 100 was selected to represent the concentration below which adverse health effects have not been observed.

■ INDOOR AIR POLLUTION

The National Academy of Sciences stresses that for a number of contaminants now found in homes and public buildings human exposures are large enough and common enough to account for substantial morbidity and premature mortality. This is especially significant because Americans spend 90% of their time indoors. Among other sources, indoor pollu-

tion is created by tobacco smoke; by combustion for cooking and other purposes; by formaldehyde used in insulation, plywood, fabrics, and many other substances used in the home; by asbestos in insulating and decorating materials; by bacteria and other organisms, some of which collect in air conditioners; and by radon from radium in construction materials and groundwater. And of no little interest is the fact that the problem has been severely exacerbated by energy conservation measures undertaken in recent years, including increased insulation. Such measures have made houses more air-tight, have reduced ventilation, and have increased concentrations of indoor contaminants.

It is difficult to assess the precise impact of indoor air pollution, and current knowledge does not permit the establishment of many federal standards governing safe exposure levels of pollution. In the instance of asbestos, however, the hazards are finally well enough understood to prevent further dangerous exposure. Inhalation of asbestos in past decades has caused tens of thousands of cancer deaths so far and is likely to result in 200,000 more cancer deaths over the next 20 years. It has also cuased thousands of others to suffer **asbestosis**, a chronic and disabling respiratory disease that is occasionally fatal. Medical experts agree that asbestos will always prove a problem, especially at the industrial level, until a substitute is found. Asbestos product manufacturers say that the problem has been eliminated by bonding asbestos into other materials or encapsulating it so that the deadly fibers cannot escape. But some medical experts expect continuing trouble even with a new generation of products, especially at the industrial and commercial level. Safe techniques for handling asbestos exist, but some workers resist them, and many more know nothing about them. The answer to asbestosis is education and, ultimately, a substitute.

■ Wood burning

Wood is a useful and increasingly popular fuel, but it is not a problem-free energy source. While wood-burning stoves provide many homeowners with an effective and economical means of space heating, wood burning does pollute both outdoor and indoor air. This pollution can affect public health, the environment, and the economy. For example, a study done in a residential area of Portland, Oregon, found that on one January day in 1978, half of the respirable particle matter in the air came from residential wood burning. Wood burning in Missoula, Montana, has occasionally resulted in pollution levels in excess of federal air quality standards. According to a 1980 EPA report, for the same energy output a wood-burning stove will produce at least 550 times more carbon monoxide than heating oil and 1000 times more carbon monoxide than is produced by heating with gas. The same report notes that the wood-burning stove produces 150 times more benzo(a)pyrene (a carcinogen) and 17 times more particulate matter than oil heat. In the view of the American Council on Science and Health we must acknowledge the drawbacks of wood-burning stoves and fireplaces and develop ways to deal with the problem. Certain difficulties of wood-burning stoves can be resolved by advanced technology, such as the use of catalytic converters to reduce pollutant emissions. Other hazards—burns and fires, for example —can be greatly reduced or eliminated by the consumer. Careful and proper installation and operation of stoves can reduce some of the basic risks associated with these heat sources.

■ ACID RAIN

Pollutants borne by rain, wind, and snow and traced to factory emissions from the heavily industralized parts of the Middle West are poisoning the lakes of the northeastern United States and parts of Canada. Specifically, sulfur oxides and nitrogen oxides chemically react with moisture to produce acids (for example, sulfuric and nitric acids)—hence, the expression **acid rain**. In many of the critical lakes, the acidity has reached pH 4.5 or below, 10 times normal atmospheric levels and 100 times more acidic than a neutral solution. Water more acidic than about pH 5.5 tends to impair the reproduction of trout and other fish and eventually kills them off. This disrupts the **web of life** in a way that scientists are striving to understand. As of 1981 there were more than 200 acid-pickled lakes in the western Adirondack Mountains (New York State) devoid of fish. Moreover, the spring-fed drinking water of the region registered three times the normal copper level and five times the normal lead level; that is, the highly acidic water was dissolving away and putting into solution otherwise insoluble hazardous metals. According to some biologists, if the acid-rain situation continues to worsen, some lands may never recover.

■ NOISE POLLUTION

Noise may be defined as a disturbing sound or, to put it another way, a sound that one does not want to hear. Excessive noise can cause hearing loss and circulatory, cardiovascular, and neurologic damage. Exposure to noise above 90 decibels in intensity will definitely impair hearing, the degree of injury depending on the duration of the exposure. The New York Department of Labor, in testing over 1000 workers, found the highest incidence of deafness in the noisiest industries. Another study involved the comparison of 7-and 8-year old children attending school in a noisy air corridor around an airport with children attending schools in quiet neighborhoods. In measuring the sound levels to which the children were exposed, the investigators found that the mean peak level of sound in the noisy school was 74

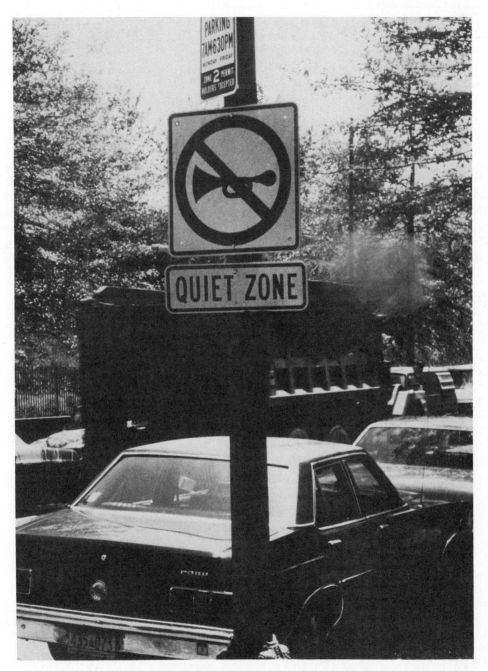

FIG. 28-12 ■ Noise control through community action.

Courtesy U.S. Environmental Protection Agency.

decibels, as opposed to 56 decibels for the quiet schools. (Ordinary conversation registers about 50 to 60 decibels.) The investigators found that the children from the noisy school had higher blood pressure than those in quiet schools. The children whose blood pressure was most affected by the noise did not become less sensitive to the noise over time, and even when these children moved into quieter schools, their increased blood pressure continued. The means by which noise exposure increases blood pressure is unknown, as is the long-term significance of any noise-induced increase. Possibly noise acts on blood pressure through some intermediate factor such as stress, which has long been debated as a cause of hypertension.

But even if there were no physically demonstrable effects of noise, the vast majority of us do not like it, and this in itself is enough to cause us to address the situation (Fig. 28-12). And the situation is getting worse, notwithstanding the Noise Control Act enacted by Congress in 1972 and its amended Quiet Communities Act of 1978. In addition to the perennial giant jet, jackhammer, motorcycle, garbage truck, pile driver, air compressor, bulldozer, vacuum cleaner, and chain saw, we now have the air conditioner, power lawn mower, loud TV, blaring radio, and acid rock. The list is endless. In short, we have a pollution problem, and the chief factors in its control involve community action and concern for the people next door.

◼◼◼◼ SELF-TEST

1. _____ groundwater
2. _____ sea water
3. _____ *Escherichia coli*
4. _____ one part per million
5. _____ trihalomethane
6. _____ boiling
7. _____ garbage and rubbish
8. _____ human excreta
9. _____ oxygen
10. _____ eutrophication
11. _____ hazardous waste
12. _____ half-life
13. _____ soot and dust
14. _____ carbon monoxide
15. _____ respiratory disease

a. refuse
b. BOD
c. chlorination
d. asbestosis
e. PCBs
f. sewage
g. wells
h. auto exhaust
i. radioisotopes
j. pollutant particulates
k. desalination
l. chloroform
m. coliform bacillus
n. algae
o. disinfection

◼◼◼◼ STUDY QUESTIONS

1. What are the sources of drinking water?
2. What does the presence of coliform organisms in water indicate?
3. What is the purpose of chlorination? Of fluoridation?
4. Chloroform has relatively few laboratory, commercial, and industrial uses, and yet it is probably the most common pollutant of drinking water. Explain.
5. When in doubt as to the safety of drinking water, what should you do?
6. What is the difference between refuse and garbage?
7. Does your home community employ recycling? If so, describe what is done.
8. What is the difference between sewage and sludge?

9. The basic idea of sewage disposal is to reduce the BOD. Explain what this means.

10. Many detergents and other washing compounds are advertized as "phosphate free." Why so?

11. What is the major concern associated with hazardous waste?

12. "Love Canal" and "Valley of the Drums" became household words in the late 1970s. Describe these "episodes," including the latest information.

13. Polychlorinated biphenyls (PCBs) and dioxin are considered the most deadly components of hazardous waste. Specifically, what is their source?

14. What is the law concerning the handling of hazardous waste in your home state?

15. What methods are employed (in your home state) to dispose of hazardous waste?

16. Would you live next door to a hazardous waste disposal facility?

17. Radioisotopes differ in two major respects. What are they?

18. What is the present situation in the United States in regard to long-term storage of radioactive waste?

19. Relative to air pollution, what is meant by "particulates"?

20. Discuss the air quality in your home community and cite examples of pollution.

21. In some areas of the United States the air quality today is much better than at the turn of the century. How do you explain this, and can you cite an example or two?

22. The complete combustion of carbon fuels produces carbon dioxide (CO_2), whereas the incomplete combustion produces carbon monoxide (CO). Based on the formulas of these two gases, what is the explanation?

23. Do you have any suggestions for air pollution control other than those cited in the text?

24. Acid rain was first noted as a major problem in 1981 after a study of the lakes of the western Adirondack Mountains (New York State). Has the problem grown worse since then? Please investigate.

25. What are your views on noise pollution and its control?

Bibliography

Chapter 1

American Cancer Society, Inc.: Cancer facts and figures, New York, 1982, The Society.

American Cancer Society, Inc.: Cancer facts for women, New York, 1977, The Society.

American Cancer Society, Inc.: The hopeful side of cancer, New York, 1976, The Society.

American Cancer Society, Inc.: Listen to your body, 71(1MM), No. 2067, LE, New York, The Society.

Anderson, W.A.D., and Scotti, T.W.: Synopsis of pathology, ed. 10, St. Louis, 1980, The C.V. Mosby Co.

Ardell, D.B.: High level wellness, Emmaus, Pa., 1977, Rodale Press, Inc.

Benenson, A., editor: Control of communicable diseases in man, ed. 13, Washington, D.C., 1981, The American Public Health Association.

Berkow, R.B., editor: The Merck manual, ed. 14, Rahway, N.J., 1982, Merck, Sharp & Dohme Research Laboratories.

Boyd, R.F., and Hoerl, B.G.: Basic medical microbiology, ed. 2, Boston, 1982, Little, Brown & Co.

Brooks, N.A., Brooks, S.M., and Pelletier, L.J.: Handbook of infectious diseases, Boston, 1980, Little, Brown & Co.

Brooks, S.M.: Integrated basic science, ed. 4, St. Louis, 1979, The C.V. Mosby Co.

Brooks, S.M.: The cancer story, Cranbury, N.J., 1973, A.S. Barnes & Co., Inc.

Brooks, S.M.: The world of the viruses, Cranbury, N.J., 1970. A.S. Barnes & Co., Inc.

Brooks, S.M., and Paynton-Brooks, N.A.: The human body: structure and function in health and disease, ed. 2, St. Louis, 1980, The C.V. Mosby Co.

Clark, R.L., and Hickey, R.C., editors: Year book of cancer, Chicago, 1982, Year Book Medical Publishers, Inc.

Dorland's illustrated medical dictionary, ed. 26, Philadelphia, 1981, W.B. Saunders Co.

Dubois, R.: The mirage of health, New York, 1979, Harper & Row, Publishers, Inc.

Dubois, R., Pines, M., and editors: Health and disease, rev. ed., New York, 1971, Time-Life Books, Inc.

Edelhart, M., and Lindenmann, J.: Interferon, Reading, Mass., 1981, Addison-Wesley Publishing Co., Inc.

Morra, M., and Potts, E.: Choices: realistic alternatives in cancer treatment, New York, 1980, Avon Books.

O'Connor, R.: Choosing for health, Philadelphia, 1980, Holt, Rinehart & Winston.

Riccardi, V.M.: Genetic approach to human disease, New York, 1977, Oxford University Press, Inc.

Smith, A.L.: Principles of microbiology, ed. 9, St. Louis, 1981, The C.V. Mosby Co.

Smith, A.L.: Microbiology and pathology, ed. 12, St. Louis, 1980, The C.V. Mosby Co.

Tortora, G.J., Funke, B.R., and Case, C.L.: Microbiology, Menlo Park, Calif., 1982, The Benjamin/Cummings Publishing Co.

Twaddle, A.C., and Hessler, R.M.: A sociology of health, St. Louis, 1977, The C.V. Mosby Co.

U.S. Department of Health and Human Services: Cancer treatment, NIH Pub. No. 80-1807, Washington, D.C., 1980.

U.S. Department of Health and Human Services: Health style: a self test, DHHS Pub. No. (PHS) 81-50155, Washington, D.C., 1981.

U.S. Department of Health and Human Services: Morbidity and mortality weekly report, Centers for Disease Control.

U.S. Department of Health, Education, and Welfare: Healthy people: the Surgeon General's report on health promotion and disease prevention 1979, DHEW (PHS) Pub. No. 79-55071, Washington, D.C., 1980.

U.S. Department of Health, Education, and Welfare: Health in America: 1776-1976, DHEW Pub. No. (HRA) 76-616, Washington, D.C., 1976.

U.S. Department of Health, Education, and Welfare: Health in the United States: chartbook, DHEW Pub. No. (PHS) 80-1233, Washington, D.C., 1980.

Waksman, S.A.: The conquest of tuberculosis, Berkeley, Calif., 1964, University of California Press.

Chapter 2

Anthony, C.P., and Thibodeau, G.A.: Textbook of anatomy and physiology, ed. 11, St. Louis, 1983, The C.V. Mosby Co.

Berkow, R.B., editor: The Merck manual, ed. 14, Rahway, N.J., 1982, Merck, Sharp & Dohme Research Laboratories.

Brooks, N.A., Brooks, S.M., and Pelletier, L.J.: Handbook of infectious diseases, Boston, 1980, Little, Brown & Co.

Brooks, S.M.: Integrated basic science, ed. 4, St. Louis, 1979, The C.V. Mosby Co.

Brooks, S.M., and Paynton-Brooks, N.A.: The human body: structure and function in health and disease, ed. 2, St. Louis, 1980, The C.V. Mosby Co.

Chaffee, E.E., and Lytle, I.M.: Basic physiology and anatomy, ed. 4, Philadelphia, 1980, J.B. Lippincott Co.

Gardner, E.J., and Snustad, D.: Principles of genetics, ed. 6, New York, 1980, John Wiley & Sons, Inc.

Guyton, A.C.: Textbook of medical physiology, ed. 6, Philadelphia, 1981, W.B. Saunders Co.

Hole, J.W.: Human anatomy and physiology, ed. 2, Dubuque, Iowa, 1982, Wm. C. Brown Co., Publishers.

Hook, E.W., et al.: Current concepts of infectious diseases, New York, 1977, John Wiley & Sons, Inc.

Landau, B.R.: Essential human anatomy and physiology, ed. 2, Glenview, Ill. 1980, Scott, Foresman & Co.

Langley, L.L., et al.: Dynamic anatomy and physiology, ed. 5, New York, 1980, McGraw-Hill Book Co.

Levine, L.: Biology of the gene, ed. 3, St. Louis, 1980, The C.V. Mosby Co.

McClintic, J.R.: Basic anatomy and physiology of the human body, ed. 2, New York, 1980, John Wiley & Sons, Inc.

Scheinfield, A.: Heredity in humans, Philadelphia, 1972, J.B. Lippincott Co.

Schottelius, B.A., and Schottelius, D.D.: Textbook of physiology, ed. 19, St. Louis, 1982, The C.V. Mosby Co.

Silverstein, A.: Human anatomy and physiology, New York, 1980, John Wiley & Sons, Inc.

Tortora, G.J., and Anagnostakos, N.P.: Principles of anatomy and physiology, ed. 3, New York, 1981, Harper & Row, Publishers, Inc.

Vander, A.J., et al.: Human physiology: The mechanisms of body function, ed. 3, New York, 1980, McGraw-Hill Book Co.

Watson, J.D.: The double helix, New York, 1968, Atheneum Publishers.

◼◼◼ Chapter 3

American Physical Therapy Association: Don't become a pain statistic! New York, 1980, The Association.

Anthony, C.P., and Thibodeau, G.A.: Textbook of anatomy and physiology, ed. 11, 1983, St. Louis, The C.V. Mosby Co.

Arthritis—the basic facts, New York, 1970, The Arthritis Foundation.

Berkow, R.B., editor: The Merck manual, ed. 14, Rahway, N.J., 1982, Merck, Sharp & Dohme Research Laboratories.

Brooks, N.A., Brooks, S.M., and Pelletier, L.J.: Handbook of infectious diseases, Boston, 1980, Little, Brown & Co.

Brooks, S.M.: Integrated basic science, ed. 4, St. Louis, 1979, The C.V. Mosby Co.

Brooks, S.M., and Paynton-Brooks, N.A.: The human body: structure and function in health and disease, ed. 2, St. Louis, 1980, The C.V. Mosby Co.

Chaffee, E.E., and Lytle, I.M.: Basic physiology and anatomy, ed. 4, Philadelphia 1980, J.B. Lippincott Co.

Dickson, F.D., and Dively, R.L.: Functional disorders of the foot, ed. 3, Philadelphia, 1953, J.B. Lippincott Co.

Guyton, A.C.: Textbook of medical physiology, ed. 6, Philadelphia, 1981, W.B. Saunders Co.

Hole, J.W.: Human anatomy and physiology, ed. 2, Dubuque, Iowa, 1982, Wm. C. Brown Co., Publishers.

Landau, B.R.: Essential human anatomy and physiology, ed. 2, Glenview, Ill. 1980, Scott, Foresman & Co.

Langley, L.L., et al.: Dynamic anatomy and physiology, ed. 5, New York, 1980, McGraw-Hill Book Co.

McClintic, J.R.: Basic anatomy and physiology of the human body, ed. 2, New York, 1980, John Wiley & Sons, Inc.

Schottelius, B.A., and Schottelius, D.D.: Textbook of physiology, ed. 19, St. Louis, 1982, The C.V. Mosby Co.

Selkurt, E.E., editor: Basic physiology for the health sciences, ed. 2, Boston, 1982, Little, Brown & Co.

Silverstein, A.: Human anatomy and physiology, New York, 1980, John Wiley & Sons, Inc.

Tortora, G.J., and Anagnostakos, N.P.: Principles of anatomy and physiology, ed. 3, New York, 1981, Harper & Row, Publishers, Inc.

U.S. Department of Health and Human Services: How to cope with arthritis, NIH Publication No. 79-1092, Washington, D.C. 1979.

Vander, A.J., et al.: Human physiology: the mechanisms of body function, ed. 3, New York, 1980, McGraw-Hill Book Co.

■■■■■ **Chapter 4**

Anthony, C.P., and Thibodeau, G.A.: Textbook of anatomy and physiology, ed. 11, St. Louis, 1983, The C.V. Mosby Co.

Berkow, R.B., editor: The Merck manual, ed. 14, Rahway, N.J., 1982, Merck, Sharp & Dohme Research Laboratories.

Brooks, N.A., Brooks, S.M., and Pelletier, L.J.: Handbook of infectious diseases, Boston, 1980, Little, Brown & Co.

Brooks, S.M.: Integrated basic science, ed. 4, St. Louis, 1979, The C.V. Mosby Co.

Brooks, S.M., and Paynton-Brooks, N.A.: The human body: structure and function in health and disease, ed. 2, St. Louis, 1980, The C.V. Mosby Co.

Chaffee, E.E., and Lytle, I.M.: Basic physiology and anatomy, ed. 4, Philadelphia, 1980, J.B. Lippincott Co.

Guyton, A.C.: Textbook of medical physiology, ed. 6, Philadelphia, 1981, W.B. Saunders Co.

Hole, J.W.: Human anatomy and physiology, ed. 2, Dubuque, Iowa, 1982, Wm. C. Brown Co., Publishers.

Landau, B.R.: Essential human anatomy and physiology, ed. 2, Glenview, Ill. 1980, Scott, Foresman & Co.

Langley, L.L., et al.: Dynamic anatomy and physiology, ed. 5, New York, 1980, McGraw-Hill Book Co.

McClintic, J.R.: Basic anatomy and physiology of the human body, ed. 2, New York, 1980, John Wiley & Sons, Inc.

Morehouse, L.E., and Miller, A.T.: Physiology of exercise, ed. 7, St. Louis, 1976, The C.V. Mosby Co.

Mountcastle, V.B., editor: Medical physiology, ed. 14, St. Louis, 1979, The C.V. Mosby Co.

Schottelius, B.A., and Schottelius, D.D.: Textbook of physiology, ed. 19, St. Louis, 1982, The C.V. Mosby Co.

Selkurt, E.E., editor: Basic physiology for the health sciences, ed. 2, Boston, 1982, Little, Brown & Co.

Tortora, G.J., and Anagnostakos, N.P.: Principles of anatomy and physiology, ed. 3, New York, 1981, Harper & Row, Publishers Inc.

Vander, A.J., et al.: Human physiology: The mechanisms of body function, ed. 3, New York, 1980, McGraw-Hill Book Co.

■■■■■ **Chapter 5**

American Heart Association cookbook, New York, 1973, David McKay Co., Inc.

Anthony, C.P., and Thibodeau, G.A.: Textbook of anatomy and physiology, ed. 11, St. Louis, 1983, The C.V. Mosby Co.

Berkow, R.B., editor: The Merck manual, ed. 14, Rahway, N.J., 1982, Merck, Sharp & Dohme Reserach Laboratories.

Berne, R.M., and Levy, M.N.: Cardiovascular physiology, ed. 4, St. Louis, 1981, The C.V. Mosby Co.

Brooks, N.A., Brooks, S.M., and Pelletier, L.J.: Handbook of infectious diseases, Boston, 1980, Little Brown & Co.

Brooks, S.M.: Integrated basic science, ed. 4, St. Louis, 1979, The C.V. Mosby Co.

Brooks, S.M., and Paynton-Brooks, N.A.: The human body: structure and function in health and disease, ed. 2, St. Louis, 1980, The C.V. Mosby Co.

Chaffee, E.E., and Lytle, I.M.: Basic physiology and anatomy, ed. 4, Philadelphia, 1980, J.B. Lippincott Co.

Folkow, B., and Neil, E.: Circulation, London, 1971, Oxford University Press, Inc.

Guyton, A.C.: Textbook of medical physiology, ed. 6, Philadelphia, 1981, W.B. Saunders Co.

Hole, J.W.: Human anatomy and physiology, ed. 2, Dubuque, Iowa, 1982, Wm. C. Brown Co., Publishers.

Landau, B.R.: Essential human anatomy and physiology, ed. 2, Glenview, Ill., 1980, Scott, Foresman & Co.

Langley, L.L., et al.: Dynamic anatomy and physiology, ed. 5, New York, 1980, McGraw-Hill Book Co.

McClintic, J.R.: Basic anatomy and physiology of the human body, ed. 2, New York, 1980, John Wiley & Sons, Inc.

Mountcastle, V.B., editor: Medical physiology, ed. 14, St. Louis, 1979, The C.V. Mosby Co.

Schottelius, B.A., and Schottelius, D.D.: Textbook of physiology, ed. 19, St. Louis, 1982, The C.V. Mosby Co.

Selkurt, E.E., editor: Basic physiology for the health sciences, ed. 2, Boston, 1982, Little, Brown & Co.

Tortora, G.J., and Anagnostakos, N.P.: Principles of anatomy and physiology, ed. 3, New York, 1981, Harper & Row, Publishers, Inc.

Vander, A.J., et al,: Human physiology: the mechanisms of body function, ed. 3, New York, 1980, McGraw-Hill Book Co.

Wintrobe, M.M.: Clinical hematology, ed. 5, Philadelphia, 1971, Lea & Febiger.

■■■■ Chapter 6

Anthony, C.P., and Thibodeau, G.A.: Textbook of anatomy and physiology, ed. 11, St. Louis, 1983, The C.V. Mosby Co.

Berkow, R.B., editor: The Merck manual, ed. 14, Rahway, N.J., 1982, Merck, Sharp & Dohme Research Laboratories.

Boyd, R.F., and Hoerl, B.G.: Basic medical microbiology, ed. 2, Boston, 1982, Little, Brown & Co.

Brooks, N.A., Brooks, S.M., and Pelletier, L.J.: Handbook of infectious diseases, Boston, 1980, Little, Brown & Co.

Brooks, S.M.: Integrated basic science, ed. 4, St. Louis, 1979, The C.V. Mosby Co.

Brooks, S.M., and Paynton-Brooks, N.A.: The human body: structure and function in health and disease, ed. 2, St. Louis, 1980, The C.V. Mosby Co.

Chaffee, E.E., and Lytle, I.M.: Basic physiology and anatomy, ed. 4, Philadelphia, 1980, J.B. Lippincott Co.

Fraser, R.G., and Pare, J.A.: Structure and function of the lung, ed. 2, Philadelphia, 1977, W.B. Saunders Co.

Guyton, A.C.: Textbook of medical physiology, ed. 6, Philadelphia, 1981, W.B. Saunders Co.

Hole, J.W.: Human anatomy and physiology, ed. 2, Dubuque, Iowa, 1982, Wm. C. Brown Co., Publishers.

Landau, B.R.: Essential human anatomy and physiology, ed. 2, Glenview, Ill., 1980, Scott, Foresman & Co.

Langley, L.L., et al.: Dynamic anatomy and physiology, ed. 5, New York, 1980, McGraw-Hill Book Co.

Maier, H.C., and Fischer, W.W.: Adenomas arising from small bronchi not visible bronchoscopically, J. Thorac. Cardiovasc. Surg. 16:398, 1947.

McClintic, J.R.: Basic anatomy and physiology of the human body, ed. 2, New York, 1980, John Wiley & Sons, Inc.

Mountcastle, V.B., editor: Medical physiology, ed. 14, St. Louis, 1979, The C.V. Mosby Co.

Schottelius, B.A., and Schottelius, D.D.: Textbook of physiology, ed. 19, St. Louis, 1982, The C.V. Mosby Co.

Selkurt, E.E., editor: Basic physiology for the health sciences, ed. 2, Boston, 1982, Little, Brown & Co.

Silverstein, A.: Human anatomy and physiology, New York, 1980, John Wiley & Sons, Inc.

Slonim, N.B., and Hamilton, L.H.: Respiratory physiology, ed. 4, St. Louis, 1981, The C.V. Mosby Co.

Tortora, G.J., and Anagnostakos, N.P.: Principles of anatomy and physiology, ed. 3, New York, 1981, Harper & Row, Publishers, Inc.

Vander, A.J., et al.: Human physiology: The mechanisms of body function, ed. 3, New York, 1980. McGraw-Hill Book Co.

Waksman, S.A.: The conquest of tuberculosis, Berkeley, Calif., 1964, University of California Press.

West, J.B.: Respiratory physiology, ed. 2, Baltimore, 1979, The William & Wilkins Co.

■■■■ Chapter 7

Anthony, C.P., and Thibodeau, G.A.: Textbook of anatomy and physiology, ed. 11, St. Louis, 1983, The C.V. Mosby Co.

Berkow, R.B., editor: The Merck manual, ed. 14, Rahway, N.J., 1982, Merck, Sharp & Dohme Research Laboratories.

Boyd, R.F., and Hoerl, B.G.: Basic medical microbiology, ed. 2, Boston, 1982, Little, Brown & Co.

Brooks, N.A., Brooks, S.M., and Pelletier, L.J.: Handbook of infectious diseases, Boston, 1980, Little, Brown & Co.

Brooks, S.M.: Integrated basic science, ed. 4, St. Louis, 1979, The C.V. Mosby Co.

Brooks, S.M.: Basic facts of body water and ions, ed. 3, New York, 1973, Springer Publishing Co., Inc.

Brooks, S.M.: The sea inside us, New York, 1968, Hawthorn Books, Inc.

Brooks, S.M., and Paynton-Brooks, N.A.: The human body: structure and function in health and disease, ed. 2, St. Louis, 1980, The C.V. Mosby Co.

Burroughs Wellcome Co.: New concepts in the control of urinary infections, New York, 1974, Science and Medicine Publishing Co., Inc.

Chaffee, E.E., and Lytle, I.M.: Basic physiology and anatomy, ed. 4, Philadelphia, 1980, J.B. Lippincott Co.

Guyton, A.C.: Textbook of medical physiology, ed. 6, Philadelphia, 1981, W.B. Saunders Co.

Hole, J.W.: Human anatomy and physiology, ed. 2, Dubuque, Iowa, 1982, Wm. C. Brown Co., Publishers.

Kilmartin, A.: Cystitis: the complete self-help guide, New York, 1981, Warner Books, Inc.

Landau, B.R.: Essential human anatomy and physiology, ed. 2, Glenview, Ill., 1980, Scott, Foresman & Co.

Langley, L.L., et al.: Dynamic anatomy and physiology, ed. 5, New York, 1980, McGraw-Hill Book Co.

McClintic, J.R.: Basic anatomy and physiology of the human body, ed. 2, New York, 1980, John Wiley & Sons, Inc.

Mountcastle, V.B., editor: Medical physiology, ed. 14, St. Louis, 1979, The C.V. Mosby Co.

Pitts, R.F.: Physiology of the kidney and body fluids, ed. 3, Chicago, 1974, Year Book Medical Publishers, Inc.

Schottelius, B.A., and Schottelius, D.D.: Textbook of physiology, ed. 19, St. Louis, 1982, The C.V. Mosby Co.

Selkurt, E.E., editor: Basic physiology for the health sciences, ed. 2, Boston, 1982, Little, Brown & Co.

Silverstein, A.: Human anatomy and physiology, New York, 1980, John Wiley & Sons, Inc.

Smith, H.W.: From fish to philosopher, Boston, 1953, Little, Brown & Co.

Strauss, M.B., and Welt, L.G., editors: Diseases of the kidney, ed. 2, Boston, 1971, Little, Brown & Co.

Sullivan, L.P., and Grantham, J.J.: Physiology of the kidney, ed. 2, Philadelphia, 1982, Lea & Febiger.

Tortora, G.J., and Anagnostakos, N.P.: Principles of anatomy and physiology, ed. 3, New York, 1981, Harper & Row, Publishers, Inc.

Vander, A.J., et al.: Human physiology: the mechanisms of body function, ed. 3, New York, 1980, McGraw-Hill Book Co.

Chapter 8

American Cancer Society: Facts on colorectal cancer, New York, 1978, The Society.

Anthony, C.P., and Thibodeau, G.A.: Textbook of anatomy and physiology, ed. 11, St. Louis, 1983, The C.V. Mosby Co.

Berkow, R.B., editor: The Merck manual, ed. 14, Rahway, N.J., 1982, Merck, Sharp & Dohme Research Laboratories.

Boyd, R.F., and Hoerl, B.G.: Basic medical microbiology, ed. 2, Boston, 1982, Little, Brown & Co.

Brooks, N.A., Brooks, S.M., and Pelletier, L.J.: Handbook of infectious diseases, Boston, 1980, Little, Brown & Co.

Brooks, S.M.: Integrated basic science, ed. 4, St. Louis, 1979, The C.V. Mosby Co.

Brooks, S.M.: Ptomaine: the story of food poisoning, Cranbury, N.J., 1974, A.S. Barnes & Co., Inc.

Brooks, S.M., and Paynton-Brooks, N.A.: The human body structure and function in health and disease, ed. 2, St. Louis, 1980, The C.V. Mosby Co.

Chaffee, E.E., and Lytle, I.M.: Basic physiology and anatomy, ed. 4, Philadelphia, 1980, J.B. Lippincott Co.

Davenport, H.W.: Physiology of the digestive tract, ed. 5, Chicago, 1982, Year Book Medical Publishers, Inc.

Guyton, A.C.: Textbook of medical physiology, ed. 6, Philadelphia, 1981, W.B. Saunders Co.

Hole, J.W.: Human anatomy and physiology, ed. 2, Dubuque, Iowa, 1982, Wm. C. Brown Co., Publishers.

Landau, B.R.: Essential human anatomy and physiology, ed. 2, Glenview, Ill., 1980, Scott, Foresman & Co.

Langley, L.L., et al.: Dynamic anatomy and physiology, ed. 5, New York, 1980, McGraw-Hill Book Co.

McClintic, J.R.: Basic anatomy and physiology of the human body, ed. 2, New York, 1980, John Wiley & Sons, Inc.

Mountcastle, V.B., editor: Medical physiology, ed. 14, St. Louis, 1979, The C.V. Mosby Co.

Schottelius, B.A., and Schottelius, D.D.: Textbook of physiology, ed. 19, St. Louis, 1982, The C.V. Mosby Co.

Selkurt, E.E., editor: Basic physiology for the health sciences, ed. 2, Boston, 1982, Little, Brown & Co.

Silverstein, A.: Human anatomy and physiology, New York, 1980, John Wiley & Sons, Inc.

Tortora, G.J., and Anagnostakos, N.P.: Principles of anatomy and physiology, ed. 3, New York, 1981, Harper & Row, Publishers, Inc.

Vander, A.J., et al.: Human physiology: the mechanisms of body function, ed. 3, New York, 1980, McGraw-Hill Book Co.

■■■■■■ **Chapter 9**

Anthony, C.P., and Thibodeau, G.A.: Textbook of anatomy and physiology, ed. 11, St. Louis, 1983, The C.V. Mosby Co.

Berkow, R.B., editor: The Merck manual, ed. 14, Rahway, N.J., 1982, Merck, Sharp & Dohme Research Laboratories.

Boyd, R.F., and Hoerl, B.G.: Basic medical microbiology, ed. 2, Boston, 1982, Little, Brown & Co.

Brooks, N.A., Brooks, S.M., and Pelletier, L.J.: Handbook of infectious diseases, Boston, 1980, Little, Brown, & Co.

Brooks, S.M.: Integrated basic science, ed. 4, St. Louis, 1979, The C.V. Mosby Co.

Brooks, S.M., and Paynton-Brooks, N.A.: The human body: structure and function in health and disease, ed. 2, St. Louis, 1980, The C.V. Mosby Co.

Chaffee, E.E., and Lytle, I.M.: Basic physiology and anatomy, ed. 4, Philadelphia, 1980, J.B. Lippincott Co.

Granit, R.: The basis of motor control, New York, 1970, Academic Press, Inc.

Greening, T., and Hobson, D., Instant relief, the encyclopedia of physiological self-help, New York, 1979, Wideview Books.

Grossman, H.J., editor: Manual on terminology and classification in mental retardation, Washington, D.C., American Association on Mental Deficiency.

Guyton, A.C.: Textbook of medical physiology, ed. 6, Philadelphia, 1981, W.B. Saunders Co.

Hales, D.: The complete book of sleep, Reading, Mass. 1981, Addison-Wesley Publishing Co., Inc.

Hole, J.W.: Human anatomy and physiology, ed. 2, Dubuque, Iowa, 1982, Wm. C. Brown Co., Publishers.

Landau, B.R.: Essential human anatomy and physiology, ed. 2, Glenview, Ill., 1980, Scott, Foresman & Co.

Langley, L.L., et al.: Dynamic anatomy and physiology, ed. 5, New York, 1980, McGraw-Hill Book Co.

Mann, F.: The ancient Chinese art of healing: acupuncture, New York, 1972, Vintage Books.

McClintic, J.R.: Basic anatomy and physiology of the human body, ed. 2, New York, 1980, John Wiley & Sons, Inc.

Mountcastle, V.B., editor: Medical physiology, ed. 14, St. Louis, 1979, The C.V. Mosby Co.

Ramacharaka, Yogi: The science of psychic healing, Chicago, 1919, Yogi Publication Society.

Schottelius, B.A., and Schottelius, D.D.: Textbook of physiology, ed. 19, St. Louis, 1982, The C.V. Mosby Co.

Selkurt, E.D., editor: Basic physiology for the health sciences, ed. 2, Boston, 1982, Little, Brown & Co.

Silverstein, A.: Human anatomy and physiology, New York, 1980, John Wiley & Sons, Inc.

Simeons, A.T.W.: Man's presumptuous brain, New York, 1962, E.P. Dutton.

Snell, R.S.: Clinical neuroanatomy, Boston, 1980, Little, Brown & Co.

Tortora, G.J., and Anagnostakos, N.P.: Principles of anatomy and physiology, ed. 3, New York, 1981, Harper & Row, Publishers, Inc.

U.S. Department of Health and Human Services: Alzheimer's disease: questions and answers, NIH Pub. No. 80-1646, Washington, D.C., 1980.

U.S. Department of Health, Education, and Welfare: Dyslexia, DHEW Pub. No. (ADM) 78-616, Washington, D.C., 1978.

Vander, A.J., et al.: Human physiology: the mechanisms of body function, ed. 3, New York, 1980, McGraw-Hill Book Co.

▰▰▰▰ Chapter 10

Anthony, C.P., and Thibodeau, G.A.: Textbook of anatomy and physiology, ed. 11, St. Louis, 1983, The C.V. Mosby Co.

Berkow, R.B.: The Merck manual, ed. 14, Rahway, N.J., 1982, Merck, Sharp & Dohme Research Laboratories.

Boyd, R.F., and Hoerl, B.G.: Basic medical microbiology, ed. 2, Boston, 1982, Little, Brown & Co.

Brooks, N.A., Brooks, S.M., and Pelletier, L.J.: Handbook of infectious diseases, Boston, 1980, Little, Brown & Co.

Brooks, S.M.: Integrated basic science, ed. 4, St. Louis, 1979, The C.V. Mosby Co.

Brooks, S.M., and Paynton-Brooks, N.A.: The human body: structure and function in health and disease, ed. 2, St. Louis, 1980. The C.V. Mosby Co.

Chaffee, E.E., and Lytle, I.M.: Basic physiology and anatomy, ed. 4, Philadelphia, 1980, J.B. Lippincott Co.

Davis, H., and Silverman, S.R., editors: Hearing and deafness, ed. 3, New York, 1970, Holt, Rinehart & Winston.

Davson, H.: Physiology of the eye, ed. 3, Boston, 1972, Little, Brown & Co.

Gearheart, B.R., and Weishahn, M.W.: The handicapped student in the regular classroom, ed. 2, St. Louis, 1980, The C.V. Mosby Co.

Gelard, F.A.: The human senses, ed. 2, New York, 1972, John Wiley & Sons, Inc.

Guyton, A.C.: Textbook of medical physiology, ed. 6, Philadelphia, 1981, W.B. Saunders Co.

Hole, J.W.: Human anatomy and physiology, ed. 2, Dubuque, Iowa, 1982, Wm. C. Brown Co., Publishers.

Landau, B.R.: Essential human anatomy and physiology, ed. 2, Glenview, Ill., 1980, Scott, Foresman & Co.

Langley, L.L., et al.: Dynamic anatomy and physiology, ed. 5, New York, 1980, McGraw-Hill Book Co.

McClintic, J.R.: Basic anatomy and physiology of the human body, ed. 2, New York, 1980, John Wiley & Sons, Inc.

Moses, R.A.: Adler's physiology of the eye, ed. 7, St. Louis, 1981, The C.V. Mosby Co.

Mountcastle, V.B., editor: Medical physiology, ed. 14, St. Louis, 1979, The C.V. Mosby Co.

Newell, F.W.: Ophthalmology: principles and concepts, ed. 5, St. Louis, 1982, The C.V. Mosby Co.

Saunders, W.H., Paparella, M.M., and Miglets, A.W.: Atlas of ear surgery, ed. 3, St. Louis, 1980, The C.V. Mosby Co.

Schottelius, B.A., and Schottelius, D.D.: Textbook of physiology, ed. 19, St. Louis, 1982, The C.V. Mosby Co.

Selkurt, E.D., editor: Basic physiology for the health sciences, ed. 2, Boston, 1982, Little, Brown & Co.

Silverstein, A.: Human anatomy and physiology, New York, 1980, John Wiley & Sons, Inc.

Tortora, G.J., and Anagnostakos, N.P.: Principles of anatomy and physiology, ed. 3, New York, 1981, Harper & Row, Publishers, Inc.

U.S. Department of Health and Human Services: The ABCs of contact lenses, DHEW Pub. No. (FDA) 80-4021, Washington, D.C., 1980.

U.S. Department of Health and Human Services: Tuning in on hearing aids, DHHS Pub. No. (FDA) 80-4024 Washington, D.C., 1980.

Vander, A.J., et al.: Human physiology: the mechanisms of body function, ed. 3, New York, 1980, McGraw-Hill Book Co.

▰▰▰▰ Chapter 11

American Cancer Society: Cancer facts and figures, New York, 1981, The Society:

American Cancer Society: Facts on skin cancer, New York, 1978, The Society.

American Cancer Society: Sense in the sun, New York, 1976, The Society.

Anthony, C.P., and Thibodeau, G.A.: Textbook of anatomy and physiology, ed. 11, St. Louis, 1983, The C.V. Mosby Co.

Arndt, K.A.: Manual of dermatologic therapeutics, Boston, 1977, Little, Brown & Co.

Berkow, R.B., editor: The Merck manual, ed. 14, Rahway, N.J., 1982, Merck, Sharp & Dhome Research Laboratories.

Boyd, R.F., and Hoerl, B.G.: Basic medical microbiology, ed. 2, Boston, 1982, Little, Brown & Co.

Brooks, N.A., Brooks, S.M., and Pelletier, L.J.: Handbook of infectious diseases, Boston, 1980, Little, Brown & Co.

Brooks, S.M.: Integrated basic science, ed. 4, St. Louis, 1979, The C.V. Mosby Co.

Brooks, S.M., and Paynton-Brooks, N.A.: The human body: structure and function in health and disease, ed. 2, St. Louis, 1980, The C.V. Mosby Co.

Chaffee, E.E., and Lytle, I.M.: Basic physiology and anatomy, ed. 4, Philadelphia, 1980, J.B. Lippincott Co.

Champion, R.H., et al., editors: An introduction to the biology of the skin, Oxford, 1970, Blackwell Scientific Publications, Ltd.

Dickson, F.D., and Dively, R.L.: Functional disorders of the foot, ed. 3, Philadelphia, 1952, J.B. Lippincott Co.

Guyton, A.C.: Textbook of medical physiology, ed. 6, Philadelphia, 1981, W.B. Saunders Co.

Hole, J.W.: Human anatomy and physiology, ed. 2, Dubuque, Iowa, 1982, Wm. C. Brown Co., Publishers.

Landau, B.R.: Essential human anatomy and physiology, ed. 2, Glenview, Ill., 1980, Scott, Foresman & Co.

Langley, L.L., et al.: Dynamic anatomy and physiology, ed. 5, New York, 1980, McGraw-Hill Book Co.

Maddin, S., editor: Current dermatologic management, ed 2, St. Louis, 1975, The C.V. Mosby Co.

McClintic, J.R.: Basic anatomy and physiology of the human body, ed. 2, New York, 1980, John Wiley & Sons, Inc.

Mountcastle, V.B., editor: Medical physiology, ed. 14, St. Louis, 1979, The C.V. Mosby Co.

Schottelius, B.A., and Schottelius, D.D.: Textbook of physiology, ed. 19, St. Louis, 1982, The C.V. Mosby Co.

Selkurt, E.E., editor: Basic physiology for the health sciences, ed. 2, Boston, 1982, Little, Brown & Co.

Silverstein, A.: Human anatomy and physiology, New York, 1980, John Wiley & Sons, Inc.

Tortora, G.J., and Anagnostakos, N.P.: Principles of anatomy and physiology, ed. 3, New York, 1981, Harper and Row, Publishers, Inc.

U.S. Department of Health and Human Services: A word of caution on tanning booths, FDA Pub. No. 80-8118, Washington, D.C., 1980.

Vander, A.J., et al.: Human physiology: the mechanisms of body function, ed. 3, New York, 1980, McGraw-Hill Book Co.

▪▪▪▪ Chapter 12

Anthony, C.P., and Thibodeau, G.A.: Textbook of anatomy and physiology, ed. 11, St. Louis, 1983, The C.V. Mosby Co.

Berkow, R.B., editor: The Merck manual, ed. 14, Rahway, N.J., 1982, Merck, Sharp & Dohme Research Laboratories.

Bernstein, R.K.: Diabetes: the GlucograF^{tm} method for normalizing blood sugar, New York, 1981, Crown Publishers, Inc.

Boyd, R.F., and Hoerl, B.G.: Basic medical microbiology, ed. 2, Boston, 1981, Little, Brown & Co.

Brooks, N.A., Brooks, S.M. and Pelletier, L.J.: Handbook of infectious diseases, Boston, 1980, Little, Brown & Co.

Brooks, S.M.: Integrated basic science, ed. 4, St. Louis, 1979, the C.V. Mosby Co.

Brooks, S.M., and Paynton-Brooks, N.A.: The human body: structure and function in health and disease, ed. 2, St. Louis, 1980, The C.V. Mosby Co.

Catt, K.J.: An ABC of endocrinology, Boston, 1972, Little, Brown & Co.

Chaffee, E.E., and Lytle, I.M.: Basic physiology and anatomy, ed. 4, Philadelphia, 1980, J.B. Lippincott Co.

Guyton, A.C.: Textbook of medical physiology, ed. 6, Philadelphia, 1981, W.B. Saunders Co.

Hole, J.W.: Human anatomy and physiology, ed. 2, Dubuque, Iowa, 1982, Wm. C. Brown Co., Publishers.

Landau, B.R.: Essential human anatomy and physiology, ed. 2, Glenview, Ill., 1980, Scott, Foresman & Co.

Langley, L.L., et al.: Dynamic anatomy and physiology, ed. 5, New York, 1980, McGraw-Hill Book Co.

Martin, C.R.: Textbook of endocrine physiology, Baltimore, 1976, The Williams & Wilkins Co.

McClintic, J.R.: Basic anatomy and physiology of the human body, ed. 2, New York, 1980, John Wiley & Sons, Inc.

Mountcastle, V.B., editor: Medical physiology, ed. 14, St. Louis, 1979, The C.V. Mosby Co.

Schottelius, B.A., and Schottelius, D.D.: Textbook of physiology, ed. 19, St. Louis, 1982, The C.V. Mosby Co.

Selkurt, E.E., editor: Basic physiology for the health sciences, ed. 2, Boston, 1982, Little, Brown & Co.

Silverstein, A.: Human anatomy and physiology, New York, 1980, John Wiley & Sons, Inc.

Tortora, G.J., and Anagnostakos, N.P.: Principles of anatomy and physiology, ed. 3, New York, 1981, Harper & Row, Publishers, Inc.

Vander, A.J., et al.: Human physiology: the mechanisms of body function, ed. 3, New York, 1980, McGraw-Hill Book Bo.

▬▬▬ Chapter 13

American Cancer Society: Cancer facts and figures, New York, 1981, The Society.

American Cancer Society: How to examine your breasts, New York, 1975, The Society.

Anthony, C.P., and Thibodeau, G.A.: Textbook of anatomy and physiology, ed. 11, St. Louis, 1983, The C.V. Mosby Co.

Ayerst Laboratories: Menopause: a time of change and choice, New York, 1979.

Barnhouse, R.T., editor: Male and female: Christian approaches to sexuality, New York, 1976, The Seabury Press, Inc.

Berkow, R.B., editor: The Merck manual, ed. 14, Rahway, N.J., 1982, Merck, Sharp & Dohme Research Laboratories.

Boston Women's Health Book Collective: Our bodies, our selves, New York, 1976, Simon & Schuster, Inc.

Boyd, R.F., and Hoerl, B.G.: Basic medical microbiology, ed. 2, Boston, 1982, Little, Brown & Co.

Brooks, N.A., Brooks, S.M., and Pelletier, L.J.: Handbook of infectious diseases, Boston, 1980, Little, Brown & Co.

Brooks, S.M.: Integrated basic science, ed. 4, St. Louis, 1979, The C.V. Mosby Co.

Brooks, S.M., and Paynton-Brooks, N.A.: The human body: structure and function in health and disease, ed. 2, St. Louis, 1980, The C.V. Mosby Co.

Carson, R.: Your menopause, Public Affairs Pamphlet No. 447, New York, 1981, Public Affairs Committee, Inc.

Chaffee, E.E., and Lytle, I.M.: Basic physiology and anatomy, ed. 4, Philadelphia, 1980, J.B. Lippincott Co.

Comfort, A.: The joy of sex, New York, 1972, Crown Publishers, Inc.

David, D.S., and Brannon, R.: The forty-nine percent majority: the male sex role, Menlo Park, Calif., 1976, Addison-Wesley Publishing Co., Inc.

Dick-Read, G.: Childbirth without fear: The principles and practices of natural childbirth, New York, 1944, Harper & Brothers, Publishers.

Gilette, P.: The pill and other birth control methods, New York, 1970, Bantam Books, Inc.

Gotwald, W.H., and Golden, G.H.: Sexuality: the human experience, 1981, New York, Macmillan, Inc.

Guyton, A.C.: Textbook of medical physiology, ed. 6, Philadelphia, 1981, W.B. Saunders Co.

Hatcher, R., et al: Contraceptive technology: 1980-1981, ed. 10, New York, 1980, Irvington Publishers, Inc.

Hendin, D., and Marks, J.: The genetic connection, New York,, 1979, The New American Library, Inc.

Hite, S.: The Hite report on male sexuality, New York, 1981, Alfred A. Knopf, Inc.

Hite, S.: The Hite report, New York, 1976, Macmillian, Inc.

Hole, J.W.: Human anatomy and physiology, ed. 2, Dubuque, Iowa, 1982, Wm. C. Brown Co., Publishers.

Kassorla, I.: Nice girls do, North Hollywood, Calif. 1981, Stratford House Publishing Co.

Kinsey, A.C., Pomeroy, W.B., and Martin, C.E.: Sexual behavior in the human male, Philadelphia, 1948, W.B. Saunders Co.

Kinsey, A.C., Pomeroy, W.B., Martin, C.E., and Gebhard, P.H.: Sexual behavior in the human female, Philadelphia, 1953, W.B. Saunders Co.

Lamaze, F.: Painless childbirth: the Lamaze method, New York, 1972, Pocket Books.

Landau, B.R.: Essential human anatomy and physiology, ed. 2, Glenview, Ill., 1980, Scott, Foresman & Co.

Langley, L.L., et al.: Dynamic anatomy and physiology, ed. 5, New York, 1980, McGraw-Hill Book Co.

Lauersen, N., and Whitney, S.: It's your body: a woman's guide to gynecology, New York, 1977, Grosset & Dunlap, Inc.

Leboyer, F.: Birth without violence, New York, 1975, Alfred A. Knopf, Inc.

Levine, L.: Biology of the gene, ed. 3, St. Louis, 1980, The C.V. Mosby Co.

Masters, W.H., and Johnson, V.E.: Human sexual inadequacy, Boston, 1980, Bantam Books, Inc.

Masters, W.H., and Johnson, V.E.: Human sexual response, Boston, 1966, Little, Brown & Co.

McClearn, G.E., and DeFries, J.C.: Introduction to behavioral genetics, San Francisco, 1973, W.H. Freeman & Co., Publishers.

McClintic, J.R.: Basic anatomy and physiology of the human body, ed. 2, New York, 1980, John Wiley & Sons, Inc.

Mountcastle, V.B., editor: Medical physiology, ed. 14, St. Louis, 1979, The C.V. Mosby Co.

National Cancer Institute: Breast exams, what you should know, NIH Pub. No. 81-2000, Washington, D.C., 1980.

Phillips, C.R., and Anzalone, J.T.: Fathering: participation in labor and birth, ed. 2, St. Louis, 1982, The C.V. Mosby Co.

Pierson, E., and D'Antonio, W.V.: Female and male: dimensions of human sexuality, Philadelphia, 1974, J.B. Lippincott Co.

Planned Parenthood Federation of America: Basics of birth control, Booklet 1253, New York, 1979, The Federation.

Reitz, R.: Menopause, a positive approach, New York, 1979, Penguin Books.

Schottelius, B.A., and Schottelius, D.D.: Textbook of physiology, ed. 19, St. Louis, 1982, The C.V. Mosby Co.

Selkurt, E.E., editor: Basic physiology for the health sciences, ed. 2, Boston, 1982, Little, Brown & Co.

Shearman, R.P., editor: Human reproductive physiology, ed. 2, Oxford, 1979, Blackwell Scientific Publications, Ltd.

Silverstein, A.: Human anatomy and physiology, New York, 1980, John Wiley & Sons, Inc.

Sorensen, R.C.: The Sorensen report: adolescent sexuality in contemporary America, New York, 1973, World Publishing Co.

Tortora, G.J., and Anagnostakos, N.P.: Principles of anatomy and physiology, ed. 3, New York, 1981, Harper & Row, Publishers, Inc.

U.S. Department of Health and Human Services: Toxic shock syndrome and tampons, DHHS Pub. No. (FDA) 81-4025, Washington, D.C., 1980.

Vander, A.J., et al: Human physiology: the mechanisms of body function, ed. 3, New York, 1980, McGraw-Hill Book Co.

Chapter 14

Alan Guttmacher Institute: Factbook on teenage pregnancy, New York, 1981, The Institute.

Alan Guttmacher Institute: Teenage pregnancy: the problem that hasn't gone away, New York, 1981, The Institute.

American Council on Science and Health: Alcohol use during pregnancy, New York, Dec. 1981, The Council.

Anthony, E.S., and Benedek, T., editors: Parenthood: its psychology and psycopathology, Boston, 1970, Little, Brown & Co.

Apgar, V., and Beck, J.: A guide to birth defects, New York, 1972, Trident Press.

Berkow, R.B., editor: The Merck manual, ed. 14, Rahway, N.J., 1982, Merck, Sharp & Dohme Research Laboratories.

Bittman, S., and Zalk, S.R.: Expectant fathers, New York, 1980, Ballantine Books, Inc.

Boston Women's Health Book Collective: Our bodies, our selves, New York, 1976, Simon & Schuster, Inc.

Brooks, N.A., Brooks, S.M., and Pelletier, L.J.: Handbook of infectious diseases, Boston, 1980, Little, Brown & Co.

Brooks, S.M.: Integrated basic science, ed. 4, St. Louis, 1979, The C.F. Mosby Co.

Brooks, S.M., and Paynton-Brooks, N.A.: The human body: structure and function in health and disease, ed. 2, St. Louis, 1980, The C.V. Mosby Co.

Chaffee, E.E., and Lytle, I.M.: Basic physiology and anatomy, ed. 4, Philadelphia, 1980, J.B. Lippincott Co.

Chesleer, P.: Women and madness, New York, 1972, Avon Books.

Cole, K.C.: What only a mother can tell you about having a baby, New York, 1980, Doubleday & Co., Inc.

Connaughton, J.F., Reeser, D.S., and Finnegan, L.P.: Pregnancy complicated by drug addiction. In Bolognese, R.J., and Schwartz, R., editors: Perinatal medicine, ed. 2, Baltimore, 1982, The Williams & Wilkins Co.

D'Augelli, F., and Weener, J.M.: Communication and parenting skills, University Park, Pa., 1976, Pennsylvania State University Press.

Ehrenreich, B., and English, D.: For her own good: 150 years of the experts' advice to women, New York, 1978, Anchor Press.

Gardner, E.J., and Snustad, D.: Principles of genetics, ed. 6, New York, 1980, John Wiley & Sons, Inc.

Guyton, A.C.: Textbook of medical physiology, ed. 6, Philadelphia, 1981, W.B. Saunders Co.

Hole, J.W.: Human anatomy and physiology, ed. 2, Dubuque, Iowa, 1982, Wm. C. Brown Co., Publishers.

Kitzinger, S.: The complete book of childbirth, New York, 1980, Alfred A. Knopf, Inc.

Kitzinger, S.: Education and counseling for childbirth, New York, 1979, Schocken Books.

Kitzinger, S.: The experience of childbirth, ed. 4, Harmondsworth, England, 1978, Penguin Books, Ltd.

Landau, B.R.: Essential human anatomy and physiology, ed. 2, Glenview, Ill., 1980, Scott, Foresman & Co.

Langley, L.L., et al.: Dynamic anatomy and physiology, ed. 5, New York, 1980, McGraw-Hill Book Co.

Levine, L.: Biology of the gene, ed. 3, St. Louis, 1980, The C.V. Mosby Co.

Lubs, H.A., and de la Cruz, F., editors: Genetic counseling, New York, 1977, Raven Press.

Lynch, H., Fain, P., and Marrero, K., editors: International directory: birth defects—genetic services, New York, 1980, March of Dimes Birth Defects Foundation.

MacFarlane, A.: The psychology of childbirth, Cambridge, Mass., 1977, Harvard University Press.

McBride, A.G.: The growth and development of mothers, New York, 1974, Barnes & Noble Books.

McClintic, J.R.: Basic anatomy and physiology of the human body, ed. 2, New York, 1980, John Wiley & Sons, Inc.

McKusick, V.A.: Mendelian inheritance in man: catalog of autosomal dominant, autosomal recessive and x-linked phenotypes, ed. 5, Baltimore, 1978, Johns Hopkins University Press.

Meade Johnson and Co.: A primer on infant nutrition, Evansville, Indiana, 1978.

National Academy of Sciences—National Research Council, Committee for the Study of Inborn Errors of Metabolism: Genetic screening: programs, principles, and research, Washington, D.C., 1975, The Academy.

National Foundation: Be good to your baby before it is born, Washington, D.C., 1977, The Foundation.

Norwood, C.: At highest risk, New York, 1980, McGraw-Hill Book Co.

Parke, R.D.: Fathers, Cambridge, Mass., 1981, Harvard University Press.

Phillips, C.R., and Anzalone, J.T.: Fathering: participation in labor and birth, ed. 2, St. Louis, 1982, The C.V. Mosby Co.

Pryor, K.: Nursing your baby, New York, 1973, Harper & Row, Publishers, Inc.

Rozdilsky, M.L., and Banet, B.: What now? A handbook for parents postpartum, New York, 1975, Charles Scribner's Sons.

Scheinfield, A.: Heredity in humans, Philadelphia, 1972, J.B. Lippincott Co.

Silverstein, A.: Human anatomy and physiology, New York, 1980, John Wiley & Sons, Inc.

Spock, B.: Baby and child care, New York, 1976, Pocket Books.

Thompson, J.S., and Thompson, M.W.: Genetics in medicine, ed. 3, Philadelphia, 1980, W.B. Saunders Co.

Tortora, G.J., and Anagnostakos, N.P.: Principles of anatomy and physiology, ed. 3, New York, 1981, Harper & Row, Publishers, Inc.

U.S. Department of Health, Education, and Welfare: Food for the teenager during pregnancy, DHEW Pub. No. (HSA) 77-5106 Washington, D.C., 1977.

Vander, A.J., et al.: Human physiology: the mechanisms of body function, ed. 3, New York, 1980, McGraw-Hill Book Co.

▬▬▬ **Chapter 15**

Benenson, A., editor: Control of communicable diseases in man, ed. 13, Washington, D.C., 1981, The American Public Health Association.

Berkow, R.B., editor: The Merck manual, ed. 14, Rahway, N.J., 1982, Merck, Sharp & Dohme Research Laboratories.

Brooks, N.A., Brooks, S.M., and Pelletier, L.J.: Handbook of infectious diseases, Boston, 1980, Little, Brown & Co.

Brooks, S.M.: Integrated basic science, ed. 4, St. Louis, 1979, The C.V. Mosby Co.

Brooks, S.M.: The v.d. story, Cranbury, New Jersey, 1971, A.S. Barnes & Co., Inc.

Brooks, S.M., and Paynton-Brooks, N.A.: The human body: structure and function in health and disease, ed. 2, St. Louis, 1980, The C.V. Mosby Co.

Chiapa, J.A., and Forish, J.J.: The VD book, New York, 1977, Holt, Rinehart & Winston.

Jerrick, S.J.: Federal efforts to control sexually transmitted diseases, Journal of School Health, Sept. 1978, pp. 428-432.

U.S. Department of Health and Human Services: Health, United States, 1980, with prevention profile, DHHS Pub. No. (PHS) 81-1232 Washington, D.C., 1980.

U.S. Department of Health and Human Services: STD fact sheet edition thirty-five, HHS Pub. No. (CDC) 81-8195 Washington, D.C., 1980.

▬▬▬ **Chapter 16**

Ackerman, N.: Treating the troubled family, New York, 1973, Basic Books.

Aguilera, D.C., and Messick, J.M.: Crisis intervention, ed. 4, St. Louis, 1982, The C.V. Mosby Co.

Alan Guttmacher Institute: Factbook on teenage pregnancy, New York, 1981, The Institute.

Alan Guttmacher Institute: Teenage pregnancy: the problem that hasn't gone away, New York, 1981, The Institute.

Alan Guttmacher Institute: 11 million teenagers, New York, 1977, The Institute.

Amonker, R.G.: What do teens know about the facts of life? Journal of School Health, Nov. 1980, pp. 527-530.

Anthony, E.J., editor: The child and his family: vulnerable children, Vol. IV, New York, 1978, Wiley Interscience.

Anthony, E.S., and Benedek, T., editors: Parenthood: its phychology and psycopathology, Boston, 1970, Little, Brown & Co.

Bach, G., and Deutsch, R.: Pairing, New York, 1970, Wyden Books.

Barnes, B.C., and Coplon, J.K.: The single-parent experience, Boston, 1980, Resource Communications, Inc.

Barnhouse, R.T., editor: Male and female: Christian approaches to sexuality, New York, 1976, The Seabury Press, Inc.

Baxandall, R., Gordon, L., and Reverby, S.: America's working women: a documentary history—1600 to the present, New York, 1976, Vintage Books.

Beckwith, J.: Make your own backyard more interesting than T.V., New York, 1980, McGraw-Hill, Inc.

Bem, S.: Sex role adaptability; one consequential psychological androgyny, Journal of Personality and Social Psychology 31:634-643, 1975.

Berger, M., editor: Beyond the double bind, New York, 1978, Brunner/Mazel, Inc.

Bernard, J.: The future of marriage, New York, 1973, Bantam Books, Inc.

Bernard, J.: Remarriage, New York, 1971, Dryden Press.

Bienvenu, M.J.: Talking it over before marriage, New York, 1980, Public Affairs Pamphlet No. 512, Public Affairs Committee.

Blau, Z.: Old age in a changing society, New York, 1973, Franklin Watts, Inc.

Blaxall, M., and Reagan, B., editors: Women in the marketplace, Chicago, 1976, University of Chicago Press.

Boston Women's Health Book Collective: Our bodies, our selves, New York, 1976, Simon & Schuster, Inc.

Brazelton, T.B.: On becoming a family, New York, 1981, Dell Publishing Co., Inc.

Brazelton, T.B.: Toddlers and parents: a declaration of independence, New York, 1974, Delacorte Press.

Briggs, D.C.: Your child's self-esteem: the key to his life, New York, 1975, Doubleday.

Bronfenbrenner, U.: Nobody home: the erosion of the American family, Psychology Today 10(12):40-47, 1977.

Bureau of the Census: 1980 census of population and housing, Pub. No. PHC80-V-1, Washington, D.C., 1982.

Calderone, M.S., and Johnson, E.W.: The family book about sexuality, New York, 1981, Harper & Row, Publishers, Inc.

Campbell, A., Converse, P., and Rogers, W.: The quality of American life, New York, 1976, Russell Sage Foundation.

Cassidy, R.: What every man should know about divorce, Washington, D.C., 1977, New Republic Books.

Cater, L., Scott, A., and Martina, W., editors: Women and men: changing roles, New York, 1976, Aspen Institute for Humanistic Studies, Praeger Publishers.

Chapman, E.: Scrambling, Los Angeles, 1981, J.P. Archer, Inc.

Chesler, P.: Women and madness, New York, 1972, Avon Books.

Comfort, A.: The joy of sex, New York, 1972, Crown Publishers, Inc.

Cox, F.D.: Human intimacy: marriage, the family and its meaning, St. Paul, Minnesota, 1978, West Publishing.

D'Augelli, F., and Weener, J.M.: Communication and parenting skills, University Park, Pa., 1976, Pennsylvania State University Press.

Davidson, T.: Conjugal crime, New York, 1978, Hawthorn Books, Inc.

Duberman, L.: The reconstituted family: a study of remarried couples and their children, Chicago, 1975, Nelson-Hall Publishers.

Edelman, A., and Stuzin, R.: How to survive a second marriage (or save a first one), Secaucus, N.J., 1981, Lyle Stuart, Inc.

Eekelaar, J.M., and Katz, S., editors: Family violence: an international and interdisciplinary study, Toronto, 1978, Butterworth and Co., Ltd.

Espinoza, R., and Newman, Y.: Stepparenting, Washington, D.C., 1979, Superintendent of Documents, U.S. Government Printing Office.

Farrell, W.: The liberated man, Des Plaines, Ill. 1975, Bantam Books, Inc.

Fraiberg, S.: Every child's birthright, New York, 1977, Basic Books, Inc., Publishers.

Getty, C., and Humphreys, W.: Understanding the family: stress and change in American family life, New York, 1981, Appleton-Century-Crofts.

Ginsberg, H., and Opper, S.: Piaget's theory of intellectual development, Englewood Cliffs, N.J., 1969, Prentice-Hall, Inc.

Glick, P.: Updating the life cycle of the family, Journal of Marriage and the Family 39:5, 1977.

Goodman, F.J.: The A,B,C's of feminine happiness, Los Angeles, 1980, gee tee bee.

Greene, S.: What bothers us about grown ups, Brattleboro, Vt., 1971, The Stephen Greene Press.

Haley, J.: Problem-solving therapy, San Francisco, 1976, Jossey-Bass, Inc., Publishers.

Hoff, L.A.: People in crisis, Menlo Park, Calif. 1978, Addison-Wesley Publishing Co., Inc.

Jones, L.Y.: Great expectations: America and the baby boom generation, New York, 1980, Coward McCann & Geohegan, Inc.

Kahn, A.U., Kamerman, S.B., and Dowling, M.: Government structure versus family policy, New York, 1979, Columbia University School of Social Work.

Keniston, K., and The Carnegie Council on Children: All our children: the American family under pressure, New York, 1977, Harcourt Brace Jovanovich, Inc.

Klemer, R.H., and Klemer, M.G.: Sexual adjustment in marriage, Public Affairs Pamphlet No. 397, New York, 1980, Public Affairs Committee.

Levinger, G., and Moles, O.: Separation and divorce, New York, 1979, Basic Books, Inc., Publishers.

Margolius, S.: Family money problems, Public Affairs Pamphlet No. 412, New York, 1980, Public Affairs Committee.

Martin, E.P., and Martin, J.M.: The extended black family, Chicago, 1978, University of Chicago Press.

McCary, J.L.: Freedom and growth in marriage, New York, 1975, John Wiley & Sons, Inc.

McCormick, M.: Stepfathers: what the literature reveals, La Jolla, Calif., 1974, Western Behavioral Sciences Institute.

Mead, M.: Male and female: a study of sexes in a changing world, New York, 1949, William Morrow & Co., Inc.

Millstone, D.: Family planning, Public Affairs Pamphlet No. 531A, New York, 1980, Public Affairs Committee.

Nass, G.: Marriage and the family, Menlo Park, Calif. 1978, Addison-Wesley Publishing Co., Inc.

Ogg, E.: One-parent families, Public Affairs Publication No. 543, New York, 1980, Public Affairs Committee.

Ogg, E.: Preparing tomorrow's parents, Public Affairs Pamphlet No. 520, New York, 1980, Public Affairs Committee.

Phillips, M.: Adopting a child, Public Affairs Publication No. 585, New York, 1980, Public Affairs Committee.

Piaget, J.: Origins of intelligence in children, New York, 1963, W.W. Norton & Co., Inc.

Pogrebin, L.C.: Growing up free: raising your child in the 80s, New York, 1980, McGraw-Hill, Inc.

Rapoport, R., and Rapoport, R., editors: Working couples, New York, 1978, Harper & Row, Publishers, Inc.

Salk, L.: What every child would like parents to know about divorce, New York, 1978, Harper & Row, Publishers, Inc.

Sorenson, R.C.: The Sorenson report: adolescent sexuality in contemporary America, New York, 1973, World Publishing Co.

Stevens, J.H., and Matthews, M., editors: Mother-child, father-child relations, Washington, D.C., 1978, National Association for the Education of Young Children.

Straus, M.A., Gelles, R.J., and Steinmetz, S.K.: Behind closed doors: violence in the American family, New York, 1980, Doubleday & Co., Inc.

Troyer, W.: Divorced kids, New York, 1979, Harcourt, Brace, Jovanovich, Inc., and Toronto, Clarke, Irwin & Company, Ltd.

U.S. Department of Health and Human Services: Single parent families, DHHS Pub No. (OHDS) 79-30247, Washington, D.C., 1981.

U.S. Department of Health and Human Services: An adolescent in your home, DHHS Pub. No. (OHDS) 80-30041, Washington, D.C., 1980.

U.S. Department of Health and Human Services: Child development in the home, DHHS Pub. No. (OHDS) 80-30042, Washington, D.C., 1980.

U.S. Department of Health and Human Services: National study of social services to children and their families, DHHS Pub. No. (OHDS) 80-30149, Washington, D.C., 1980.

U.S. Department of Health and Human Services: Serving America's children and families, DHHS Pub. No. (OHDS) 79-30229, Washington, D.C., 1980.

U.S. Department of Health and Human Services: Children and television, DHHS Pub. No. (OHDS) 81-30169, Washington, D.C., 1978.

U.S. Department of Health, Education, and Welfare: Families today: a research sampler on families and children, DHEW Pub. No. (ADM) 79-815, Washington, D.C., 1979.

U.S. Department of Health, Education, and Welfare: Education for parenthood, DHEW Pub. No. (OHDS) 78-30046, Washington, D.C., 1978.

U.S. Department of Health, Education, and Welfare: Selected recommendations of the Public Health Service advisory committee on immunization practices: vaccines for selective use in international travel, G.P.O. 1978-640-010/3965, Region No. 4, 1978.

U.S. Department of Health, Education, and Welfare: Raising a family alone, DHEW Pub. No. (OHD) 77-30101, Washington, D.C., 1977.

U.S. Department of Health, Education, and Welfare: Child care programs in nine counties, DHEW Pub No. (OHD) 76-30080, Washington, D.C., 1976.

U.S. Department of Health, Education, and Welfare: Day care for your children, DHEW Pub. No. (OHD) 74-47, Washington, D.C., 1975.

Victor, I., and Winkler, W.A.: Fathers and custody, New York, 1977, Hawthorn Books, Inc.

Weiss, R.S.: Going it alone: the family life and social situation of the single parent, New York, 1979, Basic Books, Inc., Publishers.

Weiss, R.S.: Marital separation, New York, 1977, Basic Books, Inc., Publishers.

White, B.L.: The first three years of life, Englewood Cliffs, N.J., 1975, Prentice-Hall, Inc.

Winch, R.F., editor: Selected studies in marriage and the family, New York, 1962, Holt, Reinhart & Winston.

Chapter 17

American Council on Life Insurance: Death, dying, and life extension, TAP #16, Washington, D.C., 1978, The Council.

Alsop, S.: Stay of execution, Philadelphia, 1973, J.B. Lippincott Co.

Amir, M.: Patterns of forcible rape, Chicago, 1971, University of Chicago Press.

Anderson, R.: Stress power: how to turn tension into energy, New York, 1978, Human Sciences Press, Inc.

Bellak, L., editor: The schizophrenic syndrome, New York, 1978, Grune & Stratton, Inc.

Berger, M., editor: Beyond the double bind, New York, 1978, Brunner/Mazel, Inc.

Berkow, R.B., editor: The Merck manual, ed. 14, Rahway, N.J., 1982, Merck, Sharp & Dohme Research Laboratories.

Bienvenus, M.J.: Talking it over before marriage, Public Affairs Pamphlet No. 512, New York, 1980, Public Affairs Committee.

Birren, J.E., and Schaie, K.W., editors: Handbook of the psychology of aging, New York, 1977, Van Nostrand Reinhold Co.

Blue Cross Association: Stress: blue print for health, Vol. XXV, Number 1, Chicago, 1974.

Bohannan, P., and Erickson, R.: Stepping in, Psychology Today 11(8):53-59, 1978.

Briggs, D.D.: Your child's self-esteem: the key to his life, New York, 1975, Doubleday & Co., Inc.

Brooks, N.A., Brooks, S.M., and Pelletier, L.J.: Handbook of infectious diseases, Boston, 1980, Little, Brown & Co.

Brooks, S.M.: Integrated basic science, ed. 4, St. Louis, 1979, The C.V. Mosby Co.

Brooks, S.M., and Paynton-Brooks, N.A.: The human body: structure and function in health and disease, ed. 2, St. Louis, 1980, The C.V. Mosby Co.

Brownmiller, S.: Against our will: men, women and rape, New York, 1975, Simon & Schuster, Inc.

Butler, R.N., and Lewis, M.I.: Aging and mental health, ed. 3, St. Louis, 1982, The C.V. Mosby Co.

Chapman, J., and Gates, M., editors: The victimization of women, Hollywood, Calif. 1978, Sage Publications, Inc.

Coleman, J.C.: Abnormal psychology and modern life, ed. 5, Glenview, Ill., 1976, Scott, Foresman & Co.

Datan, N., and Ginsberg, L., editors: Life-span developmental psychology: normative life crisis, New York, 1975, Academic Press, Inc.

Dubois, R.: Man adapting, New Haven, 1965, Yale University Press.

Dyer, W.: The sky's the limit, New York, 1981, Simon & Schuster, Inc.

Eddy, J.M., and Alles, W.F.: Death education, St. Louis, 1983, The C.V. Mosby Co.

Eekelaar, J.M., and Katz, S., editors: Family violence: an international and interdisciplinary study, Toronto, 1978, Butterworths.

Ehrenwald, J., editor: The history of psychotherapy, New York, 1976, Jason Aronson, Inc.

Elwell, M.E.: Sexually assaulted children and their families: social casework, The Journal of Contemporary Social Work 4(60):227-235, April, 1979.

Eysenck, H.J., and Kamin, L.: The intelligence controversy, New York, 1981, John Wiley & Sons, Inc.

Finklehor, D.: Sexually victimized children, New York, 1979, The Free Press.

Fleming, J.B.: Stopping wife abuse, Garden City, N.Y., 1979, Anchor Press.

Foreman, S.: Betrayal of innocence: incest and its devastation, New York, 1979, Penguin Books.

Freese, A.S.: Adolescent suicide: mental health challenge, Public Health Affairs Pamphlet No. 569, New York, 1979, Public Affairs Committee.

Freud, S.A.: General introduction to psychoanalysis, Garden City, N.Y., 1938, Doubleday & Co., Inc.

Freud, S.A.: New introductory lectures on psychoanalysis (standard edition), Vol. 22, London, 1933, Hogarth Press.

Friday, N.: Men in love, New York, 1980, Delacorte Press.

Friedan, B.: The feminine mystique, New York, 1963, W.W. Norton & Co., Inc.

Geiser, R.L.: Hidden victims, Boston, 1979, Beacon Press.

Gelles, R.: Family violence, Beverly Hills, Calif., 1979, Sage Publications, Inc.

Goleman, D.: The varieties of the meditative experience, New York, 1977, E.P. Dutton.

Greenfield, J.: A child called Noah: a family journey, New York, 1972, Holt, Rinehart & Winston.

Hardt, D.V.: Death: the final frontier, Englewood Cliffs, N.J., 1979, Prentice-Hall, Inc.

Hare, R.D., and Schalling, D., editors: Psychopathic behavior, New York, 1978, John Wiley & Sons, Inc.

Hilgard, E.R., Atkinson, R.C., and Atkinson, R.L.: Introduction to psychology, ed. 7, New York, 1979, Harcourt Brace Jovanovich, Inc.

Hoff, L.A.: People in crisis, Menlo Park, Calif. 1978, Addison-Wesley Publishing Co., Inc.

Hoffmann-LaRoche, Inc.: The abused child, Nutley, N.J., 1980, Public Affairs and Planning Division, The Company.

Hollister, L.E.: Chemical psychoses: LSD and related drugs, Springfield, Ill., 1968, Charles C. Thomas, Publisher.

Irwin, T.: To combat and prevent child abuse and neglect, Public Affairs Pamphlet No. 588, New York, 1980, Public Affairs Committee.

Jaffe, N.: Assaults on women: rape and wife beating, Public Affairs Pamphlet No. 579, New York, 1980, Public Affairs Committee.

Jones, H.T., and Jones, H.: Sensual drugs: deprivation and rehabilitation of the mind, New York, 1977, Cambridge University Press.

Jung, C.G.: The collected works of C.G. Jung. Vol. 1, chapt. 5, Vol. 17, Chapt. 8, Princeton, N.J., 1966, Princeton University Press.

Kastenbaum, R.J.: Death, society, and human experience, ed. 2, St. Louis, 1981, The C.V. Mosby Co.

Kopay, D., and Young, P.D.: The David Kopay story, New York, 1977, Arbor House Publishing Co., Inc.

Kübler-Ross, E.: To live until we say good-bye, Englewood Cliffs, N.J., 1978, Prentice-Hall, Inc.

Laing, R.D., and Esterson, A.: Sanity, madness and the family: families of schizophrenics, ed. 2, London, 1970, Tavistock.

Langley, R., and Levy, R.: Wife-beating: the silent crisis, New York, 1977, E.P. Dutton.

Luther, S.L., and Price, J.H.: Child sexual abuse: a review, Journal of School Health 50(3):161-165, March 1980.

Lynch, J.J.: The broken heart: the medical consequences of loneliness, New York, 1977, Basic Books, Inc., Publishers.

Maslow, A.: The farther reaches of human nature, New York, 1971, The Viking Press.

Maslow, A.: Toward a psychology of being, ed. 2, Princeton, N.J., 1968, Van Nostrand Reinhold Co.

Maslow, A.: Motivation and personality, ed. 2, New York, 1970, Harper & Row, Publishers, Inc.

Masters, W.H., and Johnson, V.E.: Homosexuality in perspective, Boston, 1979, Little, Brown & Co.

Meiselman, K.C.: Incest: a psychological study of causes and effects with treatment recommendations, San Francisco, 1978, Jossey-Bass, Inc., Publishers.

Merck, Sharp & Dohme Research Laboratories: Depression: dark night of the soul, Rahway, N.J., Health Information Services, The Laboratories.

Miles, H.S., and Harp, D.R.: Widowhood, American Journal of Nursing 75:280-282, 1975.

Mitford, J.: The American way of death, New York, 1963, Simon & Schuster, Inc.

National Hospice Organization: Hospice in America, New Haven, Conn., 1978, The Organization.

National Institute on Aging: What to do about flu, Pub. No. 335-444/5525, Washington, D.C., 1981, U.S. Government Printing Office.

National Institute on Aging: Senility: myth or madness; Pub. No. 0-327-894, Washington, D.C., 1980, U.S. Government Printing Office.

Ogg, E.: Changing views on homosexuality, Public Affairs Pamphlet No. 563, New York, 1980, Public Affairs Committee.

Ogg, E.: Partners in coping—group for self and mutual help, Public Affairs Pamphlet No. 559, New York, 1978, Public Affairs Committee.

Parkes, C.M.: Bereavement, New York, 1972, International Universities Press, Inc.

Pelletier, K.: Mind as healer, mind as slayer: a holistic approach to preventing stress disorders, New York, 1977, Delacorte Press/Seymour Lawrence (Merloyd Lawrence Book).

Piaget, J.: Memory and intelligence, New York, 1954, Basic Books, Inc., Publishers.

Sarafino, E.P.: An estimate of nationwide incidence of sexual offenses against children, Child Welfare 58(2):127-134, Feb. 1979.

Schnall, M.: Limits: a search for new values, New York, 1981, Clarkson N. Potter, Inc.

Selye, H.: Stress without distress, Philadelphia, 1974, J.B. Lippincott Co.

Sheehy, G.: Passages: predictable crises of adult life, New York, 1976, E.P. Dutton.

Stoddard, S.: The hospice movement, Briarcliff Manor, New York, 1978, Stein & Day Publishers.

Strongman, K.T.: The psychology of emotions, New York, 1973, John Wiley & Sons, Inc.

U.S. Department of Health and Human Services: Child sexual abuse: incest, assault, and sexual exploitation, DHHS Pub. No. (OHDS) 81-30166, Washington, D.C., 1981.

U.S. Department of Health and Human Services: New Light on an old problem: 9 questions and answers about child abuse and neglect, DHHS Pub. No. (OHDS) 81-31108, Washington, D.C., 1981.

U.S. Department of Health and Human Services: A consumer's guide to mental health services, DHHS Pub. No. (ADM) 80-214, Washington, D.C., 1980.

U.S. Department of Health and Human Services: Attitudes toward the mentally ill: research perspectives, DHHS Pub. No. (ADM) 80-1031, Washington, D.C., 1980.

U.S. Department of Health and Human Services: How to donate the body or its organs, NIH Pub. No. 80-776, Washington, D.C., 1980.

U.S. Department of Health and Human Services: Talking to children about death, DHHS Pub. No. (ADM) 80-838, Washington, D.C., 1979.

U.S. Department of Health, Education, and Welfare: Mental health and the elderly, recommendations for action, DHEW Pub. No. (OHDS) 80-20960, Washington, D.C., 1980.

U.S. Department of Health, Education, and Welfare: The consumer's guide to mental health and related federal programs, DHEW Pub. No. (ADM) 79-760, Washington, D.C., 1979.

U.S. Department of Health, Education, and Welfare: Federal council on aging: mental health and the elderly, DHEW Pub. No. (OHDS) 80-20960, Washington, D.C., 1979.

U.S. Department of Health, Education, and Welfare: Trends in mental health, DHEW Pub. No. (ADM) 78-407, Washington, D.C., 1978.

U.S. Department of Health, Education, and Welfare: College mental health, DHEW Publication No. (ADM) 77-457, Washington, D.C., 1977.

U.S. Department of Health, Education, and Welfare: One-parent families, DHEW Pub. No. (OHD) 74-44, Washington, D.C., 1974.

Walker, L.E.: The battered woman, New York, 1979, Harper & Row, Publishers, Inc.

Wickelgren, W.E.: How to solve problems, San Francisco, 1974, W.H. Freeman & Co., Publishers.

Weissmann, M.M., and Klerman, G.L.: Sex differences and the epidemiology of depression, Archives of General Psychiatry 34(1):98-111, 1977.

Wynne, L.C., Cromwell, R.L., and Matthysse, S., editors: The nature of schizophrenia: new approaches to research and treatment, New York, 1978, John Wiley & Sons, Inc.

Yankelovich, Skelly, and White, Inc.: The General Mills American family report, 1978-79, family health in an era of stress, Minneapolis, 1979, General Mills, Inc.

Young, L: Wednesday's children: a study of child neglect and abuse, New York, 1974, McGraw-Hill Book Co.

▬▬▬ Chapter 18

Alexander, S.: Running healthy, Brattleboro, Vt., 1980, The Stephen Greene Press.

Barney, V.S., Hirst, C.C., and Jensen, C.R.: Conditioning exercises, ed. 3, St. Louis, 1972, The C.V. Mosby Co.

Bogart, L.J., Brigg, G.M., and Calloway, D.: Nutrition and physical fitness, Philadelphia, 1973, W.B. Saunders Co.

Bucher, C.A.: Foundations of physical education, ed. 9, St. Louis, 1983, The C.V. Mosby Co.

Clark, H.H., editor: Physical fitness research digest, Washington, D.C., The President's Council on Physical Fitness and Sports, Series 6, No. 4, Oct. 1976.

Cooper, K.: New aerobics, New York, 1972, Bantum Books, Inc.

Cooper, M., and Cooper K.: Aerobics for women, New York, 1972, Bantam Books, Inc.

Dickson, F.D., and Dively, R.L.: Functional disorders of the foot, ed. 3, Philadelphia, 1952, J.B. Lippincott Co.

Dominguez, R.: The complete book of sports medicine, New York, 1979, The Scribner Book Companies, Inc.

Ferrell, J., Glashagei, J., and Johnson, M.: A family approach to youth sports, La Grange, Ill., 1978, Youth Sports Press.

Fixx, J.: Second book of running, New York, 1977, Random House, Inc.

Henderson, J.: Jog, run, race, Mountain View, Calif., 1977, World Publications.

Kaplan, J.: Women and sports, New York, 1979, The Viking Press.

Katz, J., and Bruning, N.: Swimming for total fitness, New York, 1981, Dolphin Books.

Klafs, C.E., and Lyon, M.J.: The female athlete, ed. 2, St. Louis, 1978, The C.V. Mosby Co.

Kuntzleman, C.: Rating the exercises, New York, 1980, Penguin Books.

Kuntzleman, C.: The complete book of walking, Boston, 1980, G.K. Hall & Co.

Magill, R., Ash, M., and Small, F., editors: Children in sport: a contemporary anthology, Champaign, Ill., 1978, Human Kinetics Publishers.

Metropolitan Life Insurance Company: Stay well series: exercise, New York, 1979, The Company.

Michener, J.: Sports in America, New York, 1976, Random House, Inc.

Mirkin, G.: The sports medicine book, Boston, 1978, Little, Brown & Co.

Morehouse, L.E., and Miller, A.T.: Physiology of exercise, ed. 7, St. Louis, 1976, The C.V. Mosby Co.

Morris, D.: How to change the games children play, Minneapolis, 1980, Burgess Publishing Co.

National Athletic Health Institute and Occidental Life: Exercising your right to live, Washington, D.C., 1979, Occidental Life Insurance Co. of Calif. and National Athletic Health Institute.

National Institutes of Health: Exercise your heart, Pub. No. GPO:1981-726-248, Washington, D.C., 1981.

President's Council on Physical Fitness and Sports: Exercise and weight control, Pub. No. 0-316-965, Washington, D.C., 1980, U.S. Government Printing Office.

President's Council on Physical Fitness: Adult physical fitness, Washington, D.C., U.S. Government Printing Office.

Roberts, E.H.: On your feet, Emmaus, Pa., 1975, Rodale Press, Inc.

Ryan, A.J.: The physical and sports medicine, guide to running, New York, 1980, McGraw-Hill Book Co.

Smith, R.P.: La Costa diet and exercise book, New York, 1977, Grosset & Dunlap, Inc.

United States Cycling Federation, Inc.: Bicycle safety and beyond, Colorado Springs, Colo.

U.S. Department of Health and Human Services: Aqua dynamics, Pub. No. DHHS 396, Washington, D.C., 1981.

U.S. Department of Health, Education, and Welfare: The President's council on physical fitness and sports: an introduction to physical fitness, DHEW Pub. No. (OS) 79-50068, Washington, D.C., 1979.

U.S. Department of Health, Education, and Welfare: The President's council on physical fitness and sports, DHEW Pub. No. (OS) 77-50013, Washington, D.C., 1978.

Wickstrom, R.: Fundamental motor patterns, Philadelphia, 1977, Lea & Febiger.

Wiener, H.S.: Total swimming, New York, 1980, Simon & Schuster, Inc.

Zohman, L.R., and Kattus, A.K., with Softness, D.G.: The cardiologists' guide to fitness and health through exercise, New York, 1979, Simon & Schuster, Inc.

Chapter 19

Abbott Laboratories: Vitamins: an alphabet soup for good health, North Chicago, The Laboratories.

American Council on Science and Health: ACSH News & Views, New York, Vol. 3, No. 1, Jan./Feb. 1982.

American Council on Science and Health: Food additives and hyperactivity, New York, Jan. 1982, The Council.

American Council on Science and Health: Fast food and the American diet, New York, 1981, The Council.

American Council on Science and Health: Vitamin B-15: anatomy of a fraud, New York, Sept. 1981, The Council.

American Heart Association Cookbook, New York, 1973, David McKay Co., Inc.

Bennett, W., and Gurin, J.: The dieter's dilemma, New York, 1982, Basic Books, Inc., Publishers.

Berkow, R.B., editor: The Merck manual, ed. 14, Rahway, N.J., 1982, Merck, Sharp & Dohme Research Laboratories.

Bogart, L.J., Briggs, G.M., and Calloway, D.: Nutrition and physical fitness, Philadelphia, 1973, W.B. Saunders Co.

Bricklin, M.: Lose weight naturally, Emmaus, Pa., 1979, Rodale Press, Inc.

Brody, J.E.: Jane Brody's nutrition book, New York, 1981, W.W. Norton & Company, Inc.

Brooks, N.A., Brooks, S.M., and Pelletier, L.J.: Handbook of infectious diseases, Boston, 1980, Little, Brown & Co.

Brooks, S.M.: Integrated basic science, ed. 4, St. Louis, 1979, The C.V. Mosby Co.

Brooks, S.M., and Paynton-Brooks: The human body: structure and function in health and disease, ed. 2, St. Louis, 1980, The C.V. Mosby Co.

Church, C.F., and Church, H.N.: Food values of portions commonly used, ed. 12, Philadelphia, 1975, J.B. Lippincott Co.

Clayburn, W.: Directory of salt-free foods, Chicago, 1979, Globe Communications Corp.

Fleck, H.: Introduction to nutrition, New York, 1976, Macmillan, Inc.

Food and Nutrition Board, National Research Council: Recommended dietary allowances, ed. 9, Washington, D.C., 1979, National Academy of Sciences.

Gerber, A.B.: The joy of dieting, New York, 1976, Dodd, Mead & Co.

Goldbeck, D., and Goldbeck, N.: Supermarket handbook: access to whole foods, New York, 1976, The New American Library, Inc.

Guthrie, H.A.: Introductory nutrition, ed. 5, St. Louis, 1983, The C.V. Mosby Co.

Hamilton, E.M., and Whitney, E.: Nutrition: concepts and controversies, St. Paul, 1979, West.

Hofmann, L.: The great American nutrition hassle, Palo Alto, Calif., 1978, Mayfield.

Howe, P.S.: Basic nutrition in health and disease, ed. 7, Philadelphia, 1981, W.B. Saunders Co.

Jacobson, M.: Eater's digest, New York, 1972, Doubleday & Co., Inc.

Klafs, C.E., and Lyon, M.J.: The female athlete, ed. 2, St. Louis, 1978, The C.V. Mosby Co.

Kraus, B.: The Barbara Kraus guide to fiber in foods, New York, 1981, The New American Library, Inc.

Latham, M.C., McGandy, R.B., McCann, M.B., and Stare, F.J.: Scope manual on nutrition, Kalamazoo, Mich., 1972, The Upjohn Co.

Lederle Laboratories: Vitamins, minerals, and nutrition, Pearl River, N.Y., 1978, The Laboratories.

Mayer, J.: Overweight: causes, cost and control, Englewood Cliffs, N.J., 1968, Prentice-Hall, Inc.

Metropolitan Life Insurance Company: How you can control your weight, New York, 1979, The Company.

Nidetch, J.: Weight watcher's new program cookbook, New York, 1978, The New American Library, Inc.

Roberts, H.R., editor: Food safety, New York, 1981, John Wiley Sons, Inc.

Rorty, J., and Phillip, N.: Tomorrow's food, Greenwich, Conn., 1980, Devin Adair Co.

Schottelius, B.A., and Schottelius, D.D.: Textbook of physiology, ed. 19, St. Louis, 1982, The C.V. Mosby Co.

Scriptographic Booklet: You and your weight, Greenfield, Mass., 1980, Channing L. Bete Co., Inc.

Stare, F.J., and McWilliams, M.: Nutrition for good health, Fullerton, Calif., 1974, Plycon Press.

Stare, F.J., and McWilliams, M.: Living nutrition, New York, 1973, John Wiley & Sons, Inc.

Stare, F.J., and Whelan, E.M.: Panic in the pantry, New York, 1975, Atheneum Publishers.

U.S. Department of Agriculture: Meat and poultry inspection, 1980, Pub. No. FSQS-427, Washington, D.C., 1981.

U.S. Department of Agriculture: U.S. inspected meat and poultry packing plants, Agriculture Handbook No. 570, Washington, D.C., 1981.

U.S. Department of Agriculture: Food, Home and Garden Bulletin No. 228, Stock No. 001-000-03881-8, Science and Education Administration, Washington, D.C., 1980.

U.S. Department of Agriculture: Nutrition and your health: dietary guidelines for Americans, Home and Garden Bulletin No. 232, Washington, D.C., 1980, Science and Education Administration.

U.S. Department of Agriculture: Convenience foods and home-prepared foods, Agricultural Economic Report No. 429, Washington, D.C., 1979.

U.S. Department of Agriculture: Nutrition labeling, Agriculture Information Bulletin No. 382, Washington, D.C., 1975.

U.S. Department of Agriculture: Nutritive value of American foods, in common units, Agriculture Handbook No. 456, Washington, D.C., 1975.

U.S. Department of Health and Human Services: How to read a food label, DHHS Pub. No. (FDA) 80-1063, Washington, D.C., 1980.

Williams, S.R.: Nutrition and diet therapy, ed. 4, St. Louis, 1981, The C.V. Mosby Co.

▬▬▬▬ Chapter 20

American Dental Association: Diet and dental health, Chicago, 1975, The Association.

American Dental Association: Fluoridation facts, Chicago, 1974, The Association.

American Dental Association: The decay process, Chicago, 1980, The Association.

Berkow, R.B., editor: The Merck manual, ed. 14, Rahway, N.J., 1982, Merck, Sharp & Dohme Research Laboratories.

Boyd, R.F., and Hoerl, B.G.: Basic medical microbiology, ed. 2, Boston, 1982, Little, Brown & Co.

Brooks, N.A., Brooks, S.M., and Pelletier, L.J.: Handbook of infectious diseases, Boston, 1980, Little, Brown & Co.

Brooks, S.M.: Integrated basic science, ed. 4, St. Louis, 1979, The C.V. Mosby Co.

Brooks, S.M. and Paynton-Brooks, N.A.: The human body: structure and function in health and disease, ed. 2, St. Louis, 1980, The C.V. Mosby Co.

Nolte, W.A., editor: Oral microbiology: with basic microbiology & immunology, ed. 4, St. Louis, 1982, The C.V. Mosby Co.

van Houte, J.: Characteristics of dental surfaces related to plaque adherence, growth, and pathogenicity, Ann Arbor, Mich., 1973, University of Michigan, Dental Research Institute.

World Health Organization: The mouth, threshold of health and disease, World Health, Nov. 1966.

▬▬▬▬ Chapter 21

Al-Anon: Living with an alcoholic with the help of Al-Anon, rev. ed., New York, 1977, Group Headquarters.

American Council On Science and Health: Alcohol use during pregnancy, New York, Dec. 1981, The Council.

Berkow, R.B., editor: The Merck manual, ed. 14, Rahway, N.J., 1982, Merck, Sharp, & Dohme Research Laboratories.

Berry, R.E., and Boland, J.: The economic cost of alcohol in the U.S.A., Riverside, N.J., 1977, The Free Press.

Block, M.A.: Alcohol and alcoholism, Belmont, Calif., 1970, Wadsworth, Inc.

Coudert, J.: The alcoholic in your life, New York, 1972, Stein & Day Publishers.

Diehl, H.S.: Tobacco and your health, New York, 1969, McGraw-Hill, Inc.

Goodwin, D.: Alcoholism: the facts, New York, 1981, Oxford University Press, Inc.

Green, L.W., and Anderson, C.L.: Community health, ed. 4, 1982, The C.V. Mosby Co.

Metropolitan Life Insurance Company: Alcohol and health, New York, 1979, The Company.

Ray, O.: Drugs, society, and human behavior, ed. 3, St. Louis, 1983, The C.V. Mosby Co.

Trice, H.M., and Roman, P.M.: Spirits and demons at work: alcohol and other drugs on the job, Ithaca, N.Y., 1972, Cornell University.

U.S. Department of Health and Human Services: Alcohol—some questions and answers, DHHS Pub. No. (ADM) 81-312, Washington, D.C., 1981.

U.S. Department of Health, Education, and Welfare: Clearing the air: a guide to quitting smoking, DHEW Pub. No. (NIH) 79-1647, Washington, D.C., 1979.

▬▬▬▬ Chapter 22

Akers, R.L.: Deviant behavior: a social learning approach, ed. 2, Belmont, Calif., 1977, Wadsworth, Inc.

American Council on Science and Health: ACSH news and views, vol. 3, no. 1, New York, 1982, The Council.

American Council on Science and Health: The health effects of caffeine, New York, 1981, The Council.

Bellak, L., editor: The schizophrenic syndrome, New York, 1968, Grune & Stratton, Inc.

Berkow, R.B., editor: The Merck manual, ed. 14, Rahway, N.J., 1982, Merck, Sharp & Dohme Research Laboratories.

Brooks, N.A., Brooks, S.M., and Pelletier, L.J.: Handbook of infectious diseases, Boston, 1980, Little, Brown, and Co.

Brooks, S.M.: Integrated basic science, ed. 4, St. Louis, 1979, The C.V. Mosby Co.

Brooks, S.M., editor: Nurses' drug reference, Boston, 1978, Little, Brown & Co.

Brooks, S.M., and Paynton-Brooks, N.A.: The human body: structure and function in health and disease, ed. 2, St. Louis, 1980, The C.V. Mosby Co.

Conrad, H.T.: Psychiatric treatment of narcotic addiction, New York, 1977, Springer-Verlag New York, Inc.

Ellinwood, E.H., Jr., and Kilbey, M.M., editors: Cocaine and other stimulants, New York, 1977, Plenum Publishing Corp.

Goth, A.: Medical pharmacology: principles and concepts, ed. 10, St. Louis, 1981, The C.V. Mosby Co.

Grady, D.: DMSO: the best thing since aspirin, Discover 3(1):41-43, 1982.

Graedon, J.: The people's pharmacy, ed. 2, New York, 1980, Avon Books.

Graham, J.D.P., editor: Cannabis and health, New York, 1976, Academic Press, Inc.

Green, L.W., and Anderson, C.L.: Community health, ed. 4, St. Louis, 1982, The C.V. Mosby Co.

Grinspoon, L., and Bakalar, J.B.: Cocaine: a drug and its social evolution, New York, 1976, Basic Books, Inc, Publishers.

Hawley, R.: Some unsettling thoughts on settling in with pot, Chagrin Falls, Ohio, 1978, University School Press.

Lettieri, D.J., editor: Drugs and suicide: when other coping strategies fail, Beverly Hills, Calif, 1978, Sage Publications, Inc.

Levine, R.R.: Pharmacology: drug actions and reactions, Boston, 1973, Little, Brown & Co.

McBride, A.G.: The growth and development of mothers, New York, 1974, Barnes & Noble Books.

Nahas, G.G.: Keep off the grass: a scientist's documented account of marijuana's destructive effects, Elmsford, N.Y., 1979, Pergamon Press, Inc.

National Clearinghouse for Drug Abuse Information: Phencyclidine—PCP, series 14, no. 2, Rockville, Md., 1978, The Clearinghouse.

Pawlak, V.: Conscientious guide to drug abuse, Phoenix, Ariz., 1978, Do It Now Foundation.

Platt, J.J., and Labate,: Heroin addiction: theory, research, and treatment, New York, 1976, John Wiley & Sons, Inc.

Pradhan, S.N., and Dutta, S.N., editors: Drug abuse: clinical and basic aspects, St. Louis, 1977, The C.V. Mosby Co.

Ray, O.: Drugs, society and human behavior, ed. 3, St. Louis, 1983, The C.V. Mosby Co.

Rouse, B.A.: and Ewing, J.A.: Marijuana and other drug use by women college students: associated risk taking and coping activities, Am. J. Psychiatry **130**:486-490, 1973

Saltman, J.: Children and drugs, Public Affairs Pamphlet No. 584, New York, 1980, Public Affairs Committee.

Smith, S.M., editor: The maltreatment of children, Baltimore, 1978, University Park Press.

Stephanis, C., Dornbush, R., and Fink, M., editors: Hashish: studies of long-term use, New York, 1977, Raven Press.

U.S. Department of Health and Human Services: Catching on! A drug information booklet, DHHS Pub. No. (ADM) 81-764, Washington, D.C., 1981.

U.S. Department of Health and Human Services: Drug abuse prevention: for your family, DHHS Pub. No. (ADM) 81-584, Washington, D.C., 1980.

U.S. Department of Health and Human Services: For parents only: what you need to know about marijuana, DHHS Pub. No. (ADM) 80-909, Washingtin, D.C., 1980.

U.S. Department of Health and Human Services: Parents, peers and pot, DHHS Pub. No. (ADM) 80-812, Washington, D.C., 1980.

U.S. Department of Health and Human Services: This side up, DHHS Pub. No. (ADM) 80-420, Washington, D.C., 1980.

U.S. Department of Health and Human Services: A tale of shots and drops, DHHS Pub. No. (OHDS) 79-31128, Washington, D.C., 1979.

U.S. Department of Health and Human Services: Drug abuse facts, Office of Communications and Public Affairs, National Institute on Drug Abuse, Washington, D.C., 1980.

U.S. Department of Health, Education, and Welfare: Deciding about drugs: a woman's choice, DHEW Pub. No. (ADM) 80-820, Washington, D.C., 1980.

U.S. Department of Health, Education, and Welfare: Do's and don'ts on wise drug use, DHEW Pub. no. (ADM) 78-705(e), Washington, D.C., 1979.

U.S. Department of Health, Education, and Welfare: Let's talk about drug abuse, DHEW Pub. No. (ADM) 78-706, Washington, D.C., 1979.

U.S. Department of Health, Education, and Welfare: Prescription drugs, HEW Pub. No. (FDA) 78-3059, Washington, D.C., 1979.

U.S. Department of Health, Education, and Welfare: Drug abuse prevention: for your community, DHEW Pub. No. (ADM) 78-586, Washington, D.C., 1978.

U.S. Department of Health, Education, and Welfare: A guide to the use of nonprescription drugs, DHEW Pub. No. (FDA) 76-3026, Washington, D.C., 1976.

U.S. Department of Health, Education, and Welfare and Office of Drug Abuse Policy, Executive Office of the President: Handbook on drug abuse, National Institute on Drug Abuse, Washington, D.C., 1979.

Wesson, D.R., et al., editors: Polydrug abuse: the results of a national collaborative study, New York, 1978, Academic Press, Inc.

Wolfe, S., and Coley, C.M.: Pills that don't work, Washington, D.D., 1981, Health Research Group.

Yablonsky, L.: The tunnel back: Synanon, New York, 1963, Macmillan, Inc.

Yankelovich, Skelly, and White, Inc.: The General Mills American Family Report, 1976-77: raising children in a changing society, Minneapolis, 1977, General Mills, Inc.

Young, J.H.: The toadstool millionaires: a social history of patent medicines in America before federal regulation, Princeton, N.J., 1961, Princeton University Press.

▬▬ Chapter 23

American Council on Life Insurance (TAP #19): Health care: three reports from 2030 A.D., Washington, D.C., 1980, The Council.

American Council on Science and Health: ACSH News and Views, Vol. 3, No. 1, New York, 1982, The Council.

American Health Planning Association: Second report on 1978 survey of health planning agencies, Washington, D.C., Feb. 1979, The Association.

American Health Care Association: The nursing home dilemma, Washington, D.C., 1978, The Association.

American Hospital Association: Hospital performance, Vol. 2, No. 8, Chicago, Aug. 1980, The Association

American Hospital Association: Health—a national survey of consumers and business, Chicago, 1978, The Association.

American Hospital Association: Hospital statistics, 1973-1979 editions, Chicago, 1973-1979, The Association.

Barrett, S., and Knight, G., editors: The health robbers, Philadelphia, 1976, George F. Stickley Co.

Benarde, M.A., and Mayerson, E.W.: Patient-physician negotiations, Journal of the American Medical Association **239**(14):1413-1415, 1978.

Birren, J.E., and Schaie, K.W., editors: Handbook of the psychology of aging, New York, 1977, Van Nostrand Reinhold Co.

Blau, Z.: Old age in a changing society, New York, 1973, Franklin Watts, Inc.

Breslow, L., and Somers, A.R.: The lifetime health-monitoring—a practical approach to preventive medicine, The New England Journal of Medicine **296**(11):601-608, 1977.

Brooke Army Medical Center: Your health and you, U.S. Government Printing Office: 1978-772-813 (1978).

Brooks, S.M., editor: Review of nursing, Boston, 1978, Little, Brown & Co.

Brownlee, A.T.: Community, culture, and care: a cross-cultural guide for health workers, St. Louis, 1978, The C.V. Mosby Co.

Bureau of Health Manpower: A report to the President and Congress on the status of health professions' personnel in the United States, DHEW Pub. No. (HRA) 80-53, Washington, D.C., 1980.

Butler, R.N., and Lewis, M.I.: Aging and mental health: positive social and biomedical approaches ed. 3, St. Louis, 1982, The C.V. Mosby Co.

Congress of the United States Congressional Budget Office: Profile of health-care coverage: the haves and have-nots, Washington, D.C., 1979.

Consumers Union: Health quackery, Mount Vernon, N.Y., 1980, The Union.

Cousins, N.: Anatomy of an illness, New York, 1981, Bantam Books, Inc.

Feldstein, P.: Health care economics, New York, 1979, John Wiley & Sons, Inc.

Flowers, C.: A woman with her doctor, New York, 1979, William Morrow & Co., Inc.

German, P.S.: The elderly: a target group highly accessible to health education, International Journal Health Education 21(4):267-272, 1978.

Gordon, A., and Saltman, J.: Know your medication, New York, 1981, Public Affairs Pamphlet No. 570, Public Affairs Committee.

Green, L.W., and Anderson, C.L.: Community health, ed. 4, St. Louis, 1982, The C.V. Mosby Co.

Health Insurance Institute: Source book of health insurance data, 1980-81, Washington, D.C., 1981, The Institute.

Health Insurance Institute: Health and health insurance: the public's view, Washington, D.C., 1980, The Institute.

Health Insurance Institute: What you should know about health insurance, Washington, D.C., 1980, The Institute.

Health Insurance Institute: What you should know about health insurance when you retire, Washington, D.C., 1979, The Institute.

Health Insurance Institute: Protecting people against major hospital and medical bills, Washington, D.C., 1976, The Institute.

Hendin, D.: The world almanac whole health guide, New York, 1977, The New American Library, Inc.

Insel, P.M., and Roth, W.T.: Care concepts in health, ed. 2, Palo Alto, Calif., 1979, Mayfield Publishing Co.

Johnson, G.T., and Goldfinger, S.E., editors: The Harvard medical school health letter book, Cambridge, Massachusetts, 1980, Harvard University Press.

Johnson, T.C.: Doctor! what you should know about health care before you call a physician, New York, 1975, McGraw-Hill Book Co.

Leaf, A.: Youth in old age, New York, 1975, McGraw-Hill Book Co.

Leek, S.: The story of faith healing, New York, 1973, Macmillan, Inc.

LeShan, E.J.: Mates and roommates: new styles in young marriages, Public Affairs Pamphlet, No. 468, New York, 1981, Public Affairs Committee.

Levin, L.S.: Self-care: new initiatives in health, New York, 1976, Neale Watson Academic Publications, Inc.

Lewis, C.E., Fein, R., and Mechanic, D.: A right to health: the problem of access to primary health care, New York, 1976, John Wiley & Sons, Inc.

Maple, E.: The ancient art of occult healing, New York, 1974, Samuel Weiser.

Metropolitan Life Insurance Co.: HMO—is it for you? New York, 1974, The Company.

Miller, R.L.: Economic issues for consumers, New York, 1978, West.

Monheit, A.: Research in health economics, Vol. 2, Greenwich, Conn., 1980, JAI Press, Inc.

Morgan, P.P.: The periodic health examination, Can. Med. Assoc. J. 121:3-45, 1979.

Navarro, V.: Medicine under capitalism, New York, 1976, Prodist.

Rakel, R.E.: Principles of family medicine, Philadelphia, 1977, W.B. Saunders Co.

Rees, A.M., and Young, B.A.: Consumer health information sourcebook, New York, 1981, R.R. Bowker Co.

Reichel, W., editor: Clinical aspects of aging: a comprehensive text prepared under the direction of the American Geriatric Society, Baltimore, 1978, The Williams & Wilkins Co.

Roemer, M.I.: Rural health care, St. Louis, 1976, The C.V. Mosby Co.

Russell, L.B.: Technology in hospitals, medical advances and other diffusion, Washington, D.C., 1979, The Brookings Institution.

Salkever, D.S.: Hospital-sector inflation, Lexington, Mass., 1979, D.C. Heath & Co.

Sartwell, P.E.: Preventive medicine and public health, ed. 10, New York, 1975, Appleton-Century Crofts.

Scanlon, W.: The theory of the nursing home market, Inquiry **17**(1):24-41, 1980.

Scully, D.: Men who control women's health: the miseducation of obstetricians and gynecologists, Boston, 1980, Houghton Mifflin Co.

Shapiro, I.S.: HMOs and health education, American Journal of Public Health **65**(65):469-473, 1975.

Sloan, F., and Feldman, R.: Competition in the health care sector, Washington, D.C., 1978, Federal Trade Commission.

Strauss, A.L.: Chronic illness and the quality of life, St. Louis, 1975, The C.V. Mosby Co.

Trapnell, G.R.: National health insurance issues: the cost of a national prescription program, Nutley, N.J., 1979, Roche Laboratories.

Twaddle, A.C., and Hessler, R.M.: A sociology of health, St. Louis, 1977, The C.V. Mosby Co.

Ulene, A., and Feldman, S.: Help yourself to health, New York, 1980, G.P. Putnam's Sons.

U.S. Department of Commerce: Population estimates and projections, Series P-25, No. 870, Washington, D.C., Jan. 1980, U.S. Bureau of the Census.

U.S. Department of Commerce: Statistical abstract of the United States, Washington, D.C., 1979, Bureau of the Census.

U.S. Department of Health and Human Services: Guide to health insurance for people with medicare, DHHS/HCFA Pub. No. 02110, Washington, D.C., 1980.

U.S. Department of Health and Human Services: Health care financing, DHHS/HCFA Pub. Nos. 03063 and 03089, Washington, D.C., 1981.

U.S. Department of Health and Human Services: Health care financing review, Fall 1980, DHHS/HCFA Pub. No. 03068, Washington, D.C., 1980.

U.S. Department of Health and Human Services: Keeping track of your medicines, DHHS Pub. No. (ADM) 78-705(b), Washington, D.C., 1979.

U.S. Department of Health and Human Services: Thinking of having surgery? Think about getting a second opinion, HCFA Pub. No. 02114, Washington, D.C., 1981.

U.S. Department of Health, Education, and Welfare: A brief explanation of medicare, SSA Pub. No. 10043, Washington, D.C., 1980.

U.S. Department of Health, Education, and Welfare: A student's guide to health maintenance organizations, DHEW Pub. No. (HRA) 79-3, Washington, D.C., 1979.

U.S. Department of Health, Education, and Welfare: Saving money with generic medicines: can you? should you? DHEW Pub. No. (ADM) 78-705(e), Washington, D.C., 1979.

U.S. Department of Health, Education, and Welfare: The national nursing home survey, 1977 summary for the United States, Vital and Health Statistics, series, 13, no. 43, DHEW Pub. No. (PHS) 79-1794, Washington, D.C., 1979.

U.S. Department of Health, Education, and Welfare: Using your medicines wisely: a guide for the elderly, DHEW Pub. No. (ADM) 78-705(e), Washington, D.C., 1979.

U.S. General Accounting Office: Entering a nursing home, costly implications for medicaid and the elderly, report to Congress by the Comptroller General of the United States, Washington, D.C., Nov. 16, 1979.

Vickery, D.M., and Fries, J.F.: Take care of yourself, Reading, Mass., 1976, Addison-Wesley Publishing Co., Inc.

Weaver, J.L.: National health policy and the underserved: ethnic minorities, women and the elderly, St. Louis, 1976, The C.V. Mosby Co.

Wing, K.R.: The law and the public's health, St. Louis, 1976, The C.V. Mosby Co.

▬▬▬ Chapter 24

American National Red Cross: Advanced first aid and emergency care, ed. 2, New York, 1980, Doubleday & Co., Inc.

Ashford, N.A.: A crisis in the workplace: occupational disease and injury, a report to the Ford Foundation, Cambridge, Mass., 1976, The MIT Press.

Berkow, R.B., editor: The Merck manual, ed. 14, Rahway, N.J., 1982, Merck, Sharp, and Dohme Research Laboratories.

Boston Children's Medical Center: Child health encyclopedia, New York, 1975, Delacorte Press.

Brooks, S.M., editor: Nurses' drug reference, Boston, 1978, Little, Brown & Co.

Bureau of Radiological Health: X rays: get the picture on protection, HHS Pub. No. (FDA) 80-8088, Washington, D.C., 1980.

Burroughs Wellcome Co.: Ankle, foot, spine, and hip/pelvis injuries in sports, Wellcome Medical Education Service, Research Triangle Park, N.C., 1980, The Company.

Burroughs Wellcome Co.: Sports injuries of the knee, shoulder, elbow and wrist, Research Triangle Park, N.C., 1980, The Company.

Bush, V.G.: Safety in the construction industry, Englewood Cliffs, N.J., 1975, Prentice-Hall, Inc.

Consumers Union: Health quackery, Mount Vernon, N.Y., 1980, The Union.

Green, L.W., and Anderson, C.L.: Community health, ed. 4, 1982, The C.V. Mosby Co.

Haering, F.C.: Recreation and park program safety, Urban Data Services Reports, vol. 12, no. 3, Washington, D.C., March 1980, International City Management Association.

Hendin, D.: The world almanac whole health guide, New York, 1977, The New American Library, Inc.

Hoffman-La Roche, Inc.: Protecting your family—minutes count when treating burns, Roche Health Care Guide No. 3, Nutley, N.J., 1980, The Company.

Johnson & Johnson: First aid guide, New Brunswick, N.J., The Company.

McElroy, F.E., editor: Handbook of occupational safety and health services, Chicago, 1975, National Safety Council.

Metropolitan Life Insurance Co.: First aid for the family, New York, 1981, The Company.

National Planning Council for National Poison Prevention Week: Protect your child against accidental poisoning, Washington, D.C., The Council.

National Safety Council: Accident facts, 1980 edition, Chicago, 1980, The Council.

Preger, L., editor: Induced disease: drug, irradiation, and occupation, New York, 1980, Stratton.

Sloane, E.A.: The complete book of bicycling, New York, 1974, Simon & Schuster, Inc.

Smith, R.S.: The occupational and safety act: its goal and its achievements, Washington, D.C., 1976, American Enterprise Institute for Public Policy Research.

U.S. Consumer Product Safety Commission: A handbook for public playground safety. I. General guidelines for new and existing playgrounds, U.S. Government Printing Office, 720-013/4210, Washington, D.C., 1981.

U.S. Consumer Product Safety Commission: Halloween safety, Product Safety Education, No. 9-T, Washington, D.C., 1980.

U.S. Consumer Product Safety Commission: Holiday safety, Product Safety Education, No. 7-T, Washington, D.C., 1980.

U.S. Cycling Federation, Inc.: Bicycle safety and beyond, Colorado Springs, Colo., The Federation.

U.S. Department of Health and Human Services: Aircraft accidents: emergency mental health problems, DHHS Pub. No. (ADM) 81-956, Washington, D.C., 1981.

U.S. Department of Health and Human Services: Laser light show safety—who's responsible? DHHS Pub. No. (FDA) 80-8121, Washington, D.C., 1980.

U.S. Department of Health and Human Services: Microwave oven radiation, DHHS Pub. No. (FDA) 80-8120, Washington, D.C., 1980.

U.S. Department of Health and Human Services: Sunlamps: putting safety first, DHHS Pub. No. (FDA) 78-8063, Washington, D.C., 1978.

U.S. Department of Health, Education, and Welfare: Parents: are your walls poisoning your children, DHEW Pub. No. (CDC) 79-8285, Washington, D.C., 1979.

U.S. Department of Health, Education, and Welfare: Preventing lead poisoning in children, DHEW Pub. No. (HSA) 74-113, Washington, D.C., 1974.

U.S. Department of the Interior: First aid, Safety Manual No. 3, GPO:1980o0-315-966, Washington, D.C., 1980.

U.S. Department of Labor: All about OSHA, OSHA, Pub. No. 2056, Washington, D.C., 1980.

U.S. Department of Labor: Occupational injuries and illnesses in 1978—summary, Report 586, Washington, D.C., 1980.

U.S. Department of Labor: OSHA handbook for small businesses, OSHA, Pub. No. 2209, Washington, D.C., 1979.

U.S. Nuclear Regulatory Commission: 1980 Annual report, U.S. Government Printing Office, Washington, D.C., 1980.

Williams, A.F., and Zador, P.L.: Injuries to children in automobiles in relation to seating location and restraint use, Accident Analysis and Prevention 9:69-76, 1977.

■■■■ Chapter 25

Benenson, A., editor: Control of communicable diseases in man, ed. 13, Washington, D.C., 1981, The American Public Health Association.

Boyd, R.F., and Hoerl, B.G.: Basic medical microbiology, ed. 2, Boston, 1982, Little, Brown & Co.

Brooks, N.A., Brooks, S.M., and Pelletier, L.J.: Handbook of infectious diseases, Boston, 1980, Little, Brown & Co.

de Kruif, P.: Microbe hunters, New York, 1926, Harcourt, Brace, and World.

Dowling, H.F.: Fighting infections: conquests of the twentieth century, Cambridge, Mass., 1977, Harvard University Press.

Dubos, R.J.: Louis Pasteur: free lance of science, Boston, 1950, Little, Brown & Co.

Green, L.W., and Anderson, C.L.: Community health, ed. 4, St. Louis, 1982, The C.V. Mosby Co.

Krugman, S., and Katz, S.L.: Infectious diseases of children, ed. 7, St. Louis, 1981, The C.V. Mosby Co.

Leff, S., and Leff, V.: From witchcraft to world health, New York, 1957, Macmillan, Inc.

Shattuck, L., et al.: Report of the sanitary commission of Massachusetts, 1850, facsimile edition, Cambridge, Mass., 1948, Harvard University Press.

Sigerist, H.E.: Landmarks in the history of hygiene, New York, 1956, Oxford University Press, Inc.

Tobey, J.A.: Riders of the plagues, New York, 1930, Charles Scribner's Sons.

Wehrle, P.F., and Top, F.H., editors: Communicable and infectious diseases, ed. 9, St. Louis, 1981, The C.V. Mosby Co.

■■■■ Chapter 26

Ashford, N.A.: A crisis in the workplace: occupational disease and injury, a report to the Ford Foundation, Cambridge, Mass., 1976, The MIT Press.

Bryant, J.: Health and the developing world, Ithaca, N.Y., 1969, Cornell University Press.

Bullough, B., and Bullough, V.: Poverty, ethnic identity, and health care, New York, 1972, Appleton-Century Crofts.

Bush, V.G.: Safety in the construction industry, Englewood Cliffs, N.J., 1975, Prentice-Hall, Inc.

Green, L.W., and Anderson, C.L.: Community health, ed. 4, St. Louis, 1982, The C.V. Mosby Co.

Hanlon, J.J., and Pickett, G.E.,: Public health: administration and practice, ed. 7, St. Louis, 1979, The C.V. Mosby Co.

Hutchins, B.L., and Harrison, A.: History of factory legislation, Fairfield, N.J., 1968, Augustus M. Kelley, Publishers.

McElroy, F.E., editor: Handbook of occupational safety and health series, Chicago, 1975, National Safety Council.

National Safety Council: Accident prevention manual for industrial operations, ed. 7, Chicago, 1974, The Council.

Pflanz, M., and Schach, E., editors: Cross-national sociomedical research: concepts, methods, practice, Stuttgart, 1976, Georg Thieme Verlag.

Shattuck, L., et al.: Report of the sanitary commission of Massachusetts, 1850, facsimile edition, Cambridge, Mass., 1948, Harvard University Press.

Smith, R.S.: The occupational and safety act: its goal and its achievements, Washington, D.C., 1976, American Enterprise Institute for Public Policy Research.

Smolensky, J., and Harr, F.B.: Principles of community health, ed. 4, Philadelphia, 1979, W.B. Saunders Co.

U.S. Department of Health and Human Services: 1981 NIH almanac, NIH Pub. No. 81-5, Washington, D.C., 1981.

U.S. Department of Health and Human Services: Food and drug administration acts: federal food, drug, and cosmetic act, as amended January 1980; public health service act, biological products; radiation control for health and safety act; fair packaging and labeling act, DHHS Pub. No. (FDA) 80-1051, Washington, D.C., 1980.

U.S. Department of Health and Human Services: Research, demonstration, and evaluation studies, 1979, DHHS Pub. No. (OHDS) 80-30030, Washington, D.C., 1980.

U.S. Department of Health, Education, and Welfare: A world of opportunity: programs of the public health service, DHEW Pub. No. 80-50038, Washington, D.C., 1980.

Wing, K.R.: The law and the public's health, St. Louis, 1976, The C.V. Mosby Co.

■■■■ **Chapter 27**

American Medical Association: Why health education in your school, Chicago, 1974, The Association.

American School Health Association: A pocketbook to health and health programs in school physical activities, Kent, Ohio, 1981, The Association.

American School Health Association: Growth patterns and sex education, Kent, Ohio, 1978, The Association.

American School Health Association: Guidelines for the school nurse in the school health program, Kent, Ohio, 1974, The Association.

Anderson, C.L., and Creswell, W.H.: School health practice, ed. 7, St. Louis, 1980, The C.V. Mosby Co.

Berger, L.: Falls from heights: a childhood epidemic in an urban area, American Journal Public Health **61**:90, 1971.

Florio, A.E., and Stafford, G.T.: Safety education, ed. 3, New York, 1969, McGraw-Hill, Inc.

Gearheart, B.R., and Weishahn, M.: The handicapped child in the regular classroom, ed. 2, St. Louis, 1980, The C.V. Mosby Co.

Gordon, S., and Dickman, I.R.: Schools and parents—partners in sex education, Public Affairs Pamphlet No. 581, New York, Public Affairs Committee.

Jenne, F.H., and Greene, W.H.: Turner's school health and health education, ed. 7. St. Louis, 1976, The C.V. Mosby Co.

Lewis, C.E., et al.: Children-initiated care: the utilization of school nursing services by children in a "adult-free system," Pediatrics **60**:499-507, 1977.

Mayshark, C., Shaw, D.D., and Best, W.H.: Administration of school health programs: its theory and practice, ed. 2, St. Louis, 1977, The C.V. Mosby Co.

Sex Education in the public schools (special issue), The Journal of School Health **51**(4):April 1981.

Turner, C.E.: Planning for health education in schools, Washington, D.C., 1966, UNESCO and WHO.

U.S. Department of Health and Human Services: Children and youth in action: physical activities and sports, DHHS Pub. No. (OHDS) 80-30182, Washington, D.C., 1980.

U.S. Department of Health, Education, and Welfare: School health in America, a survey of state school health programs, ed. 2, DHEW/PHS/CDS/Bureau of Health Education, Washington, D.C., 1979.

■■■■ **Chapter 28**

American Chemical Society: Cleaning our environment, ed. 2, Washington, D.C., 1979, The Society.

American Council on Science and Health: Air pollution and your health, New York, April 1981, The Council.

American Council on Science and Health: New Jersey: garden state or cancer alley? New York, April 1981, The Council.

American Council on Science and Health: Wood as home fuel: a source of air pollution, New York, Oct. 1981, The Council.

Andrews, W.: Guide to the study of environmental pollution, Englewood Cliffs, N.J., 1973. Prentice-Hall, Inc.

Barlett, R.E.: Surface water sewage, New York, 1976, Halsted Press.

Berthouex, P.M., and Rudd, D.F.: Strategy of pollution control, New York, 1977, John Wiley & Sons, Inc.

Cargo, D.B.: Solid wastes: factors influencing generation rates, Chicago, 1977, University of Chicago Press.

Carson, R.: Silent spring, Boston, 1961, Houghton Mifflin Co.

Chemical Manufacturers Association: Protecting the environment: what we're doing about it, Washington, D.C., 1980, The Association.

Culp, R.L., and Culp, G.L.: New concepts in water purification, New York, 1974, Van Nostrand Reinhold Co.

Dorfman, R., and Dorfman, N.S.: Economics of the environment, ed. 2, New York, 1977, W.W. Norton & Co., Inc.

Dubois, R.: Man, medicine and environment, New York, 1968, Praeger Publishers.

Elliott, S.M.: Our dirty water, New York, 1973, Julian Messner.

Gehm, H.W., and Bregmann, J.I., editors: Handbook of water resources and pollution control, New York, 1976, Van Nostrand Reinhold Co.

Green, L.W., and Anderson, C.L.: Community health, ed. 4, St. Louis, 1982, The C.V. Mosby Co.

Grey, J.: Noise, noise, noise, Philadelphia, 1976, The Westminister Press.

Hopkins, E.S., and Bena, E.L.: Water purification control, ed. 4, Baltimore, 1975, The Williams & Wilkins Co.

Horne, R.A.: The chemistry of our environment, New York, 1978, John Wiley & Sons, Inc.

Hunt the dump, Environmental Action Magazine, 11(3):23, 1979.

James, R.W.: Sewage sludge treatment, Park Ridge, N.J., 1972, Noyes Data Corp.

Kamlet, K.S.: Toxic substances in U.S. states and territories: how well do they work? Washington, D.C., 1979, National Wildlife Federation.

Kraybill, H.F., and Mehlman, M.A.: Environmental cancer, New York, 1977, Hemisphere Publishing Corp.

LaFond, R.E.: Cancer: the outlaw cell, Washington, D.C., 1978, American Chemical Society.

Lave, L.B., and Seskin, E.P.: Air pollution and human health, Baltimore, 1977, Johns Hopkins University Press.

League of Women Voters: Toxic substances primer, Washington, D.C., 1979, League of Women Voters Education Fund.

McCaull, J., and Croseland, J.: Water pollution, New York, 1974, Harcourt Brace, Jovanovich, Inc.

Middleton, J.T.: Plant damage: an indicator of the presence and distribution of air pollution, Bulletin WHO 34:477-80, 1966.

Moriber, G.: Environmental science, Boston, 1974, Allyn & Bacon, Inc.

National Audubon Society: Guide for citizen action, Washington, D.C., Feb. 1979, The Society.

National Wildlife Federation: The toxic substances dilemma: a plan for citizen action, 1980-60-228/4089, 1980, Washington, D.C., U.S. Government Printing Office.

National Wildlife Federation: What is happening to our water? Washington, D.C., 1979, The Federation.

National Wildlife Federation: Setting the course for clean water, Washington, D.C., 1978, The Federation.

Sinks, R.L., and Asano, T., editors: Land treatment and disposal of municipal and industrial wastes, Ann Arbor, Mich., 1976, Ann Arbor Services Science Publishers, Inc.

Smith, I.C., and Carson, B.L.: Trace metals in the environment, Ann Arbor, Mich., 1977, Ann Arbor Science Publishers, Inc.

The Amicus Journal: Will the air pollution control program survice the '80s, Vol. 2, No. 3, Winter 1981.

U.S. Environmental Protection Agency: Cleaning the air, Pub. No. 1981-720-016/5986 Region 3-1, Washington, D.C., U.S. Government Printing Office.

U.S. Environmental Protection Agency: National accomplishments in pollution control: 1970-1980, some case histories, Pub. No. EPA-PM-222, Washington, D.C., 1981.

U.S. Environmental Protection Agency: Air quality data: 1979 annual statistics including summaries with reference to standards, Pub. No. EPA-450/4-80-014, Washington, D.C., 1980.

U.S. Environmental Protection Agency: Everybody's problem: hazardous waste, Pub. No. SW-826, Washington, D.C., 1980.

U.S. Environmental Protection Agency: 1977 National emissions report, national emissions data system of the aerometric and emissions reporting system, Pub. No. EPA-150/1-80-005, Washington, D.C., 1980.

U.S. Environmental Protection Agency: Pilot national environmental profile: 1977, Office of the Administrator, Washington, D.C., 1980.

U.S. Environmental Protection Agency: The toxic substances control act, Pub. No. 1980-324-691, Washington, D.C., 1980, U.S. Government Printing Office.

U.S. Environmental Protection Agency: The toxic substances dilemma, a plan for citizen action, Washington, D.C., 1980, The National Wildlife Federation.

U.S. Environmental Protection Agency: Trends in the quality of the nation's air: a report to the people, Pub. No. OPA 16/9, Washington, D.C., October 1980.

U.S. Environmental Protection Agency, Measuring air quality, Pub. No. EPA 11/8, Washington, D.C., 1978.

U.S. Environmental Protection Agency: National air quality, monitoring, and emissions trands report, 1977, Pub. No. EPA-45 0/2-78-052, Washington, D.C., 1978.

U.S. Nuclear Regulatory Commission: 1980 annual report, Washington, D.C., 1981, U.S. Government Printing Office.

Waldbott, G.: Health effects of environmental pollutants, ed. 2, St. Louis, 1978, The C.V. Mosby Co.

Answers to self-tests

Chapter 1
1. d
2. j
3. l
4. k
5. a
6. i
7. m
8. f
9. o
10. n
11. e
12. g
13. b
14. h
15. c

Chapter 2
1. j
2. l
3. a
4. n
5. h
6. e
7. m
8. k
9. d
10. o
11. g
12. i
13. b
14. f
15. c

Chapter 3
1. e
2. l
3. a
4. g
5. f
6. m
7. o
8. n
9. i
10. k
11. c
12. h
13. d
14. j
15. b

Chapter 4
1. d
2. k
3. n
4. l
5. i
6. j
7. m
8. h
9. e
10. o
11. g
12. b
13. f
14. a
15. c

Chapter 5
1. b
2. h
3. n
4. m
5. a
6. i
7. k
8. o
9. e
10. l
11. g
12. j
13. d
14. f
15. c

Chapter 6
1. j
2. o
3. i
4. n
5. h
6. b
7. m
8. a
9. k
10. c
11. l
12. g
13. e
14. d
15. f

Chapter 7
1. d
2. j
3. l
4. m
5. o
6. i
7. k
8. c
9. n
10. h
11. e
12. g
13. a
14. b
15. f

Chapter 8
1. j
2. o
3. m
4. a
5. k
6. b
7. h
8. c
9. f
10. l
11. n
12. d
13. g
14. i
15. e

Chapter 9

1. l
2. o
3. b
4. h
5. a
6. n
7. g
8. k
9. m
10. c
11. j
12. e
13. i
14. f
15. d

Chapter 10

1. f
2. k
3. m
4. g
5. a
6. o
7. h
8. l
9. n
10. i
11. b
12. d
13. j
14. c
15. e

Chapter 11

1. j
2. a
3. l
4. o
5. h
6. n
7. k
8. f
9. b
10. m
11. d
12. i
13. g
14. e
15. c

Chapter 12

1. f
2. j
3. n
4. a
5. l
6. m
7. k
8. b
9. e
10. h
11. c
12. i
13. g
14. o
15. d

Chapter 13

1. c
2. j
3. o
4. b
5. n
6. i
7. l
8. a
9. g
10. k
11. m
12. d
13. f
14. h
15. e

Chapter 14

1. j
2. c
3. l
4. a
5. h
6. o
7. b
8. n
9. k
10. f
11. m
12. e
13. i
14. d
15. g

Chapter 15

1. b
2. g
3. m
4. k
5. o
6. a
7. e
8. i
9. d
10. h
11. f
12. c
13. j
14. l
15. n

Chapter 16

1. c
2. f
3. g
4. i
5. h
6. j
7. k
8. l
9. m
10. o
11. b
12. d
13. e
14. a
15. n

███████ **Chapter 17**

1. c
2. n
3. b
4. j
5. l
6. a
7. h
8. k
9. i
10. e
11. m
12. g
13. f
14. d
15. o

███████ **Chapter 18**

1. g
2. k
3. b
4. l
5. a
6. j
7. n
8. m
9. o
10. i
11. c
12. e
13. h
14. f
15. d

███████ **Chapter 19**

1. e
2. i
3. j
4. a
5. g
6. n
7. b
8. l
9. o
10. d
11. k
12. m
13. h
14. f
15. c

███████ **Chapter 20**

1. l
2. n
3. b
4. m
5. o
6. c
7. k
8. i
9. a
10. g
11. d
12. f
13. h
14. j
15. e

███████ **Chapter 21**

1. o
2. l
3. k
4. m
5. d
6. i
7. a
8. b
9. n
10. j
11. h
12. g
13. e
14. f
15. c

███████ **Chapter 22**

1. b
2. h
3. o
4. i
5. a
6. m
7. k
8. j
9. l
10. n
11. d
12. e
13. g
14. f
15. c

███████ **Chapter 23**

1. h
2. b
3. a
4. g
5. n
6. e
7. k
8. o
9. m
10. d
11. i
12. l
13. j
14. c
15. f

███████ **Chapter 24**

1. e
2. o
3. m
4. n
5. l
6. b
7. j
8. c
9. a
10. i
11. g
12. d
13. k
14. f
15. h

▬▬ Chapter 25	▬▬ Chapter 26	▬▬ Chapter 27	▬▬ Chapter 28
1. o	1. k	1. h	1. g
2. m	2. d	2. j	2. k
3. k	3. m	3. e	3. m
4. h	4. b	4. g	4. c
5. a	5. o	5. i	5. l
6. c	6. a	6. a	6. o
7. d	7. l	7. f	7. a
8. b	8. n	8. c	8. f
9. l	9. g	9. b	9. b
10. n	10. i	10. d	10. n
11. j	11. f		11. e
12. f	12. j		12. i
13. i	13. h		13. j
14. g	14. e		14, h
15. e	15. c		15. d

Metric system

Length

1 nanometer (nm)	= 0.000000001 meter
1 micrometer (μm)	= 0.000001 meter
1 millimeter(mm)	= 0.001 meter
1 centimeter (cm)	= 0.01 meter
1 decimeter (dm)	= 0.1 meter
Meter (m)	= 1.0 meter
1 dekameter (dkm)	= 10 meters
1 hectometer (hm)	= 100 meters
1 kilometer (km)	= 1,000 meters

Weight

1 microgram (μg)	= 0.000001 gram
1 milligram (mg)	= 0.001 gram
1 centigram (cg)	= 0.01 gram
1 decigram (dg)	= 0.1 gram
Gram (g)	= 1.0 gram
1 dekagram (dkg)	= 10 grams
1 hectogram(hg)	= 100 grams
1 kilogram (kg)	= 1,000 grams

Volume

1 microliter (μl)	= 0.000001 liter
1 milliliter (ml)	= 0.001 liter
1 centiliter (cl)	= 0.01 liter
1 deciliter (dl)	= 0.1 liter
Liter (l or L)*	= 1.0 liter
1 dekaliter (dkl)	= 10 liters
1 hectoliter (hl)	= 100 liters
1 kiloliter (kl)	= 1,000 liters

Metric-English equivalents

1 meter (m)	= 39.37 inches
1 centimeter (cm)	= 0.3937 inch
1 kilometer (km)	= 0.62 mile
1 kilogram (kg)	= 2.204 pounds
1 liter (L)	= 1.057 quarts (liquid)
1 yard (yd)	= 0.914 meter
1 foot (ft)	= 30.48 centimeters
1 inch (in)	= 2.54 centimeters
1 mile (mi)	= 1.61 kilometers
1 ounce (oz) (avoir.)	= 28.35 grams
1 pound (lb)	= 453.6 grams
1 quart (qt) (liquid)	= 0.956 liter
1 quart (dry)	= 1.101 liters

*The United States Bureau of Standards recommends the use of "L," although "l" is the official abbreviation.

Index